Disorders of Mineral Metabolism

VOLUME II

Contributors

Arnold S. Brickman
Felix Bronner
Ernesto Carafoli
Jack W. Coburn
Leonard J. Deftos
Jan A. Fischer
Mark R. Haussler
Barton S. Levine
Shaul G. Massry
Robert K. Rude
Frederick R. Singer
Marvin L. Tanzer
Marlin W. Walling

Disorders of Mineral Metabolism

VOLUME II

Calcium Physiology

Edited by

FELIX BRONNER
Department of Oral Biology
School of Dental Medicine
University of Connecticut Health Center
Farmington, Connecticut

JACK W. COBURN
Medical and Research Services
V. A. Wadsworth Hospital Center, and
Department of Medicine
UCLA School of Medicine
Los Angeles, California

1982

ACADEMIC PRESS
A Subsidiary of Harcourt Brace Jovanovich, Publishers
New York London
Paris San Diego San Francisco São Paulo Sydney Tokyo Toronto

ACADEMIC PRESS, INC.
111 Fifth Avenue, New York, New York 10003

United Kingdom Edition published by
ACADEMIC PRESS, INC. (LONDON) LTD.
24/28 Oval Road, London NW1 7DX

Library of Congress Cataloging in Publication Data
Main entry under title:

Calcium physiology.

(Disorders of mineral metabolism ; v. 2)
Includes bibliographies and index.
1. Calcium in the body. 2. Calcium--Metabolism.
3. Calcium--Metabolism--Disorders. I. Bronner, Felix.
II. Coburn, J. W., Date. III. Series. [DNLM:
1. Disorders of mineral metabolism. WD 205.5.M4 D612 (P)]
QP535.C2C264 612'.3924 81-20522
ISBN 0-12-135302-8 (v. 2) AACR2

PRINTED IN THE UNITED STATES OF AMERICA

82 83 84 85 9 8 7 6 5 4 3 2 1

Contents

2 Calcium Homeostasis

FELIX BRONNER

3 Intestinal Absorption of Calcium: Its Assessment, Normal Physiology, and Alterations in Various Disease States

BARTON S. LEVINE, MARLIN W. WALLING, and JACK W. COBURN

4 Renal Handling of Calcium

SHAUL G. MASSRY

5 Collagen Biosynthesis and Degradation

MARVIN L. TANZER

6 Parathyroid Hormone

JAN A. FISCHER

7 Vitamin D: Metabolism, Actions, and Disease States

MARK R. HAUSSLER and ARNOLD S. BRICKMAN

List of Contributors

Numbers in parentheses indicate the pages on which the authors' contributions begin.

Arnold S. Brickman (359), Mineral Metabolism Section, Veterans Administration Center, Sepulveda, California 91343

Felix Bronner (43), Department of Oral Biology, School of Dental Medicine, University of Connecticut Health Center, Farmington, Connecticut 06032

Ernesto Carafoli (1), Laboratory of Biochemistry, Swiss Federal Institute of Technology (ETH), 8092 Zurich, Switzerland

Jack W. Coburn (103), Medical and Research Services, V. A. Wadsworth Medical Center, and Department of Medicine, UCLA School of Medicine, Los Angeles, California 90073

Leonard J. Deftos (433), University of California, and San Diego VA Medical Center, La Jolla, California 92161

Jan A. Fischer (271), Research Laboratory for Calcium Metabolism, Departments of Orthopedic Surgery and Medicine, University of Zurich, 8008 Zurich, Switzerland

Mark R. Haussler (359), Department of Biochemistry, University of Arizona Health Sciences Center, Tucson, Arizona 85724

Barton S. Levine (103), V. A. Wadsworth Medical Center, and Department of Medicine, UCLA School of Medicine, Los Angeles, California 90073

Shaul G. Massry (189), Division of Nephrology, University of Southern California, Los Angeles, California 90033

Robert K. Rude (481), School of Medicine, University of Southern California, Los Angeles, California 90033

Frederick R. Singer (481), School of Medicine, University of Southern California, Los Angeles, California 90033

Marvin L. Tanzer (237), Department of Biochemistry, University of Connecticut Health Center, Farmington, Connecticut 06032

*Marlin W. Walling** (103), Research Service, V. A. Wadsworth Medical Center; Department of Orthodontics, UCLA School of Dentistry; Department of Medicine, UCLA School of Medicine, Los Angeles, California 90073

*Deceased.

Preface

"Disorders of Mineral Metabolism" is intended as a comprehensive, up-to-date treatise on the pathophysiology of calcium, phosphorus, and magnesium and of other clinically relevant minerals and elements, such as iron, copper, zinc, fluoride, and the like.

Recent years have seen major advances in our understanding of how these minerals function in the mammalian body and why they are important in medicine. Thus the failure to provide adequate concentrations of calcium in hemodialysis fluids or to regulate their fluoride or aluminum concentrations may lead to severe bone disease of patients who are being maintained on dialysis. Understanding of the metabolism of vitamin D has underscored the pivotal role played by renal tissue in providing the body with an adequate supply of 1,25-dihydroxyvitamin D_3, the metabolite active in the intestinal cell and modulating one component of calcium absorption. Indeed, what characterizes current understanding is the appreciation of what may at first appear to be remote control loops, as in the role played by the vitamin D-regulated component of bone metabolism in the body handling of cadmium.

It therefore seems entirely fitting that this treatise unites what appear to be disparate subjects whose detailed understanding differs widely. It is the editors' hope that knowledge gained in one area may serve to stimulate research in another. An example is the high intracellular concentration of magnesium whose regulation and relationship to extracellular magnesium are not understood. The total intracellular calcium is low and the intracellular free calcium concentration is carefully regulated at between 10^{-7} and 10^{-6} M. This appears to involve complicated interactions between various cellular organelles, all of which have calcium-binding proteins with an association constant of about 10^{6} M^{-1}. Yet extracellular calcium is also closely regulated at 10^{-3} M, and the body expends considerable energy in the regulation of both intra- and extracellular calcium. How are these two related and could intra- and extracellular calcium regulation serve as a model for understanding the regulation of magnesium? Such questions could be multiplied manifold. We hope this treatise will not only serve as a useful reference, but stimulate readers to reflect on parallels and distinctions between subjects.

Volume I of the treatise deals with minerals and elements whose average daily intake is under 50 mg. They are therefore conveniently termed "trace elements." While many are essential for life, the essentiality of others has not been established. Inclusion was largely a matter of clinical interest and relevance.

Volume II deals with the normal function of calcium, knowledge of which has exploded in recent years, with much emphasis on a host of intracellular functions. These have been summarized in the first chapter. In the remainder of the volume, calcium absorption, excretion, and homeostasis are discussed in detail, along with the hormonal modifiers of its metabolism. The role of connective tissue and bone, the major storehouse of body calcium, is reviewed in terms of collagen metabolism.

Volume III deals with the pathophysiology of calcium in bone and kidney and their disorders, along with detailed consideration of phosphate and magnesium metabolism. Throughout this and the other volumes the viewpoint has been that of disorders and how they arise; therapy has been discussed in terms of principles rather than from the viewpoint of specific management.

This treatise was inspired by a desire to bring up-to-date the earlier one on "Mineral Metabolism" edited by C. L. Comar and Felix Bronner. It became apparent early that comprehensive updating and expansion were no longer possible. An example is the Na^{+}-K^{+} ATPase, mentioned in a footnote in the earlier treatise, which could now easily command its own volume. Similar comments apply to iodine and the thyroid diseases, to the electrolytes Na^{+} and K^{+} and their diseases, and a host of other subjects. Not only has there been an expansion of knowledge, the approach has changed, with much greater emphasis on an understanding of the molecular basis of many events. Some subjects have not advanced as much as others. This applies in particular to the relationship between events at the cellular, tissue, and organism levels. Just as true understanding of a mechanism requires reconstitution experiments, so appreciation of the disease process ultimately demands integration of events at all levels of organization, from the molecular to the whole organism. While this treatise makes halting steps in that direction, we hope future research will bring us closer to that goal.

Felix Bronner
Jack W. Coburn

Contents of Other Volumes

VOLUME I   Trace Minerals

1

The Regulation of the Cellular Functions of Ca^{2+}

ERNESTO CARAFOLI

Disorders of Mineral Metabolism, Vol. II

ISBN 0-12-135302-8

I. INTRODUCTION—THE PHYSIOLOGICAL ROLE AND THE BIOLOGICAL FITNESS OF CALCIUM

The recognition that Ca^{2+}, in addition to playing an essential role as a structural element in mineralized tissues, may be important as a biological messenger can be traced back to the observation by Ringer (1883) that the inclusion of Ca^{2+} in the medium was essential for cardiac contractility. The observation by Ringer was made by chance and was due to the use of nondistilled water, which later was found to contain about 1 m*M* Ca^{2+}, but was quickly and correctly understood by him as due to an essential role of Ca^{2+} in cardiac contractility (Ringer, 1884). The discovery remained isolated for a long time, however, and the realization that Ca^{2+} is uniquely important as a general biological messenger is rather recent. It now appears evident that Ca^{2+} influences the generation of the electrical signals, normally due to Na^+, K^+, and, in some tissues, Ca^{2+} currents at the plasma membrane level. It is also known that Ca^{2+} carries the signals to the target activities in the interior of the cells, and it is now beginning to be recognized that in the transfer of information from the plasma membrane to some intracellular activities, Ca^{2+} may become associated with a soluble protein, capable of binding it with high specificity.

The messenger function requires (1) that Ca^{2+} be maintained inside cells at a very low activity level to prevent permanent activation of the target enzymes, and (2) that it be allowed to fluctuate widely around this low activity level to turn on and off the target activities. That the concentration of ionized Ca^{2+} inside most cells is much lower than that in the environment is now an established fact. Gradients of a factor at least 1000 have been measured. It is of interest that this situation is peculiar for the case of Ca^{2+}. The other cations commonly present in biological systems are not kept at such low activity levels inside cells, and their ionized concentration in the environment is not very different from their intracellular one (Table I).

TABLE I

Na^+, K^+, Mg^{2+} in the Environment and in the Animal Fluids[a,b]

Cation	Sea water (m*M*)	Human plasma (m*M*)	Mammalian cell (m*M*)
Na^+	490	135–145	12–20
K^+	98	5.3	150
Mg^{2+}	54	1.1	2.8

[a] From Carafoli and Crompton (1978).

[b] Values taken from Davson (1970) refer to total concentrations. The ionic activities of Na^+ and K^+ do not differ very much from the total concentraions. In the case of Mg^{2+}, only about 50–60% of the total is free (DeWeer, 1976).

A discussion of the reasons for the evolutionary choice of Ca^{2+} as a biological messenger is of necessity largely speculative and has already been treated in detail in previous reviews (Williams, 1975, 1976; Carafoli and Crompton, 1978). Basically, some of the chemical properties of Ca^{2+} make it a very suitable candidate as a biological messenger. In the context of this article, it may be sufficient to say that the messenger function requires that the chosen cation be specifically complexed by soluble ligands inside cells, and by membrane-bound systems (normally proteins) that will transport it reversibly between different cell compartments, and between the intracellular milieu and the environment. From a chemical standpoint, Ca^{2+} is indeed uniquely qualified, among the cations available in the original environment (Mg^{2+}, Na^{+}, K^{+}), to interact specifically with the irregular cavities normally offered by complex biological molecules like proteins. The polarizing power of Ca^{2+}, as resulting from its ionic size and its charge, confers on it a unique "flexibility" as a complexing agent and permits it to fit optimally into cavities of irregular dimension, where the coordinating oxygen atoms are spaced at variable bond lengths and angles. It is well known that the intracellular milieu contains many complex molecules (generally proteins) that can interact with high affinity and great specificity with Ca^{2+}, and that inside the cells there exist a variety of specific membrane Ca^{2+}-transporting systems. By contrast, for example, intracellular ligands able to complex Mg^{2+} with high specificity and affinity and specific Mg^{2+} membrane-transporting systems are almost unknown.

It is perhaps interesting to distinguish in the messenger function of Ca^{2+} the "primary" from the "secondary" function. This distinction has already been alluded to at the opening of this chapter: The regulation of the (electrical) signal production by Ca^{2+} at the level of the plasma membrane is defined as the primary messenger junction. Its existence has been established in a variety of cases (for a review, see Carafoli and Crompton, 1978). The secondary messenger function of Ca^{2+}, i.e., the transmission of the signal to the interior of the cell, has been studied much more widely, has been reviewed extensively in several articles (Rasmussen, 1970; Rasmussen *et al.*, 1972; Carafoli and Crompton, 1978), and now appears to be directed to a large series of functions, the most important of which are listed in Table II.

It would be interesting to know how Ca^{2+} interacts with target systems so as to activate them. Although the matter is currently under active investigation, definite statements can so far be made for only a few cases. One general consideration, however, is that the Ca^{2+}-modulated enzymes (Table III lists the most important of them) are activated by very low Ca^{2+} activities, and must therefore have a very high affinity for the cation.

The role of Ca^{2+} as a second messenger involves interplay with cyclic AMP, the other recognized second messenger (Sutherland, 1972). How this occurs has been vigorously debated (for reviews, see Rasmussen, 1970; Rasmussen *et al.*,

TABLE II

Targets for the Messenger Function of Ca^{2+} [a]

Action potentials (nerve and muscle cells)
Mobilization of fuels (modulation of metabolic pathways)
Contractile and motile systems
Cytoplasmic streaming
Microtubules and microfilaments function
Endocrine and exocrine secretion
Light emission
Decision to divide

[a] From Carafoli and Crompton (1978).

1972; Kretsinger and Nelson, 1976), but it is not yet known in what instances Ca^{2+} and cAMP work in series or in parallel. The discovery that Ca^{2+} influences two key enzymes involved in the metabolism of cAMP, namely phosphodiesterase (Wang *et al.*, 1975) and adenylate cyclase (Teo and Wang, 1973; Brostrom *et al.*, 1976), adds interest to the problem.

A detailed discussion on the regulation of intracellular Ca^{2+} will be presented below. The discussion will consider the role of low- and high-molecular-weight soluble ligands, an aspect of the problem which has gained considerable attention recently, largely due to the discovery and molecular characterization of several specific Ca^{2+}-binding proteins, ligands that may help maintain the ionized Ca^{2+} concentration in the cytosol at low levels. However, it is difficult to imagine how these proteins could modulate the free Ca^{2+} concentration in response to signals triggered by physiological events. The systems for reversibly transporting Ca^{2+} across membranes are a more logical target for the physiological signals demanding Ca^{2+} modulation in the cytosol and, accordingly, their role in Ca^{2+} regula-

TABLE III

Ca^{2+}-Modulated Enzymes[a]

Phosphorylase *b* kinase
Phosphodiesterase
Adenylate cyclase
α-Glycerophosphate dehydrogenase
Myofibrillar ATPase
Isocitric dehydrogenase (mitochondrial)
Pyruvate dehydrogenase phosphate phosphatase (mitochondrial)
Pyruvate dehydrogenase kinase (mitochondrial)
α-Ketoglutarate dehydrogenase (mitochondrial)

[a] Modified from Carafoli and Crompton (1978).

tion will be discussed extensively. In closing this introduction, however, and as a way of introducing the discussion on the membrane regulation of Ca^{2+}, it may be of interest to mention that one potentially important cellular action of Ca^{2+} is that on the structure and stability of membranes. This in turn, could have important consequences for metabolic regulation. As recently reviewed by Carafoli and Crompton (1978), Ca^{2+} may influence the structure of several membranes by virtue of its ability to "dehydrate" membrane components. The fluidity properties of synthetic and natural membranes are known to be profoundly influenced by Ca^{2+} (Onishi and Ito, 1974; Manery, 1966; Träuble and Eibl, 1974). Several authors have observed that Ca^{2+} induces a transition of the phospholipid bilayers from the fluid to the ordered state, an effect that could well influence the rates of transport of various solutes. The conformational changes of the axonal membrane during excitation have indeed been explained with these effects of Ca^{2+} (Tobias, 1964; Tasaki, 1968; Adam, 1970).

Also of interest is the possibility that the asymmetric distribution of Ca^{2+} across intracellular membrane boundaries may be a factor in determining the asymmetric distribution of different phospholipid species normally found in the two monolayers of membranes (Williams, 1975). Negatively charged phospholipids would thus distribute preferentially in the monolayer that faces the ambient solution having a higher Ca^{2+} concentration. Krebs *et al.* (1979) have shown that cardiolipin, the only phospholipid of the inner mitochondrial membrane able to bind Ca^{2+} with high affinity (K_d: ca 10^{-5} M), is specifically concentrated in the inner monolayer which faces a medium having a much higher Ca^{2+} concentration than the external one.

II. INTRACELLULAR CONCENTRATION OF Ca^{2+}

As mentioned above, the concentration of ionized Ca^{2+} inside cells is at least 1000 times lower than in the extracellular environment. In the cytoplasms for which direct estimates are available, it ranges between 0.13 and 1.3 μM (Baker *et al.*, 1971; Di Polo, 1976; Meech and Standen, 1975; Rose and Loewenstein, 1976; Brown and Blinks, 1974; Ridgway and Durham, 1976; see also Table IV). It is interesting that the *total* concentration of Ca^{2+} in cells may reach values as high as 8–9 mM [as, for example, in smooth muscle (Wacker and Williams, 1968)], values similar to those found in the extracellular spaces. The difference between the total and ionized Ca^{2+} concentration inside cells underscores the remarkable potential for "buffering" Ca^{2+} by soluble ligands and intracellular membranes.

As yet the role of soluble ligands in the buffering of cell Ca^{2+} is largely speculative. Most cytoplasms contain a variety of low molecular weight ligands

TABLE IV

Some Representative Values for the Ionized Ca^{2+} in the Cytoplasm[a]

	Value	Reference
Squid axoplasms	20-50 n*M*	Di Polo *et al.* (1976)
Erythrocyte	0.73-4 μ*M*	Schatzmann (1973); Quist and Roufogalis (1975); Pfleger and Wolf (1975); Scharff (1976); Ferreira and Lew (1976)
Muscle	0.1-1.0 μ*M*	Felo *et al.* (1965); Ebashi and Endo (1968); Weber (1966); Solaro *et al.* (1974) Portzehl *et al.* (1964); Hagiwara and Nakajima (1966)
Helix aspersa neurons	30-80 μ*M*	Meech and Standen (1975)
Chironomus salivary gland	<20 μ*M*	Rose and Loewenstein (1976)
Physarum polycephalum	0.1 μ*M*	Ridgway and Durham (1976)

[a] From Carafoli and Crompton (1978).

that can complex Ca^{2+}. These include inorganic phosphate, citrate, adenine nucleotides, and pyridine nucleotides. Quite conceivably, the buffering capacity of these ligands can vary with the metabolic state of the cell. For example, the levels of ATP and ADP are obviously influenced by the activity of the ATP synthesizing and the ATP utilizing systems. Since the K_d (Ca^{2+}) of ADP is about 15 times higher than that of ATP [4.5×10^{-4} *M* and 3.1×10^{-5} *M*, respectively (O'Sullivan and Perrin, 1964)], the total Ca^{2+} buffering capacity of the adenine nucleotide pool will be influenced by the metabolic state of the cell. Probably important in buffering cell Ca^{2+} are the Ca^{2+} binding proteins that occur in a number of tissues. Some of these have been studied in great detail and have provided essential information on the interaction between Ca^{2+} and complex ligands.

Several intracellular proteins are capable of binding Ca^{2+} with high affinity. Many other intracellular proteins, mostly enzymes, can also bind Ca^{2+} but with much lower affinity (K_d in the m*M* range), and therefore would appear to be less important as Ca^{2+} buffers. Of the high affinity proteins, some are present in all eukaryotic cells, some only in specialized cells (aequorin, luciferin, spasmin, parvalbumin). Troponin C, actin, myosin light chains, originally discovered and characterized as muscle-tissue proteins, are now widely recognized to be present ubiquitously in nonmuscle tissues. A special case is that of the Ca^{2+}-dependent modulator protein (CDR, or calmodulin). This molecule is now being recognized as ubiquitous and capable of mediating the transmission of the Ca^{2+} signal to many intracellular enzyme targets. Given the growing importance of this protein in the messenger function of Ca^{2+}, it will be covered in Section VIII.

In addition to the soluble ligands, the membrane-enclosed intracellular compartment are also important stores for nonionized Ca^{2+}. In mitochondria, for example, the total concentration of Ca^{2+} may exceed 0.1 *M* in some specialized tissues. The more usual mitochondrial calcium content is 10 m*M*, with most of the Ca^{2+} present in the form of insoluble deposits of phosphate salts.

III. THE TRANSPORT OF Ca^{2+} ACROSS CELLULAR MEMBRANES—GENERAL CONSIDERATIONS

At least three membranes systems have been shown to be capable of transporting Ca^{2+}: the plasma membrane, the endosarcoplasmic reticulum, and the mitochondrion. In considering the general problem of the regulation of intracellular Ca^{2+}, one may start with the observation that the cytosolic concentration of Ca^{2+} is several orders of magnitude lower than that of the environment. In the presence of a continuous influx of Ca^{2+} from the extracellular spaces (see below), this situation demands the continuous extrusion of Ca^{2+} from the cell. Therefore, the long-term maintenance of an intracellular Ca^{2+} level that is below that of the environment is due to the pumping activity of the plasma membrane. In cells where the other Ca^{2+} pumping membrane systems (mitochondria and endo- or sarcoplasmic reticulum) are absent, e.g., in the erythrocytes, the plasma membrane is by definition the only structure responsible for the intracellular homeostasis of Ca^{2+}. In most cells, however, the presence of other intracellular Ca^{2+}-transporting membrane systems suggests that the latter play a role that may be more important than that of the plasma membrane in the rapid regulation of cellular Ca^{2+}. The basis for this suggestion comes from the finding that in most cells the plasma membrane represents a comparatively minor part of the total membrane area available for the transport of calcium (see Carafoli and Crompton, 1978, for a discussion of the matter). In liver and heart, for example, it represents 11.4 and 0.8%, respectively. By contrast, the intracellular membranous network occupies up to 99% of the total cellular Ca^{2+} transporting surface. In liver and heart, the inner mitochondrial membrane contains 54.8 and 87%, and endo(sarco)plasmic reticulum 37.7 and 12.1%, respectively, of the total Ca^{2+}-transporting surface. To underscore the impressive potential of most cells for Ca^{2+} transport, one can estimate that rat hearts contain about 12 m^2 of membrane capable of transporting Ca^{2+} per gram of tissue.

IV. Ca^{2+} TRANSPORT ACROSS THE PLASMA MEMBRANE

A. Ca^{2+} Influx

In excitable tissues like heart and nerve, Ca^{2+} penetrates into the cell via specifically gated channels [reviewed by Baker (1975) and Reuter (1974)], generating a "slow inward current" which with the aid of appropriate inhibitors can be easily differentiated from the "fast inward current" generated by Na^+. The latter channel is specifically blocked by tetrodotoxin, lidocaine, or procaine, whereas the Ca^{2+} channel is blocked by verapamil, D-600, and Cd^{2+} ions (Fleckenstein *et al.*, 1969; Kohlhardt *et al.*, 1972; Kostyuk and Kristhal, 1978). In heart, the Ca^{2+} entering the cell via the specific Ca^{2+} channel seems to be essential for contractility, since the beating of heart cells stops rapidly in the absence of extracellular Ca^{2+} (Ringer, 1883; Bailey and Dresel, 1968; Rich and Langer, 1975; Shine *et al.*, 1971). Possibly, the influx of Ca^{2+} from the extracellular spaces is linked to the phenomenon of Ca^{2+}-induced Ca^{2+} release from sarcoplasmic reticulum (see below). Also interesting is the stimulation of Ca^{2+} influx into cardiac cells during excitation by catecholamines (Grossmann and Furchgott, 1964; Reuter, 1965), a phenomenon that may be connected with a cyclic AMP-dependent phosphorylation of a sarcolemmal protein (MW 24,000, Wollenberger *et al.*, 1975), that apparently increases the affinity of the membrane binding sites for Ca^{2+}. Ca^{2+} seems to diffuse passively from the extracellular spaces into nonexcitable cells such as the erythrocyte. The matter of hormonal control of the influx of Ca^{2+} into the cells is still open. Borle (1970, 1975) has presented evidence that parathyroid hormone accelerates and calcitonin inhibits the Ca^{2+} penetration. A parallel problem is that of the involvement of the vitamin D-dependent Ca^{2+}-binding protein first described in intestinal mucosa by Wasserman and Taylor (1966) and subsequently observed in a variety of other tissues. It binds Ca^{2+} at two types of sites, four of which per mole have a rather high affinity (K_d, 4 μM). Although the role of this protein is not understood, indirect evidence suggests that it may participate in the penetration of Ca^{2+} into the cell.

B. Ca^{2+} Efflux

Basically, the plasma membrane contains two systems for the ejection of Ca^{2+} into the environment. One is a Ca^{2+}-specific ATPase, the other a system that ejects Ca^{2+} in exchange for Na^+.

1. *The Ca^{2+}-ATPase*

This system was originally described, and later characterized by Schatzmann and Vincenzi for the erythrocyte (see Schatzmann, 1975, for a review). Similar systems have been subsequently described for other cell types (liver, Van Rossum, 1970; cultured L cells, Lamb and Lindsay, 1971; kidney tubules, Gmaj *et al.*, 1979). The red cell ATPase is an integral membrane protein, which splits ATP at the inner site of the plasma membrane, and becomes phosphorylated in the process. It has a high affinity for Ca^{2+}, with the K_d reported to vary between 0.73 and 4 μM. Its stoichiometry is still under discussion. Schatzmann and Vincenzi (1969) and Schatzmann (1975) have reported values of 1, whereas Quist and Roufogalis (1975), Ferreira and Lew (1976), and Sarkadi *et al.* (1977) have measured 2 ATP per Ca^{2+} transported. The maximal rate of transport has also been determined, and found to lie between 85 and 200 μmoles Ca^{2+} per liter of cells per min at 37°C (Ferreira and Lew, 1976; Sarkadi *et al.*, 1977). Very interestingly, the rate of Ca^{2+} transport by the specific ATPase can be stimulated 2 to 4 times by the Ca^{2+}-dependent modulator protein (calmodulin) (Bond and Clough, 1973; Luthra *et al.*, 1976; Gopinath and Vincenzi, 1977; Jarrett and Penniston, 1978). The specific Ca^{2+}-ATPase is inhibited by rather high concentrations of La^{3+} and ruthenium red (Watson *et al.*, 1971; Sarkadi *et al.*, 1977).

A recent series of studies (Knauf *et al.*, 1974; Dieckvoss and Wolf, 1976; Ronner *et al.*, 1977) has shown that the enzyme can be solubilized from the inner membrane domain by treatment with Triton X-100. With a partially purified preparation, Peterson *et al.* (1978) and Gietzen *et al.* (1979) have been able to reconstitute the Ca^{2+}-dependent ATPase in liposomes. In agreement with the findings of Ronner *et al.* (1977) on the specific requirement for acid phospholipids of the solubilized enzyme, the reconstituted ATPase activity (Peterson *et al.*, 1978) was optimal in the presence of acidic phospholipids. It has also been demonstrated that the Triton-solubilized enzyme can still be activated by the soluble modulator protein (Niggli *et al.*, 1979a). Indeed, using a calmodulin affinity chromatography column, Niggli *et al.* (1979b) obtained a preparation of ATPase that is practically pure. The Ca^{2+} ATPase has been studied in much less detail in other cell types; there is even a question whether it is found in liver plasma membranes (Chambaut *et al.*, 1974). Gmaj *et al.* (1979) have found the Ca^{2+} ATPase to be present in the basal-lateral membrane of kidney tubule cells, but not in the brush border. Interestingly, the basal-lateral membrane also contains a Na^+/Ca^{2+} exchange system (see next section). These authors have proposed that the Na^+/Ca^{2+} exchange system is responsible for the bulk flow of Ca^{2+} across the tubular epithelium, whereas the specific Ca^{2+} ATPase is responsible for the fine regulation of the intracellular Ca^{2+}.

2. *The Na^+/Ca^{2+}* Exchange

This Ca^{2+} extrusion system seems to be typical of excitable tissues (axons, brain, muscle, secretory cells). Squid axons and heart, indeed, are the two cell types where the system has been studied most extensively.

Thus in squid axons, the total Ca^{2+} efflux probably involves a Na^+/Ca^{2+} exchange system (Baker *et al.*, 1969; Baker, 1976; Mullins, 1976; Blaustein, 1976), a Ca^{2+}/Ca^{2+} exchange system, plus a residual efflux that is not Na^+ coupled, (Baker, 1976). The most important of these three is probably the Na^+/Ca^{2+} exchange which normally operates to extrude Ca^{2+} from the cell, but can operate in the reverse direction in the presence of excess external Ca^{2+} (Baker *et al.*, 1976). In metabolically poisoned (ATP-free) axons, the route of Ca^{2+} efflux displays a sigmoidal dependence on the external Na^+ concentration with half-maximal velocity at 120 m*M* Na^+ (Blaustein *et al.*, 1974). Kinetic data of this type have been used to infer that at least three Na^+ ions are exchanged per one Ca^{2+} ion (Baker and McNaughton, 1976; Blaustein *et al.*, 1974; Mullins and Brinley, 1975); this implies a net movement of positive charges inside the cell. Indeed, the Na^+/Ca^{2+} exchange is inhibited by depolarization. Baker and McNaughton (1976), on the other hand, have found that the exchange between internal and external Ca^{2+} (half-maximal activation at 3–8 m*M* external Ca^{2+}) is electroneutral.

An equally interesting, but as yet poorly understood, observation is that low amounts of ATP within the axon transform the Na^+-dependent Ca^{2+} efflux from a sigmoidal to a hyperbolic function, and cause the internal concentration of ionized Ca^{2+} necessary for half-maximal activation of the Na^+/Ca^{2+} exchange to drop from 10 μM to about 0.2 μM (Baker and Glitsch, 1973; Baker and McNaughton, 1976). It is not known, however, whether this requires ATP hydrolysis.

In heart, the existence of a specific Na^+/Ca^{2+} exchange system in the sarcolemma is also well documented as reviewed by Reuter (1974). The kinetic findings for that situation (Jundt *et al.*, 1975) can be interpreted to mean that an electroneutral exchange is responsible for the re-extrusion of Ca^{2+} that had entered the heart cell during the later phase of excitation on the "slow Ca^{2+} channel" (see above). Na^+ is then extruded by the membrane-bound Na^+/K^+-ATPase. Also, in the case of heart sarcolemma, ATP seems to play a role, since metabolic poisons applied to the heart preparation (Jundt and Reuter, 1977) decrease the system's affinity for Na^+. The maximum rate of Ca^{2+} extrusion by the Na^+/Ca^{2+} antiporter, normally between 0.1 and 1.0 nmoles of Ca^{2+} per mg wet muscles weight (Carafoli and Crompton, 1978), is also reduced. Very recently, vesicular preparations of heart sarcolemma have become available (Reeves and Sutko, 1979; Caroni *et al.*, 1980; Pitts, 1979). These vesicles are capable of carrying out a Na^+/Ca^{2+} exchange: very interestingly, in agreement with the squid axon data, and at variance with the kinetic findings on the intact tissue (Jundt *et al.*, 1975), the exchange seems to be electrogenic. In both nervous tissues and heart, no specific inhibitors of the Na^+/Ca^{2+} exchange have been found.

Earlier literature also suggests the existence in the cardiac plasma membrane of a Ca^{2+}-stimulated ATPase in parallel with the Na^+/Ca^{2+} exchanger (St. Louis and Sulakhe, 1978; Hui *et al.*, 1976; Anand *et al.*, 1977). The existence of this ATPase has now been conclusively demonstrated (Caroni and Carafoli, 1980). Its role would be that of extruding Ca^{2+} from the cell. The characteristics of this system, as well as its importance with respect to the Na^+/Ca^{2+} exchange in the overall ejection of Ca^{2+} from heart cells, are now being explored.

The evidence for the existence of a Na^+/Ca^{2+} exchange in secretory tissues is indirect, but convincing. It is now accepted that secretion in many cells is promoted by an increase in the concentration of ionized Ca^{2+} in the cytosol (Douglas, 1968). Viewed against this background, it is logical to attribute the secretion-inducing effect of a decrease in external Na^+ in either the endocrine pancreas (Hales and Milner, 1968a,b) or the adrenal medulla (Douglas and Rubin, 1961, 1963; Banks *et al.*, 1969; Banks, 1967) to a lowering of the activity of a plasma membrane Na^+/Ca^{2+} antiporter. Interestingly, the same effect can be achieved by the addition of ouabain, which, by inhibiting the Na^+/K^+ ATPase, causes the intracellular Na^+ to increase. By lowering the Na^+ gradient across the plasma membrane, this will lead to decreased activity of the plasma membrane Na^+/Ca^{2+} antiporter. However, the increase in intracellular Na^{2+} may also cause intracellular Ca^{2+} to go up by a different mechanism, that is, by liberating Ca^{2+} from intracellular storage sites, such as the mitochondria. This point will be discussed in more detail later on.

As mentioned in the section on the plasma membrane Ca^{2+}-ATPase, the basal–lateral membrane of kidney proximal tubular cells has been found to contain a Na^+/Ca^{2+} exchange system in which from indirect evidence there occurs an exchange of three Na^+ for one Ca^{2+}, in analogy with what happens in nervous tissues and in heart (Gmaj *et al.*, 1979). This exchange has not been found in the brush border membrane of kidney tubular cells. Costanzo *et al.* (1978) have obtained evidence for the existence of a Na^+/Ca^{2+} exchange also in the basal–lateral membranes of distal tubules. It may be interesting to recall at this point that Terepka *et al.* (1976) have obtained results compatible with the presence of a Na^+/Ca^{2+} exchange system in both the luminal *and* the basal portion of the chick chorioallantoic membrane, and of the plasma membrane of small intestine. They have proposed a model for the transcellular transport of Ca^{2+} in which endocytotic vesicles, interiorized from the plasma membrane, would migrate to the opposite pole of the cell. Into these vesicles, which contain the same Na^+ concentration as the extracellular medium, Ca^{2+} that has entered the cytosol by passive diffusion would be pumped by the Na^+/Ca^{2+} exchanger. Transcellular Ca^{2+} transport has in fact been found to depend on the presence of Na^+ in the extracellular medium (Terepka *et al.*, 1976) and the rate of the transcellular Ca^{2+} transport was found to be a sigmoidal function of the Na^+ concentration. This would indicate that also this Na^+/Ca^{2+} exchange may be electrogenic. Finally, a Na^+/Ca^{2+} exchange has also been described in the plasma membrane of toad bladder epithelia (Taylor *et al.*, 1978).

V. THE TRANSPORT OF Ca^{2+} BY ENDOPLASMIC AND SARCOPLASMIC RETICULUM

A. Sarcoplasmic Reticulum

The ability of sarcoplasmic retiulum to accumulate Ca^{2+} has been documented in skinned muscle fibers (Costantin *et al.*, 1965; Podolsky *et al.*, 1970) and in vesicular membrane fragments obtained from reticulum during muscle homogenization (for a review, see Martonosi, 1972). The "total" ability of sarcoplasmic reticulum to accumulate Ca^{2+} varies from muscle to muscle since the organelle is developed differently in different cell types, fast (white) muscle containing more than slow (red) muscles. Heart is particularly poor in sarcoplasmic reticulum. In heart, this organelle is much less active in Ca^{2+} uptake than sarcoplasmic reticulum of muscles (Suko and Hasselbach, 1976), a fact that has raised doubts on its exclusive role in the relaxation of heart myofibrils (see Carafoli, 1974, for a discussion).

Most of the studies with isolated fragments of sarcoplasmic reticulum have involved Ca^{2+} uptake. Ca^{2+} release has been studied much less, and has led to data that seem unrelated to the physiological demands for the myofibril contraction. Clearly, regulation of the contraction and relaxation of myofibrils requires Ca^{2+} to be taken up by *and* released from the sarcoplasmic reticulum by mechanisms linked to the events responsible for excitation at the level of the plasma membrane.

Ca^{2+} uptake by sarcoplasmic reticulum is catalyzed by an ATPase that is specifically activated by Ca^{2+}. This enzyme has been extracted from the membrane domain and purified to homogeneity (Martonosi, 1968; MacLennan, 1970; Ikemoto *et al.*, 1971; Warren *et al.*, 1974; Meissner *et al.*, 1973). Its MW is about 105,000 and it binds 2 nmoles of Ca^{2+} per mole of enzyme with high affinity (K_d, about $10^{-7}M$). The ATPase enzyme represents between 60 and 90% of the total protein of the membrane, depending on the portion of the sarcoplasmic reticulum network (Meissner, 1975), and since 1972 has repeatedly been reconstituted in phospholipid bilayers (Racker, 1972). The reconstituted vesicles show both Ca^{2+}-dependent ATPase activity and ATP-dependent Ca^{2+} accumulation.

The ATPase enzyme becomes phosphorylated by ATP during the Ca^{2+} transport reaction (Martonosi, 1972), with the formation of an aspartyl phosphate residue at the active site (Degani and Boyer, 1973). Some time after the formation of the phosphorylated enzyme, Ca^{2+} is transferred across the membrane, with Ca^{2+} release to the interior of the vesicle occurring prior to dephosphorylation of the enzyme (Makinose, 1973). Stoichiometrically, 2 Ca^{2+} ions are transferred per ATP hydrolyzed. In fast skeletal muscles, the V_{max} for Ca^{2+} uptake has been found to vary between 0.4 and 3.6 μmoles/mg of vesicle protein per minute (Table V). In slow muscles and in heart this rate is much slower. The mechanism of charge compensation during the influx of Ca^{2+} into the sarcoplasmic reticulum vesicles is not known. Kanazawa and Boyer (1973) have proposed that two Ca^{2+} ions exchange with one Mg^{2+} and two K^+ ions. It must be remembered, however, that the sarcoplasmic reticulum membrane is permeable to a variety of anions (Martonosi and Feretos, 1964; Duggan and Martonosi, 1970). This fact has been exploited by several authors who have used oxalate in the reaction medium to increase the total levels of Ca^{2+} accumulated in the vesicles. The penetration of oxalate precipitates Ca^{2+} in the intravesicular space, analogous to what happens in mitochondria exposed to Ca^{2+} and phosphate (see below).

A recent series of studies (Shamoo and MacLennan, 1979; see Shamoo and Goldstein, 1977, for a review) has concentrated on the proteolytic fragmentation of the ATPase molecule and on the demonstration of ionophoric activity of the proteolytic fragments in planar lipid bilayers. These and other (Thorley-Lawson and Green, 1973; MacLennan, 1970; Green *et al.*, 1977) studies have shown that trypsin treatment releases from the enzyme a fragment of 55,000 daltons, which probably corresponds to the 30–40 Å projections visible on the outer profiles of negatively stained vesicles (Ikemoto *et al.*, 1968; Inesi and Asai, 1968) and which can be phosphorylated by ATP in the presence of Ca^{2+}. Prolonged trypsin treatment splits the fragment into 20,000- and 30,000-dalton subfragments; the larger of these can still be phosphorylated by ATP, whereas the smaller shows Ca^{2+} ionophoric activity when incorporated into a planar lipid bilayer. From these studies, the picture of the molecular arrangement of the ATPase enzyme in the sarcoplasmic reticulum membrane shown in Fig. 1 has emerged (Shamoo and Goldstein, 1977).

MacLennan and Wong (1971) have isolated from sarcoplasmic reticulum fragments an extrinsic protein (calsequestrin) that can bind large amounts of Ca^{2+} with low affinity (K_d, 8×10^{-4} M; capacity, 43 moles of Ca^{2+} per mole) (Ostwald and MacLennan, 1974; Ostwald *et al.*, 1974), and is thought to be responsible for the binding of accumulated Ca^{2+} inside the vesicle, particularly in the terminal cisternal region (Meissner, 1975; Shamoo and Goldstein, 1977). Sarcoplasmic reticulum contains another Ca^{2+}-binding protein, which binds Ca^{2+} with both high (K_d, 3 μM, 1 mole/mole) and low affinity (K_d, 100 μM, 25 moles/mole) (Meissner *et al.*, 1973; Ikemoto *et al.*, 1972; Ostwald and MacLennan, 1974).

As mentioned above, the regulation of muscle contraction and relaxation requires both rapid uptake and rapid release of Ca^{2+} from the sarcoplasmic reticulum. The ATP-dependent uptake process can be reversed (Barlogie *et al.*, 1971) in the presence of ADP, P_i, and Mg^{2+}, but only when the extravesicular concentrations of Ca^{2+} and ATP are kept at very low levels. Ca^{2+} efflux from skeletal muscle sarcoplasmic reticulum has also been triggered in skinned fibers

TABLE V

Properties of Active Ca^{2+} Transport in Isolated Sarcoplasmic Reticulum[a]

Sarcoplasmic reticulum preparation	Oxalate	Maximal uptake (μmoles/mg protein)	V_{max} (μmoles Ca/min/mg)	K_m for Ca^{2+} (μ*M*)	Reference
White skeletal muscle microsomes	Present	—	0.4–0.9	0.1-1.0	Weber (1966)
	Absent	0.17	—	—	Weber (1966)
	Present	6.0	1.8	—	Sreter (1969)
	Absent	0.25	1.8	—	Sreter (1969)
	Absent	0.14	3.6	—	Inesi and Scarpa (1972)
	Present	—	2.8	10	Worsfold and Peter (1970)
	Absent	—	—	3	Martonosi (1975)
	Absent	0.14	—	0.03	Fiehn and Migala (1971)
Reconstituted pump from white skeletal muscle microsomes	Absent	—	—	25	Knowles and Racker (1975)
Red skeletal muscle microsomes	Present	1.2	0.15	—	Sreter (1969)
	Absent	0.04	0.15	—	Sreter (1969)
Cardiac microsomes	Absent	0.07	0.12	—	Besch and Schwartz (1971)
	Present	0.30	0.10	—	Fanburg *et al.* (1964)
	Present	0.42	—	—	Baskin and Deamer (1969)

[a] From Carafoli and Crompton (1978).

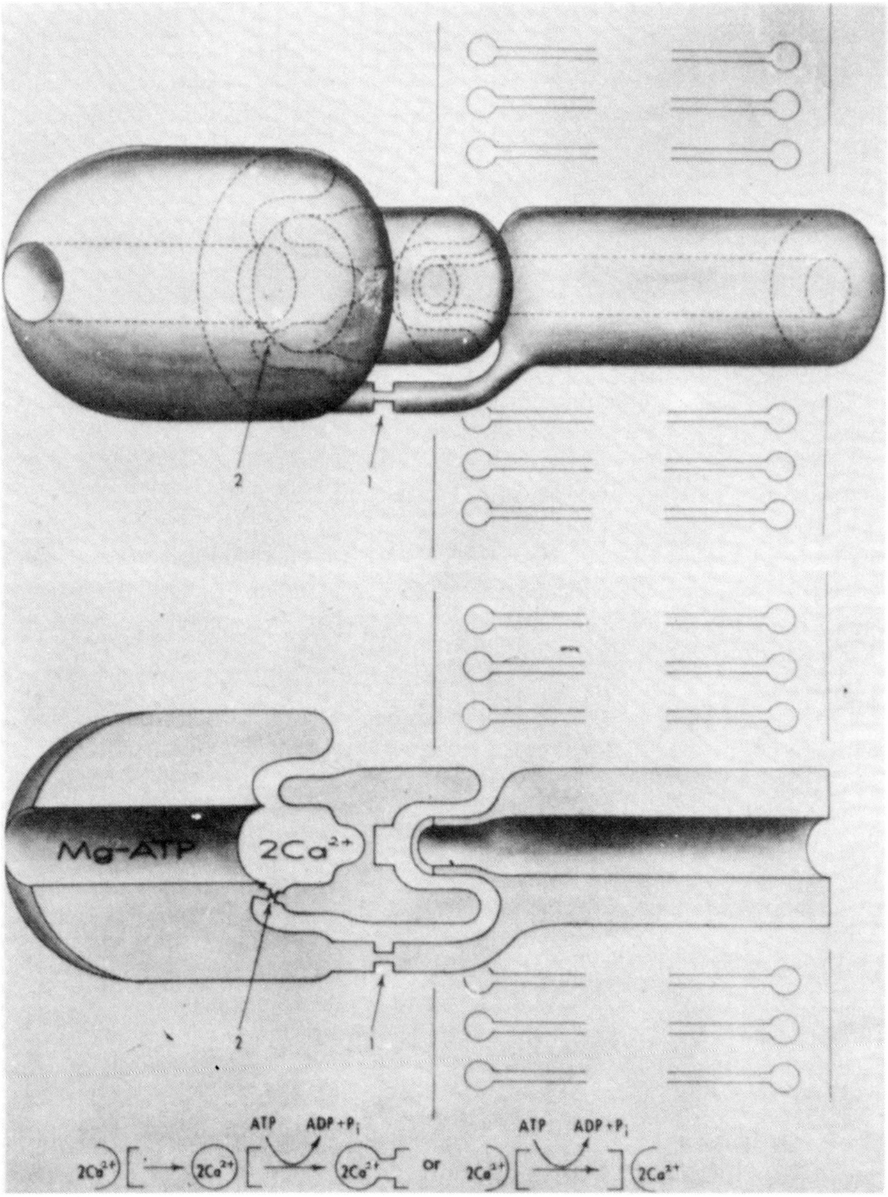

Fig. 1. Molecular arrangement of ATPase enzyme in the sarcoplasmic reticulum membrane. (From Shamoo and Goldstein, 1977.)

by an increase in the extravesicular Ca^{2+} concentration (the so-called Ca^{2+}-induced Ca^{2+} release (Ford and Podolsky, 1970, 1972a,b; Endo *et al.*, 1970), but only at unphysiologically high Ca^{2+} concentrations 10^{-5}–10^{-4} M. In skinned heart fibers, on the other hand, Ca^{2+} appears to be released from sarcoplasmic reticulum by variations in the Ca^{2+} concentration in the physiological range (Fabiato and Fabiato, 1975). Katz *et al.* (1977) have reported similar experiments on isolated fragments of cardiac sarcoplasmic reticulum.

Ca^{2+} has also been released from sarcoplasmic reticulum by inducing a membrane potential, positive outside, across the vesicle membrane (Constantin and Podolsky, 1967; Endo and Thorens, 1975; Nakajima and Endo, 1973), but the results have been criticized since the experimental conditions used induce osmotic damage to the vesicles (Meissner and McKinley, 1976).

In considering sarcoplasmic reticulum from the standpoint of the regulation of muscle Ca^{2+}, two main areas of uncertainity thus remain. One is the lack of a physiologically reasonable mechanism for the release of Ca^{2+}. Another is the fact that the Ca^{2+} uptake, so well developed in fast muscle reticulum, is much lower in slow muscles, especially in heart sarcoplasmic reticulum (see Table V). It is therefore perhaps worthwhile to extrapolate from experimental data with the help of known requirements for the concentration and relaxation of myofibrils. Solaro and Briggs (1974) have calculated that the sarcoplasmic reticulum of dog heart can bind up to 170 nmoles of Ca^{2+} per gm wet muscle, at an external Ca^{2+} concentration of 1 μM. This value is considerably in excess of the amount of Ca^{2+} exchanged between heart sarcoplasm and troponin during a contraction–relaxation cycle (25–100 nmoles Ca^{2+} per gm wet muscle weight; Solaro *et al.*, 1974; Katz, 1970). However, the maximal rate of Ca^{2+} uptake by heart sarcoplasmic reticulum is about 0.2 μmoles per mg of protein per min at 37°C (as estimated from a value of 0.1 μmoles at 25°C) (Fanburg *et al.*, 1964; Besch and Schwartz, 1971; Chiesi, 1978). Considering a maximum amount of 7 mg sarcoplasmic reticulum protein per gm of heart (wet weight; Solaro and Briggs, 1974), the maximum rate of Ca^{2+} uptake will be 1.4 μmoles per min per gm wet muscle. In 200 msec, the time required to relax the myofibrils from 90% activation (Solaro *et al.*, 1974), this would correspond to the removal of 4.7 nmoles of Ca^{2+} per gm wet muscle, an amount that is clearly insufficient when viewed against a requirement for about 35 nmoles (Solaro *et al.*, 1974). It is interesting, however, that the rate of Ca^{2+} uptake by the sarcoplasmic reticulum of heart and slow muscles (but not of fast muscles) can be stimulated by the cAMP-dependent phosphorylation of a serine residue of a 21,000-dalton protein that has been detected in the sarcoplasmic reticulum membrane (Tada *et al.*, 1974, 1975a,b; Kirchberger *et al.*, 1974; Kirchberger and Tada, 1976; Schwartz *et al.*, 1974, 1976). Also interesting is the observation that the soluble protein modulator mentioned above stimulates the transport of Ca^{2+} in heart sarcoplasmic reticulum (Katz and Remtulla, 1978).

TABLE VI

Properties of Active Ca^{2+} Transport in Isolated Endoplasmic Reticulum[a]

Source of endoplasmic reticulum	Energy source	Mg^{2+}	Oxalate	Maximal capacity (nmoles/mg protein)	K_m for Ca^{2+} (μM)	Inhibitors	Reference
Brain	ATP	Required	No stimulation	~50	—	SH reagents, oligomycin, amytal	Robinson and Lust (1968)
	ATP	Required	No stimulation	~50	—	—	Otsuka *et al.* (1965)
	ATP	Required	No stimulation	~65	50-100	—	DeMeis *et al.* (1970)
Salivary	ATP	Required	Stimulates	2750	—	Salyrgan	Selinger *et al.* (1970)
gland	ATP	Required	Stimulates	150	100	—	Alonso *et al.* (1971)
Kidney	ATP	Required	Stimulates	~50	20	—	Moore *et al.* (1974)
Liver	ATP	Required	Stimulates	~400	4.6	SH reagents, oligomycin	Moore *et al.* (1975)
Platelets	ATP	Required	Stimulates	~350	100	—	Robblee *et al.* (1973)

[a] From Carafoli and Crompton (1978).

B. Endoplasmic Reticulum

The demonstration that endoplasmic reticulum can also transport Ca^{2+} is relatively more recent. Fragments of endoplasmic reticulum from liver, kidney, brain, salivary glands, and platelets have been shown actively to accumulate Ca^{2+} (Otsuka *et al.*, 1965; Robinson and Lust, 1968; Selinger *et al.*, 1970; DeMeis *et al.*, 1970; Alonso *et al.*, 1971; Robblee *et al.*, 1973; Moore *et al.*, 1974, 1975). Table VI summarizes the most important characteristics of the process as described in the different cell types. The uptake system seems to be represented by a specific ATPase, since ATP is the necessary energizing source. The Mg^{2+} requirement is similar to that found for sarcoplasmic reticulum, and so is the generally observed potentiating effect of oxalate. The reasons for the lack of effect of oxalate on brain microsomes are unclear. However, since the effect of oxalate is artificial, the rather low maximal amounts of Ca^{2+} accumulated by brain reticulum probably represent physiological limits for brain endoplasmic reticulum. Rather interesting, however, is the fact that the affinity of the endoplasmic reticulum system of some tissues for Ca^{2+} seems to be high: K_m's of 4.6 and 20 μM, respectively, have been measured for liver and kidney. In these tissues at least, therefore, endoplasmic reticulum seems to be a system with low capacity but high affinity. It has also been found that the Ca^{2+} transport ability is higher in vesicles derived from smooth, as compared to rough, endoplasmic reticulum. A recent study by Blaustein *et al.* (1980) on Ca^{2+} metabolism in isolated nerve endings has offered convincing indication for the participation of smooth endoplasmic reticulum at low, and thus presumably physiological, Ca^{2+} concentrations.

VI. THE TRANSPORT OF Ca^{2+} BY MITOCHONDRIA

A. General Concepts

Mitochondria from all tissues studied so far can transport Ca^{2+} (Lehninger *et al.*, 1967; Carafoli, 1974; Carafoli and Crompton, 1976, 1978; Bygrave, 1977) though in some cases (yeast, blowfly flight muscle) the process exhibits peculiar characteristics (Carafoli *et al.*, 1970, 1971). In general, it is the uptake reaction, with Ca^{2+} accumulated from the environment against a concentration gradient, that has been studied most with very little attention devoted to the opposite process, i.e., Ca^{2+} release from the organelle. The need to release Ca^{2+} so as to prevent mitochondrial calcification was first postulated by Drahota *et al.* (1965), whose data were the first to indicate that Ca^{2+} may be cycled across the mitochondrial membrane, but only recently was full attention devoted to this aspect of the problem (e.g., Stucki and Ineichen, 1974), and ways and means were identified (Carafoli and Crompton, 1976; Puskin *et al.*, 1976) to release

Ca^{2+} from mitochondria. Indeed, it has become clear in the course of the last few years that the process of mitochondrial Ca^{2+} *uptake* is irreversible in a strict sense, since Ca^{2+} enters and leaves the organelle by two independent pathways. This has provided the rationale for the formulation of the concept of a "Ca^{2+} cycle" in mitochondria (Carafoli *et al.*, 1979, Carafoli, 1979).

B. Uptake of Ca^{2+} by Mitochondria

In the first few years after the discovery of the process of energy-linked uptake of Ca^{2+} by mitochondria (Vasington and Murphy, 1962), emphasis was placed on the accumulation of massive amounts of Ca^{2+} by the organelles. The process, which was observed only in the presence of simultaneous uptake of the permeant anion inorganic phosphate, was later termed "matrix loading" (Lehninger *et al.*, 1967), and led to the precipitation of amorphous deposits of hydroxylapatite within the inner mitochondrial space. It is now recognized that matrix loading *in vivo* occurs only in tissues specialized in the mobilization of large amounts of Ca^{2+} or in the early stages of cell injury (for a review, see Carafoli, 1974). In most normal tissues, however, massive loading of mitochondria with Ca^{2+} probably never takes place. The early studies of the process of "matrix loading" have established some of the essential characteristics of the process of Ca^{2+} transport, e.g., its energy requirements, its stoichiometry with the respiratory chain, and the concept that either the oxidation of substrates *or* the hydrolysis of added ATP by the action of an active mitochondrial ATPase (the "coupling" ATPase) can drive the process (Lehninger *et al.*, 1967). After the initial studies, with their emphasis on the maximum capacity of mitochondria for Ca^{2+} uptake, most investigations were directed to the so-called process of "membrane loading." In membrane loading, mitochondria are exposed to limited amounts of Ca^{2+} in the absence of permeant anions, and then do not appear to accumulate the cation in the form of insoluble matrix deposits. A large number of studies (summarized in Table VII) have characterized the process of "membrane loading." Some of the points made in Table VII require special comment, considering the emphasis of this article on the regulatory role of the process of mitochondrial Ca^{2+} uptake. Ca^{2+} loading in mitochondria can attain levels as high as 3 μmoles per mg of protein in the presence of phosphate. In a tissue like heart, which contains about 100 mg of mitochondrial protein per mg wet weight (Scarpa and Graziotti, 1973), this would correspond to the storage of about 300 μmoles of Ca^{2+} per mg of tissue. As stated above, these levels, which underscore the impressive Ca^{2+} storage ability of mitochondria, clearly represent unphysiological limits in most soft tissues, but may be realistic in specialized tissues. Osteoblasts, osteoclasts, and mitochondria of other cells involved in heavy Ca^{2+} traffic contain large numbers of electron-opaque masses that appear to be made up of insoluble Ca^{2+} and phosphate deposits. Moreover, recent findings have shown that mitochondria

TABLE VII

The Energy-Linked Uptake of Ca^{2+} by Mitochondria[a]

Requirements:	An energy source (respiration of ATP)
Inhibited by	
Indirectly	Inhibitors of energy-conservation
Directly	Lanthanides, ruthenium red, Mg^{2+}
Maximal capacity:	100-150 nmoles of Ca^{2+} per mg of protein (without phosphate) up to 3 μmoles of Ca^{2+} per mg of protein (with phosphate)
Rate:	3-10 nmoles of Ca^{2+} per mg of protein per second
K_m:	About 10 μM
Mechanism:	Electrophoretic, charge uncompensated

[a] From Carafoli and Crompton (1978).

from tissues not specialized in the transport of Ca^{2+} have been found to contain *endogenous* amounts of Ca^{2+} in excess of 0.3 μmoles per mg of protein (Vallières *et al.*, 1975; Malmström and Carafoli, 1977).

Other points of interest in Table VII are the affinity of the uptake system for Ca^{2+} and the rate of energy-linked uptake. Since many Ca^{2+}-dependent reactions in the cell are regulated by Ca^{2+} in the micromolar activity range and since the ionized Ca^{2+} concentration in the cytosol (see above) is of the order of 1 μM or less, it becomes important to establish whether mitochondria can take up Ca^{2+} from an environment that contains micromolar amounts. On this, opinions have been sharply divided in the past, but it now appears that under optimal conditions, the apparent K_m of mitochondria for Ca^{2+} is of the order of 10 μM in heart mitochondria (Crompton *et al.*, 1976a) and probably lower in liver mitochondria (Affolter and Carafoli, 1981). The kinetics of the process of active uptake is hyperbolic, at least in some tissues (Crompton *et al.*, 1976b; Wikström *et al.*, 1975), but becomes sigmoidal upon addition of Mg^{2+} to the reaction medium. Mg^{2+} inhibits the process of active uptake and does so very strongly in heart mitochondria (Sordahl, 1974; Jacobus *et al.*, 1975) and moderately in liver mitochondria (Jacobus *et al.*, 1975; Åkerman *et al.*, 1977). It is this Mg^{2+} inhibition that is responsible for the shift of the K_m in heart mitochondria toward higher values. The inhibitory effect of Mg^{2+} may be significant for physiological regulation, but this cannot be affirmed until precise data becomes available on the concentration of ionized Mg^{2+} in the cytosol (Rose, 1968). Substantial inhibition of the active Ca^{2+} accumulation in heart mitochondria is only observed at concentrations of Mg^{2+} in excess of 1 mM. Interestingly, the sigmoidal kinetics of Ca^{2+}

uptake in liver mitochondria (Gvedov *et al.*, 1973; Reed and Bygrave, 1975) is not rendered hyperbolic by the absence of Mg^{2+} (Affolter and Carafoli, 1981). The maximum rate of energy-linked Ca^{2+} uptake by mitochondria, when estimated directly, is of the order of 3–10 nmoles/mg of protein per second (Crompton *et al.*, 1976a). It may be even higher in preparations that can maintain an optimum negative potential with respect to the inner mitochondrial membrane (Vercesi *et al.*, 1978). This can be viewed against the requirements of Ca^{2+}-dependent processes in the cytosol. In heart, for example, the process of energy-linked Ca^{2+} uptake by mitochondria can mobilize up to 200 nmoles of Ca^{2+} per gram of tissue during the time of a relaxation event (200 msec). One important point brought out in Table VII is the electrogenic nature of the Ca^{2+} uptake process. Several authors (Puskin *et al.*, 1976; Rottenberg and Scarpa, 1974; Heaton and Nicholls, 1976; Crompton and Heid, 1978) have provided evidence that this process consists of a charge-uncompensated flux of Ca^{2+} that occurs in response to the membrane potential created by respiration. Others (Moyle and Mitchell, 1977a,b; Reed and Bygrave, 1975; Åkerman, 1978) have proposed partial charge compensation during the influx process, but the bulk of the experimental evidence appears now to favor the purely electrogenic nature of the reaction. A consequence of this would be that the ratio of the intra- and extramitochondrial ionized Ca^{2+} concentrations, given the probable membrane potential of about -180 mV (Mitchell, 1966), should be about 10^6 if the electrophoretic uptake process is permitted to reach equilibrium. However, this is negated by existing knowledge on the intra- and extramitochondrial ionized Ca^{2+} as derived indirectly by the arrays of activities of several Ca^{2+}-modulated enzymes in the two cellular compartments (see Carafoli and Crompton, 1978, for a discussion), and also by considerations of cell physiology: a gradient of 10^6, given the maximal ionized Ca^{2+} concentration in the mitochondria of $<< 10^{-4}$ *M*, would lower the cytosolic Ca^{2+} to intolerably low levels. These considerations have led to the proposal that the electrophoretic uptake process does not reach equilibrium *in vivo* (Carafoli and Crompton, 1976). Given the essentially irreversible nature of the electrophoretic route, which is driven by a membrane potential of -180 mV, deviation from the equilibrium can only be achieved by a separate route used exclusively for the efflux of the accumulated Ca^{2+} from mitochondria.

C. The Release of Ca^{2+} from Mitochondria

One key tool used to establish that Ca^{2+} leaves mitochondria by a route different from that for uptake is ruthenium red (see Table VII). If mitochondria are permitted to accumulate Ca^{2+} and then are treated with concentrations of ruthenium red sufficient to abolish the uptake route, any release of the cation will necessarily occur via an independent pathway. The first experimental indication for the existence of such a ruthenium-red insensitive route for Ca^{2+} efflux came from experiments of Rossi *et al.* (1973), who showed a rapid and spontaneous release of Ca^{2+} from ruthenium-red-inhibited liver mitochondria. The mechanism of the Ca^{2+} release observed by Rossi *et al.* (1973) was not investigated, but it was clear that a route different from that of the uptake was in operation.

In subsequent years, several ways and agents capable of activating a Ca^{2+} release route were described. Some of them act by collapsing the negative membrane potential responsible for maintaining the accumulated Ca^{2+} inside mitochondria and therefore promote the exit of Ca^{2+} on *both* the efflux pathway and the uptake pathway (if the latter is not inhibited by ruthenium red). In the presence of ruthenium red however, only the separate efflux pathway can be used: Recent experiments (Caroni *et al.*, 1978) have demonstrated that ruthenium red remains bound to the electrophoretic uptake route in the deenergized state. This type of release is induced by classical uncouplers, and, interestingly enough, by phosphoenolpyruvate (Roos *et al.*, 1978). From a physiological standpoint, it is unlikely that Ca^{2+} release induced by the collapse of the membrane potential plays any significant role, since many other important mitochondrial functions depend on the maintenance of this potential. The suggestion that natural substances such as prostaglandins (Kirtland and Baum, 1972; Carafoli *et al.*, 1973; Malmström and Carafoli, 1975) or other polyunsaturated fatty acids (Roman, 1978) may act as specific Ca^{2+} ionophores is more realistic, but has not been explored in detail. A recent suggestion by Lehninger *et al.* (1978) that the ratio of oxidized to reduced intramitochondrial pyridine nucleotides may determine the balance of Ca^{2+} between liver mitochondria and the medium is potentially of physiological significance. However, the mechanism by which pyridine nucleotides would exert their action is completely obscure. Hamilton and Holdsworth (1970) have obtained some evidence that the vitamin D-dependent Ca^{2+}-binding protein promotes the release of Ca^{2+} from intestinal mucosa mitochondria.

A specific mechanism for Ca^{2+} release from most (but not, significantly, from liver and kidney) mitochondria has been discovered and studied by Carafoli and associates (1974) (Crompton *et al.*, 1976a, 1977, 1978). It consists of a specific exchange between intramitochondrial Ca^{2+} and extramitochondrial Na^+, which involves a specific exchange-diffusion carrier and is activated half-maximally at about 8 m*M* external Na^+. The most important characteristics of this exchange system are summarized in Table VIII. Of particular interest is the sigmoidal character of the curve relating the velocity of Ca^{2+} release to the concentration of added Na^+. As shown in Fig. 2, more than one Na^+ is involved per cycle of exchange with Ca^{2+}. From experiments of this type, Hill coefficients of between 2.8 and 3.1 have been calculated. This indicates that the Na^+/Ca^{2+} exchange carrier is either electroneutral, or driven in the direction of Ca^{2+} release by the negative potential inside mitochondria (Crompton *et al.*, 1976a). attempts to determine the Na^+/Ca^{2+} exchange stoichiometry directly, as by measuring the

TABLE VIII[a]

General Properties of the Na^+-Induced Release of Ca^{2+}

Monovalent cation specificity	In addition to Na^+, Li^+ has some releasing effect, K^+, Rb^+, Cs^+, no effect
K_m (Na^+)	About 8 mM
K_m (Ca^{2+}, from outside)	About 13 μM
Kinetics	Strongly sigmoidal
V_{max}	About 0.2 nmoles of Ca^{2+} per mg of protein per sec
Inhibited by	La^{3+} (at high concentrations)
Present in mitochondria from	Heart, brain, skeletal muscle, exocrine and endocrine tissues
Absent in mitochondria from	Liver, kidney, lung

[a] From Carafoli and Crompton (1978).

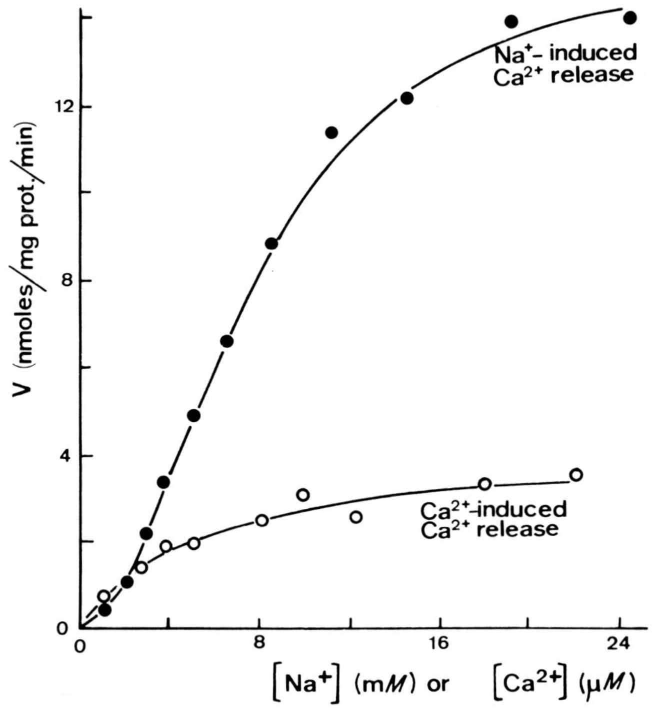

Fig. 2. Relationship of velocity of Ca^{2+} release to concentration of added Na^+.

accumulation of Na^+ consequent to Ca^{2+} release, have yielded unsatisfactory results. This is due to the presence of a very active Na^+/H^+ antiporter in the inner mitochondrial membrane (Mitchell and Moyle, 1967) which operates with a V_{max} about ten times higher that of the Na^+/Ca^{2+} exchange system (Crompton and Heid, 1978). As a result, the Na^+ that has entered the organelle in exchange for the lost Ca^{2+} will very rapidly return to the extramitochondrial medium. The sigmoidal kinetics of the Na^+-induced Ca^{2+} release is interesting also from a physiological standpoint, as it shows that relatively small changes in the concentration of Na^+ in the medium surrounding mitochondria can bring about relatively large losses of Ca^{2+} from mitochondria. When one considers (see above) the very large amounts of Ca^{2+} stored in mitochondria *in vivo,* it is clear that even minor changes in Na^+ concentration in the medium surrounding mitochondria could have profound influences on the cytosolic Ca^{2+} levels.

It is clear from Fig. 2 that the V_{max} of the Na^+-induced Ca^{2+} release is lower than that of the electrophoretic uptake process. If the Na^+-activated route is to compete efficiently with the uptake process, thus preventing excessive Ca^{2+} depletion of the cytosol, it is necessary to postulate that electrophoretic uptake normally proceeds at a suboptimal rate. How this is achieved is as yet unknown. To illustrate, consider a cytosolic calcium concentration of the order of 1 μM and a K_m of the electrophoretic Ca^{2+} uniporter of about 10 μM (Carafoli *et al.*, 1977). This would yield an approximate rate of Ca^{2+} removal from the cytoplasm of about 0.12 nmoles Ca^{2+} per mg protein per second. Under *in vivo* conditions with Mg^{2+} present, this figure would have to be much lower, about 0.02 nmoles per mg protein per second (Crompton *et al.*, 1976a). From the Ca^{2+} requirements of two intramitochondrial enzymes, i.e., isocitric dehydrogenase (Denton *et al.*, 1972, 1978) and pyruvate dehydrogenase phosphate phosphatase (Denton *et al.*, 1972; see also Carafoli and Crompton, 1978), one can calculate a probable matrix activity of about 2 μM Ca^{2+}. Since the Na^+/Ca^{2+} antiporter, when operating as a Ca^{2+}/Ca^{2+} exchanger, exhibits a K_m of 13 μM (Crompton *et al.*, 1978) and has hyperbolic kinetics, one could calculate with the aid of Fig. 2 that the actual rate of Ca^{2+} efflux at 2 μM (Ca^{2+}) would be about 0.02 nmole/mg protein per second in the presence of saturating amounts of Na^+ and Ca^{2+}. It is evident, then, that under the conditions that probably prevail *in vivo,* the rates of Ca^{2+} influx and efflux do not appear to be too far apart, at least in Na^+-sensitive mitochondria.

Much less can be said about mitochondria where the Na^+-induced Ca^{2+} release route is not present (liver, kidney, lung). In these mitochondria, Ca^{2+} release also occurs via a separate pathway (Caroni *et al.*, 1978), not yet characterized as well as the Na^+/Ca^{2+} exchange system. Recent experiments (Lötscher *et al.*, 1979) have suggested that Ca^{2+} release from liver mitochondria may be obligatorily linked to the release of inorganic phosphate.

VII. THE CONTROL AND REGULATION OF THE TRANSPORT OF Ca^{2+} ACROSS THE PLASMA AND THE INTRACELLULAR MEMBRANES

The various systems involved in the regulation of cellular Ca^{2+} are shown diagrammatically in Fig. 3. In the preceding discussion occasional mention was made of possible regulatory mechanisms. These are very important for an understanding of cellular Ca^{2+} function, but are topics on which only very little information is available. A brief survey of that knowledge, along with a discussion of some possibilities will now be presented.

That hormones like calcitonin or parathyroid hormone may control Ca^{2+} traffic across the plasma membrane of nonexcitable tissues (Borle, 1970, 1975) has already been referred to, as has the report that cathecholamines and cyclic AMP

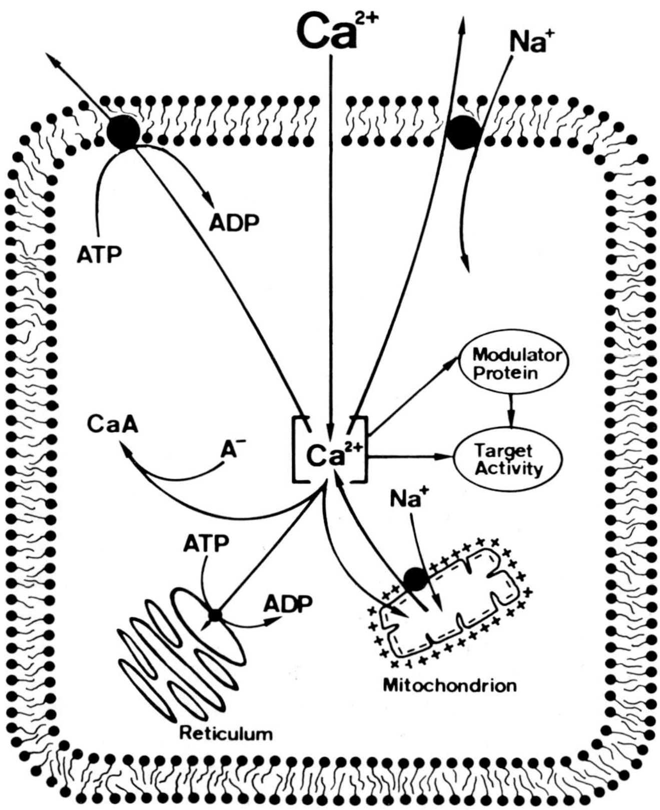

Fig. 3. Systems involved in regulation of cellular Ca^{2+}.

analogs increase the activity of the "slow Ca^{2+} channel" of heart sarcolemma (Reuter, 1974). The indirect effect of vitamin D in mediating the influx of Ca^{2+} into intestinal mucosa (and other) cells has also been mentioned.

As far as cellular calcium efflux is concerned, it is worth recalling that Parkinson and Radde (1971) have reported the activation of the red blood cell Ca^{2+}-ATPase by calcitonin. The observation is puzzling, however, since it implies that the calcitonin molecule has crossed the erythrocyte membrane in order to have induced ATP lysis. This seems rather improbable since polypeptide hormones normally do not penetrate into cells. The activation of a specific plasma membrane ATPase that leads to Ca^{2+} extrusion and that involves the modulator protein (CDR, calmodulin) is one possible means to increase the efficiency of the outward pumping of Ca^{2+} (see below).

The possible modulation of Na^+ fluxes across the plasma membrane (as by ATP, see above), along with the existence in most mitochondria of the Na^+/Ca^{2+} exchange system, suggest one way in which the plasma membrane and the mitochondrial Na^+/Ca^{2+} antiporters may function jointly in the overall regulation of cellular Ca^{2+}. Conditions that lead to increased Na^+ penetration of the cell would trigger the release of Ca^{2+} from mitochondria and increase the cytosolic Ca^{2+} concentration. This in turn would potentiate the activity of the plasma membrane Na^+/Ca^{2+} antiporter and thus lead to a depletion of *total* (i.e., cytosolic and stored) cellular calcium. Conversely, conditions limiting the penetration of Na^+ into the cell would favor Ca^{2+} retention by the mitochondria as they would inactivate the Na^+-dependent release route. This would lead to a decrease in cytosolic Ca^{2+}, but not necessarily to a decrease in "total" cellular calcium. This type of Na^+ modulated regulation of total and cytosolic cellular calcium is an attractive and reasonable model as it integrates Ca^{2+} fluxes across the plasma membrane with the "mitochondrial Ca^{2+} cycle."

A somewhat analogous situation can also be envisaged for cells containing Na^+-unresponsive mitochondria. Whenever the Ca^{2+} concentration in the cytosol decreases below the level necessary for the optimal activity of the Ca^{2+}-ejecting plasma membrane ATPase and of the electrophoretic mitochondrial uptake pathway, i.e., between 1 and 10 μM (see above) both systems will be slowed down. This will result in a buildup of the cytosolic Ca^{2+} because of entry of extracellular Ca^{2+} and because the mitochondrial Ca^{2+} release mechanism will now be potentiated more than the Ca^{2+} uptake mechanism. The presence (and possible modulation) of cytosolic Mg^{2+}, which inhibits the electrophoretic mitochondrial Ca^{2+} uptake route, may also play an additional role. The rise in cytosolic Ca^{2+} would then activate the plasma membrane Ca^{2+}-pumping ATPase, and, in turn, cause the electrophoretic mitochondrial uptake route to become more important, i.e., return the situation to "normal." In addition to Mg^{2+}, other factors affecting the Ca^{2+} balance between mitochondria and cytosol may intervene. One of these may be the mitochondrial pyridine nucleotides redox ratio (Lehninger *et al.*, 1978). Phosphoenolpyruvate has also frequently been mentioned in the past as a possible ''physiological'' inducer of Ca^{2+} release from mitochondria (Chudapongse, 1976; Chudapongse and Haugaard, 1973; Peng *et al.*, 1974). However, the recent finding by Roos *et al.* (1978) that it induces large decreases of the membrane potential makes phosphoenolpyruvate a rather unlikely candidate as a physiological calcium regulator.

To return to the integration of the Na^+/Ca^{2+} fluxes in the plasma membrane and in mitochondria, it may be interesting to cite some examples that indicate that events specifically requiring the increase in the level of cytosolic Ca^{2+} may be triggered solely by the penetration of Na^+ into the cell. In these cases, Na^+ evidently mobilizes Ca^{2+} from intracellular stores. These may indeed be the mitochondria (although proof of this is still lacking).

Using the β islet cells of Langerhans as a model, Lowe *et al.* (1976) were able to induce an impressive release of insulin even though no Ca^{2+} entered the cells from the extracellular medium. Instead Na^+ was forced into the cell with the aid of the alkaloid veratridine, which permanently opened the plasma membrane Na^+ channel. Since insulin release is well known to be calcium dependent, these observations constitute good evidence for the release of calcium from intracellular stores that must have occurred as a result of cellular Na^+ loading.

In an analogous experiment Rahamimoff *et al.* (1976) observed transmitter release from motor end plates (another Ca^{2+}-requiring process) when Na^+ was introduced into the cells in the total absence of extracellular Ca^{2+}.

The type of regulation involving mitochondrial Ca^{2+} discussed above may be considered of the ''short-term'' type. However, situations have been described where the ability of mitochondria to transport Ca^{2+} may be altered on a longer term basis as a result of hormonal stimuli. Thus, Kimberg and Goldstein (1966, 1967) have shown that steroid hormones administered *in vivo* influence the ability of liver mitochondria to transport Ca^{2+} : 17β-estradiol and dehydrocortisone enhanced the uptake (storage?) ability, whereas cortisone depressed it. Similarly Kimura and Rasmussen (1977) found that dexamethasone, acting like cortisone, depressed mitochondrial calcium uptake. Glucagon and insulin have also been investigated (Yamazaki, 1975; Hughes and Barritt, 1977; Dorman *et al.*, 1975) and found to increase the rate of Ca^{2+} uptake and retention in liver mitochondria isolated from treated animals. Of particular interest is the observation by Dorman *et al.* (1975) that there is no effect of insulin on liver mitochondrial uptake if the animal is simultaneously treated with cycloheximide, an inhibitor of protein synthesis.

Cellular calcium regulation so far has been considered the role of mitochondria, since the membranes of these organelles constitute the largest single element of the Ca^{2+}-transporting surfaces in the most frequently studied cells. Indeed, the work of Rose and Loewenstein (1975, 1976) with cells of the salivary gland of *Chironomus* has shown that mitochondria are responsible for the buffering of

Ca^{2+} injected into the cells. Thus when the mitochondrial uptake system was inhibited, the Ca^{2+}-buffering capacity of the cells was largely lost. In addition, as already discussed, mitochondria have separate mechanisms for the movement of Ca^{2+} in and out. This has an obvious advantage in terms of regulation.

The system(s) for transporting Ca^{2+} in endoplasmic reticulum is (are) as yet poorly characterized and understood. However, the above mentioned recent studies by Blaustein *et al.* (1980) on nerve endings have shown that smooth endoplasmic reticulum may possess Ca^{2+} buffering properties at physiological Ca^{2+} activity ranges. As for the sarcoplasmic reticulum, which with its very high affinity for Ca^{2+} certainly plays a key role in the fine regulation of myofibril relaxation, the key problem is the lack of a sufficiently defined mechanism for the release of Ca^{2+}. Nevertheless, the fact that Ca^{2+} uptake is markedly stimulated by a cAMP-dependent phosphorylation mechanism (see above) is of great interest, particularly since it occurs only in the sarcoplasmic reticulum from heart and slow muscles, where the ability to take up Ca^{2+} is markedly reduced. Similarly, the stimulation of Ca^{2+} uptake in cardiac sarcoplasmic reticulum by the calcium-dependent regulator protein (CDR) is of great interest (see below).

VIII. THE SOLUBLE PROTEIN ACTIVATOR (CDR, CALMODULIN) IN THE TRANSMISSION OF THE Ca^{2+} MESSAGE

The existence and some functions of the soluble Ca^{2+}-dependent modulator have already been alluded to above. A more detailed discussion of the properties of this molecule is justified by the growing importance attributed to this protein as a mediator of the Ca^{2+} message, and by reason of recent findings.

This small acidic protein (MW about 17,000) has now been sequenced (Vanaman *et al.*, 1977). It contains 148 residues, including the unusual amino acid trimethyllysine, and shows extensive homologies to troponin C. It appears to be fairly ubiquitous, and is found in variable but sometimes large amounts in the cell. Brain contains about 700 mg per kg wet weight, aorta about 150, with other cell types having intermediate values (Grand and Perry, 1979). Originally described as a specific activator of brain cyclic AMP phosphodiesterase (Kakiuchi and Yamazaki 1970; Cheung, 1970), and subsequently found to be involved in the regulation of other enzyme systems(adenylate cyclase, Brostrom *et al.*, 1975; Cheung *et al.*, 1975; phosphorylase *b* kinase, Cohen *et al.*, 1978; the Ca^{2+} pumping ATPase of the erythrocyte membrane, Bond and Clough, 1973; Luthra *et al.*, 1976; Gopinath and Vincenzi, 1977; Jarrett and Penniston, 1978), it has more recently been shown that this soluble protein activates a protein phosphorylation system present in brain membranes (Schulman and Greengard, 1978a,b), is a component of myosin light chain kinase (Dabrowska *et al.*, 1978; Yagi *et al.*, 1978; Waisman *et al.*, 1978), and activates the transport of Ca^{2+} in heart sarcoplasmic reticulum (Katz and Remtulla, 1978). Amino acid sequence studies of the activator and of troponin C (the Ca^{2+}-receptor in the troponin molecule) have shown extensive analogies (Vanaman *et al.*, 1977; Dedman *et al.*, 1978; Jarrett and Penniston, 1978). In agreement with this finding, troponin C can substitute for the soluble protein in the activation of phosphodiesterase (Amphlett *et al.*, 1976). One very recent development in this area (Cohen *et al.*, 1978) is the discovery that phosphorylase *b* kinase, previously thought to be a dodecamer consisting of 4α, 4β, and 4γ subunits, in its active form is in reality a hexadecamer, also containing 4γ subunits and Ca^{2+}. The 4γ subunits are molecules of the modulator. Also of interest is the identification of 3 other calmodulin-binding proteins in a variety of tissues (Grand and Perry, 1979), a report that underlines the possibility of still other targets for its regulatory action.

From the standpoint of the regulation of Ca^{2+} fluxes and the cellular Ca^{2+} concentration, of primary interest is perhaps the activation by calmodulin of the plasma membrane Ca^{2+}-pumping ATPase, and of the Ca^{2+}-ATPase in sarcoplasmic reticulum. The other major Ca^{2+} transporting membrane system of the cell, the mitochondrion, is insensitive to calmodulin (E. Carafoli, unpublished). Niggli *et al.* (1979a) have shown that the modulator interacts directly and with very high affinity with the plasma membrane ATPase, and does so only in the presence of Ca^{2+}. Whether this can be taken as an indication that the role of the modulator in this case is to "deliver" more Ca^{2+} to the enzyme, is an open question, and other interpretations are certainly possible.

Calmodulin (CDR) binds 4 moles of Ca with very high affinity (Dedman *et al.*, 1978). Since some tissues contain large amounts of calmodulin, this protein may well represent an important system for buffering cellular Ca^{2+}. In brain, which contains about 700 mg of calmodulin per kg wet weight (Grand and Perry, 1979), the total calcium storage capacity would correspond to about 180 nmoles of Ca^{2+} per gm wet weight. These are impressive values. Schulman and Greengard (1978b) have proposed that Ca^{2+} binding by the modulator may be a transient means to withhold calcium from the powerful pumping systems of mitochondria and sarcoplasmic reticulum.

IX. SOME GENERAL CONSIDERATIONS ON THE CELLULAR PROCESSES INVOLVING Ca^{2+}

The physiological processes modulated by Ca^{2+} (Table II) cover a large spectrum of activities: mobilization of fuels, exocrine and endocrine secretion, contractility and motility, cell division, many membrane-linked functions, and probably other as yet unidentified activities. One common feature of the modulation by Ca^{2+} is that it occurs at micromolar concentrations, a situation that underlines once again the importance of controlling cytosolic calcium activity very precisely, and justifies the existence of multiple controlling systems. At the same time these considerations make it unlikely that other intracellular enzymes, such as phosphofructokinase, creatine kinase, pyrophosphatase, or nicotinamidenucleotide transhydrogenase (Kretsinger and Nelson, 1976), play a significant role in the intracellular calcium regulation, as their calcium-binding affinities are too low to affect the cytosolic calcium concentration. It is, of course, also unlikely that the binding of Ca^{2+} plays any role in their activation. A second important concept that has emerged is that the modulator protein may be involved in mediating the Ca^{2+} signal, at least for some target activities. Some of the developments in this area are of great interest and may have far-reaching implications for the entire field of metabolic regulation. The type of interaction of the modulator protein with its targets, the role of Ca^{2+} in the process, the mechanism by which the modulator protein interacts with Ca^{2+} so as to help bring it to the target organelles—these are the problems that will undoubtedly be studied intensively in the future. The concept that the modulator protein may serve an additional role as a transient storage point for cellular Ca^{2+} is also interesting, and could be extended to other intracellular ligands such as parvalbumin.

Finally, it may be worth returning briefly to some of the concepts of molecular evolution expressed at the opening of this chapter. It should have become clear to the reader that the chemical advantages of choosing Ca^{2+} as a transmitter of information were obvious. One could say that, given the situation prevailing in the original environment, the evolutionary decision to utilize Ca^{2+} was practically obligatory. But then, it is perhaps interesting to consider other advantages resulting from the decision, and from the consequent development of systems to keep the intracellular activity of Ca^{2+} extremely low. One was to prevent the displacement (by Ca^{2+}) of Mg^{2+} from its complexes with essential metabolic fuels like ATP, which are generally only active as Mg^{2+} salts (Gomperts, 1976). But a more general and more important advantage was the possibility of orienting metabolism toward phosphate (Weber, 1976; Kretsinger, 1977; Carafoli and Crompton, 1978), which would have been clearly impossible in an intracellular environment of high Ca^{2+} activity.

REFERENCES

Adam, G. (1970). Theory of nerve excitation as a cooperative cation exchange in a 2-dimensional lattice. *In* "Physical Principles of Biological Membranes" (F. Snell, J. Wolken, G. Iverson, and J. Lam, eds.), pp. 35–67. Gordon & Breach, New York.

Affolter, H., and Carafoli, E. (1981). Hyperbolic kinetics of the electrophoretic carrier of Ca^{2+} uptake in liver mitochondria. *Eur. J. Biochem.* **119,** 199–201.

Åkerman, K.E.O. (1978). Changes in membrane potential during calcium ion influx and efflux across the mitochondrial membrane. *Biochim. Biophys. Acta* **502,** 359–366.

Åkerman, K.E.O., Wikström, M.K.F., and Saris, N.E. (1977). Effects of inhibitors on the sigmodicity of the calcium ion transport kinetics in rat liver mitochondria. *Biochim. Biophys. Acta* **464,** 287–294.

Alonso, G.L., Bazerque, P.M., Arrigo, D.M., and Tumilasci, O.R. (1971). Adenosine triphosphate-dependent calcium uptake by rat submaxillary gland microsomes. *J. Gen. Physiol.* **58,** 340–350.

Amphlett, G.W., Vanaman, T.C., and Perry, S.V. (1976). Effect of the troponin C-like protein from bovine brain (brain modulator protein) on the Mg^{2+}-stimulated ATPase of skeletal muscle actomyosis. *FEBS Lett.* **72,** 163–167.

Anand, M.B., Chauhan, M.S., and Dhalla, N.S. (1977). Calcium ion/magnesium ion ATPase of heart sarcolemma, microsomes and mitochondria. *J. Biochem. (Tokyo)* **82,** 1731–1739.

Bailey, L.E., and Dresel, P.E. (1968). Correlation of contractile force with a calcium pool in the isolated cat heart. *J. Gen. Physiol.* **52,** 969–982.

Baker, P.F. (1975). Transport and metabolism of calcium in nerve. *In* "Calcium Movements in Excitable Cells" (P.F. Baker and H. Reuter, eds.), pp. 7–53. Pergamon, Oxford.

Baker, P.F. (1976). The regulation of intracellular calcium. *Symp. Soc. Exp. Biol.* **30,** 67–69.

Baker, P.F., and Glitsch, H.G. (1973). Does metabolic energy participate directly in the sodium-dependent extrusion of calcium from squid giant axions. *J. Physiol. (London)* **233,** 44P.

Baker, P. F., and McNaughton, P.A. (1976). Kinetics and energetics of calcium efflux from intact squid axons. *J. Physiol. (London)* **259,** 103–144.

Baker, P.F., Blaustein, M.P., Hodgkin, A.L., and Steinhardt, R.A. (1969). The influence of calcium on sodium efflux in squid axons. *J. Physiol. (London)* **200,** 431–458.

Baker, P.F., Hodgkin, A.L., and Ridgeway, E.B. (1971). Depolarisation and calcium entry in squid axons. *J. Physiol. (London)* **218,** 709–755.

Banks, P. (1967). The effect of ouabain on the secretion of catecholamines and on the intracellular concentration of potassium. *J. Physiol. (London)* **193,** 631–637.

Banks, P., Biggins, R., Bishop, R., Christian, B., and Currie, N. (1969). Sodium ions and the secretion of catecholamines. *J. Physiol. (London)* **200,** 797–805.

Barlogie, B., Hasselbach, W., and Makinose, M. (1971). Activation of calcium efflux by ADP and inorganic phosphate. *FEBS Lett.* **12,** 267–268.

Baskin, R.J., and Deamer, D.W. (1969). Comparative ultrastructure and calcium transport in heart and skeletal muscle microsomes. *J. Cell Biol.* **43,** 610–617.

Besch, H.R., and Schwartz, A. (1971). Initial calcium binding rates of canine cardiac relaxing systems (sarcoplasmic reticulum fragments) determined by stopped flow spectrophotometry. *Biochem. Biophys. Res. Commun.* **45,** 286–292.

Blaustein, M.P.(1976). The ins and outs of calcium transport in squid axons: Internal and external ion activation of calcium efflux. *Fed. Proc., Fed. Am. Soc. Exp. Biol.* **35,** 2574–2578.

Blaustein, M.P., Ratzlaff, R.W., and Schweitzer, E.S. (1980). Control of intracellular calcium in presynaptic nerve terminals. *Fed. Proc., Fed. Am. Exp. Biol.* **39,** 2970–2975.

Blaustein, M.P., Russell, J.M., and De Weer, P. (1974). Calcium efflux from internally dialysed squid axons: The influx of external and internal cations. *J. Supramol. Struct.* **2,** 558–581.

Bond, G.H., and Clough, D.L. (1973). A soluble protein activator of (Mg^{2+} + Ca^{2+})-dependent ATPase in human red cell membranes. *Biochem. Biophys. Acta* **323,** 592–599.

Borle, A. (1970). Kinetic analysis of Ca^{2+} movements in cell cultures. III. Effects of Ca^{2+} and of parathyroid hormone in kidney cells. *J. Gen. Physiol.* **55,** 163–186.

Borle, A. (1975). Regulation of cellular Ca^{2+} metabolism and Ca^{2+} transport by calcitonin. *J. Membr. Biol.* **21,** 125–146.

Brostrom, C.O., Huang, Y.-C., Brechenridge, B.M., and Wolff, D.J. (1975). Identification of a calcium-binding protein as a calcium-dependent regulator of brain adenylate cyclase. *Proc. Natl. Acad. Sci. U.S.A.* **72,** 64–68.

Brostrom, M.A., Brostrom, C.O., Breckenridge, B.M., and Wolff, D.J. (1976). Regulation of adenylate cyclase from glial tumor cells by calcium and a calcium-binding protein. *J. Biol. Chem.* **251,** 4744–4750.

Brown, J.E., and Blinks, J.R. (1974). Changes in intracellular free Ca^{2+} upon illumination of invertebrate photoreceptors. *J. Gen. Physiol.* **64,** 643–665.

Bygrave, F.L. (1977). Mitochondrial calcium transport. *Curr. Top. Bioenerg.* **6,** 259–318.

Carafoli, E. (1974). Mitochondrial uptake of calcium ions and the regulation of cell function. *Biochem. Soc. Symp.* **39,** 89–109.

Carafoli, E. (1979). The calcium cycle of mitochondria. *FEBS Lett.* **104,** 1–5.

Carafoli, E., and Crompton, M. (1976). Calcium ions and mitochondria. *Symp. Soc. Exp. Biol.* **30,** 89–115.

Carafoli, E., and Crompton, M. (1978). The regulation of intracellular calcium. *Curr. Top. Membr. Transp.* **10,** 151–216.

Carafoli, E., Balcavage, W.X., Lehninger, A.L., and Mattoon, J.R. (1970). Ca^{2+} metabolism in yeast cells and mitochondria. *Biochem. Biophys. Acta* **205,** 18–26.

Carafoli, E., Hansford, R.G., Secktor, B., and Lehninger, A.L. (1971). Interaction of Ca^{2+} with blowfly flight muscle mitochondria. *J. Biol. Chem.* **246,** 964–972.

Carafoli, E., Crovetti, F., and Ceccarelli, D. (1973). Interactions between prostaglandin E, and calcium at the level of the mitochondrial membrane. *Arch. Biochem. Biophys.* **154,** 40–46.

Carafoli, E., Tiozzo, R., Lugli, G., Crovetti, F., and Kratzing, C. (1974). The release of Ca^{2+} from heart mitochondria by sodium. *J. Mol. Cell. Cardiol.* **6,** 361–371.

Carafoli, E., Crompton, M., Malmström, K., Sigel, E., Salzmann, M., Chiesi, M., and Affolter, H. (1977). Mitochondrial calcium transport and the intracellular calcium homeostasis. *In* "Biochemistry of Membrane Transport" (G. Semenza and E. Carafoli, eds.), pp. 535–551. Springer-Verlag, Berlin and New York.

Carafoli, E., Crompton, M., Caroni, P., Schwerzmann, K., and Roos, I. (1980). The cycling of Ca^{2+} across the inner mitochondrial membrane. *In* "Frontiers of Bioorganic Chemistry and Molecular Biology" (S.N. Ananchenko, ed.), pp. 405–415. Pergamon Press, Oxford.

Caroni, P., and Carafoli, E. (1980). An ATP-dependent Ca^{2+}-pumping system in dog heart sarcolemma. *Nature (London)* **283,** 765–767.

Caroni, P., Schwerzmann, K., and Carafoli, E. (1978). Separate pathways for Ca^{2+} uptake and release in liver mitochondria. *FEBS Lett.* **96,** 339–342.

Caroni, P., Reinlib, L., and Carafoli, E. (1980). Charge movements during the Na^{+}/Ca^{2+} exchange in heart sarcolemmal vesicles. *Proc. Natl. Acad. Sci. U.S.A.* **77,** 6354–6358.

Chambaut, A.-M., Leray-Pecker, F., Feldmann, G., and Hanoune, J. (1974). Calcium-binding properties and ATPase activities of rat liver plasma membranes. *J. Gen. Physiol.* **64,** 104–126.

Cheung, W.Y. (1970). Cyclic 3′,5′-nucleotide phosphodiesterase. *Biochem. Biophys. Res. Commun.* **38,** 533–538.

Cheung, W.Y., Bradham, L.S., Lynch, T.J., Lin, Y.M., and Tallant, E.A. (1975). Protein activator of cyclic 3′:5′-nucleotide phosphodiesterase of bovine or rat brain also activates its adenylate cyclase. *Biochem. Biophys. Res. Commun.* **66,** 1055–1062.

Chiesi, M. (1978). Characteristics of cardiac sarcoplasmic reticulum and of its Ca^{2+}-pumping enzyme; a comparative study with fast skeletal muscle. Ph.D. Thesis, Swiss Federal Institute of Technology (ETH), Zurich, Switzerland.

Chudapongse, P. (1976). Further studies on the effect of phosphoenolpyruvate on respiration-dependent calcium transport by rat heart mitochondria. *Biochim. Biophys. Acta* **423,** 196–202.

Chudapongse, P., and Haugaard, N. (1973). The effect of phosphoenolpyruvate on calcium transport by mitochondria. *Biochim. Biophys. Acta* **307,** 599–606.

Cohen, P., Burchell, A., Foulkes, J.G., Cohen, P.T.W., Vanaman, T.C., and Nairn, C. (1978). Identification of the Ca^{2+}-dependent modulator protein as the fourth subunit of rabbit skeletal muscle phosphorlylase kinase. *FEBS Lett.* **92,** 287–293.

Costantin, L.L., and Podolsky, R.J. (1967). Depolarization of the internal membrane system in the activation of frog skeletal muscle. *J. Gen. Physiol.* **50,** 1101–1124.

Costantin, L.L., Franzini-Armstrong, C., and Podolsky, R.J. (1965). Localization of calcium-accumulating structures in striated muscle fibres. *Science* **147,** 158–160.

Costanzo, L., Windhager, E., and Taylor, A. (1978). Sodium-calcium interaction in the distal tubule. *In* "Aspects of Renal Function" (H. Vogel and K. Ullrich, eds.), Vol. 6, pp. 147–152. Experta Medica, Amsterdam.

Crompton, M., and Carafoli, E. (1979). The application of calcium selective electrodes and inhibitor-stop techniques to the resolution of calcium fluxes in mitochondria. *In* "Detection and Measurement of Free Calcium in Cells" (C.C. Ashley and A.K. Campbell, eds.), pp. 372–382. Elsevier/North Holland Publ., Amsterdam.

Crompton, M., and Heid, I. (1978). The cycling of calcium, sodium and protons across the inner membrane of cardiac mitochondria. *Eur. J. Biochem.* **91,** 599–608.

Crompton, M., Sigel, E., Salzmann, M., and Carafoli, E. (1976a). A kinetic study of the energy-linked influx of calcium into heart mitochondria. *Eur. J. Biochem.* **69,** 429–434.

Crompton, M., Capano, M., and Carafoli, E. (1976b). The sodium induced efflux of calcium from heart mitochondria. A possible mechanism for the regulation of mitochondrial calcium *Eur. J. Biochem.* **69,** 453–462.

Crompton, M., Künzi, M., and Carafoli, E. (1977). The calcium-induced and sodium-induced effluxes of calcium from heart mitochondria. *Eur. J. Biochem.* **79,** 549–558.

Crompton, M., Moser, R., Lüdi, H., and Carafoli, E. (1978). The interrelations between the transport of sodium and calcium in mitochondria of various mammalian tissues. *Eur. J. Biochem.* **82,** 25–31.

Dabrowska, R., Sherry, J.M.F., Aromatorio, D.K., and Hartshorne, D.J. (1978). Modulator protein as a component of the myosin-light chain kinase from chicken gizzard. *Biochemistry* **17,** 253–258.

Davson, M. (1970). "A Textbook of General Physiology." Churchill, London.

Dedman, J.R., Jackson, R.L., Schreiber, W.E., and Means, A.R. (1978). Sequence homology of the Ca^{2+}-dependent regulator of cyclic nucleotide phosphodiesterase from rat testis with other Ca^{2+}-binding proteins. *J. Biol. Chem.* **253,** 343–346.

Degani, C., and Boyer, P.D. (1973). A borohydride reduction method for characterisation of the acyl phosphate linkage in proteins and its application to sarcoplasmic reticulum adenosine triphosphate. *J. Biol. Chem.* **248,** 8222–8226.

DeMeis, L., Rubin-Altschul, B.M., and Machado, R.D. (1970). Comparative data of Ca^{2+} transport in brain and skeletal muscle microsomes. *J. Biol. Chem.* **245,** 1883–1889.

Denton, R.M., Randle, P.J., and Martin, B.R. (1972). Stimulation by calcium ions of pyruvate dehydrogenase phosphate phosphatase. *Biochem. J.* **128,** 161–163.

Denton, R.M., Richards, D.A., and Chin, J.G. (1978). Calcium ions and the regulation of NAD^+-linked isocitrate dehydrogenase from mitochondria of rat heart and other tissues. *Biochem. J.* **176,** 899–906.

DeWeer, P. (1976). Axoplasmic free magnesium levels and magnesium extrusion from squid giant axons. *J. Gen. Physiol.* **68,** 159–178.

Dieckvoss, G., and Wolf, H.U. (1976). Purification of the high affinity Ca^{2+} ATPase of human erythrocyte membranes. *FEBS-Symp.* **42,** 316 (abstr.).

Di Polo, R. (1976). The influence of nucleotides on calcium fluxes. *Fed. Proc., Fed. Am. Soc. Exp. Biol.* **35,** 2579–2582.

Di Polo, R., Requena, J., Brinley, F.J., Mullins, L.J., Jr., Scarpa, A., and Tiffert, T. (1976). Ionized calcium concentrations in squid axons. *J. Gen. Physiol.* **67,** 433–467.

Dorman, D.M., Barritt, G.J., and Bygrave, F.L. (1975). Stimulation of hepatic mitochondrial calcium transport by elevated plasma insulin concentrations. *Biochem. J.* **150,** 389–395.

Douglas, W.W. (1968). Stimulus-secretion coupling: The concept and clues from chromaffine and other cells. *Br. J. Pharmacol.* **34,** 451–474.

Douglas, W.W., and Rubin, R.P. (1961). The role of calcium in the secretory response of the adrenal medulla to acetylcholine. *J. Physiol. (London)* **159,** 40–57.

Douglas, W.W., and Rubin, R.P. (1963). The mechanism of catecholamine release from the adrenal medulla and the role of calcium in stimulus-secretion coupling. *J. Physiol. (London)* **167,** 288–310.

Drahota, Z., Carafoli, E., Rossi, C.S., Gamble, R.L., and Lehninger, A.L. (1965). The steady state maintenance of accumulated Ca^{2+} in rat liver mitochondria. *J. Biol. Chem.* **240,** 2712–2720.

Duggan, P.F., and Martonosi, A. (1970). Sarcoplasmic reticulum. IX. The permeability of sarcoplasmic reticulum membranes. *J. Gen. Physiol.* **56,** 147–167.

Ebashi, S., and Endo, M. (1968). Calcium ion in muscle contraction. *Prog. Biophys. Mol. Biol.* **18,** 123–183.

Endo, M., and Thorens, S. (1975). Mechanism of release of calcium from sarcoplasmic reticulum. *In* "Calcium Transport in Contraction and Secretion" (E. Carafoli, F. Clementi, W. Drabikowski, and A. Margreth eds.), pp. 359–366. North-Holland Publ., Amsterdam.

Endo, M., Tanaka, M., and Ogawa, Y. (1970). Calcium-induced release of calcium from the sarcoplasmic reticulum of skeletal muscle fibres. *Nature (London)* **288,** 34–36.

Fabiato, A., and Fabiato, F. (1975). Contractions induced by a calcium-triggered release of calcium from the sarcoplasmic reticulum of single skinned cardiac cells. *J. Physiol. (London)* **249,** 469–495.

Fanburg, B.L., Finkel, R.M., and Martonosi, A. (1964). The role of calcium in the mechanism of relaxation of cardiac muscle. *J. Biol. Chem.* **239,** 2298–2306.

Felo, R.S., Bohr, D.F., and Ruegg, J.C. (1965). Glycerinated skeletal and smooth muscle: Calcium and magnesium dependence. *Science* **147,** 1581–1583.

Ferreira, H.G., and Lew, V.L. (1976) Use of ionophore A23187 to measure cytoplasmic Ca^{2+} buffering and activation of the Ca^{2+} pump by internal Ca^{2+}. *Nature (London)* **259,** 47–49.

Fiehn, W., and Migala, A. (1971). Calcium binding to sarcoplasmic membranes. *Eur. J. Biochem.* **20,** 245–248.

Fleckenstein, A., Tritthart, H., Fleckenstein, B., Herbst, A., and Grün, G. (1969). Eine neue Gruppe kompetitiver Ca^{2+} Antagonisten (roveratril, D 600, Prenylamin) mit starken Hemmeffekten auf die elektromechanische Kopplung Warmblütermyokard. *Pfluegers Arch.* **397,** 25–38.

Ford, L.E., and Podolsky, R.J. (1970). Regenerative calcium release within muscle cells. *Science* **167,** 58–59.

Ford, L.E., and Podolsky, R.J. (1972a). Calcium uptake and force development by skinned muscle fibres in EGTA buffered solution. *J. Physiol. (London)* **223,** 1–19.

Ford, L.E., and Podolsky, R.J. (1972b). Intracellular calcium movements in skinned muscle fibres. *J. Physiol. (London)* **223,** 21–33.

Gietzen K., Seiler, S., Fleischer, S., and Wolf, H.U. (1979). Ca^{2+}-transport by reconstituted high-affinity Ca^{2+}-ATPase of human erythrocytes. *In* "Function and Molecular Aspects of Biomembrane Transport" (E. Quagliariello, F. Palmieri, S. Papa, and M. Klingenberg, eds.), pp. 519–522. Elsvier/North-Holland Publ., Amsterdam.

Gmaj, P., Murer, H., and Kinne, R. (1979). Calcium ion transport across plasma membranes isolated from rat kidney cortex. *Biochem. J.* **178,** 549–557.

Gomperts, B.D. (1976). Calcium and cell activation. *Recept. Recognition, Ser. A* **2,** 43–102.

Gopinath, R.M., and Vincenzi, F.F. (1977). Phosphodiesterase protein activator mimics red blood cell cytoplasmic activator of ($Ca^{2+}+Mg^{2+}$) ATPase. *Biochem. Biophys. Res. Commun.* **77,** 1203–1209.

Grand, R.J.A., and Perry, S.V. (1979). Calmodulin binding proteins from brain and other tissues. *Biochem. J.* **183,** 285–295.

Green, N.M., Allen, G., Hebdon, M., and Thorley-Lawson, D.A. (1977). Structural studies on the

Ca^{2+} transporting ATPase of sarcoplasmic reticulum. *In* "Calcium Binding Proteins and Calcium Function" (R.H. Wasserman, R.A. Corradino, E. Carafoli, H.R. Kretsinger, D.H. MacLennan, and F.L. Siegel, eds.), pp. 164–172. North-Holland Publ., Amsterdam.

Grossmann, A., and Furchgott, R.F. (1964). The effects of various drugs on calcium exchange in the isolated quinea-pig left muscle. *J. Pharmacol. Exp. Ther.* **145,** 162–172.

Hagiwara, S., and Nakajima, S. (1966). Effects of intracellular calcium ion concentration on the excitability of the muscle fibre of a barnacle. *J. Gen. Physiol.* **49,** 807–818.

Hales, C.N., and Milner, R.D.G. (1968a). The role of sodium and potassium in insulin secretion from rabbit pancreas. *J. Physiol. (London)* **194,** 725-743.

Hales, C.N., and Milner, R.D.G. (1968b). Cations and secretion of insulin from rabbit pancreas in vitro. *J. Physiol. (London)* **199,** 177–187.

Hamilton, J.W., and Holdsworth, E.S. (1970). The release of ^{45}Ca from mitochondria of chicken intestinal mucosa by calcium binding protein. *Biochem. Biophys. Res. Commun.* **40,** 1325-1330.

Heaton, G.M., and Nicholls, D.G. (1976). The calcium conductance of the inner membrane of rat liver mitochondria and the determination of the calcium electrochemical gradient. *Biochem. J.* **156,** 635-646.

Hughes, B.P., and Barritt, G.J. (1977). The effects of glucagon adrenalin, and dibutyryl adenosine 3′,5 monophosphate on calcium transport in rat liver mitochondria. *Proc. Aust. Biochem. Soc.* **10,** 36-45.

Hui, C., Drummond, M., and Drummond, G.I. (1976). Calcium accumulation and cyclic AMP-stimulated phosphorylation in plasma membrane-enriched preparations of myocardium. *Arch. Biochem. Biophys.* **173,** 415-427.

Ikemoto, N., Sreter, F.A., Nakamura, A., and Gergely, J. (1968). Trypic digestion and localisation of calcium uptake and ATPase activity in fragments of sarcoplasmic reticulum. *J. Ultrastruct. Res.* **23,** 216-232.

Ikemoto, N., Bhatnagar, G.M., and Gergely, J. (1971). Fractionation of solubilised sarcoplasmic reticulum. *Biochem. Biophys. Res. Commun.* **44,** 1510-1515.

Ikemoto, N., Bhatnagar, G.M., Nagy, B., and Gergely, J. (1972). Interaction of divalent cations with the 55,000 dalton protein component of the sarcoplasmic reticulum. Studies of fluorescence and circular dichroism. *J. Biol. Chem.* **247,** 7835–7837.

Inesi, G., and Asai, H. (1968). Trypsin digestion of fragmented sarcoplasmic reticulum. *Arch. Biochem. Biophys.* **126,** 469–481.

Inesi, G., and Scarpa, A. (1972). Fast kinetics of adenosine triphosphate dependent Ca^{2+} uptake by fragments sarcoplasmic reticulum. *Biochemistry* **11,** 356–359.

Jacobus, W.E., Tiozzo, R., Lugli, G., Lehninger, A.L., and Carafoli, E. (1975). Aspects of energy linked Ca^{2+} accumulation by rat-heart mitochondria. *J. Biol. Chem.* **250,** 7863–7870.

Jarrett, H.W., and Penniston, J.T. (1978). Purification of the Ca^{2+} stimulated ATPase activator from human erythrocytes. *J. Biol. Chem.* **253,** 4676–4682.

Jundt, H., and Reuter, H. (1977). Is sodium activated calcium efflux from mammalian cardiac muscle dependent on metabolic energy? *J. Physiol. (London)* **266,** 78P–79P.

Jundt, H., Prozig, H., Reuter, H., and Stucki, J.W. (1975). The effect of substances releasing intracellular calcium ions on sodium-dependent calcium efflux from guinea-pig auricles. *J. Physiol. (London)* **246,** 229-253.

Kakiuchi, S., and Yamazaki, R. (1970). Calcium dependent phosphodiesterase activity and its activation factor (PAF) from brain. Studies on cyclic 3′,5′-nucleotide phosphodiesterase (III). *Biochem. Biophys. Res. Commun.* **41,** 1104–1110.

Kanazawa, T., and Boyer, P.D. (1973). Occurrence and characteristics of a rapid exchange of phosphate oxygens catalyzed by sarcoplasmic reticulum. *J. Biol. Chem.* **248,** 3163-3172.

Katz, A.M. (1970). Contractile proteins of the heart. *Physiol. Rev.* **50,** 63–158.

Katz, A.M., Repke, E.I., Dunnett, J., and Hasselbach, W. (1977). Dependence of calcium permeability of sarcoplasmic reticulum vesicles on external and internal ion concentrations. *J. Biol. Chem.* **252,** 1950–1956.

Katz, S., and Remtulla, M.A. (1978). Phosphodiesterase protein activator stimulates calcium transport in cardiac microsomal preparations enriched in sarcoplasmic reticulum. *Biochem. Biophys. Res. Commun.* **83,** 1373–1379.

Kimberg, D.V., and Goldstein, S.A. (1966). Binding of calcium by liver miotchondria of rats treated with steroid hormones. *J. Biol. Chem.* **241,** 95–103.

Kimberg, D.V., and Goldstein, S.A. (1967). Binding of calcium by liver mitochondria: An effect of steroid hormones in Vitamin D-depleted and parathyroid-ectomized rats. *Endocrinology* **80,** 89–98.

Kimura, S., and Rasmussen, H. (1977). Adrenal glucocorticoids, adenine nucleotide translocation and mitochondrial calcium accumulation. *J. Biol. Chem.* **252,** 1217–1225.

Kirchberger, M.A., and Tada, M. (1976). Effects of adenosine 3′:5′-monophosphate-dependent protein kinase on sarcoplasmic reticulum isolated from cardiac and slow and fast contracting muscle. *J. Biol. Chem.* **251,** 725–729.

Kirchberger, M.A., Tada, M., and Katz, A.M. (1974). Adenosine 3′:5′-monophosphate-dependent protein kinase catalysed phosphorylation reaction and its relationship to calcium transport in cardiac sarcoplasmic reticulum. *J. Biol. Chem.* **249,** 6166–6173.

Kirtland, S.J., and Baum, H. (1972). Prostaglandin E, may act as a "calcium ionophore." *Nature (London)* **236,** 47–49.

Knauf, P.A., Proverbio, F., and Hoffman, J.F. (1974). Electrophoretic separation of different phosphoproteins associated with Ca-ATPase and Na, K-ATPase in human red cells ghosts. *J. Gen. Physiol.* **63,** 324–336.

Knowles, A.F., and Racker, E. (1975). Properties of a reconsituted calcium pump. *J. Biol. Chem.* **250,** 3538–3544.

Kohlhardt, M., Bauer, B., Krause, H., and Fleckenstein, A. (1972). Differentiation of the transmembrane Na and Ca channels in mammalian cardiac fibres by the use of specific inhibitors. *Pfluegers Arch.* **355,** 309–322.

Kostyuk, P.G., and Krishthal, O.A., (1978). Ionic and qating currents in the membrane of nerve cells. *Mem. Transp. Processes* **2,** 101–123.

Krebs, J.J.R., Hauser, H., and Carafoli, E. (1979). Asymmetric distribution of phospholipids in the inner membrane of beef heart mitochondria. *J. Biol. Chem.* **254,** 5308–5316.

Kretsinger, R.H. (1977). Evolution of the formational role of calcium in eukaryotes. *In* "Calcium Binding Proteins and Calcium Function" (R.H. Wasserman, R.A. Corradino, E. Carafoli, R.H. Kretsinger, D.H. MacLennan, and F.L. Sigel, eds.), pp. 63–72. Elsevier/North-Holland Publ., Amsterdam.

Kretsinger, R.H., and Nelson, D.J. (1976). Calcium in biological systems. *Coord. Chem. Rev.* **18,** 29–124.

Lamb, J.F., and Lindsay, R. (1971). Effect of Na metabolic inhibitors and ATP on Ca movements in L cells. *J. Physiol. (London)* **218,** 691–708.

Lehninger, A.L., Carafoli, E., and Rossi, C.S. (1967). Energy-linked ion movements in mitochondrial systems. *Adv. Enzymol. Relat. Areas Mol. Biol.* **29,** 259–320.

Lehninger, A.L., Vercesi, A., and Bababunmi, E.A. (1978). Regulation of Ca^{2+} release from mitochondria by the oxidation-reduction state of pyridine nucleotides. *Proc. Natl. Acad. Sci. U.S.A.* **79,** 1690–1694.

Loetscher, H.R., Schwerzmann, K., and Carafoli, E. (1979). The transport of Ca^{2+} in a purified population of inside-out vesicles from rat liver mitochondria. *FEBS Lett.* **99,** 194–198.

Lowe, D.A., Richardson, B.P., Taylor, P., and Donatsch, P. (1976). Increasing intracellular sodium triggers calcium release from bound pools. *Nature (London)* **260,** 337–338.

Luthra, M.G., Hildenbrandt, G.R., and Hanahan, D.J. (1976). Studies on an activator of the (Ca^{2+} + Mg^{2+})-ATPase of human erythrocyte membrane. *Biochem. Biophys. Acta* **419,** 164–179.

MacLennan, D.H. (1970). Purification and properties of an adenosine triphosphatase from sarcoplasmic reticulum. *J. Biol. Chem.* **245,** 4508–4518.

MacLennan, D.H., and Wong, P.T.S. (1971). Isolation of a calcium-sequestring protein from the sarcoplasmic reticulum. *Proc. Natl. Acad. Sci. U.S.A.* **68,** 1231–1235.

Makinose, M. (1973). Possible functional states of the enzyme of the sarcoplasmic calcium pump. *FEBS Lett.* **37,** 140–143.

Malmström, K., and Carafoli, E. (1975). Effects of Prostaglandins on the interaction of Ca^{2+} with mitochondria. *Arch. Biochem. Biophys.* **171,** 418–423.

Malmström, K., and Carafoli, E. (1977). The interaction of Ca^{2+} with mitochondria from human myometrium. *Arch. Biochem. Biophys.* **182,** 657–666.

Manery, J.F. (1966). Effects of Ca ions on membranes. *Fed. Proc., Fed. Am. Soc. Exp. Biol.* **25,** 1804–1810.

Martonosi, A. (1968). Sarcoplasmic reticulum. IV. Solubilization of microsomal adenosine triphosphatase. *J. Biol. Chem.* **243,** 71–81.

Martonosi, A. (1972). Biochemical and clinical aspects of sarcoplasmic reticulum function. *Curr. Top. Memb. Transp.* **3,** 83–197.

Martonosi, A. (1975). The mechanism of calcium in sarcoplasmic reticulum. *In* "Calcium Transport in Contraction and Secretion" (E. Carafoli, E. Clementi, W. Drabikowski, and A. Margreth, eds.), pp. 313–327. North-Holland Publ., Amsterdam.

Martonosi, A., and Feretos, R. (1964). Sarcoplasmic reticulum. I. The uptake of Ca^{2+} by sarcoplasmic reticulum fragments. *J. Biol. Chem.* **239,** 648–658.

Meech, R.W., and Standen, N.B. (1975). Postassium activation in Helix aspersa neurones under voltage-clamp. *J. Physiol. (London)* **249,** 211–239.

Meissner, G. (1975). Isolation and characterization of two types of sarcoplasmic reticulum vesicles. *Biochim. Biophys. Acta* **389,** 51–68.

Meissner, G., and McKinley, D. (1976). Permeability of sarcoplasmic reticulum membrane. The effect of changed ionic environments of Ca^{2+} release. *J. Membr. Biol.* **30,** 79–80.

Meissner, G., Conner, G.E., and Fleischer, S. (1973). Isolation of sarcoplasmic reticulum by zonal centrifugation and purification of Ca^{2+} pump and Ca^{2+}-binding proteins. *Biochim. Biophys. Acta* **298,** 246–269.

Mitchell, P. (1966). "Chemiosmotic Coupling in Oxidative and Photosynthetic Phosphorylation." Glynn Res. Ltd., Bodmin, England.

Mitchell, P., and Moyle, J. (1967). Respiration driven proton translocation in rat liver mitochondria. *Biochem. J.* **105,** 1147–1162.

Moore, L., Fitzpatrick, D.F., Chen, T.S., and Landon, E.J. (1974). Calcium pump activity of the renal plasma membrane and renal microsomes. *Biochim. Biophys. Acta* **345,** 405–418.

Moore, L., Chen, T.S., Knapp, H.P., and Landon, E.J. (1975). Energy-dependent calcium sequestration activity in rat liver microsomes. *J. Biol. Chem.* **250,** 4562–4568.

Moyle, J., and Mitchell, P. (1977a). Electric change stoichiometry of calcium translocation in rat liver mitochondria. *FEBS Lett.* **73,** 131–136.

Moyle, J., and Mitchell, P. (1977b). The lanthanide-sensitive calcium phosphate porter of rat liver mitochondria. *FEBS Lett.* **77,** 136–145.

Mullins, L.J. (1976). Steady state calcium fluxes: Membrane versus mitochondrial control of ionized calcium in axoplasm. *Fed. Proc., Fed. Am. Soc. Exp. Biol.* **35,** 2583–2588.

Mullins, L.J., and Brinley, F.J. (1975). Sensitivity of calcium efflux from squid axons to change in membrane potential. *J. Gen. Physiol.* **65,** 135–152.

Nakajima, Y., and Endo, M. (1973). Release of calcium by depolarisation of the sarcoplasmic reticulum membrane. *Nature (London), New Biol.* **246,** 216–218.

Niggli, V., Ronner, P., Carafoli, E., and Penniston, J.T. (1979a). Effects of calmodulin on the (Ca^{2+} + Mg^{2+})-ATPase partially purified from erythrocyte membranes. *Arch. Biochem. Biophys.* (in press).

Niggli, V., Penniston, J.T., and Carafoli, E. (1979b). Purification of the Ca^{2+}, Mg^{2+} ATPase from human erythrocyte membranes using a calmodulin affinity column. *J. Biol. Chem.* **254,** 9955-9957.

Ohnishi, S., and Ito, T. (1974). Calcium-induced phase separations in phosphatidylserine-phosphatidylcholine membranes. *Biochemistry* **13,** 881-887.

Ostwald, T.J., and MacLennan, D.H. (1974). Isolation of a high affinity calcium-binding protein from sarcoplasmic reticulum. *J. Biol. Chem.* **249,** 974-979.

Ostwald, T.J., MacLennan, D.H., and Dorrington, K.H. (1974). Effects of cation-binding on the conformation and the high affinity calcium-binding proteins of sarcoplasmic reticulum. *J. Biol. Chem.* **249,** 5867-5871.

O'Sullivan, W.J., and Perrin, D.D. (1964). The stability constants of metal-adenine nucleotide complexes. *Biochemistry* **3,** 18-26.

Otsuka, M., Ohtsuki, I., and Ebashi, S. (1965). ATP-dependent Ca-binding of brain microsomes. *J. Biochem. (Tokyo)* **58,** 183-190.

Parkinson, D.K., and Radde, I.C. (1971). Properties of a Ca^{2+}-and Mg^{2+}-activated ATP-hydrolyzing enzyme in rat kidney cortex. *In* "Cellular Mechanism for Calcium Homeostasis" (G. Nicholls, Jr. and R.H. Wasserman, eds.), pp. 506-511. Academic Press, New York.

Peng, C.F., Price, C.W., Bhuvaneswaran, C., and Wadkins, C.L. (1974). Factors that influence phosphoenolpyruvate-induced calcium efflux from rat liver mitochondria. *Biochem. Biophys. Res. Commun.* **56,** 134-141.

Peterson, S.W., Ronner, P., and Carafoli, E. (1978). Partial purification and recombination of the (Ca^{2+} + Mg^{2+})-ATPase of erythrocyte membranes. *Arch. Biochem. Biophys.* **186,** 202-210.

Pfleger, H., and Wolf, H.U. (1975). Activation of membrane-bound high affinity calcium ion-sensitive adenosine triphosphatase of human erythrocytes by bivalent metal ions. *Biochem. J.* **147,** 359-361.

Pitts, B.J.R. (1979). Stoichiometry of sodium-calcium exchange in cardiac sarcolemmal vesicle. *J. Biol. Chem.* **254,** 6232-6235.

Podolsky, R.J., Hall, T., and Hatchett, S.L. (1970). Identification of oxalate precipitates in striated muscle fibres. *J. Cell Biol.* **44,** 699-702.

Portzehl, H., Caldwell, P.C., and Rüegg, J.C. (1964). The dependence of contraction and relaxation of muscle fibres of the crab Maia Squinado on the internal concentrations of free calcium ions. *Biochim. Biophys. Acta* **74,** 581-591.

Puskin, J.S., Gunter, T.E., Gunter, K.K., and Russell, P.R. (1976). Evidence for more than one Ca^{2+} transport mechanism in mitochondria. *Biochemistry* **15,** 3834-3842.

Quist, E.E., and Roufogalis, B.P. (1975). Determination of the stoichiometry of the calcium pump in human erythrocytes lanthanum as a selective inhibitor. *FEBS Lett.* **50,** 135-139.

Racker, E. (1972). Reconstitution of a calcium pump with phospholipids and a purified Ca^{2+} adenosine triphosphatase from sarcoplasmic reticulum. *J. Biol. Chem.* **247,** 8198-8200.

Rahamimoff, R., Erulkav, S.D., Anals, E., Meiri, H., Rotsenkev, S., and Rahamimoff, H. (1976). Modulation of transmitter release by calcium-ions and nerve impulses. *Cold Spring Harbor Symp. Quant. Biol.* **40,** 107-116.

Rasmussen, H. (1970). Cell communication, calcium ion, and cyclic adenosine monophosphate. *Science* **170,** 404-411.

Rasmussen, H., Goodman, D.B.P., and Tenenhouse, A. (1972). The role of cyclic AMP and calcium in cell activation. *CRC Crit. Rev. Biochem.* **1,** 95-148.

Reed, K.C., and Bygrave, F.L. (1975). A kinetic study of mitochondrial calcium transport. *Eur. J. Biochem.* **55,** 497-504.

Reeves, J.P., and Sutko, J.L. (1979). Sodium-calcium exchange in cardiac membrane vesicles. *Proc. Natl. Acad. Sci. U.S.A.* **76,** 590–594.

Reuter, H. (1965). Ueber die Wirkung von Adrenalin auf den Cellulä-nalin ren Ca-Umsatz des Meerschweinchenvorhofs. *Naunyn-Schmiedebergs Arch. Exp. Pathol. Pharmakol.* **251,** 401–412.

Reuter, H. (1974). Exchange of calcium ions in the mammalian myocardium. Mechanisms and physiological significance. *Circ. Res.* **34,** 399–605.

Rich, T.L., and Langer, G.A. (1975). A comparison of excitation contraction coupling in heart and skeletal muscle: An examination of "calcium induced calcium release." *J. Mol. Cell. Cardiol.* **7,** 747–765.

Ridgway, E.B., and Durham, A.C.H. (1976). Oscillation of calcium concentrations in physarum polycepharum. *J. Cell Biol.* **69,** 223–226.

Ringer, S. (1883). Regarding the action of hydrate of soda, hydrate of ammonia, and hydrate of potash on the ventricle of the frog's heart. *J. Physiol. (London)* **3,** 195–202.

Ringer, S. (1884). A further contribution regarding the influence of the different constituents of the blood on the contraction of the heart. *J. Physiol. (London)* **4,** 29–42.

Robblee, L.S., Shepro, D., and Belamarich, F.A. (1973). Calcium uptake and associated ATPase activity of isolated platelets membranes. *J. Gen. Physiol.* **61,** 462–481.

Robinson, J.D., and Lust, W.D. (1968). Adenosine triphosphate dependent calcium accumulation by brain microsomes. *Arch. Biochem. Biophys.* **125,** 286–294.

Roman, I. (1978) Regulation of transport of Ca^{2+} in rat kidney mitochondria by unsaturated fatty acids and Na^{+} ion. Ph.D. Thesis, Medical Academy, Gdansk, Poland.

Ronner, P., Gazzotti, P., and Carafoli, E. (1977). A lipid requirement of the (Ca^{2+} + Mg^{2+}) activated ATPase of erythrocyte membranes. *Arch. Biochem. Biophys.* **179,** 578–583.

Roos, I., Crompton, M., and Carafoli, E. (1978). The effect of phosphoenolpyruvate on the retention of calcium by liver mitochondria. *FEBS Lett.* **94,** 418–421.

Rose, B., and Loewenstein, W.R. (1975). Calcium ion distribution in cytoplasm visualized by aequorin. Diffussion in the cytosol is restricted due to erergised sequestering. *Science* **190,** 1204–1206.

Rose, B., and Loewenstein, W.R. (1976). Permeability of a cell junction and the local cytoplasmic free ionized calcium concentration. A study with aequorin. *J. Membr. Biol.* **28,** 87–119.

Rose, I.A. (1968). The state of magnesium in cells as estimated from the adenylate kinase equilibrium. *Proc. Natl. Acad. Sci. U.S.A.* **59,** 1079–1086.

Rossi, C.S., Vasington, F.D., and Carafoli, E. (1973). The effect of ruthenium red on the uptake and release of Ca^{2+} by mitochondria. *Biochem. Biophys. Res. Commun.* **50,** 846–852.

Rottenberg, H., and Scarpa, A. (1974). Calcium uptake and membrane potential in mitochondria. *Biochemistry* **13,** 4811–4819.

St. Louis, P.J., and Sulakhe, P.V. (1978). Protein analysis of cardiac sarcolemma: Effects of membrane-perturbing agents on membrane proteins and calcium transport. *Biochemistry* **17,** 4540–4556.

Sarkadi, B., Szász, I., Gerlóczy, A., and Gárdos, G. (1977). Transport parameters and stoichiometry of active calcium ion extrusion in intact human red cells. *Biochim. Biophys. Acta* **464,** 92–107.

Scarpa, A., and Graziotti, P. (1973). Mechanisms for intracellular calcium regulation in heart. *J. Gen. Physiol.* **62,** 756–772.

Scharff, O. (1976). Ca^{2+} activation of membrane-bound (Ca^{2+} + Mg^{2+})-dependent ATPase from human erythrocytes prepared in the presence or absence of Ca^{2+}. *Biochim. Biophys. Acta* **443,** 206–218.

Schatzmann, H.J. (1973). Dependence on Ca^{2+} concentration and stoichiometry of the Ca^{2+} pump in human red cells. *J. Physiol. (London)* **235,** 551–569.

Schatzmann, H.J. (1975). Active calcium transport and Ca^{2+}-activated ATPase in human red cells. *Curr. Top. Membr. Transp.* **6,** 126–168.

Schatzmann, H.J., and Vincenzi, F.F. (1969). Ca^{2+} movements across the membrane of human red cells. *J. Physiol. (London)* **201,** 369-395.

Schulman, H., and Greengard, P. (1978a). Stimulation of brain membrane protein phosphorylation by calcium and an endogenous heat-stable protein. *Nature (London)* **271,** 478–479.

Schulman, H., and Greengard, P. (1978b). Ca^{2+}-dependent protein phosphorylation system in membranes from various tissues, and its activation by "calcium-dependent regulator." *Proc. Natl. Acad. Sci. U.S.A.* **75,** 5432–5436.

Schwartz, A., Entman, M.L., Kaniike, K., and Bornet, E. (1974). Phosphorylase b kinase and c-AMD-dependent protein kinase effects on sarcoplasmic reticulum: Cardiac, fast and slow skeletal muscle. *Fed. Proc., Fed. Am. Soc. Exp. Biol.* **33,** Abstr. 1583.

Schwartz, A., Entman, M.L., Kaniike, K., Lane, L.K., van Winkle, W.B., and Bornet, E.P. (1976). The rate of calcium uptake into sarcoplasmic reticulum of cardiac muscle and skeletal muscle. Effects of cyclic AMP-dependent protein kinase and phosphorylase b kinase. *Biochim. Biophys. Acta* **426,** 57–72.

Selinger, Z., Nains, E., and Lasser, M. (1970). ATP-dependent calcium uptake by microsomal preparations from rat parotid and submaxillary glands. *Biochim. Biophys. Acta* **203,** 326–334.

Shamoo, A., and Goldstein, D.A. (1977). Isolation of ionophores from ion transport systems and their role in energy transduction. *Biochim. Biophys. Acta* **472,** 13–53.

Shamoo, A., and MacLennan, D.H. (1974). A Ca^{2+}-dependent and - selective ionophore as part of the Ca^{2+} + Mg^{2+}-dependent adenosientriphosphatase of surcoplasmic reticulum. *Proc. Natl. Acad. Sci. U.S.A.* **71,** 3522–3526.

Shine, K.I., Serena, S.P., and Langer, G.A. (1971). Kinetic localisation of contractile calcium in rabbit myocardium. *Am J. Physiol.* **221,** 1408–1417.

Solaro, R.J., and Briggs, F.N. (1974). Estimating the functional capabilities of sarcoplasmic reticulum in cardiac muscle. *Circ. Res.* **34,** 531–540.

Solaro, R.J., Wise, R.M., Shiner, J.S., and Briggs, E.N. (1974). Calcium requirements for cardiac myofibrilliar activation. *Circ. Res.* **34,** 525–530.

Sordahl, L.A. (1974). Effects of magnesium, ruthenium red and the antibiotic ionophore A23187 on initial rates of calcium uptake and release by heart mitochondria. *Arch. Biochem. Biophys.* **167,** 104–115.

Sreter, F.A. (1969). Temperature, pH and seasonal dependence of Ca^{2+}-uptake and ATPase activity of white and red muscle microsomes. *Arch. Biochem. Biophys.* **134,** 25–33.

Stucki, J.W., and Ineichen, E.A. (1974). Energy dissipation by Calcium recycling and the efficiency of calcium transport in rat-liver mitochondria. *Eur. J. Biochem.* **48,** 365–375.

Suko, J., and Hasselbach, W. (1976). Characterization of cardiac sarcoplasmic reticulum ATP-ADP phosphate exchange and phosphorylation of the calcium transport adenosine triphosphatase. *Eur. J. Biochem.* **64,** 123–130.

Sutherland, E.W. (1972). Studies on the mechanism of hormone action. *Science* **177,** 401–408.

Tada, M., Kirchberger, M.A., Repke, D.I., and Katz, A.M. (1974). The stimulation of calcium transport in cardiac sarcoplasmic reticulum by adenosine 3′,5′-monophosphate-dependent protein kinase. *J. Biol. Chem.* **249,** 6174–6180.

Tada, M., Kirchberger, M.A., and Katz, A.M. (1975a). Phosphorylation of a 22,000 dalton component of the cardiac sarcoplasmic reticulum by adenosine 3′:5′-monophosphate-dependent protein kinase. *J. Biol. Chem.* **250,** 2640–2647.

Tada, M., Kirchberger, M.A., Li, H.C., and Katz, A.M. (1975b). Interrelationships between calcium and cyclic AMP in the mammalian heart. *In* "Calcium Trasnport in Contraction and Secretion" (E. Carafoli, F. Clementi, W. Drabikowski, and A. Margreth, eds.), pp. 373–382, North-Holland Publ., Amsterdam.

Tasaki, I. (1968). "Nerve Excitation." Thomas, Springfield, Illinois.

Taylor, A., Eich, E., and Pearl, M. (1978). Cytosolic calcium and action of vasopressin in toad bladder. *In* "Proceedings of the International Union of Physiological Sciences" (Pitié-Salpetriére, ed.), Vol. XIII, Abstr. 2217. Cedex 1300, Paris.

Teo, T.S., and Wang, J.H. (1973). Mechanism of activation of a cyclic adenosine 3′:5′-monophosphate phosphodiesterase from bovine heart by calcium ions. Identification of the protein activator as Ca^{2+} binding protein. *J. Biol. Chem.* **248,** 5950–5955.

Terepka, A.R., Coleman, J.R., Armbrecht, H.J., and Gunter, T.E. (1976). Transcellular transport of calcium. *Symp. Soc. Exp. Biol.* **30,** 117–140.

Thorley-Lawson, D.A., and Green, N.M. (1973). Studies on the location and orientation of proteins in the sarcoplasmic reticulum. *Eur. J. Biochem.* **40,** 403–413.

Tobias, J.M. (1964). A chemically specified nolecular mechanism underlying excitation in nerve: A hypothesis. *Nature (London)* **203,** 13–17.

Träuble, H., and Eibl, H. (1974). Electrostatic effects on lipid phase transition: Membrane structure and ionic environment. *Proc. Natl. Acad. Sci. U.S.A.* **71,** 214–219.

Vallières, J., Scarpa, A., and Somlyo, A.P. (1975). Subcellular fractions of smooth muscle. Isolation, substrate utilization and calcium transport by main pulmonary artery and mesenteric vein mitochondria. *Arch. Biochem. Biophys.* **170,** 659–669.

Vanaman, T.C., Sharief, F., and Watterson, D.M. (1977). Structural homology between brain modulator protein and muscle TnCs. *In* "Calcium Binding Proteins and Calcium Function" (R.H. Wasserman, R.A. Corradino, E. Carafoli, R.H. Kretsinger, D.H. MacLennan, and F.L. Siegel eds.), pp. 107–116. Elsevier/North Holland Publ., Amsterdam.

Van Rossum, G.D.V. (1970). Net movements of Ca^{2+} and Mg^{2+} in slices of rat liver. *J. Gen. Physiol.* **55,** 18–32.

Vasington, F.D., and Murphy, J.V. (1962). Ca^{2+} uptake by rat kidney mitochondria and its dependence on respiration and phosphorylation. *J. Biol. Chem.* **237,** 2670–2672.

Vercesi, A., Reynafarje, B., and Leheninger, A.L. (1978). Stoichiometry of H^+ ejection and Ca^{2+}-uptake coupled to electron transport in rat heart mitochondria. *J. Biol. Chem.* **253,** 6379–6385.

Wacker, W.E.C., and Williams, R.J.P. (1968). Magnesium/calcium balances and steady state of biological systems. *J. Theor. Biol.* **20,** 65–78.

Waisman, D.M., Singh, T.J., and Wang, J.H. (1978). The modulator-dependent protein kinase. *J. Biol. Chem.* **253,** 3387–3390.

Wang, J.H., Teo, T.S., Ho, H.C., and Stevens, F.C. (1975). Bovine heart protein activator of cyclic nucleotide phosphodiesterase. *Adv. Cyclic Nucleotide Res.* **5,** 179–194.

Warren, G.B., Toon, P.A., Birdsall, N.J.M., Lee, A.G., and Metcalfe, J.C. (1974). Reconstitution of a calcium pump using defined membrane components. *Proc. Natl. Acad. Sci. U.S.A.* **71,** 622–626.

Wasserman, R.H., and Taylor, A.N. (1966). Vitamin D_3-induced calcium binding protein in chick intestinal mucosa. *Science* **152,** 791–793.

Watson, E.L., Vincenzi, F.F., and Davies, P.W., (1971). Ca^{2+} activated membrane ATPase: Selective inhibition by ruthenium red. *Biochim. Biophys. Acta* **249,** 606–610.

Weber, A. (1966). Energized calcium transport and relaxing factors. *Curr. Top. Bioenerg.* **1,** 203–254.

Weber, A. (1976). Synopsis of the presentations. *Symp. Soc. Exp. Biol.* **30,** 445–455.

Wikström, M., Ahonen, P., and Luukkainen, T. (1975). The role of mitochondria in uterine contraction. *FEBS Lett.* **56,** 120–123.

Williams, R.J.P. (1975). The binding of metal ions to membranes and its consequences. *In* "Biological Membranes: Twelve Assays on Their Organization, Properties, and Functions" (D.S. Parsons, ed.), pp. 106–121. Oxford Univ. Press (Clarendon), London and New York.

Williams, R.J.P. (1976). Calcium chemistry and its relation to biological function. *Symp. Soc. Exp. Biol.* **30,** 1–17.

Wollenberger, A., Will, H., and Krause, E.G. (1975). Adenosine 3′.5′-monophosphate, the myocardial cell membrane, and calcium. *Recent Adv. Stud. Card. Struct. Metab.* **5,** 81–93.

Worsfold, M., and Peter, J.B. (1970). Kinetics of calcium transport by fragmented sarcoplasmic reticulum. *J. Biol. Chem.* **245,** 5545–5552.

Yagi, K., Yazawa, M., Kakiuchi, S., Oshima, M., and Uenishi, K. (1978). Identification of an activator protein for myosin light chain kinase as the Ca^{2+}-dependent modulator protein. *J. Biol. Chem.* **253,** 1338–1340.

Yamazaki, R.K. (1975). Glucagon stimulation of mitochondrial respiration. *J. Biol. Chem.* **250,** 7924–7930.

2

Calcium Homeostasis

FELIX BRONNER

List of Symbols and Abbreviations

$[Ca_s]$	Plasma calcium concentration (mg/dl, m*M*)
$[U]$	Plasma calcium reference value (same units as $[Ca_s]$)
ϵ	Plasma calcium error, $[Ca_s] - [U]$
S_i	Disturbing signal, i.e., the steady-state net calcium load from the intestine (mg/day)
v_i	Calcium ingested (mg/day)
v_F	Calcium excreted in stool (mg/day)
v_a	Calcium absorbed from intestine (mg/day)
v_{ndo}	Endogenous fecal calcium (mg/day) Note: $S_i = v_i - v_F = v_a - v_{ndo}$
v_u	Calcium excreted in urine (mg/day)

(*Continued*)

Disorders of Mineral Metabolism, Vol. II

ISBN 0-12-135302-8

List of Symbols and Abbreviations (*Continued*)

v_{fi}	Calcium filtered at glomerulus
v_r	Calcium reabsorbed along nephron
v_s	Calcium "secreted" into nephron
	Note: $v_u = v_{fi} - v_r + v_s$
Δ	Body calcium balance = skeletal calcium balance (mg/day)
v_{o+}	Calcium deposited in bone (mg/day)
v_{o-}	Calcium removed (resorbed) from bone (mg/day)
	Note: $\Delta = v_i - v_u - v_F = v_{o+} - v_{o-}$
v_T	Calcium pool turnover rate (mg/day)
	Note: $v_T = v_{o-} + v_a = v_{o+} + v_u + v_{ndo}$
g	Rate at which [Ca_s] returns to [U]
$\dot{g}$	dg/dt
+D	Vitamin D-replete state[7a]
−D	Vitamin D-deficient state
PTH	Parathyroid hormone
PTX	Parathyroidectomized
$1,25(OH)_2D_3$	1,25-dihydroxyvitamin D_3
EDTA	Disodium ethylenediaminetetraacetic acid
$S_{e(max)}$	Maximum error of plasma calcium
[L]	The plasma calcium concentration when PTH release is at a minimum
[H]	Plasma parathyroid hormone concentration
[CT]	Plasma calcitonin concentration
CT	Calcitonin
CX or TX	Calcitoninectomized
$K, K_1, K', K_2, K_3, k_1, k_2, k_3$	Various constants

[a] For footnote 7, see p. 86.

List of Equations[a]

Equation	Special condition	Species
(1) $v_u = 114 + 0.23\ S_i$		Adult women
(2) $\Delta = -114 + 0.77\ S_i$		Adult women
(3) $v_u/S_i = 0.23 + 114/S_i$		Adult women
(4) $\Delta/S_i = 0.77 - 114/S_i$		Adult women
(5) $v_a = 3.4 + 0.51\ v_i$		Rat
(6) $v_a = -8.6 + 0.55\ v_i$	−D	Rat
(7) $v_{ndo} = 0.4 + 0.05\ v_i$		Rat
(8) $v_u = v_{fi} - (\Sigma v_{in} - \Sigma v_{out})$		
(9) $F_r = \dfrac{(\Sigma v_i - \Sigma v_{out})}{v_{fi}}$		
(10) $v_u = 28.3 + 0.047\ S_i$	Renal failure	Patients
(11) $v_{o+} = 354 + 0.13\ S_i$		Adult women
(12) $v_{o+} = 67.2 + 0.11\ S_i$		Rat

List of Equations (*Continued*)

Equation	Special condition	Species
(13) $v_{o-} = v_{o+} - \Delta = v_{o+} + v_u + v_{ndo} - v_a$		
(14) $v_{o-} = 14 - 1.0\ v_a$		Cow
(15) $v_{o-} = 468 - 0.64\ S_i$		Adult women
(16) $v_{o-} = 67.5 - 0.87\ S_i$		Rat
(17) $v_{o+} = 36.5 + 0.29\ S_i$	PTX	Rat
(18) $v_{o-} = 36.9 - 0.69\ S_i$	PTX	Rat
(19) $v_T = 3.3 + 5.3\ \mathrm{PTH}$		Cow
(20) $v_u = 0.30 + 0.02\ S_i$		Rat
(21) $v_u = 0.36 + 0.02\ S_i$	PTX	Rat
(22) $\Delta = -0.3 + 0.98\ S_i$		Rat
(23) $\Delta = -0.4 + 0.98\ S_i$	PTX	Rat
(24) $\epsilon = [\mathrm{Ca_s}] - [\mathrm{U}]$		
(25) $S_{\epsilon(\max)} = [\mathrm{Ca_s}]_{\lim \to S_i} - [\mathrm{U}]$		
(26) $S_{\epsilon(\max)} = S_i/K$	PTX	
(27) $S_{\epsilon(\max)} = \dfrac{S_i\ [\mathrm{L}] - [\mathrm{U}]}{K'\ [\mathrm{L}] - \beta]\mathrm{U}]}$		
(28) $[\mathrm{Ca_s}] = 6.02 + 0.021\ S_i$	PTX	Rat
(29) $[\mathrm{Ca_s}] = 10.80 + 0.0021\ S_i$		Rat
(30) $v_{o+} = 0.3\ \mathrm{K}\ [\mathrm{Ca_s}]$	PTX	Rat
(31) $v_{o-} = 0.7\ \mathrm{K}\ (2\beta\ [\mathrm{U}] - [\mathrm{Ca_s}])$	PTX	Rat
(32) $v_{o+} = 0.3\ K'\ [\mathrm{Ca_s}] - 0.1\ K_3\ [\mathrm{H}]$		Rat
(33) $v_{o-} = 0.7\ K'\ (2\beta\ [\mathrm{U}] - [\mathrm{Ca_s}] + 0.9\ K_3\ [\mathrm{H}])$		Rat
(34) $d[\mathrm{CT}]/dt = k_1\epsilon + k_2 d\epsilon/dt - k_3\ [\mathrm{CT}]$		
(35) $v_{o+} = 50.5 + 0.29\ S_i$		Rat
(36) $v_{o-} = 50.1 - 0.68\ S_i$		Rat
(37) $v_{o+} = 32 + 0.50\ S_i$	−D	Rat
(38) $v_{o-} = 32 - 0.49\ S_i$	−D	Rat

[a] None of the above equations have been normalized for body weight and age. A first approach toward such an analysis has been presented elsewhere (Bronner, 1973a). The rats were males, weighed 100–250 gm and were 6–12 weeks old, the women were aged 37–70 years, with a mean body weight of about 60 kg, and the cows were 4.5–8 years old and weighed about 400 kg. PTX, parathyroidectomized state; −D, vitamin D-deficiency.

I. INTRODUCTION

Homeostasis is a term introduced by Cannon (1932) to designate the maintenance of the *milieu interne,* a concept originally developed by Claude Bernard (1865).[1] Often the term "homeostasis" is used to refer to the steady-state level of

[1]For interesting historical reviews of the term "homeostasis" see Langley (1965) and Fulton (1966).

plasma constituents and their maintenance. Use of the term in this sense implies that the steady state plasma level of ions and minerals is regulated, i.e., that the organism attempts to maintain a given plasma level in the face of variations in input or output. However, the plasma level of most minerals or ions varies significantly with dietary input. For example, when rats are placed on very low phosphate or magnesium inputs, plasma levels of inorganic phosphate or magnesium will drop dramatically overnight; repletion or shifts to high intakes will produce an equally rapid rise in the corresponding plasma level. These rapid changes, leading to marked variations in steady state plasma levels, may be accompanied by over- or undershoots (Watkins *et al.*, 1976), i.e., transient rises above or drops below the ultimate steady-state levels. If a plasma concentration is a direct and sensitive function of dietary input, then the term homeostasis may not apply, since there is no operational indication that the organism is making an effort at maintaining the plasma and extracellular fluid concentration at a level other than that determined by dietary input. This, however, is not true for either calcium or sodium. In the case of calcium, in particular, drastic changes in dietary calcium input have only a minor immediate effect on plasma calcium levels and mammalian organisms must be maintained on a low calcium diet for relatively long periods (i.e., weeks) before the steady-state calcium level is altered appreciably. There can be little doubt, therefore, that maintenance of the plasma and extracellular calcium concentration, like that of sodium and bicarbonate, is a prime example of ion homeostasis in the mammalian body.

It is important to differentiate between ion regulation as a whole and regulation of the plasma and extracellular ion concentration. A major functional characteristic of all cells is their ability to maintain an identity distinct from their environment. As a result inputs are generally transformed, and one definition of physiology is the study of the nature of input transformation. For example, the intracellular free calcium ion concentration is thought to lie between 10^{-7} to 10^{-6} *M*, substantially below the calcium ion concentration in most environments of unicellular populations. Consequently, as discussed in the preceding chapter, cellular energy must be expended on intracellular calcium homeostasis. It is interesting yet puzzling that cells regulate both intracellular and extracellular calcium concentrations, i.e., that cells, acting in concert as tissues, make what is undoubtedly a major metabolic expenditure to maintain the extracellular calcium concentration so precisely. In addition cells appear to regulate their intracellular calcium ion concentration. Whether maintenance of a 1000-fold gradient between intra- and extracellular calcium requires close control of both intra- and extracellular calcium is not known, nor is it known how the two are related.

In what follows, we shall describe extracellular calcium homeostasis, its mechanisms, and how it may be altered in disease. Emphasis throughout will be on acute regulation with only limited discussion of the mechanisms leading to

TABLE I

Distribution of Calcium in Normal Plasma[a]

	mM	% Total
Ionized [Ca^{2+}]	1.18	47.5
Protein-bound calcium	1.14	46.0
$CaHPO_4$	0.04	1.6
Calcium citrate	0.04	1.7
Unidentified complexes	0.08	3.2
Total	2.48	100

[a] From Walser (1961).

chronic changes. However, the effect of chronic changes, as in disease, on acute regulation will be discussed in detail.

II. PLASMA CALCIUM

1. *Biological Description*

The calcium in the blood is found principally in the plasma, only about 3% of the total blood calcium occurring in the red blood cells. Of the calcium in plasma, about 45% is bound to protein, mostly albumin. The remainder is diffusible largely in the form of ionized calcium with small amounts of diffusible calcium also occurring as complexes of citrate, phosphate, and other organic or inorganic complexes (see Table I).

The total amount of calcium in plasma [Ca_S] is 2.5 m*M* (10 mg/dl)[2] and this concentration seems typical of vertebrates. In man, detailed studies of plasma calcium have shown that values in males tend to be higher than in females (Roof *et al.*, 1976) and that plasma calcium tends to decrease with age (Ryckewaert *et al.*, 1974; Frank *et al.*, 1973; Table II). Conceivably, these age- and sex-dependent variations reflect in imprecise fashion the differences in turnover of the parameters of calcium metabolism, i.e., of the rates at which skeletal calcium turns over.

While there can be little doubt that the plasma calcium [Ca_S] drops with age, the rate at which it drops is less certain. Ryckewaert *et al.* (1974) report a slope in 5978 men of −0.0062 mg/dl/year between the ages of 20 and 75. From the data

[2]Since most clinical data have been expressed as mg Ca/dl, this notation will be used along with m*M*. The latter is more universally understood; the former tends to be more precise as data are commonly reported to two decimals, whether as mg/dl or m*M*, even though 0.01 mg/dl equals 0.0025 m*M*. There is no analytical difficulty in measuring calcium within ± 0.1 μg/ml.

TABLE II

Plasma Calcium Values as a Function of Age in U.S. Men, Women, and Children[a]

Age range (years)	Adults			
	Men		Women	
	Black	White	Black	White
20-29	5.17 (0.04)	5.28 (0.04)	5.00 (0.06)	5.09 (0.04)
30-39	5.25 (0.05)	5.19 (0.03)	5.13 (0.06)	5.10 (0.04)
40-49	5.35 (0.07)	5.16 (0.05)	5.15 (0.04)	5.09 (0.03)
50-59	5.15 (0.10)	5.08 (0.03)	5.20 (0.05)	5.07 (0.03)
60-69	5.12 (0.04)	5.07 (0.01)	5.10 (0.02)	5.10 (0.01)
70-79	5.13 (0.09)	5.03 (0.02)	5.22 (0.04)	5.07 (0.02)
80-89	—	5.08 (0.06)	—	5.04 (0.05)

Age (years)	Children	
	Male	Female
<1	5.45 (0.08)	5.47 (0.08)
1	5.39 (0.09)	5.41 (0.06)
2	5.15 (0.08)	5.40 (0.10)
3	5.48 (0.11)	5.28 (0.07)
4	5.27 (0.07)	5.13 (0.07)
5	5.28 (0.06)	5.15 (0.03)
6	5.05 (0.06)	5.16 (0.10)
7	5.10 (0.06)	5.31 (0.05)
8	5.23 (0.05)	5.19 (0.05)
9	5.23 (0.10)	5.38 (0.07)
10	5.08 (0.08)	5.26 (0.04)
11	5.23 (0.07)	5.14 (0.05)
12	5.31 (0.05)	5.28 (0.05)
13	5.22 (0.06)	5.07 (0.16)
14	5.16 (0.06)	5.21 (0.03)
15	5.37 (0.08)	5.14 (0.07)
17	5.32 (0.08)	5.15 (0.05)

[a] [Ca_5], mEq/liter (standard error). To convert mEq/liter to mg Ca/dl, multiply by 2; to convert to m*M*, divide by 2 (From Roof *et al.*, 1976).

of Roof *et al.* (1976), on the other hand, the corresponding slope in 400 white men, aged 20–89 years, can be calculated to be −0.0092, substantially larger. In women, the age-dependent drop appears to be much smaller, perhaps −0.0030 mg/dl/year (Roof *et al.*, 1976). Table II shows that in adults, the values for white women are lower than those for white men, except in the 60–80 year range. In female children, they are lower in only about half the cases.

It is generally accepted that ionized calcium is the vector that is regulated and in turn effects regulation. Yet the dynamic equilibrium between ionized and bound calcium is established so rapidly in the blood (< 5 sec; Carr, 1953) that under nearly all circumstances total plasma calcium is a satisfactory experimental measure of the ionized calcium level (Edmondson and Li, 1976; Larsson and Ohman, 1979). Nevertheless, as pointed out by Ladenson *et al.* (1978), there is no simple satisfactory way of predicting the true free serum calcium level from total serum calcium, even when the latter is corrected for protein, albumin, and pH. While the ionized calcium is inorganic, not all inorganic calcium need be ionized. Infusions of the sulfate ion have been showed to lead to hypercalcemia without symptoms, presumably because the sulfate ion served as a counter-ion to calcium, but caused only a negligible increase in the ionic calcium level (Walser and Browder, 1959). Moreover, until recently the determination of the ionized calcium level was cumbersome and substantially less accurate than the determination of total calcium. The advent of reliable calcium ion electrodes will permit experimental studies to be based on the calcium ion level. Studies already published (Edmondson and Li, 1976) have shown that in hyperparathyroidism the proportion of ionized to total calcium is unchanged from the normal state. Larsson and Ohman (1979) have reported a normal ionized Ca^{2+} concentration of 1.1 m*M*, while Li and Piechocki (1971) reported a value of 1.2 m*M*. The total $[Ca_s]$ averaged 2.3 m*M* in the case of Li and Piechocki (1971) and 2.4 m*M* in the study of Larsson and Ohman (1979), so that the percentage of ionized calcium in human plasma reported by these two groups of investigators brackets the value shown in Table I.

Rodan and Katz (1973) have studied the effect of increasing plasma calcium on calcium binding in the rat, using an experimental model of extracorporeal circulation. They found that as the calcium concentration rose from 2.36 to 5.02 m*M*, the dialyzable calcium rose from 1.44 to 3.60 m*M*. Although the proportion of dialyzable calcium rose from 61 to 72%, the mean dialyzable fraction in 23 normocalcemic rats was 0.66 ± 0.05 (SD). The authors therefore concluded that any process that introduces calcium ions into the blood or removes them will cause a corresponding change in dialyzable calcium, with calcium binding contributing little to plasma calcium regulation. In other words, the calcium ligands of the plasma exert no added buffering action when there is an independent rise in the ionic calcium. On the other hand, the relative independence of the concentration of unbound calcium means that a relatively small change in the "free" calcium could bring about a calcium-dependent change, as might occur in a calcium-induced conformational change of a membrane protein.

For the plasma calcium to remain constant, the rates of calcium entry into and removal from the blood must remain equal, since calcium is not stored in blood cells. In a growing rat, the net daily calcium balance can readily attain 60 mg/day (Sammon *et al.*, 1970) or 5 mg/hr, on the assumption that rats feed largely at night. Therefore the turnover of the plasma calcium pool must exceed 5 mg/hr if the plasma calcium is to remain constant. The size of the plasma calcium pool may be estimated from the plasma volume, approximately 3.5% of the body weight. However, from load and radiocalcium studies the actual volume of distribution appears to be much larger. Bronner *et al.* (1968) injected a calcium load (3.8 mg) intravenously into 182 gm rats whose plasma calcium was 10.86 mg/dl and measured plasma calcium beginning at 0.5 min after injection. Extrapolation to zero time yielded an apparent initial plasma calcium level of about 26 mg/dl, corresponding to a volume of distribution of 25 ml. If, on the other hand, the injected calcium had been distributed only in the plasma volume (6.4 ml), the plasma calcium concentration immediately after injection would have amounted to 70 mg/dl.

Using a defined mathematical approach, Riggs (1966) and Hausmann and Riggs (1966) studied the effect of calcium infusions on the plasma calcium level of normal and thyroparathyroidectomized dogs. They found that by the eighth hour of infusion, a steady-state value had been reached in both groups of animals, but that the rate of approach to the steady state, which was describable by a simple exponential function, was much faster in the euparathyroid dogs. Riggs (1966) concluded that the infused calcium behaved as if it became distributed throughout a single compartment whose apparent volume was 258 ml/kg body wt, or about 25% of body wt.

Rodan (1970), studying an isolated dog limb, concluded from an analysis of experiments utilizing radiocalcium, radiosodium, or EDTA, that the distribution of these substances could be described by a bicompartmental model. The first compartment was equal for all substances and measured about 200 ml, about three times the plasma volume as determined by radioiodine-labeled serum albumin. These findings thus confirm Riggs (1966) and indicate what has been observed by many investigators utilizing intravenously injected radiocalcium: The zero time specific activity value estimated by extrapolation is consistently smaller than the estimate arrived at by dividing the injected dose by the plasma calcium. Inasmuch as the circulation time in many mammals is under 0.5 min, and since, as also shown by Rodan (1970), calcium crosses the compartmental barriers very rapidly, it is not surprising that the volume of distribution is much greater than the plasma volume into which radioisotope is injected.

It is difficult to know the anatomical identity of the volume of distribution following a calcium load. Bronner *et al.* (1968), in addition to the intravenous load studies, also administered calcium to rats by intraperitoneal injection and measured plasma calcium at varying times after dosing. Plasma calcium peaked at about 30 min and thereafter decreased curvilinearly to reach the preinjection value in 2–3 hr, depending on the endocrine status of the animal (see below). The apparent volume of distribution at the time of the peak varied between 125 and 160 ml, with no obvious effect due to the size of the load. This volume is of course much larger than the extracellular volume and would come closer to the total body water.

When radiocalcium is injected, the so-called "pool," i.e., the amount of calcium in the body that has become labeled in the course of the experiment, is much larger than an anatomically identifiable calcium store. Bronner and Lemaire (1969), using a two-compartment model, calculated that the size of the first compartment was about 1.6 gm calcium in 7 women, aged 41–63 years, three of whom were clinically normal, with the others diagnosed to have post-menopausal osteoporosis. In these studies, ^{45}Ca was injected intravenously and the time-course of the drop in plasma specific activity ($^{45}Ca/Ca$, cpm/mg) was expressed as the sum of two exponential terms. It can be shown (Hart, 1967) that by the end of the experiment (148 hr) virtually all of the radiocalcium that will return to the pool, made up of the two compartments, will have done so. In other words, isoionic exchanges will have been completed and the size of the two compartments making up the pool can be calculated (Bronner and Lemaire, 1969) by assuming that the isotope had been distributed instantaneously in the first compartment. The size of the second compartment is determined by the rates of entry and exit of the system, which in turn are derived from the time-course of the plasma specific activity (Bronner, 1973a). The volume of distribution of the first compartment depends on the mean calcium concentration and would lie between 16 and 32 liters. These subjects weighed 60 kg on the average and their extracellular fluid would have been about 16 liters (S.H. Cohn, personal communication). Yet the calcium concentration of the extracellular fluid is about 50 mg/liter. In other words, the first compartment of a two-compartment model necessarily includes skeletal calcium. In fact as much as half of the calcium in compartment 1 may be skeletal in origin. These considerations make clear that skeletal calcium must play an intimate role in the regulation of plasma calcium.

While remarkably constant, plasma calcium is subject to variation over a 24-hr period. Talmage *et al.* (1975a) have reported that in rats allowed continuous access to food, plasma calcium reached a low of about 9 mg/dl at around 5 A.M., rose thereafter to a maximum of about 11 mg/dl at around 2 P.M., and then began dropping. The excursion about the mean was therefore ± 10%. When the animals were allowed access to food only at night (9 P.M.–9 A.M.), the daytime peak was spread out more but the overall trend of the circadian variation was the same. Interestingly, when the animals were fasted at night and fed during the day, plasma calcium still dropped at night, but less so. Finally, when animals were trained to consume their feed between 3 P.M. and 9 P.M., with light provided from 7 A.M. to 7 P.M., the light cycle having been unchanged from the earlier experiments, the drop in plasma calcium occurred just before feeding independently of the onset of light or dark. Thyroidectomy diminished but did not abolish the circadian variation in plasma calcium. Talmage *et al.* (1975a), who discuss their results in relation to findings by Milhaud and associates

(Milhaud *et al.*, 1972; Perault-Straub *et al.*, 1974), do not believe the variations they have observed are diurnal in nature, as they seemed more dependent on food intake than on the light cycle (Talmage *et al.*, 1975b).

Staub *et al.* (1979) have confirmed the existence of a circadian rhythm in total or ionized plasma calcium. This rhythm was similar whether the animals were fed a diet normal (0.7%) or deficient (< 0.03%) in calcium. The amplitude of the variation about the mean was about ± 6% in the animals fed a normal calcium intake. In the animals that had been fed the deficient diet for two weeks before the experiments, the excursions about the daily mean became greater, reaching 30% as the mean plasma calcium dropped to 7.42 mg/dl. There were no differences in the amplitude of variation in the ionized as compared to the total calcium. Staub *et al.* (1979), like Talmage *et al.* (1975a), found the maximum $[Ca_s]$ value at around 2 P.M.; but in their experiments, the nadir occurred at around 11 P.M. rather than at 5 A.M., as was the case in the studies by Talmage *et al.* (1975a).

In their study Talmage *et al.* (1975a) also studied the fate of radioactive calcium that had been administered to the animals 5 days before the experiments. The excursions about the mean were much greater for the radioactive calcium, whether the animals were intact or thyroidectomized. Total plasma calcium fell at night whether or not the animals had been calcium-fasted or calcium-fed, but the radiocalcium rose at night in the calcium-fasted rats. These data clearly indicate that bone calcium that entered the plasma was not labeled homogeneously. The data also confirm that calcium that has entered the skeleton relatively recently can be mobilized more readily than calcium that had been deposited earlier. This has been known since the early days of skeletal experiments with radioactive calcium (Hevesy, 1955). However no experiments have been reported beyond those by Talmage *et al.* (1975a) in which this inhomogeneity has been utilized to evaluate plasma calcium regulation.

2. *Regulatory Description*

Plasma calcium regulation may be analyzed in terms of three characteristics: the "set value" around which the calcium level is regulated and which has been termed [U] by Aubert and Bronner (1965); the precision with which the set value is maintained and which can conveniently be expressed as the coefficient of variation of the set value; and the rate with which a positive or negative calcium load is overcome. The return to [U] from a new plasma calcium value resulting from an exogenous load is a time-dependent function which we shall term g; its derivative will be symbolized by $\dot{g}$.

As is well known, the steady-state plasma calcium differs in various conditions. It is low in hypoparathyroidism or vitamin D deficiency and elevated in hyperparathyroidism and certain lytic bone diseases. One may ask whether the body attempts regulation about the steady-state value found in a given condition, e.g., 12 mg/dl in a case of hyperparathyroidism, or whether regulation is toward the "normal" value of 10 mg/dl. An operational definition is that regulation is around the value maintained in the absence of a load, i.e., the steady state value characteristic of a condition and an individual. Therefore the actual value for [U] differs from individual to individual and is characteristically low for hypoparathyroidism and high for hyperparathyroidism.

Inasmuch as [U] may differ in different endocrine states, it is not surprising that the precision with which [Ca_s] is maintained around [U] also differs. For example, in parathyroidectomized animals, the precision with which the steady-state plasma calcium is maintained is less than half that encountered in euparathyroid animals (Hausmann and Riggs, 1966; Sammon *et al.*, 1970). This is also true in the hypocalcemia of vitamin D deficiency (Hurwitz *et al.*, 1969). On the other hand, when parathyroidectomized animals were placed on a low-phosphate diet, causing their steady-state plasma calcium levels to rise, the precision with which they maintained the new steady-state plasma calcium levels was as good as that of the sham-operated controls that had become hypercalcemic (Cuisinier-Gleizes *et al.*, 1975). These findings, along with others (e.g., Staub *et al.*, 1979), suggest that the coefficient of variation may be smaller when plasma calcium is in the 10–12 mg/dl range than when it is low (<8 mg/dl). The relationship between [U] and its coefficient of variation is complicated and may be related to the absolute value of [U] as well as to the endocrine and nutritional status associated with a given steady-state plasma calcium value. This is a topic that needs further study.

The third characteristic of plasma calcium regulation is its response to an acute load. In contrast with [U] and its coefficient of variation, which are steady-state measures, g and $\dot{g}$ are dynamic measures of the system response and therefore should reveal much about the system. Unfortunately few studies have utilized these parameters. One example is the report by Parfitt (1969) who, on the basis of the rate at which the plasma calcium returned to the preinjection level following a negative load—induced with an EDTA infusion—was able to classify a patient population into three groups and associate the three classes of response with a rate at which a bone calcium pool was mobilized. As might be expected, patients who were severely hypoparathyroid were least able to induce rapid recovery; the slow partial recovery was attributed to "passive rearrangement of the pool calcium."

As already discussed, Hausmann and Riggs (1966) have shown that in both euparathyroid and parathyroidectomized dogs[3] the time-dependent approach to the (new) steady-state plasma calcium that resulted when the animals received positive or negative loads (Ca or EDTA infusions, respectively) was the same

[3]The dogs were thyroparathyroidectomized; their diet was supplemented daily with 10 gm calcium lactate and 30 mg thyroid powder.

and could be described by a one-term exponential expression. Rodan (1970) has also shown that both negative and positive loads provoke an exponential-like drop from the under- or overshoot provoked by the load. However, in his isolated dog limb system, there was no return to the preinjection value; instead new plateau values were maintained.

King *et al.* (1965) infused EDTA (50 mg/kg body weight) into ten normal volunteers and found the plasma calcium had returned to the preinfusion level by 12 hr after the infusion had been stopped. The time course resembled that of a single exponential but measurements were made at only three time points. In patients with operated goiters the rate of return seemed slower; in hypoparathyroid patients, as in parathyroidectomized dogs (Hausmann and Riggs, 1966), both return and plateau levels were lower than in euparathyroid individuals.

Waron and Rich (1969) used an approach like that of Hausmann and Riggs (1966) in that they analyzed the rate by which plasma calcium returned to normal in dogs after an EDTA infusion. These investigators report that treating dogs with imidazole markedly depressed this rate, while treating the animals with parathyroid extract (Lilly) for 1 hr before the infusion raised this rate. The mean rate of recovery in puppies was nearly four times that in mature dogs. To calculate the rate, Waron and Rich assumed a constant volume of distribution, larger than the plasma volume; they also assumed that the return to the preinjection value was described by a simple exponential expression.

Argenzio *et al.* (1974) studied the time required for infusion-induced hypercalcemia in horses to return to the preinjection level and found that thyroidectomy markedly increased this "tolerance time," but that thyroxine treatment overcame this increase.

Bronner and associates have studied the effect of intraperitoneal calcium loads in rats on different calcium intakes with or without endogenous supplies of parathyroid hormone and/or calcitonin (Bronner *et al.*, 1967, 1968; Sammon *et al.*, 1969, 1970; Fig. 10). They observed that plasma calcium peaked at about 0.5 hr after load administration and thereafter dropped in an exponential-like function to the preinjection value. When the calcium load was 4.1 mg/100 gm body weight, the relative peak value was the same in all animals studied; in other words, neither dietary intake nor endocrine status had an effect on the relative peak value. On the other hand, the rate at which the preinjection value was approached ($\dot{g}$) differed considerably with endocrine status. In animals lacking endogenous parathyroid hormone and/or calcitonin plasma calcium returned to the preinjection value in about 3 hr, whereas in normal animals the preinjection value was attained in 2 hr, though no mathematical expression was derived. Dietary calcium intake did not seem to have an effect on the time in which the preinjection plasma calcium value was attained (Bronner *et al.*, 1968).

When the calcium load was doubled to 8.2 mg/100 gm body wt, the peak value was still attained in about 0.5 hr after load administration, but it took 4 hr or more to reach the preinjection value, regardless of calcium intake or endocrine status. On the other hand, peak values seemed higher in PTX or TPTX animals than in either normal or calcitonin-deprived rats.

Many more detailed studies of the type outlined above are needed to delineate the mechanisms of plasma calcium homeostasis in quantitative terms.

III. SYSTEMS REGULATING CALCIUM HOMEOSTASIS

1. General

Total body calcium in a 70-kg person is between 1 and 1.5 kg, with more than 99% of this residing in the skeleton. In these terms bone is the only significant storage system, since the calcium content of most extraskeletal tissues is relatively constant throughout life, whereas the skeletal calcium concentration varies with age, sex, dietary intake, and physiological state. Consider a growing male rat weighing 150 gm whose body calcium balance is +50 mg/day. In 100 days on that intake its body will have gained 5 gm Ca and its body weight will have gone up by about 200 gm. If the calcium were distributed uniformly throughout the body, the new tissue would have had to have a calcium concentration of 2.5%, whereas soft tissue averages only about 3–4 mg/100 gm or 0.003–0.004%. In other words, the skeleton whose weight will have increased by 30 gm in that period of time would have gained 4.99 gm Ca. A skeletal calcium concentration of 16–17% has in fact been reported for 250-day-old male rats (Widdowson and Dickerson, 1964).

The preceding description implies that dietary calcium (entering via the intestine) constitutes a major input into the plasma (and the volume of calcium distribution) and that the intestine is a major gateway for body calcium. The description also implies that the skeleton constitutes a major sink for calcium that leaves the plasma (and the calcium distribution volume). The third system is the kidney which modulates losses from the plasma.

Figure 1 shows a simple regulatory scheme with net inputs or outputs from the three system—gut, kidney, and bone. In that scheme net intestinal calcium input would tend to raise plasma calcium and the net kidney and bone responses would tend to lower plasma calcium. As discussed above, the actual volume of calcium distribution is much larger than the plasma, but the equilibrium between plasma calcium and the calcium of the volume of distribution appears to be so rapid that the plasma calcium may be considered representative of the calcium content of the volume of distribution. Moreover, the plasma calcium is the only readily accessible body calcium compartment.

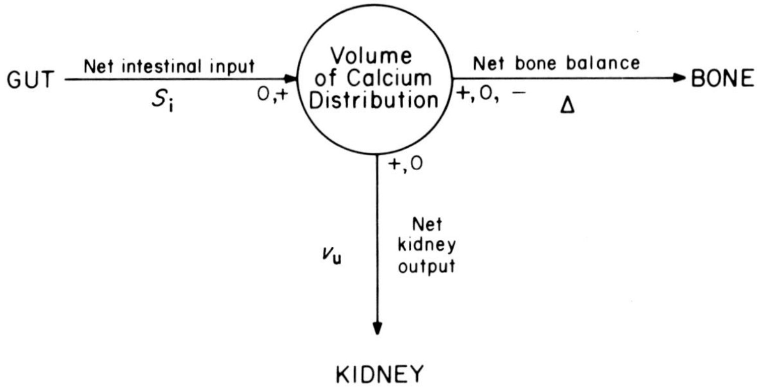

Fig. 1. A simple regulatory scheme of plasma calcium regulation. The ionic calcium concentration is the same in the plasma and in the much larger volume of distribution. In order for it to remain unchanged, with an unchanging volume of distribution, the sum of the input and output vectors must equal zero, i.e., $S_i = \Delta - v_u$. The units are rates, milligrams calcium per day, and the vectors are defined as follows: $S_i = v_a - v_{ndo} = v_i - v_F$, where v_a = calcium absorption, v_{ndo} = fecal endogenous output; $\Delta = v_{o+} - v_{o-}$, where v_{o+} = bone calcium deposition and v_{o-} bond calcium removal; $v_u = v_{fi} - v_r + v_s$, where v_{fi} = filtered calcium, v_r = reabsorbed calcium, v_s = secreted calcium. The plus, minus, and zero signs indicate direction of flow. A more detailed description of the three systems, intestine, bone, and kidney is given in Figs. 2, 4, and 5.

In the scheme in Fig. 1, the body calcium balance, i.e., intake (v_i) minus excretion ($v_u + v_F$, where v_u = urinary calcium and v_F = fecal calcium) equals the calcium balance of the skeleton. The reasons for this have been stated above.

In adult humans and other nongrowing organisms, the body calcium balance approximates zero; in other words, there is no net calcium gain or loss. Under those conditions, net calcium entry from the intestine, obviously equal to the difference between input into the intestine and net excretion, must equal net urinary loss.

It has been argued (Nordin *et al.*, 1972) that since in the adult the net body balance of calcium is zero, the major regulatory role is that exerted by the kidney. However, the relative importance of a given system can be assessed only under conditions of load. When an acute positive load is introduced into the mammalian body, it is the body calcium balance that goes up. Hence the major response to an acute positive load is exerted by the skeleton. There is a rise in urinary calcium output but it is relatively small in relation to the increase in calcium retention (Talmage and Grubb, 1977).

The effect of a chronic increase in net calcium absorption (S_i, Fig. 1) on urinary calcium excretion and net bone calcium retention can be predicted from the equations of Hall *et al.* (1969) derived for a group of postmenopausal women:

$$v_u = 114 + 0.23\ S_i \tag{1}$$

$$\Delta = -114 + 0.77\ S_i \tag{2}$$

where v_u = urinary Ca excretion, Δ = body or skeletal Ca balance, and S_i = net intestinal absorption, in milligrams calcium per day.

The equations can be rewritten as follows:

$$v_u/S_i = 0.23 + 114/S_i \tag{3}$$

and

$$\Delta\ /S_i = 0.77 - 114/S_i \tag{4}$$

Here v_u/S_i expresses the proportion of the net intestinal input that is handled by the kidney and Δ/S_i is the proportion of the net intestinal input handled by the skeleton. Equations (3) and (4) predict that as S_i goes up, both ratios approach their respective limits, i.e., 0.23 for v_u/S_i and 0.77 for Δ/S_i, but from opposite directions. In other words, as input from the gut increases, the kidney will handle a decreasing proportion of that input and the skeleton will handle an increasing proportion. According to Eq. 2, the subjects do not begin having a positive balance until $S_i \simeq 148$ mg Ca/day, corresponding to calcium intakes of $\geqslant 600$ mg/day. At lower intakes these subjects would lose calcium from their skeleton. As calcium intake increases from 600 to 1000 mg/day, a probable upper limit, the ratio of v_u/S_i decreases from 1 to 0.69 and the ratio of Δ/S_i increases from 0 to 0.31. These considerations show that in a situation of increased calcium input from the gut, an increasing proportion of this input would find its way to the skeleton. Whether under conditions of high chronic calcium intake one could reach a situation of skeletal saturation, so that other excretory routes would have to handle a greater proportion of the load has not been studied as such. Talmage and Grubb (1977) have shown that when normal male rats (>200 gm body wt) were subjected to the same intravenous calcium load (0.01 mg Ca/gm body wt/hr) on two successive days, the urinary calcium output during the 4 hr infusion increased by 37% (1.86 →2.54 mg) on the second day. Yet 2.54 mg represents less than 40% of the load. Whether a major portion of an intravenous calcium load can be excreted via the kidney in an adult rat reared on a high calcium diet, when its skeleton can be presumed near saturation, has not been tested.

Jaros *et al.* (1979) have developed an analog-digital computer simulation of calcium homeostasis and estimated the rate at which plasma calcium is restored after extracellular calcium is removed at −8 mmol/hr. The slope of calcium return is 0.18 mmol/liter/hr which in a 70-kg man would amount to 0.18 × 15 or 2.7 mmol/hr, a rate far in excess of what could be supplied by the intestine and by shutting off the renal calcium output. Therefore, rapid calcium efflux from bone appears the only feasible explanation. Parfitt (1979) and Talmage *et al.* (1978) have argued along the same lines and suggested mechanisms of how this occurs (see also below and Powell, 1972).

R.V. Talpaz *et al.* (personal communication) have studied regulation of the plasma calcium concentration in chicks following a calcium load by indwelling catheters and have used these and other data to study by a modeling approach the relative contribution of bone and kidney to plasma error minimization. They showed that the kidney overcomes the initial error, but that bone can account for the remainder of the error, doing so by a combination of proportional, derivative, and integral modes, as originally suggested by Aubert and Bronner (1965).

The above considerations thus show that the skeleton plays a major role in handling either chronic or acute calcium loads, whether these loads are positive or negative and whether they are transient or chronic. The kidney does, however, play a significant role in modifying the effects of transient or chronic loads.

The regulatory role of the intestine is less obvious. From the viewpoint of plasma calcium homeostasis, net intestinal calcium input has been treated (Aubert and Bronner, 1965; Bronner, 1973a,b; Fig. 1) as the disturbing signal, i.e., as the input that tends to raise plasma calcium above the point maintained in the absence of a load. This classification can be justified since a step shift in dietary calcium input leads to a prompt rise in the amount of calcium absorbed. Such a rise could imply that regulation at the intestinal level is sluggish and/or inefficient. However, the biological function of the intestine is to extract calcium from the environment via the food eaten. Transepithelial calcium transport involves two processes, one that is saturable, metabolically driven and regulatable, and another that is nonsaturable, with calcium movement down its chemical gradient. The proportion of calcium moved by the regulatable process is a function of calcium intake, vitamin D intake, other nutrient intake, physiological or endocrine state, age, etc., but under few conditions exceeds half of the absorbed calcium. Thus from a regulatory viewpoint there is an obligatory calcium input from the gut that cannot be shut off except by lowered intake.

This is illustrated in the computer simulation study of Hurwitz *et al.* (1979). These authors predict that in chickens a shift in calcium intake from 900 to 1300 mg/kg/day would within 24 hr result in a 15% decrease of calcium flow from the intestine, whereas the net calcium flow into bone would double. In a downward shift from 900 to 100 mg/kg/day, the intestinal calcium inflow would increase by about 12%, while the bone balance would become severely negative because of increased negative flow. Therefore, the predicted adaptive responses of the intestine would be quite modest.

The full response was not predicted to occur until 24 hr after the dietary shift. In reality this delay may be much shorter, as Hurwitz *et al.* (1979) based their analysis on absorption and $1,25(OH)_2D_3$ data from Holick *et al.* (1976), which had been obtained in vitamin D-deficient animals. Buckley and Bronner (1980) have shown that vitamin D-replete rats on a high calcium diet respond to exogenous $1{,}25(OH)_2D_3$ much more rapidly than vitamin D-deficient animals. The regulatory response of the saturable component of calcium absorption, thought to be vitamin D-dependent (Ambrecht *et al.*, 1979; Pansu *et al.*, 1981), may therefore occur more rapidly and in this way could play a role in acute plasma calcium homeostasis. However, since the rate of response probably does not modify its extent, the role of the intestine in acute plasma calcium regulation appears small and its major function in an analysis of plasma calcium homeostasis remains that of providing the net disturbing signal.

The preceding section provides a regulatory classification of the net outputs of the three major organ systems involved in calcium metabolism, i.e., intestine, kidney, and skeleton. Since net output of each system is the resultant of calcium inflows and outflows, these will now be analyzed in regulatory terms. To do that each system will be briefly described; for more detailed description of a given system, the reader is referred to the relevant chapters of this treatise.

Before this is done, it may be useful to differentiate between mass flows and signals. In a simple flow system, regulation is typically effected by gating, e.g., pressure-sensitive controls. Mass flow thus acts as a signal for the control which usually effects regulation by other means, e.g., electrical or mechanical. In the case of calcium regulation in the body, there is no known central coordinator or master control that regulates calcium flows. Rather, all cells in some way respond to variations in calcium concentration at the plasma membrane, at the same time modifying calcium extrusion. Cells also act in concert in tissues. The tissues in turn may exert direct action, as kidney cells that reabsorb and excrete calcium specifically, or the cardiovascular system that profoundly affects calcium handling via the blood and lymph but by itself has only a modest effect on the calcium economy of the body. Mechanisms involved in cellular calcium handling and regulation are beginning to be understood (see Chapter 1, this volume), but the manner in which cells interact and effect directed action at the tissue level is virtually unknown. In a description, therefore, of the role played by specific tissues in calcium homeostasis, very little can as yet be said of mechanisms, i.e., of how calcium flow is sensed and then modified. One can postulate calcium-dependent conformational changes in membrane and organelle proteins that in turn directly or indirectly modify calcium entry and release in the cell and ultimately in the tissue. Many cellular and subcellular calcium-dependent processes have been and are being discovered, some of which may utilize calcium without affecting the body's calcium economy. Others undoubtedly will be found to affect calcium flows profoundly, but these studies are still in a very early stage. In addition to the direct effect of calcium flow on calcium handling by the major organ systems, there is an effect of calcium on specific regulators, e.g., the kidney cells making 1,25-dihydroxyvitamin D_3, the parathyroid gland cells, and the C cells of the thyroid gland, to name only primary regulators. These respond to calcium flows by releasing specific regulator molecules, which in turn modify the calcium handling of their respective target tissues. In the descriptions to follow, an attempt will be made to differentiate signal from mass flow, but in most instances this distinction will necessarily be conceptual rather than experimental.

2. *Intestine (See Chapter 3, This Volume)*

Figure 2 summarizes current views of intestinal calcium absorption in symbolic terms. As ingested calcium moves by peristaltic action from the proximal to the distal end of the intestine, it is subjected to transepithelial movement. The movement is bidirectional with a net amount retained by the body in the

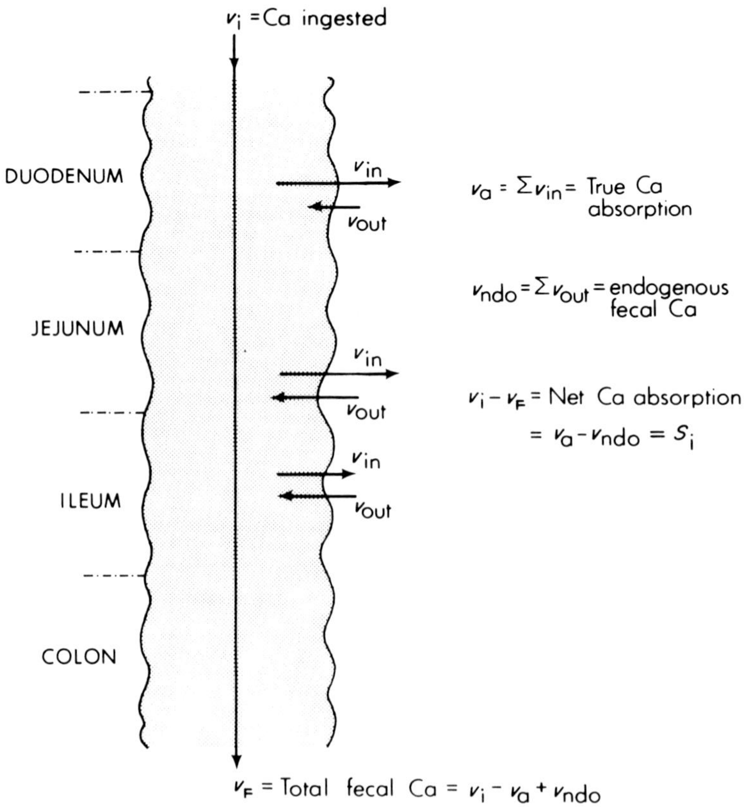

Fig. 2. Symbolic scheme of intestinal calcium absorption. Units for all vectors are mass per unit time, e.g., mg/day. In young males on a typical Western diet, v_i = 1000 mg Ca/day, v_F = 825 mg Ca/day, v_a = 325 mg Ca/day, v_{ndo} = 150 mg Ca/day.

duodenum and jejunum, while there is a tendency toward net loss in the ileum. In most situations the net intestinal balance is positive, i.e., $v_a > v_{ndo}$ and S_i (= $v_a - v_{ndo} = v_i - v_F$) is positive.

In the duodenum, transepithelial calcium movement may be described as the sum of a saturable and a nonsaturable process (Fig. 3). The saturable process appears regulatable and related to the vitamin D status of the animal. It varies inversely with calcium intake and status, is small in animals on high and relatively important in animals on low calcium intakes (Ambrecht *et al.*, 1979; Pansu *et al.*, 1981). It is absent in vitamin D deficiency, is significant in the young, and relatively insignificant in the older animal (Zornitzer and Bronner, 1971).

The proportion of calcium absorbed by each of the two processes varies with many factors. If one extrapolates from the usual calcium intakes encountered in man or the rat to the luminal calcium concentration, one can estimate (Zornitzer and Bronner, 1971; see also Fig. 3) that the saturable component rarely accounts for more than half of the total absorbed in the duodenum.

In the jejunum, the proportion of calcium moved by the saturable process is much less than in the duodenum, while in the ileum the saturable component is, for all practical purposes, absent (D. Pansu, C. Bellaton, and F. Bronner, unpublished). Moreover, as shown by Walling and Kimberg (1973), the net amount of calcium absorbed in the ileum may become negative, i.e., the vector of calcium movement may be in the direction of the lumen.

From the viewpoint of regulation, only the saturable component can be modified. This means that calcium absorption cannot be stopped completely. The report by Hurwitz *et al.* (1969) illustrates this conclusion. These investigators found that in vitamin D-deficient rats on an adequate mineral intake (0.6% Ca, 0.6% P) absorption can be described by the following equations:

$$v_a = 3.4 + 0.51\ v_i \qquad (+\text{D}) \qquad (5)$$

$$v_a = -8.6 + 0.55\ v_i \qquad (-\text{D}) \qquad (6)$$

where v_a = true calcium absorption, v_i = calcium intake, in milligrams calcium per day, +D = vitamin D-replete state, and −D = vitamin D-deficient state.

Equations (5) and (6) show that the major difference in the two groups was in the intercept, but that the slope was similar. Although the absorption function in the whole animal probably cannot be analyzed as directly as transepithelial movement alone (Fig. 3), the intercept undoubtedly reflects the saturable component, while the linear component of the equations, which was similar regardless of vitamin D status, must be related to the nonsaturable processes. Thus, with sufficient dietary calcium, the absolute amount of calcium absorbed was not much lower in the vitamin D-deficient than in the vitamin D-replete rat, even though the saturable absorption process was found only in vitamin D-replete

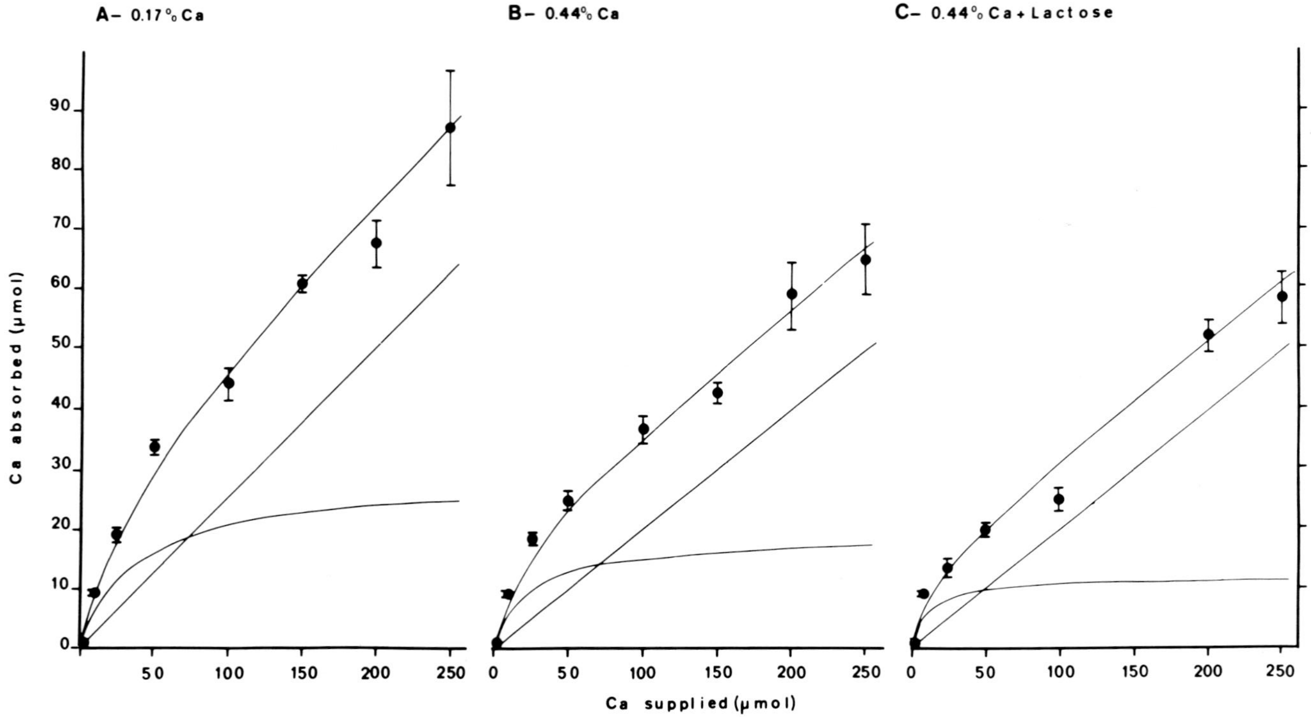

Fig. 3. Saturable and nonsaturable calcium movement in the duodenum. Calcium absorption was measured by an *in situ* loop method (Zornitzer and Bronner, 1971), where the amount of absorbed calcium, ordinate, was determined after 1 hr when the rate of calcium loss from the loop had reached a plateau. The line connecting the experimental points is the sum of the straight-line and curvilinear functions, thought to represent saturable and nonsaturable transfer, respectively (Wasserman and Taylor, 1969). Note that the maximum of the saturable transfer, $J_{\max}$, varied inversely with calcium intake; the slope of the nonsaturable function was similar in all three diet groups. The animals had been raised on the respective diets (0.17% Ca, 0.44% Ca, 0.44% Ca + lactose) from weaning and were studied 5 weeks later. The addition of 30% lactose acted as if calcium intake had been raised to 0.7%. $J_{\max}$ and calcium-binding protein content of the duodenum varied positively and linearly. (From Pansu *et al.,* 1981, reproduced by permission.)

animals. These considerations add to the justification for considering intestinal calcium entry as a signal that disturbs plasma calcium (Fig. 1).

Even if total calcium absorption, v_a, were relatively insensitive to the physiological state, because a significant component of v_a is not subject to regulation, endogenous fecal calcium, v_{ndo}, might be subject to regulation so that net intestinal absorption, $S_i = v_a - v_{ndo}$, could vary to a greater extent than v_a. Sammon *et al.* (1970) evaluated S_i, v_a, and v_{ndo} as a function of calcium intake, v_i, in euparathyroid and parathyroidectomized rats. Over an intake range of 2–260 mg Ca/day, v_{ndo} varied according to the equation,

$$v_{ndo} = 0.4 + 0.05\ v_i \qquad (7)$$

Parathyroidectomy had no effect on the slope, but led to a lower intercept. Although the linear fit was adequate, an exponential-type function is not excluded. Endogenous fecal calcium may therefore be a regulated parameter, but its overall contribution in the rat seems small. At the highest intakes, v_{ndo} approached 14 mg/day while v_a approached 80 mg/day, so that the net loss from the body calcium pool to the intestine accounted for less than 20% (14/80) of the input from intestine to the body pool.

In humans, the endogenous fecal calcium has been found to average 102 mg/day in 207 studies of premenopausal women (aged 40–45 years), with calcium absorption averaging 202 mg/day (Heaney *et al.,* 1978a). Thus in the human, endogenous fecal calcium represents a much larger fraction of the total intestinal calcium input. This may also be true in the older rat (Bronner and Lemaire, 1969). Kales and Phang (1971) found that in patients who, as a result of ingesting calcium in divided doses, absorbed 20% more than when the same amount was ingested in a single dose, v_{ndo} rose by about 12%. Heaney *et al.* (1977) have shown that in perimenopausal women the slope relating total endogenous calcium output ($v_u + v_{ndo}$) to absorbed calcium, v_a, was 0.64 (r = 0.7), with v_{ndo} accounting for about half of the total endogenous output. The findings suggest that the endogenous fecal route may assume a minor regulatory role. Brodan *et al.* (1975) have constructed a theoretical model in which the backflow of calcium from the plasma into the intestine plays an important role.

In experimental phosphate deficiency, characterized in the rat by hypercalcemia and in all species by marked hypercalciuria, one might imagine that the body's attempt to get rid of the large amounts of calcium that result from skeletal destruction (Bronner, 1976) would lead to a relative increase in v_{ndo}, but this was not the case in one report (Hurwitz *et al.,* 1969). For these reasons the endogenous fecal calcium does not seem to play an important regulatory role and S_i may be classified as a disturbing signal. A full understanding of the regulatory importance of the intestine for plasma calcium regulation, however, must await loading studies in which the acute and long-term responses of v_{ndo} and v_a are evaluated in response to experimentally induced variations in plasma calcium.

3. *Kidney (See Chapter 4, This Volume)*

Figure 4 is a symbolic representation of current views of renal calcium handling. Calcium in the cirrculation is filtered in the glomerulus, with the filtrate constituting about 60% of plasma calcium and containing inorganic ionized or complexed calcium, but normally no protein-bound calcium. A little over half of the filtered calcium undergoes transtubular reabsorption in the proximal tubule. Most of the proximal calcium reabsorption is thought to be passive, secondary to water and sodium movements, but Ullrich *et al.* (1976) have concluded that perhaps one-third of proximal calcium movement is due to active movement. Calcium is absorbed in the *pars recta* with about 10% of filtered calcium reabsorbed between the end of the proximal convoluted tubule and the ascending limb of the loop of Henle. Another 20% of the filtered calcium is reabsorbed in the

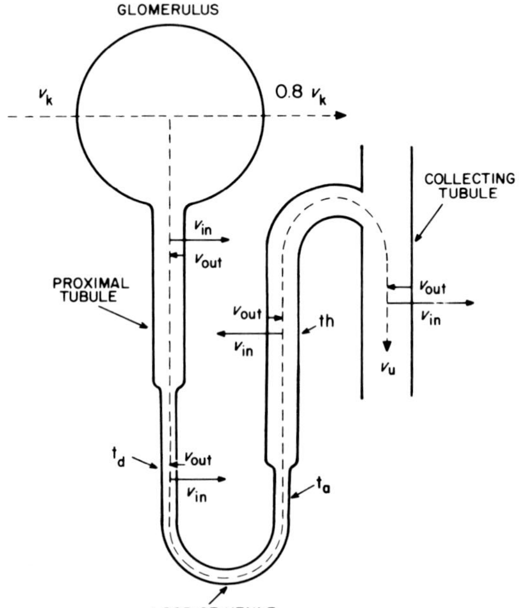

Fig. 4. Symbolic model of calcium movement in the kidney, shown as a nephron with glomerulus, proximal tubule, thin descending (t_d) limb of loop of Henle, thin (t_a) and thick (th) ascending limbs of loop of Henle and collecting tubule. The symbol v refers to an average rate, mass per time, and subscripts define the rates as follows: v_K = the calcium presented by the circulation to the kidney for filtration, approximately one-fourth of the cardiac output; v_{fi} = the amount of calcium filtered, approximately $0.2v_K$. The arrows indicating transtubular movement of calcium are placed in the segments where calcium movement is thought to occur (see text). $\Sigma v_{in} - \Sigma v_{out} = v_r$, calcium reabsorbed in the kidney. The urinary calcium output, v_u, is defined as $v_u = v_{fi} - v_r + v_s$, where v_s is the "secreted" calcium, the existence of which is in doubt. If v_s exists, it would necessarily be part of v_{out} and would have to occur at a site where $v_{in} < v_{out}$.

thick ascending limb of the loop of Henle. There calcium transport is probably passive in the cortical and perhaps active in the medullary segment. Calcium reabsorption is active in the distal nephron and this is probably the major site of direct regulation. Calcium is also reabsorbed actively in the collecting ducts.

Constanzo (1978) has shown that efflux of calcium from lumen to blood is a function of the luminal calcium concentration and that the net backflux of calcium across the distal renal epithelium is insignificant. Constanzo (1978) has also shown that calcium reabsorption in the distal nephron is proportional to the load when the load is varied between 10 and 20 μmol/min, with reabsorption approximately 70%.

From the viewpoint of regulation, it is the active components of tubular calcium reabsorption that are of interest. An increase in intestinal calcium input is known to increase urinary calcium output [Hall *et al.*, 1969, Eq. (1); Sammon *et al.*, 1970, Eq. (20); Clark and Rivera-Cordero, 1973] and intravenous calcium infusions have been shown to increase urinary calcium excretion (Talmage and Grubb, 1977), as might be expected.[4] What is not known is how the load affects the individual parameters that make up urine calcium. One can write

$$v_u = v_{fi} - (\Sigma v_{in} - \Sigma v_{out}) \tag{8}$$

where v_u = rate of urinary calcium excretion, v_{fi} = rate of glomerular calcium filtration, Σv_{in} = the sum of all movements from tubule to the blood, and Σv_{out} = the sum of all movements from blood to tubule (units are mass per time, e.g., milligrams calcium per hour).

The fraction of calcium that is reabsorbed can then be defined as:

$$F_r = \frac{(\Sigma v_{in} - \Sigma v_{out})}{v_{fi}}$$

and net renal calcium reabsorption, v_r, is $(\Sigma v_{in} - \Sigma v_{out})$. v_r over the entire kidney is measured in clearance studies. As pointed out above, v_r has also been measured in different tubular segments. To assert that calcium reabsorption is active implies that v_r is saturable or at least contains a saturable component, as illustrated for the intestine in Fig. 3. Moreover, v_{in} is probably a function of v_{fi} (Constanzo, 1978). If v_{in} is made up of a saturable and nonsaturable function, the saturable function could be subject to regulation. In addition v_{out} might be a function of the cellular calcium and therefore be indirectly, albeit insensitively, related to v_{in} and ultimately to v_{fi}. Moreover, v_{out} could be independently regulated. Until these underlying relationships have been elucidated quantitatively, only qualitative predictions are possible.

[4]C.F. Ramberg (personal communication) has observed that when cows received intravenous calcium infusions of 14 gm/day for many days, their urinary calcium output increased from a base level of 0.8 gm/day to 6.1 gm/day. A similar response was observed in the parathyroidectomized cow.

Whether or not true renal calcium secretion, v_s, occurs is moot. If in a given segment, $v_{out} > v_{in}$, this would be equivalent to v_s. The regulatory diagrams (see Figs. 6, 7, and 9) include v_s to reflect the possibility that $v_{out} > v_{in}$. In that case, v_{out} (or a part of it) would be subject to regulation.

For these reasons the constituent signals that make up v_u will also be classified as regulatory, even though in theory v_{in} or v_{out}, but not both, could function as disturbing signals. The filtered calcium, v_{fi}, is a special case, as it is directly proportional to the plasma calcium and there is no evidence that glomerular filtration of calcium is regulated by the plasma calcium.

The many factors that affect v_u are detailed in Chapter 4, this volume, and in Chapters 3 and 4, Vol. III. Whether direct or indirect, their action must be presumed to alter the active components of renal calcium transport, since only these by definition are regulatable. The mechanisms by which these processes respond to variations in calcium input, alter renal calcium output, and thus contribute to plasma calcium regulation are not yet understood. The effect of the known hormonal regulators will be discussed below, but overall knowledge of cellular calcium transport is even more rudimentary in the kidney than in the intestine. Probably the fullest description is that of Borle (1978).

Quantitative description of how v_u varies in different conditions also is rudimentary. Equation (1) predicts that as net intestinal calcium absorption increases in adults, 23% of the load is handled by the kidney. The report by Kales and Phang (1971) confirms this. No systematic studies have been published, however, to show how this relationship is altered in the many conditions known to alter calcium metabolism. For example, from published balance studies for patients with renal failure the following relationship has been calculated (Bronner, 1979):

$$v_u = 28.3 + 0.047\ S_i \tag{10}$$

Comparison with Eq. (1) shows that the slope, i.e., the fraction of the intestinal load handled by the kidney, is only about one-fifth that found in normal individuals. This may be the result of a decrease in renal tissue or a decrease in the filtered load.

In experimental phosphate deficiency, when urinary calcium output is very large, the slope of the relationship between v_u and S_i is about six times that in phosphate-replete rats (Bronner, 1979). If the slope is a measure of the nonsaturable components (as analyzed for the intestine in Fig. 3), then this would reflect tissue alteration and a consequent tubular "leak."

It would be useful to compile relationships like Eq. (10) for a variety of conditions and diseases because they may provide a guide to possible mechanisms. If urinary calcium output is the resultant of saturable and nonsaturable processes, then the slope of the linear relationship between v_u and S_i reflects nonsaturable events and the apparent intercept[5] reflects the saturable component. In the intestine, the nonsaturable component does not appear to vary widely (Zornitzer and Bronner, 1971; Pansu *et al.*, 1981); this may not be the case for the kidney (Constanzo, 1978). The nature of renal calcium transport therefore is still open.

4. Bone

a. The Rate of Bone Calcium Deposition To evaluate the effect of bone calcium handling on plasma calcium homeostasis, it is necessary to be able to measure calcium flows into and out of the skeleton and to dissect these into active and passive processes. There is no direct experimental approach by which a bone calcium clearance can be evaluated. The only available method for measuring calcium flow into the whole skeleton is by kinetic means. In this approach radioactive calcium is injected into the organism, usually by the intravenous route, and the time-dependent decrease in specific radioactivity of the plasma calcium is analyzed. In essence, the decrease in specific activity results from dilution by unlabeled calcium that enters the blood compartment either from the intestine or bone, plus redistribution of calcium within the pool. It is the latter process that leads to complication in the analysis, since analysis of redistribution requires formulation of a specific model. From the earliest whole organism studies with labeled calcium it became clear that the time-dependent decrease in specific radioactivity of the blood calcium cannot be described by a single exponential term. In other words, the radiocalcium had not been injected into a single, well-mixed compartment, but into one that communicated with one or more compartments. Moreover the size of the pool, i.e., the sum of these compartments, was such that a major portion of the pool calcium had to be skeletal in origin (see above). Consequently, in trying to solve for a clearance value, it became difficult to differentiate between redistribution and net loss, even though it is only the latter that can play a regulatory role.

The analytical problem of arriving at a value for the unidirectional loss of calcium from blood to skeleton (here termed v_{o+}) is compounded by the difficulty of determining if and when the pool approaches an isotopic equilibrium. If that were to occur relatively soon after administration of radiocalcium, the entire system would thereafter behave as a well-mixed single compartment and all unidirectional losses could be readily calculated. Instead, even in studies that have lasted for 3–4 weeks, it is not clear whether a dynamic equilibrium has been

[5]Although urinary calcium loss may never equal zero, it is likely to drop appreciably when net calcium absorption S_i is maintained at zero for a period of time. The intercept is also "apparent" if it is considered to reflect the saturable component of urinary calcium reabsorption, which, in analogy with the intestine, may be a hyperbolic function of the filtered calcium.

reached or whether labeled calcium is already being returned to the pool by bone resorption.

In practice, most human studies have been based on experimental periods of 4–20 days, with the largest number of studies (Heaney *et al.*, 1978a,b) made on perimenopausal women who were on an 8-day study period. In these subjects the rate of total bone calcium deposition, v_{o+}, also termed accretion, was on the order of 350 mg/day. The absolute value of this parameter is a function of the length of study and of the model used to analyze the disappearance equation—the shorter the period, the bigger the value. If a two-compartment model is used as by Heaney *et al.* (1978b), the values tend to be larger than in a four-compartment model, but the differences are not very great (Bronner and Lemaire, 1969).

The rate of bone calcium deposition, v_{o+}, is a function of age. In boys under 16 years of age it approximates 1200 mg/day (Bronner *et al.*, 1956; Hall *et al.*, 1969); some time thereafter it begins to drop gradually, reaching about 400 mg/day in 71-year-old men (Cohn *et al.*, 1965). In cows, v_{o+} decreased from 11.7 to 4.2 gm/day as their age increased from 4.8 to 7 years (Ramberg *et al.*, 1976). Women probably have lower values than men, especially after menopause, but quantitative comparisons with age-matched male controls have not been published. In female rats, v_{o+} values are lower than in comparably aged males (Bronner and Lemaire, 1969; Sammon *et al.*, 1970).

The effect of increased calcium intake on v_{o+} is relatively modest, with most of the effect of an increase in calcium intake and balance reflected by a decrease in the rate of bone calcium removal (v_{o-}, see below). This is true in man (Schwartz *et al.*, 1965; Phang *et al.*, 1969; Hall *et al.*, 1969), the rat (Sammon *et al.*, 1970), cows (Ramberg *et al.*, 1976), as well as in most other mammals studied (e.g., ponies, Schryver *et al.*, 1970). Over a range of net calcium absorption of 0–650 mg Ca/day, Hall *et al.* (1969) found that in 23 studies with 16 women, 37–70 years old, the relationship between v_{o+} and S_i can be described by

$$v_{o+} = 354 + 0.13\ S_i \tag{11}$$

in milligrams calcium per day.

In that group of subjects a zero calcium balance would have been attained when $S_i = 148$ mg/day and v_{o+} would then equal 373 mg/day. This value agrees remarkably well with the mean value of 387 mg calcium/day (SD: 126) found in a large group of women (5.3 years postmenopausal, untreated) studied by Heaney *et al.* (1978a). Although the slope of Eq. (11) was not statistically significant, it was comparable in magnitude to the modest, but statistically significant slope found by Sammon *et al.* (1970) for growing male rats:

$$v_{o+} = 67.2 + 0.11\ S_i \tag{12}$$

in milligrams per day.

The similarities in the slopes of Eqs. (11) and (12) suggest that approximately 10% of the calcium brought into the body by net intestinal absorption may go to increase the rate of calcium deposition into the skeleton.

Hall *et al.* (1969) also found [Eqs. (1) and (2)] that in these women 23% of the net calcium absorption is handled by the kidney, so that over half of the disturbing signal ($0.64\ S_i = 0.77\ S_i - 0.13\ S_i$) must be overcome by a decrease in bone calcium removal (v_{o-}). In cows this proportion is closer to unity (Ramberg *et al.*, 1976).

No studies have been published to evaluate v_{o+} as a function of calcium input into the skeleton. C.F. Ramberg (personal communication) has studied the effect of constant calcium infusions on the parameters of calcium metabolism in two cows, one of which had been on a high and the other on a low calcium diet. Calcium was infused into the circulation at a rate to exceed the total plasma calcium clearance ($v_T = v_{o+} + v_u + v_{ndo}$). This caused plasma calcium to increase, with the increase greater in the animal that had been on a high calcium diet. In both animals, v_u increased; bone calcium resorption, v_{o-}, appeared to decrease. There was, however, no reliable change in v_{o+}. The increases in v_u were greater in the cow that had been on the high calcium diet. Parathyroidectomy appeared to have no effect on these responses.

Because v_{o+} is a steady-state parameter, measured over a period of several days, its acute regulatory role is difficult to evaluate. To approach this question it will be necessary to develop acute methods, as in the perfused limb system. Using such a system, Rodan (1970) has evaluated the unidirectional loss of calcium as a function of the calcium load. The addition of from 0.2 to 0.5 mmol calcium to the perfusion system had no obvious effect on the unidirectional loss of calcium into bone. More such studies are required before one may conclude that v_{o+} (or its equivalent) either has or does not have a regulatory effect on plasma calcium. If v_{o+} were to vary with a load, as v_a appears to in relation to the luminal calcium (Fig. 3), then this response could be analyzed in analogous fashion. As yet, however, it is not possible to state whether v_{o+} is a homogeneous or heterogeneous process with a specific regulatable component.

b. The Rate of Bone Calcium Removal Bone calcium removal, v_{o-}, is the net rate of loss of calcium from the bone compartment, with the difference between v_{o+} and v_{o-} necessarily equal to the bone calcium balance. The latter in turn must equal the body calcium balance, if there is no significant extraskeletal storage. Formally v_{o-} is defined as follows:

$$v_{o-} = v_{o+} - \Delta = v_{o+} + v_u + v_{ndo} - v_a \qquad (13)$$

in milligrams calcium per day.

Lauffenburger *et al.* (1977) have evaluated v_{o-} in their human studies from $\Delta - v_{o+}$ and estimated the error associated with v_{o-} was 23%, while that of v_{o+} was only 10%. Heaney *et al.* (1978b), on the other hand, who estimated v_{o-} from the difference between turnover ($v_T = v_{o+} + v_u + v_{ndo}$) and v_a, report the same magnitude for the error of both parameters, approximately 14% (SE).

Qualitatively speaking, v_{o+} and v_{o-} vary in parallel, though the parallelism cannot be strict. When, as a result of some treatment or condition, bone turnover is increased, both v_{o+} and v_{o-} will increase, though not necessarily to the same extent. Therefore v_{o+} and v_{o-} like v_a, rise with age in childhood and, beginning in young adulthood, gradually decrease with age. Like v_{o+}, v_{o-} is high in conditions of high bone turnover (hyperthyroidism, hyperparathyroidism, Paget's disease, lytic bone disease) and low in conditions of low bone turnover (hypothyroidism, hypoparathyroidism, hypogonadism, etc.) However, from a regulatory viewpoint, in response to positive or negative calcium loads, v_{o+} and v_{o-} vary in opposite directions, inasmuch as increased calcium intake that leads to an increased calcium balance brings about no or a small positive change in v_{o+} (see above), while effecting a marked drop in v_{o-}. Thus in cows Ramberg *et al.* (1976) report that

$$v_{o-} = 14 - 1.0\ v_a \tag{14}$$

in grams calcium per day, whereas in women Hall *et al.* (1969) found that

$$v_{o-} = 468 - 0.64\ S_i \tag{15}$$

in milligrams calcium per day, and in rats Sammon *et al.* (1970) report the relationship as

$$v_{o-} = 67.5 - 0.87\ S_i \tag{16}$$

in milligrams calcium per day. Similar findings for humans were also reported by Schwartz *et al.* (1965) and Phang *et al.* (1969).

Even though v_{o-} clearly plays a much larger regulatory role than does v_{o+} in overcoming the disturbance to calcium homeostasis represented by an increase in steady state calcium input from the gut, no data are available on the response of v_{o-} (or its acute signal equivalent) to acute variations in bone calcium inflow. Phenomenologically, we do not know whether the v_{o-} response is the result of a single or of several processes and whether one or more are saturable and therefore presumably regulatable. Indeed the nature of v_{o-} (or v_{o+}) is not understood. Although by definition v_{o-} represents a unidirectional loss of calcium from bone into the circulation, it is not known whether this calcium originates only from enzymatically directed bone destruction or whether it comprises also calcium that has remained in the fluid phase. If bone resorption involves the release and/or activation of exoenzymes (as by extrusion of lysosomal enzymes; Vaes, 1966), then increased inflow of calcium into the bone compartment might inhibit enzyme release and/or activation. However, such a response might be initiated less rapidly than changes in calcium flows that do not involve a change in phase. As bone cell cultures become available, studies to elucidate these problems can be undertaken.

From the viewpoint of regulation, it is interesting that nearly total regulation by the skeleton is effected via v_{o-}. The simplest situation to imagine is one where v_{o+} would have varied directly and proportionately with input (e.g., S_i); indeed, when this was not found by early investigators, the nature of the measurement was questioned. Another intuitively simple regulatory possibility is that v_{o+} and v_{o-} vary symmetrically and in opposite direction. This is what early rat studies suggested (Aubert *et al.*, 1961). However, subsequent rat studies (Bronner and Aubert, 1965; Sammon *et al.*, 1969, 1970) have shown that in rats fed ample protein and vitamin D, i.e., in rats growing rapidly and probably at a maximum rate, major regulation is exerted by v_{o-}, and the regulatory role of v_{o+} becomes negligible. If, therefore, the optimum situation is represented by relationships such that $v_{o+} = a - bS_i$ and $v_{o-} = a - (1-b)\,S_i$, with $b \simeq 0.1$, it is not surprising that any alteration of the calcium metabolism of the organism will lead

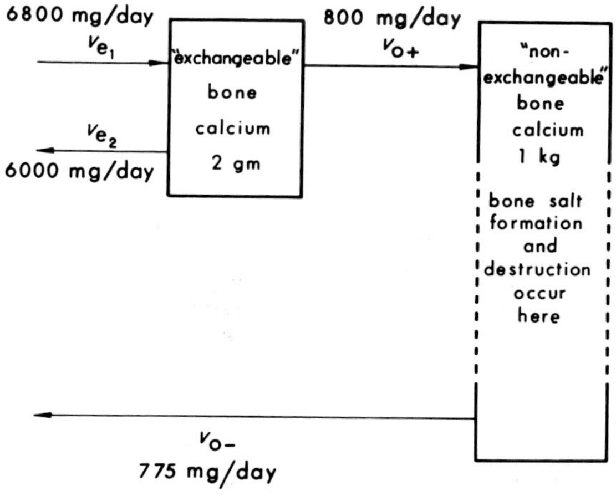

Fig. 5. Symbolic model of calcium movement in the skeleton. The symbol *v* refers to an average rate, milligrams of calcium per day, and the subscripts define the rates as follows: v_{e_1}: rate of calcium movement into bone; v_{o+}: rate of calcium deposition in bone, where deposition implies a sojourn time greater than the period of observation. Normally the period of observation is on the order of days, whereas sojourn times associated with deposition are of the order of weeks, months, years, or even lifetimes. v_{e_2}: the rate of movement of calcium out of the skeleton with sojourn times on the order of days or less. v_{o-}: the rate of calcium resorption, where resorption implies a sojourn time of weeks or more. The model shows a return of calcium removed by v_{o-} directly into plasma or ECF. Regulation involves only v_{o+} and v_{o-}. To the extent that the body stores calcium only in the nonexchangeable bone calcium, the calcium balance of bone equals that of the whole organism. The numbers are typical of a young male adult. (From Bronner, 1973b, by permission.)

to an increase in the numerical value of *b* and a corresponding decrease in the regulatory role by v_{o-}. No systematic studies have been published that have attempted to relate changes in *b* to nutritional or physiological conditions. Such studies could provide useful insights into the modulation of calcium metabolism from a regulatory viewpoint. A symbolic model of calcium flows into and out of bone is shown in Fig. 5.

5. *Organs Other Than Intestine, Kidney, or Bone*

Some organ-related processes such as lactation can serve to disturb plasma calcium. Indeed, reproductive events like pregnancy, giving birth, and lactation all represent severe challenges to the calcium metabolism of the mother. It is obvious that calcium that has crossed the placenta and become incorporated in the fetus or calcium that is excreted in the milk is lost to the mother, with calcium loss through lactation quantitatively much more important than calcium deposited in the fetus (Payne, 1970). With adequate intake, enough dietary calcium can be diverted to these processes that the drain on the mother's endogenous calcium is minimized and plasma calcium can be maintained. In rats, only about 10–15% of the calcium in the mother's milk or the skeleton of the offspring is derived from the body stores of the mother, while the remainder is dietary in origin (Bronner, 1960).

Pregnant dairy cows are known to develop hypocalcemia when beginning to lactate, a condition known as parturient hypocalcemia. When the hypocalcemia is low enough to lead to symptoms, the condition is termed parturient paresis or milk fever. Payne (1970) has discussed some of the factors thought to predispose to milk fever, i.e., high milk yield, age, inappetance, high calcium diets, and perhaps stress and exercise. However, actual causes are not known.

Ramberg *et al.* (1970a) did a combined balance and radiokinetic analysis of cows before and after calving and found that the major initial effect of lactation was a decrease in v_{o+}, in Δ, a small decrease in v_{o-}, and a marked increase in v_a and absorption efficiency. Indeed, the increase in total calcium turnover was almost totally accounted for by an increase in v_a, most of which found its way into the milk. Thus it was the gastrointestinal tract that responded to the increased body need for calcium. Bone calcium removal, v_{o-}, did not rise significantly until 2–3 weeks postpartum. These observations extend and complement the observations on the rat and indicate that in both cows and rats on normal calcium intakes milk calcium, at least in the first 2–3 weeks postpartum, is largely derived from dietary calcium. As lactation proceeds in the cow, intestinal absorption drops and there occurs a corresponding increase in bone calcium turnover, mostly accounted for by an increase in v_{o-} (Ramburg *et al.*, 1970b).

The effect on plasma calcium maintenance of the added disturbance represented by the drain of lactational calcium is relatively complicated. In the cow and probably most mammals the mammary gland very efficiently transfers calcium from the plasma to the milk. Plasma calcium can therefore be maintained only if net intestinal input is increased and/or net calcium input into the skeleton and/or net renal loss is reduced. The work by Ramberg and colleagues (1970a,b) indicates that the cow maintained on a low calcium intake before calving more readily adapts to the calcium stress of lactation than the cow on a high calcium diet. The onset of lactation leads to a significant rise in calcium absorptive efficiency, but this response may be delayed by 24 hours. Modern dairy cows, bred to produce maximum amounts of milk, are in negative calcium balance in early lactation. In other words, they lose skeletal calcium, at least in the early period. When pregnant cows on a high calcium intake give birth and start giving milk, even a marked rise in the total calcium absorbed may be insufficient to balance the efficient transfer of calcium from plasma to milk and their ability to cause increased skeletal turnover is delayed by about two weeks. They therefore develop hypocalcemia. Pregnant cows on a low calcium diet, on the other hand, receive so little dietary calcium, relatively speaking, that they must rely on skeletal calcium to maintain plasma calcium even before the onset of lactation. Therefore their ability to adapt to the sudden onset of lactational calcium drain does not seem impaired.

Details of the mechanisms by which the onset of lactation leads to increased calcium absorption and turnover and by which calcium flows within the body pool are altered are not known.

IV. CALCIUM-REGULATING HORMONES

1. General

Regulation depends on the transmission of information. Within biological systems, information is largely chemical, i.e., molecular in nature. Information regarding physical changes involving heat, light, or a change in field is generally transformed into chemical information that is then propagated within the system. Information flow is of two types: flow of mass, as of calcium circulating in the blood to which organs like kidney or bone respond by excretion or deposition, and flow of specific messenger molecules, such as parathyroid hormone. As organisms evolved, specific messengers must have been developed to effect more rapid changes than brought about solely by changes in flow. In turn the development of specific messengers also opened up the possibility of modulating the nature of the change. However, communication can and does occur in the absence of specific messengers. For this reason, calcium metabolism continues to be regulated in the parathyroidectomized animal, though less efficiently.

Messenger molecules, particularly in the case of steroids, are associated with carriers that help deliver the messenger to target organs. These may be specific, as in the vitamin D-binding protein (Bouillon and Van Baden, 1979; Van Baden *et al.*, 1980) which, by binding the biologically active metabolite with a lower affinity than the precursor(s), may also contribute to regulating the supply of active metabolites when vitamin D input varies.

How messenger molecules interact with their target cells and cause them to respond is one of the most active fields of investigation. Of the three major calcium-regulating hormones, parathyroid hormone and calcitonin are polypeptides that interact with specific membrane receptors and elicit a response that is mediated by the adenyl cyclase system. 1,25-Dihydroxyvitamin D_3, the most active metabolite of vitamin D, interacts with a cellular receptor in the intestinal cell to induce synthesis of the calcium-binding protein by a transcriptional route (Norman, 1979), though a posttranscriptional route has also been postulated (Buckley and Bronner, 1980). For none of these three hormones, however, is it known how the responses become transformed into changed calcium flows. Parathyroid hormone acts on bone cells that in turn are stimulated to modify their extracellular milieu, i.e., bone, presumably by the release of lysosomal enzymes (Vaes, 1966). Enzymatic action would then cause calcium and phosphate to be released into the circulation. Parathyroid hormone may also have a direct effect on the calcium flux of bone cells (Bronner *et al.*, 1978), but this changed flux probably plays but a minor role in the altered calcium flow from bone that results from the action of parathyroid hormone. In the case of vitamin D, on the other hand, interaction with the target cell probably affects cellular calcium transport directly (Freund and Bronner, 1975b; Bronner *et al.*, 1976a), which, at least in the case of the duodenal cell, markedly alters the proportion of calcium translocated actively. Molecular details of the vitamin-D-stimulatable calcium transport process are not known.

While vitamin D and parathyroid hormone differ in terms of the mechanisms by which they effect changes in calcium flows—one acting at the cell membrane via the adenylate cyclase system, the other probably acting via protein synthetic mechanisms—differences also reside in the nature of calcium flow in the different regulatory systems. In the intestine and kidney, calcium flows through the two organs that regulate this flow. In bone, calcium is deposited and much becomes highly insoluble (Fig. 5). Thus in bone, calcium flow is either followed or preceded by a change in phase (from solid to liquid or vice versa) and the cells of that organ exert their major control at the point of solubilization. It is generally accepted that parathyroid hormone acts at that point, perhaps via lysosomal enzymes, but how and whether vitamin D acts at that control point is unclear. In turn, it is generally accepted that vitamin D acts to increase calcium absorption by a mechanism that enhances active transport in the duodenum, but whether and how parathyroid hormone acts in the intestinal cell is moot. Finally, parathyroid hormone is known to act and vitamin D may act to increase renal tubular calcium reabsorption (see Chapters 6 and 7, this volume), but sites of action and mechanisms may well differ.

In what follows, details of how these agents modify calcium metabolism will be discussed from a regulatory viewpoint.

2. *Parathyroid Hormone*

Parathyroidectomy has several effects on plasma calcium: There is a drop in the steady-state reference level [U] from 2.5 m*M* to about 1.5 m*M*, and the precision with which [Ca_s] is maintained around [U] is lower (Hausmann and Riggs, 1966; Sammon *et al.*, 1970). Moreover, the exponential rate of return to the steady-state value is slower in parathyroidectomized animals (Hausmann and Riggs, 1966; Sammon *et al.*, 1970). This is illustrated by the experiments of Grubb *et al.* (1977), who maintained rats without food for 21 hr and found that in thyroparathroidectomized (TPTX) animals [Ca_s] dropped 35%, from 7.4 to 4.8 mg/dl in the last 13 hr, while in the euparathyroid animals [Ca_s] had dropped less than 5% from a base value of 10.8 mg/dl. The percent standard error in the TPTX animals also was twice that in the intact rats. Sammon *et al.* (1970) found that when PTX rats received an intraperitoneal load of calcium, the overshoot in [Ca_s] produced by the load was corrected in about 3 hr, whereas the correction took only 2 hr in euparathyroid animals (see Fig. 10). Thus, parathyroid hormone improves the efficiency and accuracy of plasma calcium regulation, permitting positive and negative errors to be overcome more readily and minimizing the extent of these errors.

How then are the systems regulating calcium homeostasis modified by parathyroid hormone?

a. Bone As already discussed, the major regulator of plasma calcium is bone. Parathyroidectomy can therefore be expected to have a major effect on bone calcium deposition and removal. In growing rats, parathyroidectomy was found (Sammon *et al.*, 1970) to depress bone turnover by about half and to alter the regulatory relationship between v_{o+} and v_{o-}, leading to a somewhat greater role for v_{o+} and depressing the regulatory importance of v_{o-}. This is illustrated by comparing Eqs. (12) and (16), derived for euparathyroid animals:

$$v_{o+} = 67.2 + 0.11\ S_i \tag{12}$$

$$v_{o-} = 67.5 - 0.87\ S_i \tag{16}$$

with Eqs. (17) and (18) derived for PTX rats:

$$v_{o+} = 36.5 + 0.29\ S_i \tag{17}$$

$$v_{o-} = 36.9 - 0.69\ S_i \quad \text{(units: mg Ca/day)} \tag{18}$$

Ramberg *et al.* (1976) have shown that total calcium inflow ($v_T = v_{o+} + v_u + v_a$) in the cow is directly proportional to the PTH level:

$$v_T = 3.3 + 5.3 \text{ PTH} \tag{19}$$

in which v_T is in grams calcium per day, and PTH is in nanograms per milliliter.

In other words, the steady-state circulating level of PTH in adult cows determines in large part the intensity of calcium turnover in the body. Equation (19) therefore provides independent experimental confirmation for the difference in the baseline levels of v_{o+} and v_{o-} between normal and PTX rats [Eqs. (12) and (16) versus Eqs. (17) and (18)].

In addition to the quantitative difference due to PTH, Eqs. (12), (16), (17), and (18) also indicate a qualitative difference, since in the euparathyroid animal v_{o-} accounts for 0.87 S_i, i.e., for nearly 90% of the disturbing signal, while in the PTX rat, v_{o-} overcomes only 0.69 S_i; in other words, v_{o-} in the PTX animals is only 80% as effective as in the normal animal. On the other hand, v_{o+} handles a larger proportion of the disturbing signal in the PTX as compared to the euparathyroid rat.

No detailed model has been proposed of how parathyroid hormone acts on bone so as to increase bone calcium turnover and to alter the regulatory importance of v_{o-} with respect to v_{o+}. Parathyroid hormone is known to act via the adenyl cyclase system and appears to alter the release and/or activation of exoenzymes via extrusion of lysosomes (Vaes, 1966), but whether and how the hormone acts directly on v_{o+}, i.e., on the rate of calcium incorporation in the extracellular phase, is not known. Moreover, at the mechanistic level no distinction has been made between long-term hormonal effects that may involve alterations in the number and proportion of the various bone cells (osteoblasts, osteoclasts, and osteocytes) and acute effects, more likely to be expressed in terms of relative enzymatic and cellular activities. Until cultured bone cells have been studied in detail and mechanisms of bone formation and resorption are better understood, a symbolic model as shown in Fig. 5 can be based only on available whole animal data.

b. Kidney The effect of PTH on urinary calcium handling and the regulatory role played by the kidney is much less clear. To be sure, hyperparathyroidism is associated with hypercalciuria and hypoparathyroidism with hypocalciuria. In regulatory terms, however, it is unclear how parathyroid hormone alters the relationship between the disturbing signal, net calcium absorption, S_i, and the controlling signal, urinary calcium output, v_u.

Sammon *et al.* (1970) have studied this in normal (N) and PTX rats and found virtually no difference in the relationship between v_u and S_i in the two states, i.e.,

$$v_u = 0.30 + 0.02\ S_i \qquad \text{(N)} \tag{20}$$

$$v_u = 0.36 + 0.02\ S_i \qquad \text{(PTX)} \tag{21}$$

in milligrams calcium per day.

Equations (20) and (21) indicate that the proportion of the disturbing signal handled by the urinary calcium output was the same in the normal and ablated animals. Moreover, the base level of urinary calcium output was statistically the same in the two groups. However, the proportion of urinary calcium to total calcium flow, i.e., v_u/v_T, was much greater in the PTX than in the normal animals (0.99% versus 0.44%), undoubtedly reflecting the calcium conserving action of PTH in the kidney. Furthermore, while the PTX animal handled the same low proportion of the disturbing signal via the kidney as did the normal animal, it is not known whether the proportion of constituent signals is altered in the PTX state. When one expresses the effect of parathyroidectomy on total bone handling by combining Eqs. (12) and (16) and Eqs. (17) and (18), one obtains

$$\Delta = v_{o+} - v_{o-} = -0.3 + 0.98\ S_i \qquad \text{(N)} \tag{22}$$

$$\Delta = v_{o+} - v_{o-} = -0.4 + 0.98\ S_i \qquad \text{(PTX)} \tag{23}$$

Equations (22) and (23) are comparable to Eqs. (20) and (21) and imply no effect of parathyroidectomy on the overall regulatory role of bone, whereas a significant effect is revealed when the constituent signals are analyzed separately. Until this is done also for the renal handling of calcium, no firm quantitative statements can be made as to how parathyroid hormone acts on kidney regulation of calcium homeostasis. As already pointed out, the regulatory importance of renal calcium handling differs with age and species.

c. Intestine From the viewpoint of plasma calcium regulation, net intestinal calcium absorption, S_i, is treated as the disturbing signal (Fig. 1). For this reason an effect of PTH on calcium absorption would not be reflected in the analysis of homeostasis which examines the result of a given signal on regulation, i.e., on how the disturbing signal is overcome by the two regulatory organs, bone and kidney. Of course it is of interest to know whether the parathyroprivic state is associated with lower intensity of the disturbing signal and whether this is due to a change in true calcium absorption, v_a, and/or in endogenous fecal output, v_{ndo}. Sammon *et al.* (1970) found that in PTX rats, both S_i and v_a were lower at intakes above, but not below 80 mg/day. Differences in v_{ndo} were negligible. Although no data are available on the effect of parathyroidectomy on the saturable and nonsaturable components of calcium absorption, the decrease in v_a that becomes evident at high calcium intakes could be brought about by a decrease in the saturable component. Current data (reviewed by Haussler *et al.*,

1977; Norman, 1979) indicate that parathyroidectomy is associated with lowered $1{,}25(OH)_2D_3$ levels and probably also with lowered calcium-binding protein levels in the duodenum (Thomasset *et al.*, 1979). Conceivably, therefore, the saturable component is depressed in the parathyroprivic organism, perhaps because less vitamin D metabolite is produced in such an individual. It is interesting that in the parathyroprivic state the decreased ability to overcome positive or negative errors in plasma calcium regulation is associated with a lower intensity disturbing signal.

d. Regulatory Aspects of Parathyroid Hormone Action What is the nature of parathyroid control? Aubert and Bronner (1965) have proposed that the presence of parathyroid hormone can be likened to the addition of an integral to a proportional control in man-made linear control systems. In this model plasma calcium homeostasis in the thyroparathyroidectomized animals is considered to be a proportional control system, i.e., the control is proportional to the error ϵ defined as the difference between steady-state plasma calcium in the absence and presence of a load

$$\epsilon = [Ca_s] - [U] \tag{24}$$

in milligrams calcium per deciliter.

In PTX animals the error is proportional to the steady-state calcium load and is reduced in euparathyroid animals due to the action of parathyroid hormone. The maximum error, $S_{\epsilon(max)}$ can then be defined as

$$S_{\epsilon(max)} = [Ca_s]_{\lim \to S_i} - [U] \tag{25}$$

$S_{\epsilon(max)}$ therefore represents the difference between the value the plasma calcium reaches with a maximum net intestinal load and the reference value around which plasma calcium is regulated in the absence of a load. Accordingly, the expression for $S_{\epsilon(max)}$ in the parathyroidectomized and euparathyroid states can be written as

$$S_{\epsilon(max)} = \frac{S_i}{K} \qquad \text{(PTX)} \tag{26}$$

$$S_{\epsilon(max)} = \frac{S_i}{K'} \, \frac{[L] - [U]}{[L] - \beta[U]} \tag{27}$$

where K and K' are proportionality constants and β is a coefficient less than 1. [L] is the plasma calcium concentration when parathyroid hormone release ceases or is at a minimum.

Sammon *et al.* (1970) have shown that in growing male rats plasma calcium varies with net calcium absorption, S_i, as follows:

$$[Ca_s] = 6.02 + 0.021\, S_i \qquad \text{(PTX)} \tag{28}$$

$$[Ca_s] = 10.80 + 0.0021\ S_i \qquad (N) \tag{29}$$

where $[Ca_s]$ is in milligrams calcium per deciliter, and S_i is in milligrams calcium per day.

In terms of Eq. (24), the value of [U] for normal animals therefore is 10.8. $S_{\epsilon(max)}$ in PTX animals can be set by equal to 0.021 S_i and $S_{\epsilon(max)}$ in normal animals would then be one-tenth smaller for a given load. If we assume that K $\simeq$ K′ in Eqs. (26) and (27), then ([L] − [U])/([L] − β [U]) would equal 0.1. Substitution of the experimental values for PTX animals from Sammon *et al.* (1970) in the appropriate equations of Aubert and Bronner (1965) yields a numerical value of $\beta = 0.36$ and [L] would equal 11.6 mg/dl, a value consistent with that reported by Bronner *et al.* (1976b) who measured the immunoreactive PTH level in similar rats at various $[Ca_s]$ levels.

The diminution of the plasma calcium error due to the action of parathyroid hormone must largely be due to the differential effect of parathyroid hormone on bone. In the PTX animal, the bone response to a steady state load is $v_{o+} = 0.3\ S_i$ and $v_{o-} = 0.7\ S_i$ [Eqs. (17) and (18)]. If, as a first approximation, it is assumed that the renal contribution to plasma calcium regulation is negligible, then in accordance with Aubert and Bronner (1965) and on the assumption that mass and signals behave equivalently one can write

$$v_{o+} = 0.3\ K\ [Ca_s] \tag{30}$$

$$v_{o-} = 0.7\ K\ (2\beta[U] - [Ca_s]) \tag{31}$$

Substitution in the equations of the mean values reported for PTX animals by Sammon *et al.* (1970) yields a value for K of approximately 2.3 liter/day.

Since the presence of parathyroid hormone reduces the regulatory importance of v_{o+} and increases that of v_{o-} [compare Eq. (12) with Eq. (17) and Eq. (16) with Eq. (18)], one should be able to write for euparathyroid rats that:

$$v_{o+} = 0.3\ K'\ [Ca_s] - 0.1\ K_3[H] \tag{32}$$

$$v_{o-} = 0.7\ K'\ (2\beta[U] - [Ca_s] + 0.9\ K_3[H]) \tag{33}$$

where [H] refers to the level of circulating parathyroid hormone and K_3 is a proportionally constant. K′ is a constant like K and as a first approximation may be considered equal to it. If, as in the cow (Ramberg *et al.*, 1976), v_{o+} does not respond at all to an increased load, then the term relating to the parathyroid hormone level, K[H], would appear only in Eq. (33) or its equivalent. When data on rat parathyroid hormone levels become available, it will be possible to evaluate the equations and to determine their validity. Numerical predictions made so far seem reasonable.

The regulatory diagram shown in Fig. 6 is based on the above considerations. In the model, calcium input from the intestine, in the form of S_i, will tend to raise plasma calcium. The circle is a comparator in which plasma calcium is compared with a set value, [U]. The error, i.e., the difference between [Ca_s] and [U], acts directly on the two regulators, bone and kidney, causing changes in the constituent signals, v_{o+} and v_{o-} in bone, and $v_{fi} + v_s$ and v_r in the kidney. If the error is negative, i.e., [Ca_s] < [U], as might occur in the absence of a positive input from the intestine, v_{o-} would increase, v_{o+} would decrease a little and, in the kidney, v_r would increase. The net effect would be a decrease in the bone calcium balance, Δ, and in v_u, the urinary calcium output. A negative error would also cause release of parathyroid hormone which would act on bone so as to further increase v_{o-} in accordance with Eq. (33) and decrease v_{o+} in accordance with Eq. (32). Parathyroid hormone would act in the kidney, presumably to increase v_r (or at least the saturable component of v_r), but, as suggested above, not enough is known to permit writing even a tentative equation.

In the diagram, the plus, minus, and zero symbols are used to indicate direction of flow. For example, v_{o-} is positive with respect to plasma and negative with respect to bone. A positive error does not, however, necessarily provoke a positive signal or flow. On the contrary, the direction of flow may be opposite to the sign of the error.

The model necessarily contains formulations for which there is as yet no direct experimental evidence. For example, although comparators are known in physiology (pressure- or volume-sensitive receptors), no plasma calcium comparator is known to exist, nor need it exist as a direct cellular aggregate. Instead one can imagine a molecular mechanism, such as a conformational change in a widespread calcium-sensitive membrane-bound protein molecule, that could serve as a comparator. In recent years cytosolic and now membrane-bound calcium-binding proteins have been described (Siegel *et al.*, 1980), some of which may ultimately come to be recognized as fulfilling the role of a comparator.

One could also object to the model as being too simple or propose a model that does not respond to an error, but to a specific signal like [Ca_s].

Aubert and Bronner (1965) have proposed that the functioning of the parathyroid control can be likened to the presence of an integral error correction, added to the proportional error correction system represented by bone and kidney. The suggestion is based on the virtual absence of an error in plasma calcium in the euparathyroid animal [cf. Eq. (29)] and the greater efficiency achieved by an integral control, as compared with that achieved by the addition of a second proportional control. For example, it is difficult to adjust the error correction in two concerted proportional control systems so as to avoid over- or undershoots. The absence of over- or undershoots in the plasma calcium correction system of normal rats (Bronner *et al.*, 1968) is consistent with, but constitutes no proof for, an integral control. Evidence that parathyroid hormone exerts an integral control over plasma calcium could come from experiments in which plasma calcium is raised in stepwise fashion and the systemic release of parathyroid hormone is

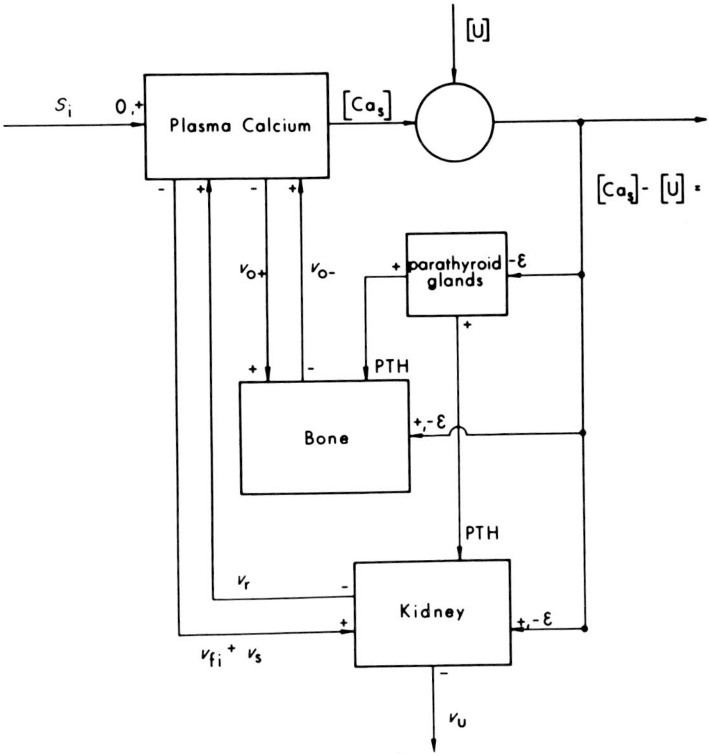

Fig. 6. Regulatory scheme of plasma calcium regulation with parathyroid hormone (PTH) control only. Other hormonal controls omitted. S_i is the net amount of calcium that enters from the intestine and disturbs the steady-state plasma calcium, whose concentration [Ca_s], is compared with [U], the plasma calcium reference value. The plasma calcium error, $\epsilon = [Ca_s] - [U]$, activates the two controlling systems, kidney and bone, in a proportional manner. A positive error leads to an increase in v_u, effected mostly by a decrease in v_r and perhaps an increase in v_s. A negative error leads to an increase in v_r, perhaps a decrease in v_s and a decrease in v_u. In bone, a positive error leads mostly to a decrease in v_{o-} and a modest increase in v_{o+}; as a result the net bone signal, $\Delta = v_{o+} - v_{o-}$, increases. A negative error leads to a marked increase in v_{o-} and a modest decrease in v_{o+} resulting in a decrease in Δ. A negative error also stimulates the release of PTH. The hormone acts in kidney and bone so as to magnify their response to a negative error, i.e., v_u and Δ are further decreased. The plus, minus, and zero signs indicate direction of flow. For example, v_{o-} brings calcium from bone to plasma. For further quantitative description and explanation of symbols, see text. (From Bronner, 1973b, by permission.)

measured. The major advantage of the model shown in Fig. 6 is that it can be tested experimentally. When that is done, a more refined model will undoubtedly emerge.

One problem that has not yet been dealt with is how parathyroid hormone causes the various parameters of calcium metabolism to assume higher base levels, e.g., for $[Ca_s]$ to rise from 6.0 to 10.8 mg/dl or for v_{o+} to increase from 37 to 67 mg Ca/day. Perhaps a future model will account for this as well.

3. *Calcitonin*

Calcitonin is a polypeptide, MW $\simeq$ 3600 daltons, secreted by the parafollicular cells of the thyroid gland. These cells arise from the ultimobranchial glands which retain their identity in the lower vertebrates, but migrate to become part of the thyroid gland in mammals. The cells, also known as C ("clear") cells because of their differential staining characteristics, are mesothelial in origin and respond to gastrin or pentagastrin, powerful secretagogues. Injection of calcitonin produces transient hypocalcemia in mammals, but not in the lower vertebrates (Clark and Wideman, 1980), even when the latter receive homologous calcitonin (Clark, 1968).

Interestingly, an infusion of two international units calcitonin per hour produced a mild hypocalcemia in parathyroidectomized starlings, but a larger dose was without effect (Clark and Wideman, 1980).

Because calcitonin produces hypocalcemia, it was thought to play a role in calcium metabolism analogous to, but opposite in direction to, parathyroid hormone. However, calcitoninectomy has been shown to have virtually no effects on the steady-state parameters of calcium metabolism (Bronner *et al.*, 1967; Sammon *et al.*, 1969). Thus calcitoninectomized (CX) animals have plasma calcium levels that do not differ significantly from appropriate controls (C) at all calcium intake levels studied (Sammon *et al.*, 1969). The response of net and constituent signals to the disturbing signal, S_i, also does not differ in the ablated from that in the control animals. Bone calcium deposition (v_{o+}) and removal rates (v_{o-}) were the same in CX and control animals and urinary calcium output also was unchanged as a result of calcitoninectomy.

The major difference in plasma calcium homeostasis between the normal and calcitoninectomized animal is that the latter takes longer to overcome a positive error. In other words, when calcitoninectomized rats were given an interperitoneal injection of calcium (as the gluconate), it took 3 hr before the plasma calcium returned to the preinjection level, whereas it took only 2 hr in control animals (Sammon *et al.*, 1969; see Fig. 10). In the rat, there were no differences in either the preinjection or peak plasma calcium levels of the control and calcitoninectomized animals (Bronner *et al.*, 1968; Sammon *et al.*, 1969) and only the rate of return differed. In man, on the other hand, peak levels and $\Delta[Ca_s]$ have been reported as higher (Coen and Palagi, 1976); the rate of return to the preinjection value was slower, as in lower mammals.

Recent studies (Austin *et al.*, 1979) have shown that oral calcium loads in 10 healthy young adults led to a rise in immunoreactive calcitonin. This rise reached a maximum at 2–3 hr after the meal and was proportional to the rise in plasma calcium. Immunoreactive gastrin also responded in a dose-like fashion; that response was pulse-like and completed when plasma calcium and calcitonin were still rising. Earlier work by the same group (Owyang *et al.*, 1978) had shown that ingestion of a mixed meal that led to a marked stimulation in gastrin secretion without raising serum calcium, had no effect on immunoreactive calcitonin levels. The authors therefore conclude that calcium rather than gastrin is the normal secretagogue for calcitonin.

Later work by Freed *et al.* (1979) suggests that calcitonin inhibits feeding by acting directly on the central nervous system. It is conceivable that the release of calcitonin is triggered by gastrin or pentagastrin as also suggested by Talmage *et al.* (1975b); on the other hand, the time course of calcitonin response was relatively slow in the experiments by Freed *et al.* (1979).

Just as the total absence of calcitonin has been shown to have little effect on the steady-state parameters of calcium metabolism (Sammon *et al.*, 1969), so large excess of circulating calcitonin, as characteristic of medullary carcinoma of the thyroid, seems also to be without a demonstrable effect on the calcium metabolism of these patients (Melvin *et al.*, 1973).

The only demonstrable effect of the lack of calcitonin on calcium metabolism remains faster error correction.

Norimatsu *et al.* (1979) injected small doses of calcitonin into neonatal rats and were able to detect changes in the cells lining the endosteum of the tibia within 5 min of drug administration. The changes included increased numbers of microvilli and surface blebs, cell contraction and enlargement of intracellular channels. Within 15 min the appearance of the cells began returning to normal. The authors interpret these changes as consistent with the possibility that the cells act to store in their microenvironment excess calcium, presumably of dietary origin, which does not become mineralized and is available to maintain plasma calcium during nonfeeding periods. Regardless of mechanism, the rapid bone cell response to calcitonin is consistent with a transient pulse-like calcitonin action in inhibiting bone calcium efflux, as demonstrated in early studies (Milhaud *et al.*, 1965; O'Riordan and Aurbach, 1968).

Detailed studies relating plasma calcitonin appearance in the circulation to plasma calcium changes have not appeared. It is therefore difficult to know whether calcitonin release is proportional only to the positive error, $[Ca_s]$-[U], or, as proposed earlier (Bronner, 1973a,b), also to the derivative of the positive error. The advantage of a derivative error control is that it permits very rapid release of calcitonin when plasma calcium is rising, but can be turned off promptly. There is moreover evidence that the glandular store of calcitonin is large in relation to the amount released and is difficult to deplete (Shah *et al.*, 1968; Bronner *et al.*, 1968). Therefore, the active hormone molecule must be degraded rapidly and its plasma concentration may be described as follows:

$$d[\mathrm{CT}]/dt = k_1\epsilon + k_2 d\epsilon/dt - k_3[\mathrm{CT}] \tag{34}$$

where [CT] is the plasma calcitonin concentration and k_1, k_2, and k_3 are constants such that when the plasma calcium error is large, $k_1\epsilon + k_2 d\epsilon/dt > k_3[C]$, but when the error is small, $k_1\epsilon > k_2 d\epsilon/dt$. The reason for introducing a term proportional to the derivative of the error is that without it it would be difficult to effect a rapid and large increase in circulating bioactive calcitonin without the danger of substantial overshoot.

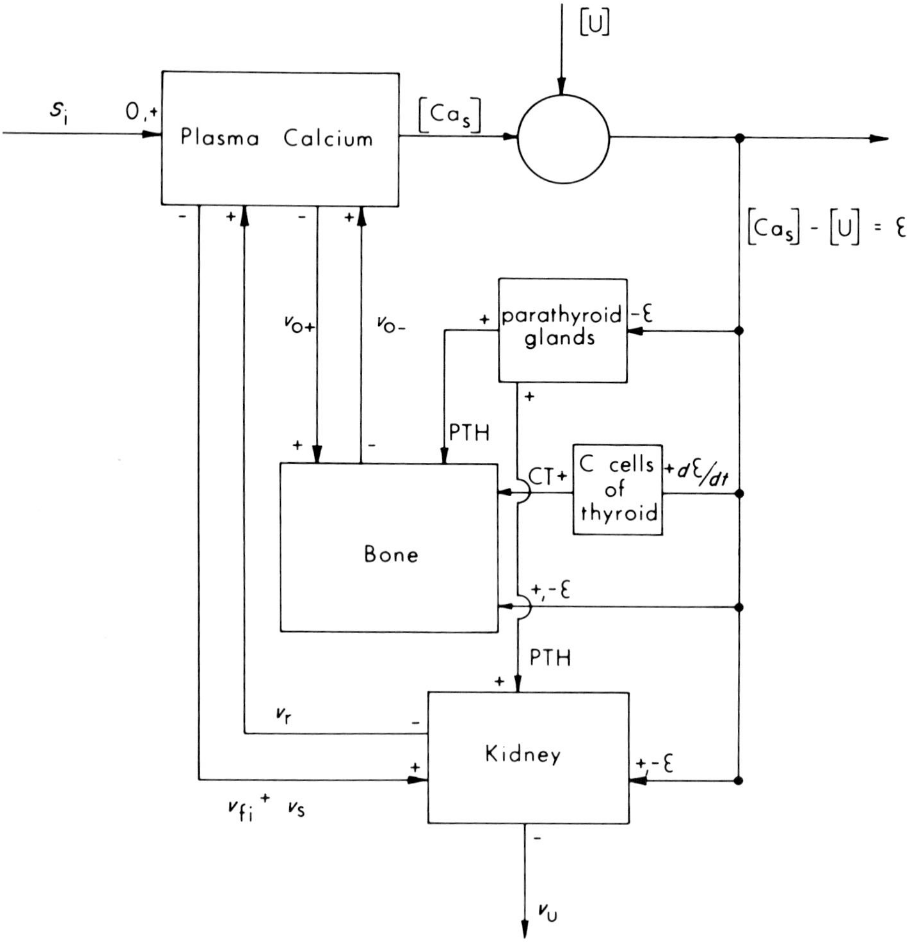

Fig. 7. Regulatory scheme of plasma calcium regulation, with parathyroid hormone (PTH) and calcitonin (CT) control. Other hormonal controls omitted. The system is explained in the legend of Fig. 6. CT is released in response to the positive derivative of the plasma calcium error and transiently magnifies the response of bone to the error by diminishing v_{o-}. However, as explained in the text, there is no steady-state effect on v_{o+} and v_{o-} in the calcitoninectomized animal. For further quantitative description and explanation of symbols, see text. (From Bronner, 1973b, by permission.)

Figure 7 is a regulatory diagram of plasma calcium regulation that includes the derivative control due to calcitonin. It shows that parafollicular cells of the thyroid responding to the plasma calcium error according to Eq. (34) by releasing calcitonin, which is then shown to act only on bone. Calcitonin, like other peptide hormones, acts via the adenylate cyclase system. There is now increasing evidence (Wong and Cohn, 1975) that only specialized and not all bone cells respond to calcitonin stimulation. This differential response is receptor-mediated. The molecular nature of the cellular response is not known; if it involves a transient decrease in calcium flow from the skeleton into the blood, this does not necessarily mean action on calcium in the solid phase. It can simply mean a slowing of the transfer of calcium ions from the bone to the blood compartment. These mechanistic questions are as yet unresolved. If, however, it were to be shown that calcitonin does not act directly by diminishing calcium transfer from the solid to the fluid phase, it may be necessary to indicate bone transfer vectors in the diagram (Fig. 7) other than v_{o+} and v_{o-}.

Even though the model shown in Fig. 7 conforms to what has been learned about the regulatory role of calcitonin, it is not clear what benefit an organism derives from faster correction of the plasma calcium error. Freed *et al.* (1979) speculate that the release of endogenous calcitonin could subsequently bring about diminished feeding activity and thereby contribute to appetite regulation. If so, this would occur only if the initial meal had some hypercalcemic effect. In the study by Austin *et al.* (1979) ingestion of 0.5 gm calcium as the gluconate after an overnight fast raised plasma calcium in volunteers by 0.2 mg/dl and calcitonin by 5 pg/ml. Freed *et al.* (1979) report that subcutaneous injection of 2 units/kg calcitonin, which for a 70-kg person would correspond to a maximum plasma calcitonin increase of 24 pg/ml, caused a significant reduction in body weight 24–36 hr later. Even if it were shown that stimulation of calcitonin release as occurs when animals are fed on high calcium diets helps keep their body weight down,[6] one wonders what benefit is conferred by the faster correction of the plasma calcium error when calcitonin is released.

4. *Vitamin D*

Simple vitamin D deficiency leads to a drop in the steady-state plasma calcium reference level, [U], from 2.5 m*M* to about 1.5 m*M*, and to a decrease in the precision with which [Ca_s] is maintained around [U] (Hurwitz *et al.*, 1969). Indeed, from the viewpoint of steady-state regulation of plasma calcium, the vitamin D-deficient rat behaves very much like a parathyroidectomized animal. Yet vitamin D deficiency in the presence of an adequate mineral intake leads to elevated parathyroid hormone levels (Bronner *et al.*, 1976b). Since, moreover,

[6]In this writer's experience, Sprague-Dawley rats fed on semi-synthetic diets containing 1.5% Ca and 1.5% P tend to weigh somewhat less than comparable animals fed on the same diet but containing 0.5% Ca and 0.5% P.

vitamin D-deficient animals exhibit a limited or no hypercalcemic response when treated with exogenous parathyroid hormone, it was suggested some time ago that vitamin D is needed for full expression of parathyroid hormone activity (Harrison, 1966). No relevant experiments have been published, however, to indicate whether vitamin D deficiency and parathyroid deficiency are quatitatively equivalent in terms of their effect on steady-state plasma calcium regulation.

Because of the similarity in response by parathyroidectomized and vitamin D-deficient animals to a steady-state calcium load from the intestine, one would predict that the ability of vitamin D-deficient organisms to overcome an intraperitoneally administered calcium load would also be delayed. Such data are unavailable. Whether the ability of vitamin D-deficient animals to regulate plasma calcium acutely is impaired therefore is not known.

Vitamin D deficiency diminishes the ability of the kidney to reabsorb calcium. In regulatory terms, therefore, the kidney plays a somewhat larger role in overcoming a disturbing signal in the deficient as compared to the replete[7] organism. This is brought out in Fig. 8 which shows that the relative urinary calcium clearance is greater in vitamin D deficiency, whether or not accompanied by phosphorus deficiency. Since vitamin D deficiency diminishes intestinal calcium absorption, the absolute output of urinary calcium is lower than in the replete animal, but the regulatory role of vitamin D can be evaluated by equalizing S_i and correcting for differences in the plasma calcium pool (see legend, Fig. 8).

Lack of vitamin D, since it alters the regulatory importance of the kidney, is likely also to have such an effect on bone.

Analysis of the regulatory role played by v_{o+} and v_{o-} shows [Eqs. (35–38)] that in vitamin D deficiency a larger proportion of the disturbing signal is handled by v_{o+} and a smaller proportion by v_{o-}:

$$\left.\begin{aligned} v_{o+} &= 50.5 + 0.29\, S_i \quad (35) \\ v_{o-} &= 50.1 - 0.68\, S_i \quad (36) \end{aligned}\right\} +\mathrm{D}$$

$$\left.\begin{aligned} v_{o+} &= 32 + 0.50\, S_i \quad (37) \\ v_{o-} &= 32 - 0.49\, S_i \quad (38) \end{aligned}\right\} -\mathrm{D}$$

in milligrams calcium per day.

[7]The term "vitamin D-replete" is used to designate organisms that have a nutritionally adequate intake of vitamin D. For the rat, this amounts to 2200 IU vitamin D_2 per kg dry diet, equivalent to a daily intake of 33–44 IU or 0.8 to 1.2 μg. Where milk is fortified with 400 IU (=10μg)/quart, as in the United States, typical human intakes are 5–10 μg/day. The term "repleted" refers to organisms that had been experimentally depleted of vitamin D and then restored to a normal intake. A "replete" animal, on the other hand, has never been deprived of its vitamin D supply.

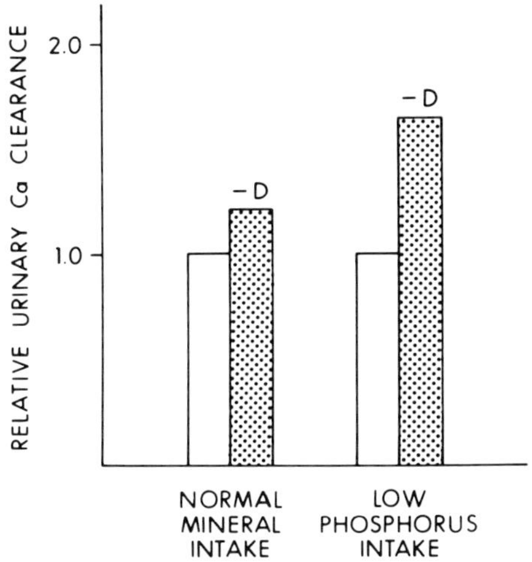

Fig. 8. The effect of vitamin D deficiency on the relative urinary calcium clearance. The urinary calcium output, v_u, was calculated from the experimentally determined relationship between v_u and S_i [as in Eq. (1)] in each of the four groups, i.e., control, D-deficient, P-deficient, and P- plus D-deficient. The clearance was then estimated by dividing v_u by the plasma calcium pool. The values (per day) were

Normal mineral intake		Low phosphorus intake	
+D	−D	+D	−D
0.33	0.40	15.4	25.2

Note that the absolute values were much higher in the low phosphorus group. To obtain the relative clearance, shown in the ordinate, the values of the −D groups were divided by the respective +D values. (From Bronner, 1979, by permission).

These equations, previously unpublished, were derived for one group of replete and deficient animals, raised from weaning on a normal mineral intake (0.5% Ca, 0.5% P; Table 3, Hurwitz *et al.*, 1969). They show a near-doubling in the fraction of the disturbing signal, S_i, handled by v_{o+} in the deficient as compared to the replete animal. This increase in the regulatory role of v_{o+} is also typical of parathyroidectomy [cf. Eqs. (17) and (18) with Eqs. (12) and (16)]. However, as pointed out above, all changes in calcium metabolism are likely to lead to a decrease in the relative importance of v_{o-} in overcoming a disturbing signal. Therefore the effect of vitamin D repletion in increasing the regulatory importance of v_{o-} is consistent with, but does not necessarily stem from the reputed "osteolytic" action of vitamin D.

In simple vitamin D deficiency, even if the kidney handles a larger proportion of the disturbing signal than in the replete animal, most of the disturbing signal is still overcome by bone. This can be verified by solving for $\Delta(\equiv v_{o+} - v_{o-})$ in the vitamin D-replete and -deficient situations. In both instances Δ still handles well over 95% of the disturbing signal. The ash content and proximal mineral composition of the long bones also is not much altered in simple vitamin D deficiency (Hurwitz *et al.*, 1969). However when vitamin D deficiency was imposed along with severe phosphate deficiency, the animal, unable to form anything like near-normal bone, appeared also unable to have bone tissue exert its normal regulatory role and less than 20% of the disturbing signal was handled by the skeleton of the doubly deficient rat (Hurwitz *et al.*, 1969). Vitamin D repletion restored to bone its regulatory primacy so that it overcame 84% of the disturbing signal, even though the phosphate content of the diet had remained at 0.14% (Hurwitz *et al.*, 1969). This may have resulted from the markedly improved phosphate absorption. In the vitamin D-replete phosphate-depleted animal net phosphate absorption was ten times greater than in the comparable vitamin D-deficient animal; net calcium absorption, on the other hand, had only doubled, from 11.2 to 23.1 mg/day.

The action of vitamin D has been likened to that of a hormone (Norman, 1979; DeLuca, 1981), inasmuch as the sterol undergoes hydroxylation at the 25-carbon in liver and then at the 1-carbon in the kidney. The 1,25-dihydroxy-vitamin D_3 made in the kidney acts on the kidney, as well as on two more distant target organs, the duodenum and bone. In the kidney $1{,}25(OH)_2D_3$ appears to regulate renal calcium reabsorption (Puschett *et al.*, 1972a,b) but how this is accomplished and whether it involves the renal calcium-binding protein, the synthesis of which is dependent on vitamin D (Hermsdorf and Bronner, 1975) is not known. In the duodenal cell, $1{,}25(OH)_2D_3$ stimulates the synthesis of the calcium-binding and other specific proteins (Freund and Bronner, 1975a,b; Norman, 1979). It also acts on calcium transport, but whether the stimulation of calcium transport involves protein synthesis is controversial. In the bone cell neither the molecular action nor the function of vitamin D is shown. The hydroxylation step in the kidney is closely regulated, with the amount of $1{,}25(OH)_2D_3$ produced inversely related to the plasma calcium concentration (Boyle *et al.*, 1973).

Vitamin D or its biologically active metabolites may therefore intervene in plasma calcium regulation in several ways: Changes in plasma calcium may lead to inverse changes in the 25-hydroxyvitamin D_3-1-hydroxylase activity in the kidney, with low plasma calcium stimulating the enzyme. The enzyme product, $1{,}25(OH)_2D_3$, would then act on the three target organs, kidney, intestine, and bone, so as to cause an increase in plasma calcium. Detailed quantitative studies relating enzyme to product and product to target organ activity have not been published. Parfitt *et al.* (1979) have proposed a model for man in which the hydroxylation of 25-hydroxyvitamin D is related to vitamin D intake; the model does not relate these predictions to plasma calcium. Moreover, since $1{,}25(OH)_2D_3$ acts intracellularly, feedback loops involving calcium and vitamin D-dependent intracellular pathways seem likely. One for which some experimental evidence exists is the inhibition by calcium of full expression of the $1,25(OH)_2D_3$ stimulated synthesis of the calcium-binding protein (Singh and Bronner, 1980).

The regulatory diagram shown in Fig. 9 embodies the action of vitamin D on plasma calcium homeostasis, but in contrast with the actions presumed for PTH and calcitonin, includes no hypothesis concerning plasma calcium error control by

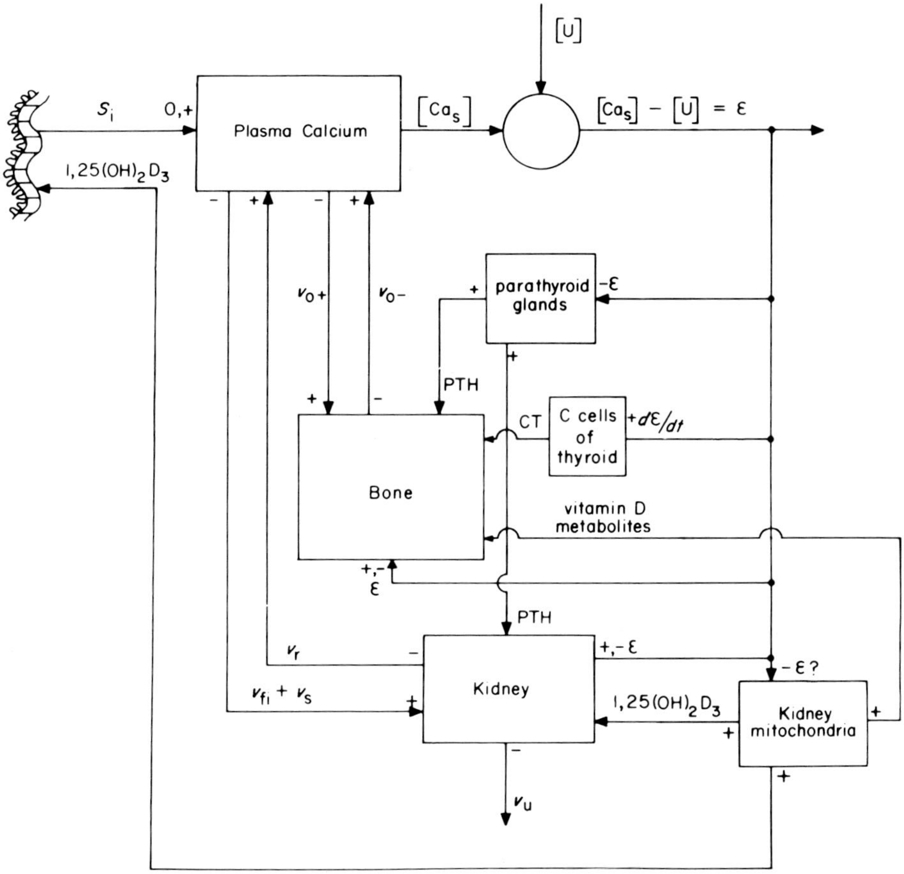

Fig. 9. Regulatory scheme of plasma calcium regulation, including parathyroid hormone (PTH), calcitonin (CT) and vitamin D control. Other possible hormonal controls omitted. The system is explained in the legends of Figs. 6 and 7. 1,25-dihydroxyvitamin D_3, $1,25(OH)_2D_3$, is released from kidney mitochondria in response to the negative plasma calcium error, but it is not known whether this release is proportional to the error, its derivative, or its integral. $1,25(OH)_2D_3$ is shown as acting on the kidney to magnify its response to a negative error, i.e. by decreasing v_u, largely because of an increase in v_r. $1,25(OH)_2D_3$ is also shown to act on the intestinal cell to increase S_i, although from a regulatory viewpoint S_i is a disturbing signal. Vitamin D metabolites act on bone to magnify its response to a negative plasma calcium error, i.e., by increasing v_{0-} and decreasing v_{0+} (see text).

vitamin D. Because quantitative information is unavailable, there is no way of knowing whether the 25(OHD$_3$-1-hydroxylase responds to the plasma calcium error in a proportional, derivative or integral manner and how the increased enzyme activity is reflected in target organ response to the enzyme products, 1,25(OH)$_2$D$_3$ or other metabolites. Also, in contrast with PTH and calcitonin, the response to 1,25(OH)$_2$D$_3$ has not been studied quantitatively, nor have detailed comparisons been made between deficient and replete animals or organs. For this reason, our knowledge of the regulatory role of vitamin D is far sketchier than that of the other two calcium-regulating hormones.

5. Calcium-Regulating Hormones Other Than PTH, CT, and Vitamin D

As detailed in Chapter 9, this volume, many hormones have some effect on calcium metabolism. These include notably the sex hormones and gonadotrophins, the thyroid hormones and also gastric hormones (which may act independently of calcitonin, Kaplan *et al.*, 1977). However, very few studies have compared the capacity to regulate the plasma calcium in two states, e.g., castrated and intact animals, so that it is difficult to analyze the calcium homeostatic role played by these hormones. King *et al.* (1965), in a study referred to previously, have shown that thyroidectomized patients as a group exhibited impaired ability to mobilize calcium in response to a 1-hr infusion of trisodium EDTA. Since patients with unoperated goiters behaved like normal controls, the impaired response may have been due to the absence of calcitonin; excess thyroid hormone is known to alter calcium metabolism (Krane *et al.*, 1956) and thyroidectomy is associated with an impaired ability to overcome a negative error (Argenzio *et al.*, 1974; see below).

Waron and Rich (1969) analyzed the data of Gershberg *et al.* (1967) to show that human growth hormone administered to adults markedly enhanced the rate of plasma calcium recovery from an EDTA infusion. Waron and Rich (1969) also showed that young dogs overcame the hypocalcemic effects of an EDTA infusion much faster than older dogs, an observation made earlier by Alexander (1965) on dogs and rats.

There is increasing evidence for a close relationship between glucose and calcium metabolism. Intestinal calcium retention is increased by lactose (Pansu *et al.*, 1979) and oral glucose loading leads to significant changes in urinary calcium excretion (DeFronzo *et al.*, 1976). Monnier *et al.* (1978) showed that insulin therapy of patients with severe endogenous insulin deficiency led to a near-halving of urinary calcium excretion and that the untreated patients exhibited higher intestinal calcium absorption, which was reduced as a result of treatment. However, neither this nor earlier papers report studies of plasma calcium regulation.

Many reports have dealt with the effect of the menopause on various parameters of calcium metabolism, but studies of calcium homeostasis have not been reported other than that the plasma calcium level was statistically unchanged by either estrogen or calcium carbonate treatment (Recker *et al.*, 1977). Nevertheless, estrogen treatment depressed urinary calcium, from 129 to 49 mg/day, whereas $CaCO_3$ treatment increased urinary calcium to 175 mg/day (Recker *et al.*, 1977). The same investigators (Heaney *et al.*, 1978a) report that the untreated postmenopausal women excretes 17.2 mg Ca/day more in her urine than does a premenopausal or estrogen-treated postmenopausal woman. Thus the ability to reabsorb calcium in the kidney appears impaired in the postmenopausal woman. A similar conclusion was also reached by Young and Nordin (1967) who also reported a statistically significant rise in the plasma calcium levels of postmenopausal women. Whether these individuals also have an impaired response to positive or negative calcium loads is unknown, but seems likely. Oophorectomy in the rat has been shown to lead to lighter bones with lower ash weight and lower calcium and phosphorus content (Hodgkinson *et al.*, 1978); orchidectomy has an even greater effect (Hodgkinson, 1979). How gonadal hormones act on bone and kidney to alter their capacity for regulation of calcium metabolism is not known.

V. DISTURBANCES OF CALCIUM HOMEOSTASIS

A. Classification

The traditional classification of disorders of calcium metabolism is exemplified by the approach of Thomas and Howard (1964), who discuss calcium deficiency with normocalcemia, as well as hypocalcemic and hypercalcemic states. Sometimes hypo- and hypercalcemia are defined numerically, as by Root and Harrison (1976), but more often they are not. Theoretically hypo- and hypercalcemia may be defined as the lower and upper limits of the plasma calcium level for a given normal population. These populations should be defined in terms of age and sex, with age groups defined in terms of functional ages, i.e., infants, prepuberal children, puberal youths, young adults. The overall population norm probably is found within a range of 2.0–3.0 m*M* (8–12 mg/dl). The norm for a given individual is probably much narrower, perhaps within ± 5% of an individual's mean. Since reliable and efficient methods for plasma calcium determination are only about 20 years old and have been in widespread use even less time, it is not surprising that only a limited amount of information on the distribution by sex and functional age groups is available (Roof *et al.*, 1976; Ryckewaert *et al.*, 1974; Franke *et al.*, 1973). Moreover, detailed statistical analysis often fails to reveal statistically significant differences between sexes of a given age or in adjoining age groups (Table II).

From the viewpoint of regulation, the plasma calcium at any time may be considered the sum of some base value plus the error, which is a function of the disturbing signal, i.e.,

$$[Ca_s] = [U] + \epsilon \tag{24}$$

In terms of Eq. (24), [U] would necessarily be low in conditions characterized by hypocalcemia and high in conditions with hypercalcemia, since the error can equal zero. One could get around this by setting $Ca_s = \alpha[U] + \epsilon$, as did Aubert and Bronner (1965). This formulation implies that [U] is a constant ($\simeq$ 10–11 mg/dl) and that α, which normally is close to unity, would decrease in conditions with hypocalcemia and increase in hypercalcemia. The advantage of a formulation like Eq. (24) is that it separates out acute from steady state regulation and permits investigating whether the error (or error correction) is altered in various pathological conditions, since error correction is at present more amenable to study. It also permits distinguishing between the steady-state situation, of which [U] or α[U] is characteristic, and the acute response, which is a more direct reflection of error control. It is possible and even likely that the mecahnisms that underlie [U] and ϵ are similar, but the relationship between these two parameters is not obvious.

The advantage of a formulation like Eq. (24) becomes evident from a comparison of two conditions that both lead to hypercalcemia, i.e., thyroidectomy (Argenzio *et al.*, 1974) and phosphate deficiency (Cuisinier-Gleizes *et al.*, 1975). Thyroidectomized horses had a mean $[Ca_s]$ of 12.1 ($\pm$ 0.3) mg/dl, compared with control values of 11.4 ($\pm$ 0.3) mg Ca/ml. Following an intravenous load of calcium glucontate, the ablated animals took 173 $\pm$ 24 min before $[Ca_s]$ returned to normal, while the controls took only 63 $\pm$ 8 min. Phosphate-deficient rats had a $[Ca_s]$ of 11.4 ($\pm$ 0.2) mg/dl, compared with a value of 10.6 ($\pm$ 0.2) mg/dl for the controls. Here, as for the horses, the difference was statistically significant. However, in contrast with the situation in thyroidectomy, an intraperitoneal calcium gluconate load evoked virtually the same rate of return to the preinjection $[Ca_s]$ as in the controls.

It is therefore apparent that while disease classification into normocalcemic, hypocalcemic, and hypercalcemic states may be of some help, it does little to distinguish between acute and long-term error correction, nor does it necessarily indicate whether the reference values are the same in two conditions with the same average $[Ca_s]$. In terms of the preceding comparison of thyroidectomy and phosphate deficiency—assuming the differences to be species or age-unrelated—[U] is probably higher than normal in the athyroid state, but normal or near-normal in the phosphopryvic state. Experiments to assess [U] in these two or other conditions have not been published.

Argenzio *et al.* (1974) also have reported that, following an EDTA infusion, thyroidectomized horses showed a slower return of $[Ca_s]$ to the preinjection value than did controls. The impaired ability to overcome either a positive or a negative error was overcome by thyroxine administration. It is therefore clear that thyroxine has a direct effect on calcium homeostasis (see also Jowsey and Detenbeck, 1969).

The effects of parathyroidectomy and vitamin D deficiency on plasma calcium regulation have already been discussed. To recapitulate, in parathyroidectomy [U] is clearly lower and the ability to overcome an acute positive (Sammon *et al.*, 1970) or an acute negative error (Alexander, 1965; Hausmann and Riggs, 1966) is impaired. In vitamin D-deficiency, [U] also is lower; whether the ability to overcome acute errors is also impaired has not been determined, but seems probable.[8] It would be interesting to know whether the likely impairment of acute error correction in vitamin D deficiency is quantitatively or qualitatively similar to the impairment resulting from parathyroidectomy.

As a further illustration consider the difference in plasma calcium regulation in the parathyroidectomized (PTX) and calcitoninectomized (CX) states. From the point of view of acute error regulation, the two states appear similar, inasmuch as PTX as well as CX rats take 3 hr to overcome an experimentally induced hypercalcemia that is overcome in two hours by the normal animal (Fig. 10). Yet the reference levels of the two groups of experimental animals differ widely, the PTX animals being clearly hypocalcemic, while the CX animals are essentially normocalcemic. From the viewpoint of differential diagnosis of calcium homeostasis the PTX state can therefore be presumptively identified on the basis of a steady-state [Ca_S] measurement, while the CX state requires an error analysis for presumptive diagnosis.

Thus at the level of plasma calcium regulation, a disorder can manifest itself either by a variation in the reference level [U] alone, e.g., in phosphate deficiency, by a variation in acute error (ϵ) correction only, e.g., in calcitonin deficiency or (and probably more commonly) by variations in both [U] and ϵ, e.g., in parathyroid hormone deficiency. Until a nosology of [U] and ϵ and their relationship has been established, it is difficult to know how commonly a change in [U] is accompanied by a change in ϵ and whether a changed capacity for error correction always means impairment, regardless of whether [U] goes up or down.

From the viewpoint of differential diagnosis, a load test is more efficient than repeated steady-state [Ca_S] determinations, but may be more difficult to defend under clinical conditions, especially in hypercalcemic states. For an understanding of mechanisms, however, a load test is indispensable.

[8]Thus Sereni and Vaccari (1966) found that in infants with rachitic tetany with normal serum protein and calcium, but elevated phosphorus, the plasma calcium response to an EDTA infusion was impaired in comparison with a normal infant control group. However, the report states that the infants with rachitic tetany were tested at the end of their hospitalization, "when their serum calcium had already increased substantially by vitamin D_2 administration". The impairment of their response before treatment might well have been greater.

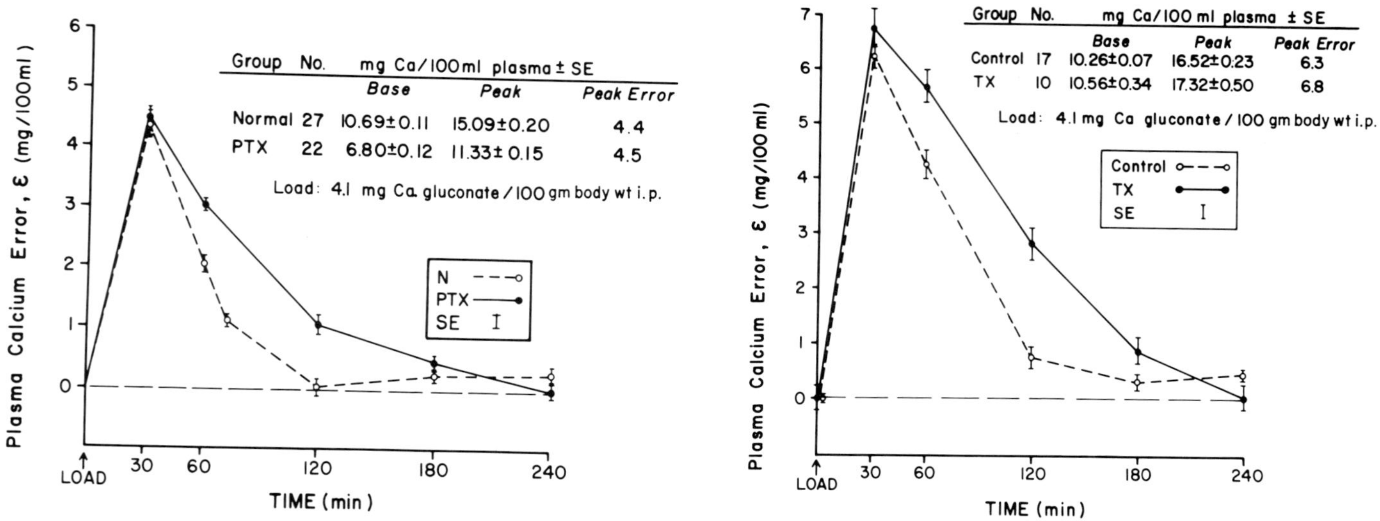

Fig. 10. Acute plasma calcium error correction in normal or control, parathyroidectomized (PTX) and calcitoninectomized (TX) rats. The animals received an intraperitoneal injection of 4.1 mg calcium (as the gluconate)/100 mg body wt. The experimental points represent the mean values of three successive loading experiments, done about 4 weeks after surgery. The control and TX groups had functional parathyroid autografts and the TX group received L-thyroxine in its diet. (From Sammon *et al.*, 1969, 1970, reproduced by permission).

TABLE III

Disorders of Calcium Homeostasis Classified According to Changes in the Reference Value [U] or Acute Error Control (ϵ)

- Normocalcemia with altered error control
  - Calcitonin deficiency—error increased[a]
- Hypocalcemia with altered error control
  - Parathyroid deficiency—error increased[b]
  - Simple vitamin D deficiency—error increased?[c]
  - Phosphate excess—error increased[d]
- Hypocalcemia with unchanged error control
  - Prolonged calcium deficiency[e]
- Hypercalcemia with altered error control
  - Hyperparathyroidism?[f]
  - Thyroid deficiency—error increased[g]
- Hypercalcemia with unchanged error control
  - Long-term high calcium intake[e]
  - Low phosphate intake[h]

[a] Sammon *et al.*, 1969; King *et al.*, 1965; Coen and Palagi, 1976.
[b] Sammon *et al.*, 1970; Parfitt, 1975.
[c] Sereni and Vaccari (1966) on the assumption that the infants with rachitic tetany were hypocalcemic prior to admission.
[d] Schryver *et al.* (1971) demonstrated an increased positive error, but claim a decreased negative error following EDTA infusion. Their Figure 7 does not bear this out, however.
[e] Bronner *et al.* (1968).
[f] Parfitt (1979) suggests this may be the case for type I hyperparathyroidism, but no data are quoted.
[g] Argenzio *et al.* (1974).
[h] Cuisinier-Gleizes *et al.* (1975).

Table III summarizes those conditions where either the reference value or the acute error control or both have been shown to be altered. It is obviously incomplete in that it does not list all states of hypo- or hypercalcemia and the conditions that give rise to them. These have been summarized often, e.g., by Thomas and Howard (1964), Bijvoet and van der Sluys Veer (1968), Isgreen (1976), Root and Harrison (1976), and Parfitt (1979), to name a few. Such lists are also found in standard texts.

B. Therapy

The traditional aim of therapy is to return the patient to normocalcemia. When the underlying disorder is understood, as when a parathyroid adenoma has been verified, normocalcemia is achieved by tumor ablation, provided care is taken to leave some residual functional tissue and to manage the patient so as to avoid initial hypocalcemia, as by appropriate vitamin D or calcium therapy.

The situation is less obvious in the case of hypoparathyroidism. Short of a homologous transplant that is not rejected or some other hormone replacement therapy, the treating physician is faced with the question of whether to return the patient to near-normocalcemia by therapy with hypercalcemic agents such as dihydrotachysterol, high calcium intake, vitamin D or its metabolites, etc. While severe hypocalcemia has undesirable effects like tetany and therefore should be avoided, raising the plasma calcium by drugs alone probably has no effect on error control. Indeed, the difficulty of maintaining a stable $[Ca_s]$ in parathyroprivic patients is undoubtedly related to the absence of this major controlling hormone. Therefore from the viewpoint of managing a hypocalcemic patient, it is probably more prudent to try to maintain $[Ca_s]$ in the low to low-normal range, than to run the risk of hypercalcemic overshoots.

In cases of hypercalcemia where error control has not been studied, it is probably more prudent to assume impairment of error control and to aim for slight hypercalcemia than to force the plasma calcium to a point where hypocalcemia might supervene.

If after sufficient search the cause of a moderate, largely symptom-free hypo- or hypercalcemia cannot be determined, and if error correction is not impaired, it may be prudent not to treat the condition, rather than risk upsetting what is the resultant of the complicated interaction of three major organ systems and a host of regulatory agents, acting on these and perhaps other organs.

ACKNOWLEDGMENT

The experimental work of the author has been generously supported by the National Institutes of Health, the National Science Foundation, the U. S. Department of Agriculture, the National Dairy Council, the U. S. Atomic Energy Commission, and the University of Connecticut Research Foundation.

REFERENCES

Alexander, R.L., Jr. (1965). Calcium homeostasis in the thyroparathyroidectomized dog. *Endocrinology* **77,** 985–990.

Argenzio, R.A., Lowe, J.E., Hintz, H.F., and Schryver, H.F. (1974). Calcium and phosphorus homeostasis in horses. *J. Nutr.* **104,** 18–27.

Armbrecht, H.J., Zenser, T.V., Bruns, M.E.H., and Davis, B.B. (1979). Effect of age on intestinal calcium absorption and adaptation to dietary calcium. *Am. J. Physiol.* **236,** E769–E774.

Aubert, J.-P., and Bronner, F. (1965). A symbolic model for the regulation by bone metabolism of the blood calcium level in rats. *Biophys. J.* **5,** 349–358.

Aubert, J.-P., Moukhtar, M.S., and Milhaud, G. (1961). Etude du métabolisme du calcium chez le rat à l'aide de calcium^{45}. III. Les relations entre les différents processus chez le rat normal. *Rev. Fr. Etud. Clin. Biol.* **6,** 1034–1043.

Austin, L.A., Heath, H., III, and Go, V.L.G. (1979). Regulation of calcitonin secretion in normal man by changes of serum calcium within the physiologic range. *J. Clin. Invest.* **64,** 1721-1724.

Bernard, C. (1865). "Introduction à l'étude de la médecine expérimentale." Baillière et Fils, Paris.

Bijvoet, O.M., and van der Sluys Veer, J. (1968). The homeostasis of plasma calcium and phosphate. *Folia Med. Neerl.* **11,** 161-178.

Borle, A.B. (1978). Cellular aspects of renal calcium transport. *Fed. Proc., Fed. Am. Soc. Exp. Biol.* **37,** 2112-2119.

Bouillon, R., and Van Baden, H. (1979). The transport of vitamin D. In "Vitamin D: Basic Research and Its Clinical Applications" (A.W. Norman, K. Schaefer, D. von Herrath, H.-G. Grigoleit, J.W. Coburn, H.F. DeLuca, E.B. Mawer, and T. Suda, eds.), pp. 129-135. de Gruyter, Berlin.

Boyle, I.T., Gray, R.W., Omdahl, J.L., and DeLuca, H.F. (1972). Calcium control of the *in vivo* biosynthesis of 1,25 dihydroxyvitamin D_3: Nicolaysen's endogenous factor. *Endocrinol. Proc. Int. Symp. 3rd 1971* pp. 468-476.

Brodan, V., Hajek, M., and Kocian, J. (1975). Analog model of kinetics of calcium in healthy subjects during alimentary Ca absorption. *Comput. Biol. Med.* **4,** 257-267.

Bronner, F. (1960). Transfer of maternal calcium to the offspring via the milk. *Science* **132,** 472-473.

Bronner, F. (1973a). Kinetic and cybernetic analysis of calcium metabolism. *In* "Calcium and Phosphorus" (J.T. Irving, ed.), pp. 149-186. Academic Press, New York.

Bronner, F. (1973b). Calcium homeostasis. *In* "Engineering Principles in Physiology" (J.H.U. Brown and D.S. Gann, eds.), Vol. 1, pp. 227-248. Academic Press, New York.

Bronner, F. (1976). Vitamin deficiency and rickets. *Am. J. Clin. Nutr.* **29,** 1307-1314.

Bronner, F. (1979). Clinical investigations of calcium metabolism. In "Skeletal Research: An Experimental Approach" (D.J. Simmons and A.S. Kunin, eds.), pp. 243-261. Academic Press, New York.

Bronner, F., and Aubert, J.-P. (1965). Bone metabolism and regulation of the blood calcium level in rats. *Am. J. Physiol.* **209,** 887-890.

Bronner, F., and Lemaire, R. (1969). Comparison of calcium kinetics in man and the rat. *Calcif. Tissue Res.* **3,** 238-248.

Bronner, F., Harris, R.S., Maletskos, C.J., and Benda, C.E. (1956). Studies in calcium metabolism. The fate of intravenously injected radiocalcium in human beings. *J. Clin. Invest.* **42,** 898-905.

Bronner, F., Sammon, P.J., Stacey, R.E., and Shah, B.G. (1967). Role of thyrocalcitonin in the regulation of the blood calcium level. *Biochem. Med.* **1,** 261-279.

Bronner, F., Sammon, P.J., Nichols, C., Stacey, R.E., and Shah, B.G. (1968). Thyrocalcitonin and plasma calcium homeostasis in the rat. *In* "Parathyroid Hormone and Thyrocalcitonin (Calcitonin)" (R.V. Talmage and L.F. Bélanger, eds.), pp. 353-369. Excerpta Medica, Amsterdam.

Bronner, F., Charnot, Y., Golub, E.E., and Freund, T. (1976a). Calcium binding protein and regulation of calcium transport. *Proc. Eur. Symp. Calcif. Tissue, 11th, 1975* pp. 27-38.

Bronner, F., Golub, E.E., and Fischer, J. (1976b). The effect of vitamin D on renal calcium clearance. *In* "Urolithiasis Research" (H. Fleisch, W.G. Robertson, L.H. Smith, and W. Vahlensieck, eds.), pp. 383-388. Plenum, New York.

Bronner, F., Golub, E.E., Reid, M., Eilam, Y., and Ehrenberg, E. (1978). Calcium transport in bone and intestinal cells. *Ann. N.Y. Acad. Sci.* **307,** 440-441.

Buckley, M., and Bronner, F. (1980). Calcium-binding protein biosynthesis in the rat: Regulation by calcium and 1,25-dihydroxyvitamin D_3. *Arch. Biochem. Biophys.* **202,** 235-241.

Cannon, W.B. (1932). "The Wisdom of the Body." Norton, New York.

Carr, C.W. (1953). Studies on the binding of small ions in protein solutions with the use of membrane electrodes. II. The binding of calcium ions in solutions of bovine serum albumin. *Arch. Biochem. Biophys.* **43,** 147–156.

Clark, J., and Rivera-Cordero, J. (1973). Effects of endogenous parathyroid hormone on calcium, magnesium and phosphate metabolism in rats. *Endocrinology* **92,** 62–71.

Clark, N.B. (1968). Calcitonin studies in turtles. *Endocrinology* **83,** 1145–1148.

Clark, N.B., and Wideman, R.F., Jr. (1980). Calcitonin stimulation of urine flow and sodium excretion in the starling. *Am. J. Physiol.* **238,** R406–R412.

Coen, G., and Palagi, B. (1976). Calcitonin and blood calcium homeostasis during intestinal calcium absorption. *Calcif. Tissue Res.*, **21,** Suppl. 294–298.

Cohn, S.H., Bozzo, S.R., Jesseph, J.E., Constantinides, C., Huene, D.R., and Gusmano, E.A. (1965). Formulation and testing of a compartmental model for calcium metabolism in man. *Radiat. Res.* **26,** 319–333.

Constanzo, L.S. (1978). The distal tubule in renal handling of calcium. A symposium report by R.A.L. Sutton and J.H. Dirks. *Fed. Proc., Fed. Am. Soc. Exp. Biol.* **37,** 2112–2119.

Cuisinier-Gleizes, P., Thomasset, M., and Mathieu, H. (1975). Homeostasis of phosphate and calcium in phosphorus deprivation. *In* "Phosphate Metabolism. Kidney and Bone (L. Avioli, P. Bordier, H. Fleisch, S. Massry, and E. Slatopolsky, eds.), pp. 381–386. Armour Montagu, Paris.

DeFronzo, R.A., Goldberg, M., and Agus, Z.S. (1976). The effects of glucose and insulin on renal electrolyte transport. *J. Clin. Invest.* **58,** 83–90.

DeLuca, H.F. (1981). The vitamin D story. *Harvey Lect.* **75,** 333–379.

Edmondson, J.W., and Li, T.-K. (1976). The relationship of serum ionized and total calcium in primary hyperparathyroidism. *J. Lab. Clin. Med.* **87,** 624–629.

Franke, H., Gall, L., Gross, W., Moll, E., and Weisshaar, D. (1973). Klinisch-chemische Befunde bei 41 Hundertjährigen im Vergleich mit jüngeren Altersstufen. *Klin. Wochenschr.* **51,** 183–190.

Freed, W.J., Perlow, M.J., and Wyatt, R.J. (1979). Calcitonin: Inhibitory effect on eating in rats. *Science* **206,** 850–852.

Freund, T., and Bronner, F. (1975a). Regulation of intestinal calcium-binding protein by calcium intake in the rat. *Am. J. Physiol.* **228,** 861–869.

Freund, T., and Bronner, F. (1975b). Stimulation *in vitro* by 1,25-hydroxyvitamin D_3 of intestinal cell calcium uptake and calcium-binding protein. *Science* **190,** 1300–1302.

Fulton, J.F. (1966). "Selected Readings in the History of Physiology" (completed by L.G. Wilson), 2nd ed., Chapter VIII. Thomas, Springfield, Illinois.

Gershberg, H., Hecht, A., and Javier, Z. (1967). Growth hormone and blood calcium homeostasis. *J. Clin. Endocrinol. Metab.* **27,** 1492–1494.

Grubb, S.A., Edwards, G., and Talmage, R.V. (1977). Effect of endogenous and infused parathyroid hormone on plasma concentrations of recently administered ^{45}Ca. *Calcif. Tissue Res.* **24,** 209–214.

Hall, B.D., MacMillan, D.R., and Bronner, F. (1969). Vitamin D-resistant rickets and high fecal endogenous calcium output. A report of two cases. *Am. J. Clin. Nutr.* **22,** 448–457.

Harrison, H.E. (1966). Parathyroid hormone and vitamin D. *Yale J. Med.* **38,** 393–409.

Hart, H.E. (1967). Analysis of tracer experiments. VIII. Integrodifferential equation treatment of partly accessible, partly injectable multicompartment systems. *Bull. Math. Biophys.* **9,** 319–333.

Hausmann, E., and Riggs, D.S. (1966). The effectiveness of negative feedback in regulating plasma calcium in the dog. *J. Theor. Biol.* **12,** 350–363.

Haussler, M., Hughes, M., Baylink, D., Littledike, E.T., Cork, D., and Pitt, M. (1977). Influence of phosphate depletion on the biosynthesis and circulating level of 1α,25-dihydroxyvitamin D.

In "Phosphate Metabolism" (S.G. Massry and E. Ritz, eds.), pp. 233–250. Plenum, New York.

Heaney, R.P., Recker, R.R., and Saville, P.D. (1977). Calcium balance and calcium requirement in middle-aged women. *Am. J. Clin. Nutr.* **30,** 1603–1611.

Heaney, R.P., Recker, R.R., and Saville, P.D. (1978a). Menopausal changes in calcium balance performance. *J. Lab. Clin. Med.* **92,** 953–963.

Heany, R.P., Recker, R.R., and Saville, P.D. (1978b). Menopausal changes in bone remodeling. *J. Lab. Clin. Med.* **92,** 964–970.

Hermsdorf, C.L., and Bronner, F. (1975). Vitamin D-dependent calcium binding protein from rat kidney. *Biochim. Biophys. Acta* **379,** 553–561.

Hevesy, G. (1955). Conservation of skeletal calcium atoms through life. *Dan. Biol. Medd.* **22,** No. 9.

Hodgkinson, A. (1979). Effects of calcium deprivation and orchidectomy on bone composition in the rat. *Horm. Metab. Res.* **11,** 493–532.

Hodgkinson, A., Aaron, J.E., Horsman, A., MacLachlan, M.S.F., and Nordin, B.E.C. (1978). Effect of oophorectomy and calcium deprivation on bone mass in the rat. *Clin. Sci. Mol. Med.* **54,** 439–446.

Holick, S.A., Holick, M.F., Tavela, T.E., Schnoes, H.K., and DeLuca, H.F. (1976). Metabolism of 1α-hydroxyvitamin D_3 in the chick. *J. Biol. Chem.* **251,** 1025–1028.

Hurwitz, S., Stacey, R.E., and Bronner, F. (1969). Role of vitamin D in plasma calcium regulation. *Am. J. Physiol.* **216,** 254–262.

Hurwitz, S., Talpaz, H., and Bar, A. (1979). Vitamin D and calcium absorption: Computer simulation. *In* "Vitamin D: Basic Research and Its Clinical Applications" (A.W. Norman, K. Schaefer, D. von Herrath, H.-G. Grigoleit, J.W. Coburn, H.F. DeLuca, E.B. Mawer, and T. Suda, eds.), pp. 735–742. deGruyter, Berlin.

Isgreen, W.P. (1976). Normocalcemic tetany. A problem of erethism. *Neurology* **26,** 825–834.

Jaros, G.G., Coleman, T.G., and Guyton, A.C. (1979). Model of short-term regulation of calcium-ion concentration. *Simulation* **32,** 193–204.

Jowsey, J., and Detenbeck, L.C. (1969). Importance of thyroid hormones in bone metabolism and calcium homeostasis. *Endocrinology* **85,** 87–95.

Kales, A.N., and Phang, J.M. (1971). Effect of divided calcium intake on calcium metabolism. *J. Clin. Endocrinol. Metab.* **32,** 83–87.

Kaplan, E.L., North, P.T., Norberg, H.P., Schulak, J.A., and Hill, B.J. (1977). Evidence for a role of the stomach in serum calcium regulation. *J. Surg. Res.* **22,** 237–241.

King, L.R., Portnoy, R.M., and Goldsmith, R.E. (1965). Serum calcium homeostasis following thyroid surgery as measured by ethylene diamine tetra-acetate infusion. *J. Clin. Endocrinol. Metabl.* **25,** 577–584.

Krane, S.M., Brownell, G.L., Stanbury, J.B., and Corrigan, H. (1956). The effect of thyroid disease on calcium metabolism in man. *J. Clin. Invest.* **35,** 874–887.

Ladenson, J.H., Lewis, J.W., and Boyd, J.C. (1978). Failure of total calcium corrected for protein, albumin, and pH to correctly assess calcium status. *J. Clin. Endocrinol. Metab.* **46,** 986–993.

Langley, L.L. (1965). "Homeostasis." Van Nostrand-Reinhold, Princeton, New Jersey.

Larsson, L., and Ohman, S. (1979). Serum calcium ion activity. Some aspects of methodological differences and intraindividual variation. *Clin. Biochem. (Ottawa)* **12,** 138–141.

Lauffenburger, T., Olah, A.J., Dambacker, M.A., Guncaga, J., Lentner, C., and Haas, H.G. (1977). Bone remodeling and calcium metabolism: A correlated histomorphometric, calcium kinetic, and biochemical study in patients with osteoporosis and Paget's disease. *Metab., Clin. Exp.* **26,** 589–606.

Li, T.-K., and Piechocki, J.T. (1971). Determination of serum ionic calcium with an ion-selective electrode: Evaluation of methodology and normal values. *Clin. Chem. (Winston-Salem, N.C.)* **17,** 411–416.

Melvin, K.E.W., Tashijian, A.H., Jr., and Bordier, P. (1973). The metabolic significance of calcitonin-secreting thyroid carcinoma. *In* "Clinical Aspects of Metabolic Bone Disease" (B. Frame, A.M. Parfitt, and H. Duncan, eds.), pp. 193-201. Excerpta Medica, Amsterdam.

Milhaud, G., Perault, A.-M., and Moukhtar, M.S. (1965). Etude du mécanisme de l'action hypocalcémiante de la thyrocalcitonine. *C. R. Hebd. Seances Acad. Sci.* **261,** 813-816.

Milhaud, G., Perault-Staub, A.-M., and Staub, J.F. (1972). Diurnal variations of plasma calcium and calcitonin function in the rat. *J. Physiol. (London)* **222,** 559-567.

Monnier, L., Colette, C., Aguire, L., Sarry, C., and Mirouze, J. (1978). Intestinal and renal handling of calcium in human diabetes mellitus: Influence of acute oral glucose loading and diabetic control. *J. Clin. Invest.* **8,** 225-231.

Nordin, B.E.C., Peacock, M., and Wilkinson, R. (1972). The relative importance of gut, bone and kidney in the regulation of serum calcium. *In* "Calcium, Parathyroid Hormone and the Calcitonins" (R.V. Talmage and P.L. Munson, eds.), pp. 262-272. Excerpta Medica, Amsterdam.

Norimatsu, H., Vander Wiel, C.J., and Talmage, R.V. (1979). Electron microscopic study of the effect of calcitonin on bone cells and their extracellular milieu. *Clin. Orthop. Relat. Res.* **139,** 250-258.

Norman, A.W. (1979). "Vitamin D: The Calcium Homeostasis Steroid Hormone." Academic Press, New York.

O'Riordan, J.L.H., and Aurbach, G.D. (1968). Mode of action of thyrocalcitonin. *Endocrinology* **82,** 377-383.

Owyang, C., Heath, H., III, Sizemore, G.W., and Go, V.L.W. (1978). Comparison of the effects of pentagastrin and meal stimulated gastrin on plasma calcitonin in normal man. *Am. J. Dig. Dis.* **23,** 1084-1088.

Pansu, D., Bellaton, C., and Bronner, F. (1979). Effect of lactose on duodenal calcium binding protein and calcium absorption. *J. Nutr.* **109,** 508-512.

Pansu, D., Bellaton, C., and Bronner, F. (1981). The effect of calcium intake on the saturable and nonsaturable components of duodenal calcium transport. *Am. J. Physiol.* **240,** G32-G37.

Parfitt, A.M. (1969). Study of parathyroid function in man by EDTA infusion. *J. Clin. Endocrinol. Metab.* **29,** 569-580.

Parfitt, A.M. (1975). Effect of cellulose phosphate on calcium and magnesium in homeostasis: Studies in normal subjects and patients with latent hypoparathyroidism. *Clin. Sci. Mol. Med.* **49,** 83-90.

Parfitt, A.M. (1979). Equilibrium and disequilibrium hypercalcemia. New light on an old concept. *Metab. Bone Dis. Relat. Res.* **1,** 279-293.

Parfitt, A.M., Mathews, M., Rao, D.S., and Kleere-Koper, M. (1979). The regulation of 25-hydroxylation by vitamin D intake in man: A theoretical model. In "Vitamin D: Basic Research and Its Clinical Applications" (A.W. Norman, K. Schaefer, D. Von Herrath, H.-G. Gringoleit, J.W. Coburn, H.F. DeLuca, E.B. Mawer, and T. Suda, eds.), pp. 497-500. de Gruyter, Berlin.

Payne, J.M. (1970). Some recent work on the pathogenesis and prevention of milk fever. *In* "Parturient Hypocalcemia" (J.J.B. Anderson, ed.), pp. 1-13. Academic Press, New York.

Perault-Staub, A.M., Staub, J.F., and Milhaud, G. (1974). A new concept for plasma calcium homeostasis in the rat. *Endocrinology* **94,** 480-484.

Phang, J.M., Berman, M., Finerman, G.A., Neer, R., Rosenberg, L.E., and Hahn, T.J. (1969). Dietary perturbation of calcium metabolism in normal man: Compartmental analysis. *J. Clin. Invest.* **48,** 67-77.

Powell, T. (1972). A mathematical model for calcium homeostasis. *Bull. Math. Biophys.* **34,** 483-502.

Puschett, J.B., Fernandez, P.C., Boyle, I.T., Gray, R.W., Omdahl, J.L., and DeLuca, H.F. (1972a). The acute renal tubular effects of 1,25-dihydroxycholecalciferol. *Proc. Soc. Exp. Biol. Med.* **141,** 379-384.

Puschett, J.B., Moranz, J., and Kurnick, W.S. (1972b). Evidence for a direct action of cholecalciferol and 25-hydroxycholecalciferol on the renal transport of phosphate, sodium and calcium. *J. Clin. Invest.* **51,** 373–385.

Ramberg, C.F., Mayer, G.P., Kronfeld, D.S., Phang, J.N., and Berman, M. (1970a). Calcium kinetics in cows during late pregnancy, parturient and early lactation. *Am. J. Physiol.* **219,** 1166–1177.

Ramberg, C.F., Phang, J.M., and Kronfeld, D.S. (1970b). A compartmental model of calcium metabolism in cows. *In* "Parturient Hypocalcemia" (J.J.B. Anderson, ed.), pp. 119–134. Academic Press, New York.

Ramberg, C.F., Mayer, G.P., Kronfeld, D.S., and Potts, J.T., Jr. (1976). Dietary calcium, calcium kinetics and plasma parathyroid hormone concentration in cows. *J. Nutr.* **106,** 671–679.

Recker, R.R., Saville, P.D., and Heaney, R.P. (1977). Effect of estrogens and calcium carbonates on bone loss in postmenopausal women. *Ann. Intern. Med.* **87,** 649–655.

Riggs, D.S. (1966). A quantitative hypothesis concerning the action of the parathyroid hormone. *J. Theor. Biol.* **12,** 364–372.

Rodan, G.A. (1970). Blood-bone calcium fluxes in the perfused dog limb and the hormonal control of calcium homeostasis. Ph.D. Thesis, p. 114. Weizmann Institute of Science, Rehovot, Israel.

Rodan, G.A., and Katz, E.P. (1973). Calcium binding to nondialyzable components of rat blood under in vivo conditions. *Am. J. Physiol.* **225,** 1082–1088.

Root, A.W., and Harrison, H.E. (1976). Recent advances in calcium metabolism. II. Disorders of calcium metabolism. *J. Pediatr.* **88,** 177–199.

Roof, B.S., Piel, C.F., Hansen, J., and Fudenberg, H.H. (1976). Serum parathyroid hormone levels and serum calcium levels from birth to senescence. *Mech. Ageing Dev.* **5,** 289–304.

Ryckewaert, A., Richet, G., Lemaire, V., Begue, M.C., and Fenelon, J.P. (1974). Etude de la calcémie dans une population de 6048 hommes. Variation avec l'âge. Correlations avec d'autres valeurs biologigues. *Rev. Rhum. Mal. Osteo-Articulaires* **41,** 473–478.

Sammon, P.J., Stacey, R.E., and Bronner, F. (1969). Further studies on the role of thyrocalcitonin in calcium homeostasis and metabolism. *Biochem. Med.* **3,** 252–270.

Sammon, P.J., Stacey, R.E., and Bronner, F. (1970). Role of parathyroid hormone in calcium homeostasis and metabolism. *Am. J. Physiol.* **218,** 479–485.

Schryver, H.F., Craig, P.H., and Hintz, H.F. (1970). Calcium metabolism in ponies fed varying levels of calcium *J. Nutr.* **100,** 955–964.

Schryver, H.F., Hintz, H.F., and Craig, P.H. (1971). Calcium metabolism in ponies fed a high phosphorus diet. *J. Nutr.* **101,** 259–264.

Schwartz, E., Panariello, V.A., and Saeli, J. (1965). Radioactive calcium kinetics during high calcium intake in osteoporosis. *J. Clin. Invest.* **44,** 1547–1560.

Sereni, F., and Vaccari, A. (1966). Efficiency of calcium homeostatic mechanisms in newborns and infants measured by the edetic acid test. *Schweiz. Med. Wochenschr.* **96,** 374–377.

Shah, B.G., Sammon, P.J., and Bronner, F. (1968). Effect of calcium intake levels on the response to exogenous rat thyrocalcitonin. *In* "Calcitonin, Proceedings of the Symposium on Thyrocalcitonin and the C Cells" (S. Taylor, ed.), pp. 282–289. Heinemann, London.

Siegel, F., Carafoli, E., Kretsinger, R.H., MacLennan, F., and Wasserman, R.H., eds. (1980). "Calcium Binding Proteins: Structure and Function." Elsevier/North Holland Publ., Amsterdam and New York.

Singh, R.P., and Bronner, F. (1980). Stimulation of in vitro synthesis of calcium-binding protein (CaBP) by 1,25-dihydroxyvitamin D_3 (1,25-$(OH)_2$-D_3). *Fed. Proc., Fed. Am. Soc. Exp. Biol.* **39,** 661 (abstr).

Staub, J.-F., Perault-Staub, A.-M., and Milhaud, G. (1979). Endogenous nature of circadian rhythms in calcium metabolism. *Am. J. Physiol.* **237,** R311–R317.

Talmage, R.V., and Grubb, S.A. (1977). The influence of endogenous or exogenous calcitonin in daily urinary calcium excretion. *Endocrinology* **101,** 1351–1357.

Talmage, R.V., Roycroft, J.H., and Anderson, J.J.B. (1975a). Daily fluctuations in plasma calcium, plasma phosphate, and their radionuclide concentrations in the rat. *Calcif. Tissue Res.* **17,** 91–102.

Talmage, R.V., Doppelt, S.H., and Cooper, C.W. (1975b). Relationships of blood concentrations of calcium, phosphate, gastrin and calcitonin to the onset of feeding in the rat. *Proc. Soc. Exp. Biol. Med.* **149,** 855–859.

Talmage, R.V., Grubb, S.A., Vander Wiel, C.J., Doppelt, S.H., and Norimatsu, H. (1978). The demand for bone calcium in maintenance of plasma calcium concentrations. *In* "Mechanisms of Localized Bone Resorption" (J.M. Horton, T.M. Tarpley, and W.F. Davis, eds.), pp. 73–92. Information Retrieval, Inc., Washington, D.C.

Talpaz, H., Hurwitz, S., and Risenfeld, G. Regulation of plasma calcium concentration: Initial approach at computer simulation. (Unpublished manuscript.)

Thomas, W.C., and Howard, J.E. (1964). Disturbances of calcium metabolism. *In* "Mineral Metabolism. An Advanced Treatise" (C.L. Comar and F. Bronner, eds.), Vol. 2, Part A, pp. 445–482. Academic Press, New York.

Thomasset, M., Cuisinier-Gleizes, P., Mathieu, H., Golub, E.E., and Bronner, F. (1979). Regulation of intestinal calcium binding protein in rats: role of parathyroid hormone. *Calcif. Tissue Int.* **29,** 141–145.

Ullrich K.J., Rumrick, G., and Kloss, S. (1976). Acute Ca^{2+} reabsorption in the proximal tubule of the rat kidney. Dependence on sodium and buffer transport. *Pflüger's Arch.* **364,** 223–228.

Vaes, G. (1966). La resorption osseuse et l'hormone parathyroidienne. Thesis, Université Catholique de Louvain, Warny, Louvain.

Van Baden, H., Bouillon, R., and DeMoor, P. (1980). Vitamin D-binding protein (Gc Globulin) binds actin. *J. Biol. Chem.* **255,** 2270–2272.

Walling, M.W., and Kimberg, D.V. (1973). Active secretion of calcium by adult rat ileum and jejunum in vitro. *Am. J. Physiol.* **225,** 415–422.

Walser, M. (1961). Ion association. VI. Interaction between calcium, magnesium, inorganic phosphate, citrate and protein in normal human plasma. *J. Clin. Invest.* **40,** 723–730.

Walser, M., and Browder, A.A. (1959). Ion association. III. The effect of sulfate infusion on calcium excretion. *J. Clin. Invest.* **38,** 1404–1411.

Waron, M., and Rich, C. (1969). Rate of recovery from acute hypocalcemia as a measure of calcium homeostatic efficiency in the dog. *Endocrinology* **85,** 1018–1027.

Wasserman, R.H., and Taylor, A.N. (1969). Some aspects of the intestinal absorption of calcium, with special reference to vitamin D. *In* "Mineral Metabolism. An Advanced Treatise" (C.L. Comar and F. Bronner, eds.), Vol. 3, pp. 321–403. Academic Press, New York.

Watkins, G.W., Johnson, T.D., Golub, E.E., and Bronner, F. (1976). Regulation of plasma phosphate in the rat. *In* "Phosphate Metabolism. Kidney and Bone" (L. Avioli, P. Bordier, H. Fleisch, S. Massry, and E. Slatopolski, eds.), pp. 317–328. Armour Montagu, Paris.

Widdowson, E.M., and Dickerson, J.W.T. (1964). Chemical composition of the body. *In* "Mineral Metabolism. An Advanced Treatise" (C.L. Comar and F. Bronner, eds.), Vol. 2, Part A, pp. 1–247. Academic Press, New York.

Wong, G.L., and Cohn, D.V. (1975). Target cells in bone for parathormone and calcitonin are different: Enrichment for each cell type by sequential digestion of mouse calvaria and selective adhesion to polymeric surfaces. *Proc. Natl. Acad. Sci. U.S.A.* **72,** 3167–3171.

Young, M.M., and Nordin, B.E.C. (1967). Effects of natural and artificial menopause on plasma and urinary calcium and phosphorus. *Lancet* **ii,** 118–120.

Zornitzer, A.E., and Bronner, F. (1971). In situ studies of calcium absorption in rats. *Am. J. Physiol.* **220,** 1261–1265.

3

Intestinal Absorption of Calcium: Its Assessment, Normal Physiology, and Alterations in Various Disease States

BARTON S. LEVINE, MARLIN W. WALLING, AND
JACK W. COBURN

Disorders of Mineral Metabolism, Vol. II

ISBN 0-12-135302-8

I. INTRODUCTION

The metabolism of calcium (Ca) is regulated in part via changes in its intestinal absorption. This chapter will review general aspects of Ca absorption, the methods for measuring overall intestinal absorption and the transport of Ca, various hormonal and other factors that may alter Ca absorption, and common physiologic events and clinical disorders that modify the intestinal Ca absorption.

In the United States, the average diet consumed by an adult contains approximately 600–1000 mg of Ca. Unlike other elements in the diet such as sodium and potassium, which are almost entirely absorbed, only a fraction of dietary Ca is absorbed by the intestine of adult humans. The net absorption of Ca represents the vectoral sum of two processes, the transfer of Ca from the intestinal lumen into the blood and the transfer of Ca from the plasma into the lumen. Thus, fecal Ca consists not only of unabsorbed Ca that was ingested in the diet but also the quantity of Ca that is endogenously secreted into the gastrointestinal tract and not reabsorbed later. In man, the total quantity of Ca in the feces is approximately 700–1000 mg; of this, approximately 130 ± 50 mg/day represents "endogenous fecal Ca" or Ca secreted from the blood into the lumen and not reabsorbed (Heaney and Skillman, 1964). For this estimate, it is assumed that approximately 15% of total intestinal Ca secreted is nonabsorbable, even under conditions when dietary Ca is completely absorbed. Such observations are based on the assumption that dietary Ca is mixed homogeneously with endogenously secreted Ca and that the absorptive efficiencies are identical for both. Also, a portion of the endogenous fecal Ca is nonabsorbable because it enters the intestine distal to the absorptive sites and/or perhaps because endogenous Ca is precipitated more readily with co-secreted phosphate within the intestinal lumen than is dietary Ca (Schedl *et al.*, 1968).

There are a number of factors that have a major effect on intestinal Ca absorption; thus, Ca absorption is much greater in children during periods of skeletal growth; on the other hand, Ca absorption decreases with advancing age. The fraction of intestinal Ca absorbed is known to increase in patients ingesting a diet low in Ca content; also, there are several hormones, agents, and constituents in the diet that may alter the intestinal absorption of Ca.

II. METHODS FOR MEASUREMENTS OF CALCIUM ABSORPTION

Numerous methods have been utilized to measure intestinal Ca absorption; each has certain limitations and advantages, and the results obtained may differ somewhat with various methods. In this discussion, overall methods of Ca absorption will be reviewed followed by a consideration of methods for the evaluation of Ca transport. When Ca absorption is discussed, we refer to the "efficiency" of absorption as the fraction of dietary Ca that is absorbed, whereas net absorption refers to the absolute quantity absorbed (i.e., the product of fractional absorption and dietary intake).

A. Calcium Absorption in Man

A classic method that is still utilized is the metabolic balance technique. With this method, overall net Ca absorption is measured, but this method provides no insight into the sources of fecal Ca, which arises from Ca that is secreted into the intestine and dietary and secreted Ca that are not absorbed. Also, this method does not measure "true" absorption, which is net absorption plus the Ca that was absorbed but is resecreted into the intestinal lumen. This method has the disadvantages that it requires a metabolic kitchen to prepare a constant diet, and it requires several days for fecal collection; variation or irregularities in fecal flow have a profound effect on the results; correction for such irregularities in fecal flow with the use of exogenous (Whitby and Lang, 1960) or endogenous (Samachson, 1965) fecal markers can add to the accuracy but also to the complexity of this procedure.

With the availability of radioisotopes of Ca, ^{45}Ca, and ^{47}Ca, various tracer methods have been utilized for the study of Ca absorption in man. ^{47}Ca, which is a gamma emitter, has the advantage that it has a short half-life ($t_{\frac{1}{2}}$ = 4.7 days), but is expensive and not always available; ^{45}Ca is a beta emitter and has a very long half-life. The use of such a "bone-seeking" isotope has limited applicability in man.

The absorption of Ca can be determined from the quantity of radiocalcium recovered in the feces after an oral dose of the isotope (Blau *et al.*, 1954; Bronner, 1962; Rich and Ivanovich, 1964). The major disadvantage is the need to obtain the total and accurate collection of feces for several days until the unabsorbed isotope is passed. This method does not measure "true" absorption, since some radiocalcium recovered in the feces represents that which was absorbed and then secreted into the intestinal lumen; this error is small, representing only 6–8% of absorbed Ca (Rich and Ivanovich, 1964).

Another approach utilizes the whole body counter to determine the quantity of ^{47}Ca retained in the body after its ingestion (DeGrazia *et al.*, 1965; Deller *et al.*, 1965). This method is relatively simple, but it requires a whole body counter; also, sufficient time must elapse to allow for fecal excretion of the radiocalcium that was not absorbed. This technique would obviously not be appropriate when radiocalcium is removed by another route, i.e., in a patient undergoing hemodialysis. Also, there is a small error similar to that for the fecal recovery method.

Several methods employ the administration of two separate isotopes, ^{45}Ca and ^{47}Ca, one given orally and the other intravenously (Birge *et al.*, 1969; DeGrazia *et al.*, 1965; Szymendera *et al.*, 1972; Mautalen *et al.*, 1969). It is assumed that the radiocalcium absorbed from the intestine is distributed within the body in the same manner as that given intravenously. The radioactivity derived from each isotope is determined in either blood or urine samples and the results are calculated from the fraction of the two doses present in the blood or urine: The fraction of Ca absorbed (α) is derived from this ratio, with the formula:

$$\alpha = \frac{\text{Fraction of orally administered isotope/sample}}{\text{Fraction of intravenously administered isotope/sample}}$$

This ratio is usually obtained 6–24 hr after the administration of the isotopes (DeGrazia *et al.*, 1965). In addition, the disappearance curve of the intravenous radiocalcium and the simultaneous appearance curve of the oral tracer can be analyzed utilizing deconvolutional analysis (Birge *et al.*, 1969; Szymedera *et al.*, 1972). With this technique, both absolute and fractional rates of absorption can be calculated for frequent intervals following the ingestion of the isotope. These methods that employ two radioisotopes can measure "true" absorption; their disadvantages include contamination of ^{47}Ca with a small amount of ^{45}Ca and the necessity of allowing time for the decay of the short-lived ^{47}Ca before the activity from administered ^{45}Ca can be determined. Also, the estimation of ^{45}Ca in the urine can be cumbersome, although simplified techniques have been reported (Kapitola *et al.*, 1979).

A modification of the double isotope method involves administration of two doses of ^{47}Ca on two separate occasions, one dose orally and the other intravenously (Curtis *et al.*, 1967; Lutwak, 1969). Radioactivity can be assessed with the use of an external counting technique, i.e., with measurement of ^{47}Ca accumulated in the forearm utilizing external detectors rather than from blood samples. This method is simple, can be done with a small quantity of ^{47}Ca, and does not require the collection of blood or urine; its major disadvantage is the lack of availability of the instrument needed for detection of the ^{47}Ca.

"True" Ca absorption can be measured by combining the metabolic balance technique with kinetic studies after the intravenous injection of radiocalcium (Heaney and Whedon, 1958; Bronner *et al.*, 1963; Heaney and Skillman, 1964). With this method, endogenous fecal Ca is calculated from fecal radioactivity and a knowledge of the specific activity of Ca in either serum or urine; the theoretical considerations of this method were reviewed in detail by Aubert *et al.* (1964). The "true" absorption of Ca is then determined from the net absorption, which is determined from the metabolic balance technique, and the measured endogenous fecal Ca. Also, this approach measures the fraction of Ca absorbed from the diet rather than from a "test dose" of stable Ca. Unfortunately, this method requires a constant dietary intake on a metabolic unit, with all the errors and disadvantages intrinsic to the metabolic balance technique. It should be noted that the measurement of Ca absorption is done ideally under conditions when dietary Ca has been constant for 3–4 weeks prior to its measurement. Thus, this technique has somewhat limited applicability except under rigid research conditions.

Another method utilizes the sequential injection of ^{47}Ca followed in 2 hr by the ingestion of an oral dose of the isotope. Several blood samples are obtained, and the log plasma radioactivity is plotted against the log time following the injection of the ^{47}Ca. The fraction of Ca absorbed is calculated from the distance between the two parallel lines, divided by the average quantity of isotope in blood after the IV dose. The value obtained is then corrected for the ratio of the doses of radioisotope given intravenously and orally (Chanard *et al.*, 1974). This method has not been utilized widely, and further data may be needed to substantiate its accuracy and broad applicability.

Several of the techniques described above measure "total" Ca absorption. However, there has been a wide variation in the results obtained for Ca absorption in normal subjects employing these methods (Mautalen *et al.*, 1969; Lutwak and Shapiro, 1964; Coburn *et al.*, 1973a). Two factors that can affect the results obtained include the quantity of nonradioactive, stable Ca added as a carrier and the accompanying anion given with the Ca salt. When radiocalcium is administered without added stable carrier, 90–100% of the administered dose may be absorbed (Kaye and Silverman, 1965). On the other hand, when the stable Ca carrier is 500 mg or more, the fraction of Ca absorbed falls below 20% (Rich and Ivanovich, 1964). Calcium absorption also varies with the Ca salt given; data indicate that the absorption of calcium chloride exceeds that of calcium lactate, which is somewhat greater than that for calcium carbonate (Mautalen *et al.*, 1969). In studies carried out in man, even when the Ca salt and dose of carrier used are not varied, there is a wide variation in the fractional absorption of Ca between individual subjects. However, Ca absorption varies only slightly in the same individual when it is measured on two or more occasions utilizing the same method (Wensel *et al.*, 1969; Rich and Ivanovitch, 1964; Coburn *et al.*, 1973a). The reason for this inter-subject variation is not clear; recent studies suggest that variations in the "steady-state," circulating level of plasma 1,25-dihydroxyvitamin D may be related to the variation in Ca absorption (Wilz *et al.*, 1979).

Other methods provide only an index of Ca absorption rather than a measure of true absorption of Ca. Thus, the measurement of radiocalcium in the blood following its oral administration can provide a simple method to estimate Ca absorption. Plasma levels are obtained at various intervals from 30 min to 4 hr after ingestion of the radiocalcium (Bhandarkar *et al.*, 1961; Jaworski *et al.*, 1963; Avioli *et al.*, 1965a; Nordin *et al.*, 1968). The quantity of stable Ca given as a carrier is usually relatively small (0–50 mg) to insure absorption of adequate amounts of radiocalcium into the blood. The method cannot be utilized beyond 2–4 hr after ingestion of the isotope because absorbed radiocalcium disappears from the blood. Opinions as to the reliability of this method as a measure of absorption vary widely (Mautalen *et al.*, 1969; Jaworski *et al.*, 1963; Avioli *et al.*, 1965a; Tothill *et al.*, 1970; Parsons *et al.*, 1968).

Another indirect method for the assessment of Ca absorption involves the administration of an oral load of stable Ca and the measurement of urinary Ca excretion (Pak *et al.*, 1975; Broadus *et al.*, 1978; Sakhaee *et al.*, 1979). These methods have been utilized to detect an intestinal absorptive cause of hypercalciuria and are not suitable in situations where other factors affect the renal handling of Ca independent of its absorption. In this procedure, one utilizes either the absolute rate of urinary Ca excretion following an oral Ca load or measures an increment in urinary Ca excretion following the load; urine collections are corrected for creatinine excretion making accurate estimation of urine volume less important. These techniques do not require the use of radioisotopes, and they can be repeated frequently. Therefore, they may be applicable to a broader population.

Intestinal Ca absorption can also be evaluated *in situ* in different segments of the intestine in subjects who have been intubated with a triple-lumen tube. The intestinal segment is perfused at a known rate with a solution containing Ca and a nonabsorbable volume marker to estimate the water absorbed. At a more distal point, the perfusate is aspirated and the fraction of Ca absorbed/unit of time in the segment is determined (Wensel *et al.*, 1969; Parker *et al.*, 1974). This method can yield information about Ca transport in various segments of the intestine; also, different Ca concentrations can be added to the perfusate providing a means for assessing the kinetics of Ca transport.

B. Calcium Transport in Experimental Animals

In experimental animals, metabolic balance and Ca kinetic methods similar to those already described in man have been utilized (Aubert *et al.*, 1964). In addition, several other methods have been utilized to study Ca transport, both *in vivo* and *in vitro*. An early *in vivo* method involved injection of Ca, either stable or radioactive, into various segments of intestine with subsequent evaluation of Ca recovered and presumably not absorbed (Nicolaysen, 1937a). Also, *in situ* perfusion techniques and isolated gut loops remaining *in situ* have been utilized (Zornitzer and Bronner, 1971). These techniques have the advantage that they are carried out *in vivo* and can be used to measure Ca transport in different intestinal segments. Moreover, with perfusion techniques it is possible to evaluate transport kinetics by varying the Ca concentration within the perfusate.

Various *in vitro* gut sac techniques have also been utilized to evaluate Ca transport. Everted gut sacs, with the mucosal surface on the outside, have been used to evaluate the transport of Ca from the external or mucosal surface to the internal or serosal surface; also, it can be used to evaluate the mucosal uptake of Ca (Wilson and Wiseman, 1954). These techniques are simple and can be carried out in large numbers; also they allow for the measurement of uptake or transport in different segments of the intestine. Moreover, the results correlate with more refined measures of Ca transport (Fig. 1). The disadvantages of these techniques include problem arising from unstirred layers, lack of prolonged viability of the preparation, difficulties in measuring potential differences across the mucosal and serosal layers, and variable pool sizes of intracellular and extracellular spaces. Thus, steady-state conditions are impossible to achieve with this preparation. Everted gut sac preparations may serve as a useful screening procedure prior to the performance of more sophisticated transport studies described below (Walling *et al.*, 1977a). Another useful *in vitro* technique involves assessment of the mucosal uptake of Ca (O'Donnell and Smith, 1973a), with only the mucosal

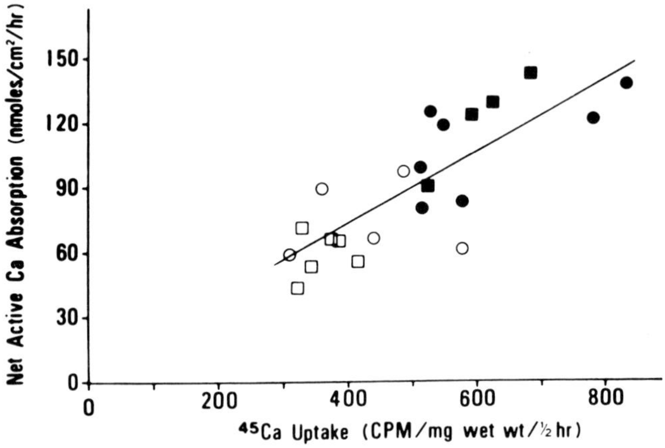

Fig. 1. The relationship between active duodenal Ca absorption, measured with the Ussing technique, and ^{45}Ca uptake by everted duodenal sacs from vitamin D-deficient rats receiving vehicle (open symbols) or 1,25$(OH)_2D_3$ (closed symbols); the Ca absorption and ^{45}Ca uptake were studied using adjacent segments of the duodenum from the same animal. Circles represent untreated sham-operated rats, and squares indicate the nephrectomized animals ($r = 0.81$). (From Walling *et al.*, 1977a, with permission of *Arch. Biochem. Biophys.)*

surface exposed to the bathing media and the uptake of radioisotope measured over a short interval of time. This method provides insight into initial transport events occurring across the brush border membrane.

Another *in vitro* technique involves the use of the Ussing chamber (Ussing and Zerahn, 1951); with this procedure a segment of intestinal mucosa is mounted in a lucite chamber designed to allow control of both electrical and chemical gradients (Fig. 2). This technique is particularly useful for the evaluation of active transport. The measurement of short-circuit current can provide both an indication of epithelial viability and serves as an event marker that confirms the effect of experimental manipulations on the mucosa. A modification of this technique, whereby widely varying voltages are applied across the epithelial surface, has recently been applied to the study of Ca transport (Nellans and Kimberg, 1978). Most of the flux that is voltage-dependent is believed to occur via paracellular routes, while non-voltage-dependent flux is thought to represent transcellular movement. By varying the transepithelial voltage and simultaneously measuring changes in Ca flux, it is possible to estimate the degree of paracellular, or voltage-dependent flux, compared to transcellular or voltage-independent Ca movement. Special modifications of the Ussing chamber have also been devised to evaluate the mucosal uptake of Ca and study the effect of voltage clamping (Nellans and Kimberg, 1978).

More recently, brush border membrane preparations have been utilized for the measurement of Ca uptake (Rasmussen *et al.*, 1979). With this method, Ca uptake is studied across an isolated membrane with both the intravesicular and

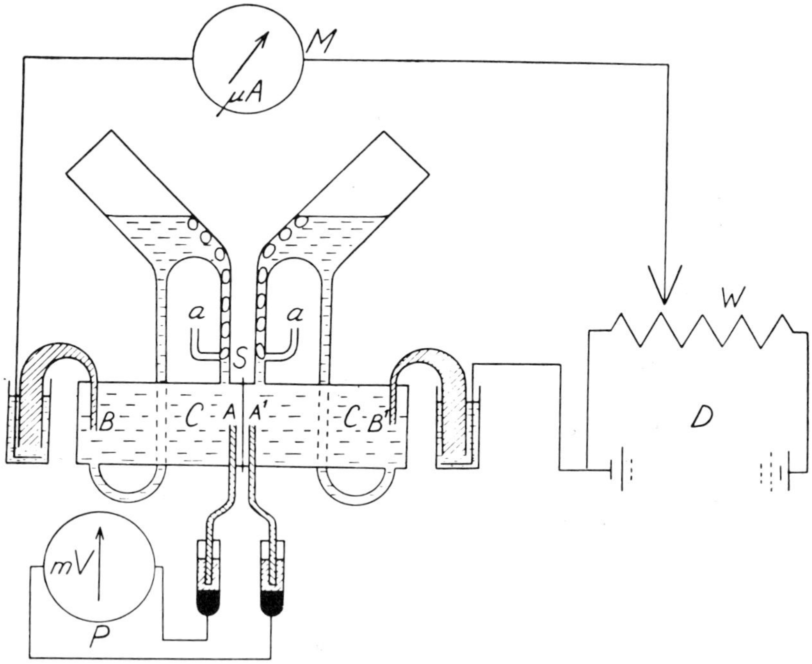

Fig. 2. Diagram of the apparatus utilized for measuring active Ca transport across the intestinal epithelium. With this apparatus, both electrical and chemical gradients can be eliminated. C, the lucite chamber containing bathing solution; S, the epithelial mucosa or other membrane being studied; a, inlets for bubbling the CO_2-O_2; A and A^1, Agar-Ringer bridges which connect the inside and outside solutions, respectively, with electrodes; B and B^1, Agar-Ringer bridges used for applying outside electromotive force; D, battery; W, potential divider; M, microammeter; P, tube potentiometer. (Reproduced from Ussing and Zerahn, 1951, with permission of the publisher.)

extravesicular milieu controlled by the investigator. This method allows assessment of the first step of Ca transport, i.e., the entry of Ca across the brush border membrane. A major problem with this method is a high degree of binding of Ca to the brush border surface and hence difficulty in discerning between Ca transport, per se, and its nonspecific binding (Rasmussen *et al.*, 1979).

III. MECHANISMS OF INTESTINAL CALCIUM TRANSPORT

There are two major means by which nutrients cross the intestinal epithelium: passive diffusion or carrier-mediated transport processes that involve the expenditure of metabolic energy, directly or indirectly. The processes involving direct expenditure of energy may be considered "active transport," while those carrier-mediated processes, which indirectly involve energy expenditure, may be referred to as facilitated diffusion. Furthermore, solutes can cross the epithelial membranes either across the cells (transcellularly) or may move paracellularly through channels between the cells. This discussion will consider the various processes whereby Ca may move across the intestinal epithelium.

A. Passive versus Active Mechanisms of Transepithelial Transport

1. *Transepithelial Passive Diffusion*

Before reviewing the mechanisms whereby Ca moves either through or between the cells across the epithelium, a general discussion of the general forces that operate to produce net Ca movement across the entire epithelial membrane will be presented. Measurements of the transepithelial electrical potential indicate the existence of a potential difference of 5–6 mV, with the blood or serosal (S) surface positive relative to the luminal or mucosal (M) surface (Okada *et al.*, 1975). Calculations, based on this observed potential difference and a Ca concentration of 1.3 m*M* in extracellular fluid, indicate that net passive diffusion will occur from the lumen into the blood only when the luminal concentration exceeds 2 m*M*. The Ca concentration in the intestinal lumen of man can reach 8.5 m*M* following a meal (Fordtran and Locklear, 1966). Thus, it has generally been assumed that absorption occurs primarily by diffusion when the luminal Ca concentration is high; on the other hand, active absorption is assumed to be the predominant mode of Ca transport with Ca concentrations below 2 m*M*.

Indeed, evidence suggests that a certain fraction of Ca transport occurs via simple passive diffusion with another portion transported via carrier-mediated and presumably active transport. Studies of isolated intestinal loops, perfused *in vivo* (Wasserman and Taylor, 1969), and Ca fluxes across the intestine, measured *in vitro* (Walling and Rothman, 1969), are consistent with this concept. With both types of studies, the flux of Ca from either lumen to blood or from the mucosal to serosal (M–S) surface could be defined by an equation with (a) a saturable component that may be defined by Michaelis–Menton kinetics and (b) a diffusional component that can be predicted by the Ussing equation. Further data obtained from *in vitro* transport studies and from radiocalcium studies in humans (Heany *et al.*, 1975) from the perfusion of human jejunum (Ireland and Fordtran, 1973) are consistent with part of Ca flux occurring by simple diffusion, the other by carrier-mediated transport. More recently, attempts have been made to determine the fraction of Ca absorption that occurs via each of these two processes with the use of the Ussing chamber. It is generally considered that paracellular or intercellular transport occurs via simple diffusion, while transcellular transport arises both by a carrier-mediated process and by simple diffusion. In an attempt to distinguish carrier-mediated from passive Ca flux, Nellans and Kimberg

(1978) applied a voltage clamp technique across the rat ileum. With this technique, Ca flux is measured across the epithelium at varying applied transepithelial voltages that produce specific potential differences. The relationship between the change in Ca flux and the voltage applied is then derived. Under these conditions, Nellans and Kimberg (1979a) found that unidirectional Ca flux conforms to a modified Goldman equation (1943), an observation that indicates that a passive relationship exists between the change in Ca flux and the applied electrical gradients. The equation for this is as follows:

$$J_i = J_c i + {}_0J_p i \left[\frac{\chi}{[(\exp(\chi) - 1]} \right]$$

where

$$\chi = \frac{ZF\Delta\Psi ms}{RT}$$

Z = valence of ion, F = Faraday constant, $\Delta\Psi ms$ = potential imposed across the tissue, R = gas constant, T = absolute temperature; J_i = total unidirectional flux of species i, $J_c i$ = a voltage-independent component, and ${}_0J_p i$ = a voltage-dependent component. In this equation, the voltage-independent component, measured by $J_c i$, represents the intercept, while the voltage-dependent portion of Ca flux is indicated by the slope between the net flux and voltage. Nellans and Kimberg (1978) provided extensive evidence for a significant diffusional component of Ca movement across the epithelium of the distal small intestine utilizing this technique. They measured the effects of varying an externally generated voltage from −22 to +22 mV on the flux of ^{45}Ca. When the data were analyzed according to the formula of Frizzell and Schultz (1972), the kinetics of Ca flux appeared to fit the model. However, a surprising finding was the observation that the M–S flux was nearly twice that of the voltage-dependent Ca flux in the serosal to mucosal (S–M) direction with luminal Ca concentrations of 0.05 and 1.25 m*M*. This observation suggested that the applied voltage may also affect Ca movement across the basolateral membrane of the cell and would indicate that the voltage dependent flux includes both cellular and paracellular components. Therefore, the voltage-dependent flux cannot be used entirely as a measure of paracellular flux. In a further attempt to distinguish between paracellular and cellular Ca flux, Nellans and Kimberg (1978) used the same voltage clamp technique to study mucosal uptake of Ca. To measure paracellular flux they used [^{3}H]-labeled polyethyleneglycol (PEG), which distributes only in the extracellular space of the mucosal surface, as a marker. While applying a wide range of voltages, they found that extracellular flux of Ca was approximately 25% of total influx. At a Ca concentration of 1.25 m*M*, the influx from the mucosal surface was equal to total M–S flux, an observation suggesting that little efflux had occurred. Under circumstances when there is little or no efflux, it seems reasonable that the ratio between cellular and paracellular influx is similar to the distribution of total M–S flux; i.e., about 25% of transmural absorption of Ca occurs via the paracellular pathway when a gradient for net diffusion exists. In these studies, Nellans and Kimberg (1978) estimated that less than 10% of the voltage-driven flux of Ca, i.e., the passive flux, would occur through the cells. It should be noted that these observations of transcellular/paracellular movement of Ca were carried out in the ileum, where vitamin D-dependent and presumably carrier-mediated Ca transport is relatively insignificant; it is possible that other segments of the intestine differ with regard to paracellular movement. Thus, there are observations to indicate that transport characteristics of the intestine vary substantially from one portion to another (Walling, 1977a; Lee *et al.*, 1980).

2. *Transepithelial Solvent Drag*

Another mechanism that may be involved in the passive transepithelial movement of Ca is that arising due to "solvent drag." Thus, the flow of water can carry with it solutes that are present in solution if the solutes can permeate either the membrane or porous structure through which the water is moving. Behar and Kerstein (1976) studied the effect of D-glucose on Ca absorption in the duodenum of vitamin D-treated and vitamin D-deficient rats. There was a 15% increase in the lumen to plasma flux of Ca in the D-deficient animals, but there was no augmentation in rats treated with vitamin D. In the ileum, urea and glucose increased the lumen to plasma flux of Ca, while vitamin D did not stimulate Ca transport. They concluded that the active cellular absorption of Ca in the duodenum was independent of glucose or other stimuli for water absorption. On the other hand, they suggested that solvent drag was a major force for Ca absorption in the ileum. A number of studies, which are described below, indicate that the active transport of Ca may be the major means for Ca absorption under certain conditions; on the other hand, solvent drag may be a means for absorption that predominates when a hormonally regulated, cellular-mediated component of transport is not required (i.e., under conditions with low metabolic needs for Ca).

3. *Transepithelial Carrier-Mediated Processes*

Despite evidence that Ca may be absorbed by passive diffusion when the luminal concentrations of Ca are sufficiently high, it is well established that carrier-mediated transport processes contribute significantly to the intestinal absorption of Ca in man and other animal species. Moreover, under circumstances of increased Ca need, such as pregnancy, growth, or lactation, and under circumstances when dietary Ca is markedly reduced, there is evidence that carrier-mediated transport of Ca provides the major mechanism for increasing Ca absorption. Many of the earlier experimental methods precluded an unequivocable interpretation in favor of a carrier-mediated Ca transport process. Thus, early studies which measured the S/M ratios of radiocalcium concentration in everted gut sacs suggested that the uptake of Ca increased and became saturated as the concentration of Ca in the mucosal fluid was increased (Schachter and Rosen, 1959; Rasmussen, 1959; Schachter *et al.*, 1960a,b, 1961). Moreover, it was found that treatment with vitamin D greatly increased Ca uptake, while it was reduced by metabolic inhibitors (Schachter *et al.*, 1960b). These data obtained using everted gut sacs probably indicate the presence of a carrier-mediated process for Ca absorption; however, the results are difficult to analyze in terms of a kinetic model because flux rates were not measured under steady-state conditions but during dynamic distribution of radiocalcium between mucosal and serosal compartments. As has been alluded to above, studies of Ca absorption utilizing intestinal loops, perfused *in situ*, have shown that changes in Ca absorption were linear when perfusate Ca concentrations exceeded 10 m*M* (Nicolayson, 1937a; Dumont *et al.*, 1960; Wasserman and Kallfelz, 1962; Zornitzer and Bronner, 1971). On the other hand, data obtained at lower luminal Ca concentrations demonstrated curvilinear relationships between Ca absorption and luminal Ca concentrations (Wasserman and Kallfelz, 1962; Cramer and Dueck, 1962; Pansu *et al.*, 1981). Similar observations were found *in situ* in the human jejunum during perfusion experiments (Ireland and Fordtran, 1973). In order to show the nonlinear relationship and saturation kinetics, it is necessary to substract the rate of Ca absorption that theoretically could have occurred through simple diffusion from the observed total rates of absorption (Ireland and Fordtran, 1973). The use of such a method might very likely result in the detection of saturation kinetics from data that were previously thought to be linear in an "uncorrected" form, particularly at high luminal Ca concentrations (Nicolayson, 1937a; Dumont *et al.*, 1960; Wasserman and Kallfelz, 1962; Zornitzer and Bronner, 1971).

Data obtained with the Ussing system have provided the most definitive evidence for a carrier-mediated or saturable process for Ca absorption. Although initial studies of Helbock *et al.* (1966) failed to demonstrate saturation kinetics for Ca flux in the rat duodenum, subsequent studies by Walling and Rothman (1969) provided evidence for a carrier-mediated process; M–S Ca flux approached a maximum rate, while the S–M rate increased in proportion to the change in Ca concentration. Kinetic analysis applied to such data suggested an apparent affinity constant with a K_a of 1-2 m*M* (Walling and Rothman, 1968, 1970). It was found that Ca deprivation caused a decrease in the apparent K_a by approximately 50% (Walling and Rothman, 1970). Subsequent studies carried out in the ileum of the adult rat could not demonstrate saturation unless the animal had previously received a low Ca diet (Walling and Kimberg, 1974). Such changes, as will be noted later, probably arose via activation of vitamin D to $1,25(OH)_2D_3$. Differences between the earlier results of Helbock *et al.* (1966) and those of Walling and Rothman (1969) may have arisen because of the wider range of Ca concentrations utilized in the latter study. Subsequent studies with the human jejunum have provided evidence for a saturable process for Ca transport with a K_a of 1.3–5.6 mM. Moreover, Nellans and Kimberg (1978) found that the voltage-independent component of Ca transport across the ileum demonstrated saturation when the Ca concentration exceeded 1 mM; presumably, this voltage-independent flux is transcellular, and these observations suggest that this component of Ca transport is carrier mediated.

There is good evidence that this carrier-mediated process is, in large part, an active process. The development of various procedures that utilize isotopic tracers and the everted intestinal sac technique developed by Wilson and Wiseman (1954) have provided tools for identifying this process. Schachter and colleagues (Schachter and Rosen 1959; Schachter *et al.*, 1960a, 1961; Kimberg *et al.*, 1961) carried out numerous studies measuring the accumulation of radiocalcium from the M–S surface. Fortunately, the transmural potential difference is polarized such that the blood or serosal surface of the gut sac is relatively positive, a situation that should retard the flux of Ca from the M–S surface. This is fortuitous because the effect of the potential difference on Ca flux was not measured when the greater part of this work was done. These studies of Schachter and his colleagues showed that the S–M ratio of ^{45}Ca in the rat intestine was increased by vitamin D treatment, dietary Ca deprivation, and pregnancy. It was also noted that the ^{45}Ca S–M ratios achieved differed from one segment of the intestine to another, with the highest ratios found in the duodenum. The S–M ratios were decreased by vitamin D deficiency, the presence of various metabolic inhibitors, and the addition of other divalent cations. Subsequently, these investigators provided evidence that the S–M ratios for stable ^{40}Ca were the same as those for ^{45}Ca. These comprehensive studies provided strong evidence that the transepithelial transport of Ca must involve an active process. However, the experiments did not rigorously demonstrate the existence of an active process according to the criteria established by Ussing (1949) and by which ion transport is generally evaluated. Subsequently, Asano (1960) and Wasserman *et al.* (1961) measured the unidirectional or bidirectional fluxes of radiolabeled Ca and the potential difference across the membrane; they found the M–S flux of Ca to exceed values predicted for passive diffusion from the Ussing equation (Ussing, 1949).

Subsequent experiments that utilized more sophisticated *in vitro* techniques provided data, which were initially considered contradictory, on the existence of active Ca transport. Helbock *et al.* (1966) studied the transport of Ca across the duodenum of rat using a short-circuit technique (Ussing and Zerahn, 1951) and found that Ca was transported actively only in the presence of inorganic phosphate; they concluded that Ca transfer itself was not an active process. Subsequently, Walling and Rothman (1969), who studied duodena from young rats, observed a steady-state M–S flux of Ca that exceeded the S–M flux even when inorganic phosphate (Pi) was removed. Thus, there was net absorption of Ca against a transmural electrochemical gradient of 3–5 mV (Walling and Rothman, 1968, 1969). Furthermore, the active transport was stimulated by vitamin D or prior low Ca intake. Walling and Rothman could not detect "active" Ca transport in adult rats, observations similar to those of Helbock *et al.* (1966). Earlier observations by Schachter *et al.* (1960a,b) of S–M ratios of ^{45}Ca had shown a reduced Ca uptake with increasing age of the rats. Martin and DeLuca (1969a) also provided evidence for active Ca absorption by the duodenum of growing rats; this transport was abolished by the addition of dinitrophenol or the removal of oxygen, procedures that depress cellular metabolism. A variety of subsequent experiments have provided firm evidence for the existence of an active transport system for Ca in the duodenum of growing rats (Walling and Kimberg, 1975a,b; Walling, 1977a; Walling *et al.*, 1974, 1977a; Favus *et al.*, 1974). Other studies that have evaluated the intestinal response to $1,25(OH)_2D_3$ (Lee *et al.*, 1980), have suggested that the intestine of older rats transported Ca in a manner which suggested such animals were "deficient" in 1,25-dihydroxyvitamin D, with a lesser degree of active Ca transport. Studies utilizing the chick ileum and duodenum have provided evidence for active transport of Ca in this species, as well (Adams and Norman, 1970).

B. Transcellular Transport

A major component of transepithelial Ca transport involves the movement of Ca across the intestinal cell. It is convenient to think of transcellular movement in terms of three steps: (1) the influx of Ca across the brush border membrane into the cell; (2) the movement of Ca across the cell; and finally (3) the extrusion of Ca across the basolateral membrane into the extracellular fluid.

1. Cellular Uptake of Calcium

Considerable interest has focused on the mechanism of Ca entry into the cell, since this is believed to be the rate-limiting step for Ca transport, and there are data to indicate that Ca influx is the process that is stimulated during adaptation, i.e., with intake of a low Ca diet or with administration of vitamin D (O'Donnell and Smith, 1973a; Walling and Rothman, 1973; Martin and DeLuca, 1969a). Because the electrochemical gradients favor the passive movement of Ca into the cell, the clear demonstration of a process that leads to the active uptake of Ca at the brush border membrane of the cell is difficult. Major problems in evaluating the uptake of Ca by the cell relate to methodologic difficulties: thus, radiocalcium uptake by the cell may be affected by (1) nonspecific binding, (2) the diffusional characteristics of "unstirred layers," or (3) trapping in the glycocalyx. Thus, in evaluating results obtained from "short-term," rapid uptake studies, it becomes difficult to separate the component of Ca that is merely bound to the membrane, that component of Ca uptake that diffuses back into the lumen, and that component of Ca uptake that is actually taken up by the cell and transported. There has been considerable disagreement about the appropriate timing for such studies. Studies of Martin and DeLuca (1969a,b) evaluated the rapid intestinal uptake of radiocalcium by gut sacs between 1 and 5 min; on the other hand, Papworth and Patrick (1970) and O'Donnell and Smith (1973b) measured the mucosal uptake of radiocalcium at 5 min and 12 min, respectively. These studies provided data suggesting that the uptake occurring after 1 min was saturable, and the apparent K_t values obtained by each investigator were of similar magnitude. Of interest, these values were similar to the K_t value for M–S flux obtained by Walling and Rothman (1968, 1969, 1970). However, there are data suggesting that the cellular uptake of Ca measured after the first 1–2 min involves processes other than mere Ca influx. Thus, Wasserman *et al.* (1961) were able to detect lumen-to-blood and blood-to-lumen fluxes of ^{47}Ca across the duodenum of chicks and rats within two and one-half min, observations suggesting that "uptake" measured over this time period represents Ca movement out of as well as into the cell. There is compelling evidence that the uptake of other cations, such as sodium, by the brush border of the small intestine begins to decline significantly at times in excess of one minute (Frizzell and Schultz, 1972); this suggests that significant back diffusion can already occur at this early time period. Indeed, the mucosal uptake rates reported by Martin and DeLuca (1969a) were more than forty times the extrapolated transepithelial rate of net Ca flux, a finding which is grossly inconsistent with a rate-limiting function of influx, per se. Walling and Rothman (1973), who preincubated gut sacs in a medium containing Ca, found a linear rate of Ca uptake for 60–80 sec (Fig. 3); moreover, the uptake rate at 1 min was nearly doubled by previous feeding with a low Ca diet. However, at 1 min they could not demonstrate saturation kinetics, while uptake measurements at 3 min did demonstrate saturation kinetics for animals on a low Ca diet (Fig. 4). More recently, Nellans and Kimberg (1978) utilized [^{3}H]polyetheleneglycol to correct for radiocalcium remaining in extracellular fluid and found that uptake of Ca by ileum remained linear for periods up to at least 4 min. Also, the data could be extrapolated to zero at zero time when corrected for extracellular contamination. The kinetics of uptake indicated a K_t of 1.9 mM. They interpreted these data to suggest that trapping of Ca in the media may account for the major portion of the initial rapid uptake (Nellans and Kimberg, 1978).

Rasmussen *et al.* (1979) studied the uptake of radiocalcium by brush border membrane vesicles from the duodenum of vitamin D-deficient chicks. Ca uptake was biphasic, with an initial rapid binding and a slower uptake into an osmotically active space. Prior treatment with 1α-hydroxyvitamin D_3 led to a 2.5- to 5.3-fold increase in the rate of Ca accumulation.

Studies using the lipophilic polyene antibiotic filipin (Wong and Norman, 1975; Adams *et al.*, 1970; Demel and van Deenen, 1965; Norman *et al.*, 1972;

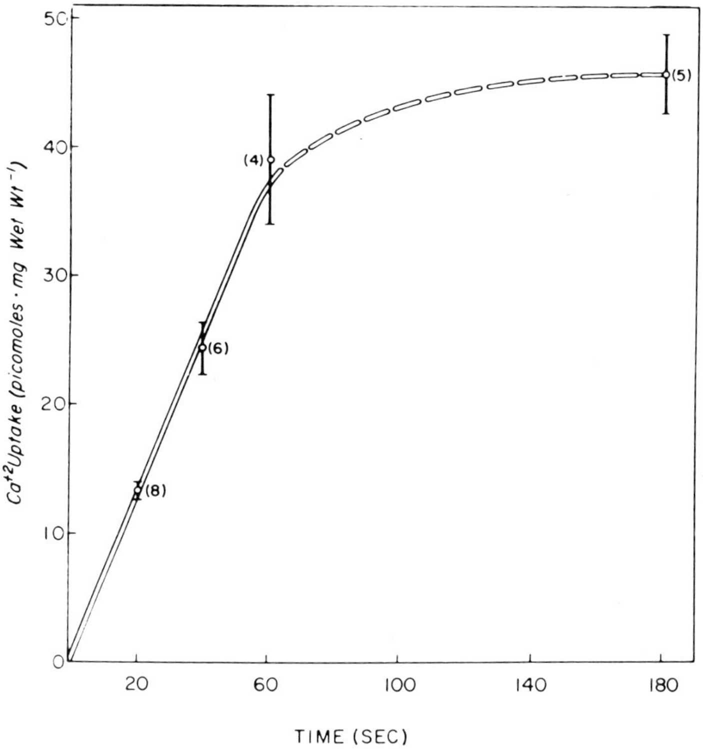

Fig. 3. Duodenal Ca uptake shown in relation to time in normal rats. Ca concentration is 1.25 m*M;* the initial rate was calculated utilizing the least-squares fit. Data are mean ± SE, with the values in parentheses indicating the number of observations. (Reproduced from Walling and Rothman, 1973, with permission of *Am. J. Physiol.)*

Rasmussen *et al.*, 1979) provide evidence that a major effect of vitamin D is to enhance Ca entry into the cell. This antibiotic, when applied to the brush border surface of the ileum of vitamin D-deficient chicks, enhanced the M–S flux of Ca with somewhat less effect on the flux of Ca in the intestine from vitamin D-replete chicks. When the filipin was removed from the media bathing mucosa, the effect was reversed. Also, the effect was rather specific for Ca, as there was no effect of filipin on the fluxes of water, rubidium, sulfate, phosphate, serine, or thiourea.

Thus, it appears that a large component of the initial mucosal uptake of Ca, particularly that occurring within 1 min, represents nonspecific binding; after this time, there is evidence for continued uptake that occurs in part by a carrier-mediated process; moreover, the studies with brush border vesicles (Rasmussen *et al.*, 1979) and the data of Nellans and Kimberg (1979a) suggest that this

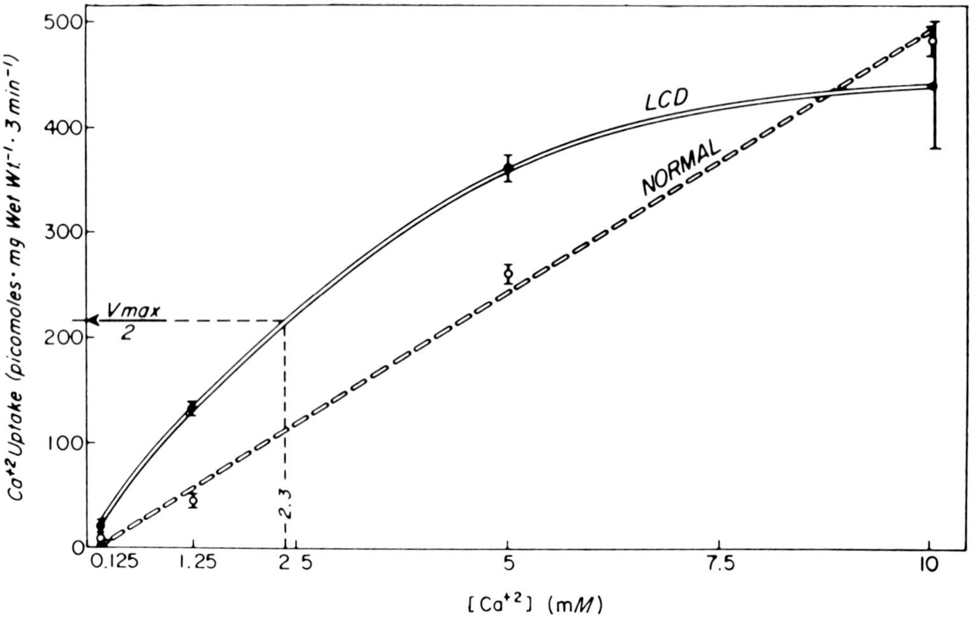

Fig. 4. Relationship between Ca uptake by the everted duodenal gut sac at 3 min and Ca concentration in the bathing media; rats were fed either a normal or a low Ca diet (LCD). The apparent K_t of 2.3 m*M* is extrapolated from $V_{max}/2$. Data are mean ± SE. These data provide evidence for saturation kinetics in the animals fed the low Ca diet (see text). (Reproduced from Walling and Rothman, 1973, with permission of *Am. J. Physiol.)*

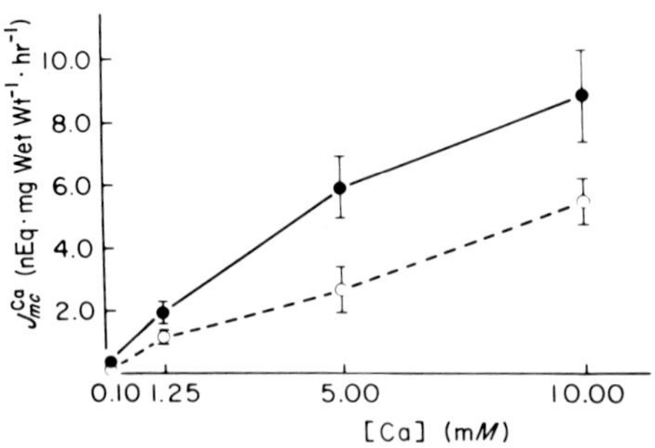

Fig. 5. The relationship between the mucosal influx of Ca, J^{Ca}_{mc} in the ileum, and the concentration of Ca in the bathing medium; the rats received either a low Ca, 0.02%, (●) or high Ca, 2.0%, (○) diet. Each point represents the mean ± SE. There are higher rates of Ca influx in animals fed the low Ca diet. (Reprinted from Nellans and Kimberg, 1978, with permission of *Am. J. Physiol.)*

process may be stimulated by vitamin D or a low calcium diet (Fig. 5) and, hence, may take part in the adaptation process.

2. *Intracellular Movement of Calcium*

For net absorption of Ca to occur, it is apparent that the Ca, which has entered the cell, must move across the cytoplasm to reach the basolateral membrane. While such intracellular movement occurs, the ionized Ca in the cystosolic fluid must be maintained at a very low level to avoid gross distortion of metabolic processes. A number of observations indicate that the Ca in transit is not free but is present in a complexed form and may be sequestered in an intracellular organelle. An electron microscopic study of the rat duodenum indicates that electron-dense granules occur within the microvillus membrane and within mitochondria (Sampson *et al.*, 1970). In vitamin D-deficient rats, such granules were found almost exclusively within the microvillus membrane. Treatment with vitamin D reduced the number of granules in this region and increased their appearance within the mitochondria. Analysis of Ca within the duodenum from both rat and chick utilizing the electron probe has revealed high concentrations of Ca within the goblet cells and in discrete packets along the inner surface of the basolateral membranes (Warner and Coleman, 1975). Vitamin D-dependent calcium-binding protein, discussed below, may participate in the intracellular binding of Ca.

It is well established that there is mitochondrial uptake of Ca, which is enhanced as cytosolic Ca increases (Sampson *et al.*, 1970). However, the role of mitochondrial uptake of Ca in the translocation of Ca across the cell remains uncertain. Mitochondria are unable to accumulate Ca in concentrations believed to exist in the cytosol. Furthermore, increased numbers of mitochondrial granules are absent after the initial period of increased Ca transport. These two facts suggest that mitochondria are not prime movers of Ca across the cell (Bikle *et al.*, 1979).

Other intracellular organelles, such as smooth endoplasmic reticulum and the Golgi apparatus, might also be involved in the compartmentalization of Ca. Freedman *et al.* (1977) provided evidence that the Golgi apparatus may function in the sequestration of Ca; in subcellular fractions of basolateral membranes and the Golgi apparatus, treatment with vitamin D led to a greater initial rate of Ca uptake and a higher equilibrium level. Moreover, the Golgi apparatus exhibited substantially greater uptake than did the basolateral membranes. They suggested that the Golgi apparatus may function by sequestering Ca and keeping it compartamentalized until it is transported across the basolateral membranes and out of the cell. The basolateral membranes are believed to be synthesized by the Golgi apparatus, and the uptake of Ca by the Golgi apparatus may reflect an activity related to a pre-plasma membrane activity rather than by a subcellular compartment. Davis *et al.* (1979) have described a lysosome-like structure, perhaps originating from the Golgi apparatus, which appears to shuttle from the luminal to the basolateral membrane. Thus, the actual means by which Ca is transferred across the intestinal cell is far from being understood.

3. *Extrusion of Calcium from the Cell*

Although Ca may move into the cell down an electrochemical gradient, its extrusion from the cell cytosol into the extracellular fluid must involve active transport against significant chemical and electrical gradients. Thus, the interior of the cell has a potential difference of -50 mV, whereas that in the extracellular fluid is $+5$ mV; moreover, the Ca activity within the cell is probably less than 10^{-5} *M*, whereas that in extracellular fluid is 1.3 m*M*.

Although little is known about the mechanism for active extrusion of Ca from the cell, there is considerable evidence to indicate that this process is stimulated by factors that enhance the movement of Ca into the cell. Also, there are certain enzymes that have been largely localized to the basolateral membrane and that have been implicated in Ca transport. These include calcium-activated and sodium-activated ATPases, which are considered in more detail later. Birge *et al.* (1972) found that ethacrynic acid inhibited both sodium and Ca transport presumably by its inhibition of a specific ATPase. On the other hand, ouabain, which is thought to inhibit sodium transport by blocking sodium-activated ATPase, had no effect on the movement of Ca. Studies of Nellans and Kimberg (1978), who measured ^{45}Ca flux in the ileum with the Ussing method, suggested that a major component of Ca flux was linked to sodium transport. Moreover, the sodium-dependent portion of Ca flux was largely independent of voltage change, i.e., occurred via a transcellular flux, perhaps at the basolateral membrane. Thus, available data suggest the existence of a sodium-dependent component of Ca transport, which probably involves the extrusion of Ca from the cell.

C. Intestinal Calcium Secretion

The luminal surface of the intestine is negatively charged with respect to the serosal surface, resulting in an electrical gradient that favors the movement of Ca from the blood to the lumen. When the Ca content of the fluid within the intestinal lumen is low, there are both concentration and electrical gradients for the net diffusion of Ca into the lumen. Results of metabolic balance studies in man (Steggerda and Mitchell, 1946) and experimental animals (Harris and Innes, 1931; Nicolayson, 1934, 1956; Henry *et al.*, 1960) indicate that the Ca content of the feces may actually exceed that ingested in the diet under certain circumstances; this Ca added to the feces is termed ''endogenous fecal Ca.''

The mechanism whereby Ca is secreted into the intestinal lumen is not entirely clear; it may involve passive diffusion, active secretion, or a combination of both. It has generally been assumed that Ca secretion does not occur by an active process because of the presence of both electrical and chemical gradients, which favor the passive movement of Ca from the blood into the lumen of the small intestine. However, Dumont *et al.* (1960), in a study of Ca flux utilizing the Ussing apparatus, found that the Ca flux from mucosal to serosal surface was lower than predicted when the luminal Ca concentration exceeded 5 m*M*, data indicating active secretion of Ca. They suggested that such secretion may occur by ''exchange diffusion'' via a carrier process. Subsequently, Wasserman and Kallfelz (1962) and Walling and Kimberg (1973, 1974) provided strong evidence that the S–M flux of Ca occurring in the jejunum and ileum of the adult rat and in the duodenum of the chick fulfilled all the criteria for active secretion. Evidence for active secretion is shown in Fig. 6. This process was blocked by various inhibitors of metabolism, i.e., gassing with nitrogen or the addition of iodoacetate, while a low Ca diet increased net Ca absorption without an effect on the

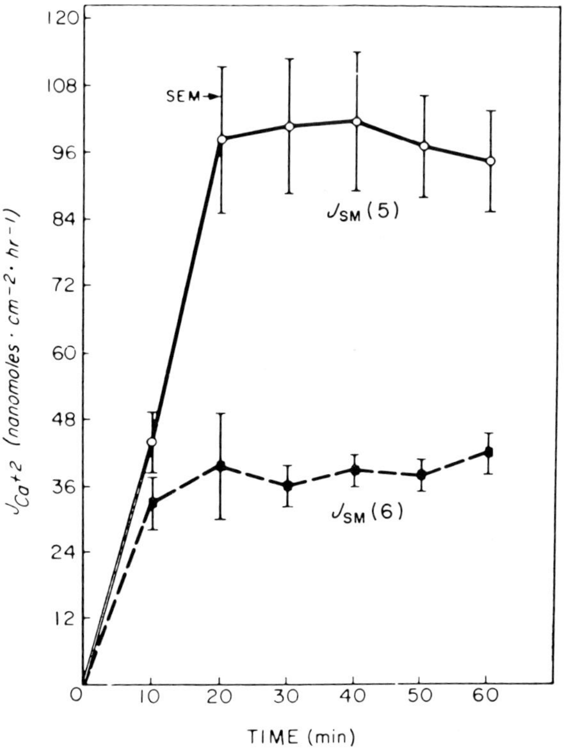

Fig. 6. Steady-state rates of Ca flux across the ileum of the adult rat, studied utilizing a Ca concentration of 1.25 and with the potential difference nulled utilizing a short circuit current; J_{SM} exceeded J_{MS}, $p < 0.001$. These experiments, carried out with the Ussing technique, provide strong evidence for active Ca secretion by the rat ileum. (Reproduced from Walling and Kimberg, 1973, with permission of *Am. J. Physiol.*)

S–M flux. When rats were fed a high Ca diet (2%), active secretion into the lumen occurred, while the ileum from animals fed a low Ca diet had active absorption of Ca. Thus, with changes in dietary Ca, the regulation of the direction of net Ca movement appeared to be achieved by changes in M–S flux rather than through S–M flux. It was concluded that active ileal secretion occured whenever the animal was in a "adequately positive" balance for Ca, while active ileal absorption occurred when there was sufficient metabolic need for Ca. These observations are consistent with earlier studies of Wallace *et al.* (1951), who found that 15% of parenterally administered ^{45}Ca appeared in the feces of young growing rats, whereas 42% of administered ^{45}Ca was lost in the feces of mature rats. It was estimated that the active secretion of Ca by the lower small intestine contributed significantly to the production of "endogenous fecal Ca," and the value calculated from the data of Walling and Kimberg (1974) agreed well with values for endogenous fecal Ca obtained from metabolic balance studies in adult rats (Steggerda and Mitchell, 1946; Henry *et al.*, 1960). In a study with growing male rats fed either 0.05%, 0.5%, or 1.4% Ca diets and utilizing balance techniques and radiocalcium kinetics, Sammon *et al.* (1970) noted progressive increments in endogenous fecal Ca as the dietary Ca was increased; parathyroidectomy led to a small but significant decrease in endogenous fecal Ca.

Although the previously cited data are consistent with an active secretory process for Ca, recent observations of Nellans and Kimberg (1979b) suggest that a net S–M flux of extracellular fluid can occur and lead to the net secretion of Ca by bulk flow. Thus, in studies carried out with the rat ileum under short circuit conditions and with [^{3}H]mannitol as an extracellular marker, there was a net secretory flux of mannitol with S–M flux greater M–S flux. Further, it was suggested that glucose stimulated the transport of sodium from the lumen into the cell, increasing the extrusion of sodium with water from the cell into the paracellular channel. Theoretically, this would increase the hydrostatic pressure in the lateral paracellular space and lead to water movement from the paracellular space into both the serosal and mucosal compartments. The water transported transcellularly into the intercellular space would be free of extracellular fluid markers such as mannitol and PEG; however, water that flowed back into the lumen from the intercellular compartment would carry with it extracellular marker-solutes via solvent-drag. Such an event would lead to a net secretory flux of such molecules. Whether such asymmetric flow of water would cause net secretion of solutes such as sodium and Ca is not clear.

Curiously in the studies by Nellans and Kimberg (1978), glucose failed to stimulate an asymmetrical flux of [^{3}H] PEG (molecular weight, 900) which is believed to be a more precise marker of extracellular fluid than is mannitol. Contrary to their conclusions, this would suggest that glucose-stimulated, asymmetric flow of water may not occur across the tight junction, but rather occurs via an active Ca secretory pump, as was originally proposed by Walling and Kimberg (1973, 1974). Further studies are needed to clarify the exact mechanism of Ca secretion.

D. Calcium-Binding Protein

There are several proteins present in the intestinal mucosa that can specifically bind Ca and that have been implicated as playing a role in intestinal Ca absorption. Under many conditions, the quantities of these Ca-binding proteins correlate closely with various indices of Ca absorption, observations suggesting that they may be intimately involved in the transport of Ca. Wasserman and his co-workers (Wasserman *et al.*, 1968; Taylor and Wasserman, 1967) first identified an intestinal Ca-binding protein (CaBP) in the chick; this protein had a molecular weight of 26,000 and it was induced by vitamin D or feeding a low Ca diet. Greater concentrations were observed in younger animals and larger amounts were present in the duodenum than ileum. Under various conditions with alterations either in the needs for Ca and changes in intestinal Ca absorption, including growth, low Ca diets, egg-laying status in hens, ingestion of a low phosphate diet or excessive strontium and treatment with diphenylhydantoin or cortisone, there were very close correlations between intestinal Ca transport and the intestinal concentrations of CaBP (Bar *et al.*, 1978; Wasserman and Taylor, 1969; Corradino *et al.*, 1971; Corradino, 1977; Feher and Wasserman, 1979; Freund and Bronner, 1975; Morrissey and Wasserman, 1971; Thomasset *et al.*, 1976; Villereale *et al.*, 1974). Such observations provide strong evidence that CaBP is involved in Ca transport.

The Ca-binding proteins identified in several species are substantially different from one species to another; thus, the molecular weight of CaBP in the chick is approximately 28,000, while those in the cow and pig are 9700 and 9000, respectively, and the value in the rat is 13,000. Also, the binding characteristics for Ca^{2+} varies from species to species (Wasserman *et al.*, 1968; Bredderman and Wasserman, 1974; Fullmer and Wasserman, 1973; Fullmer *et al.*, 1977; Dorrington *et al.*, 1974, 1978; Hitchman and Harrison, 1972). Thus, information about the characteristics of CaBP from one species may not necessarily relate to those in another.

Despite the strong association between the rates of Ca transport and the quantities of CaBP found in the intestine, certain discrepancies have been found to exist. It has been shown by Spencer *et al.* (1976) and Morrissey *et al.* (1978) that treatment with $1,25(OH)_2D_3$ stimulated Ca absorption before any increase in CaBP could be detected, but Wasserman (1980) has suggested that highly sensitive methods could disclose an increased CaBP before Ca transport was stimulated by vitamin D therapy. On the other hand, several investigators have shown that the intestinal content of CaBP remains elevated for many hours after intestinal Ca transport has decreased to control levels following a single dose of

$1,25(OH)_2D_3$ (Spencer *et al.*, 1976; Wasserman, 1980). Furthermore, studies by Bikle *et al.* (1978) have shown that treatment with actinomycin D or cycloheximide, which block the synthesis of CaBP, do not inhibit the stimulation of Ca absorption by $1,25(OH)_2D_3$. Further dissociation between CaBP and Ca transport was reported by Ueng *et al.* (1979), who were unable to detect CaBP in suckling rats, which presumably were absorbing Ca. Feher and Wasserman (1979) reported that treatment with vitamin D_3 causes a greater increase in CaBP than did $1,25(OH)_2D_3$, while the effects on intestinal Ca transport were similar. Thus, there are certain data that do not fit with the theory that CaBP is an absolutely essential element in the process of Ca transport.

The localization of intestinal CaBP has been considered to be a key factor for establishing its biological role in Ca transport. Initially, Taylor and Wasserman (1970), utilizing an immunofluorescent technique, found CaBP localized within the goblet cells of the epithelieum and along the microvillar surface of the intestinal epithelial cells. It was suggested that CaBP might be secreted by the goblet cells with subsequent localization along the external surface of the epithelial cells (Wasserman and Taylor, 1973). Subsequently, more refined techniques have localized CaBP to the cytoplasm and nuclei of absorptive cells, and none could be found in goblet cells (Arnold *et al.*, 1976; Morrissey *et al.*, 1978a,b). Moreover, it has been suggested that the intracellular accumulation of CaBP may lead to greater binding of Ca during its transcellular movement, thereby preventing the accumulation of or the extrusion of free Ca^{2+} (Bikle *et al.*, 1979). Other studies (Bronner *et al.*, 1976) indicate that the level of CaBP may be depressed as Ca transport increases, and it was suggested that there may be a feedback relationship between the quantity of CaBP and the intracellular Ca concentration.

Thus, considerable evidence indicates a strong relationship between the quantity of various Ca-binding proteins in the intestinal mucosa and the intestinal transport of Ca. In many instances, these proteins are stimulated by vitamin D and are augmented with increased Ca needs when the endogenous synthesis of $1,25(OH)_2D_3$ would most likely be increased. Nonetheless, the mechanism whereby Ca-binding protein participates in increased Ca transport, particularly in relation to that stimulated by vitamin D, is uncertain.

Kowarski and Schachter (1975) have described a very large complex molecule, molecular weight of 0.5–1 million, in the brush border of the rat intestine; they described this as a "calcium binding complex." The presence of this complex protein correlated well with the activities of Ca transport by various parts of the intestine and with alterations in Ca transport produced by vitamin D treatment and with changes in diet, and age. They suggested that this calcium-binding complex might facilitate the passage of Ca across the brush border membrane into the cell. Evidence for this was provided by observations that preparations of calcium-binding complex, which were loaded with ^{45}Ca and then incubated with a CaBP soluble preparation led to transfer of ^{45}Ca from the particulate calcium-binding complex to the soluble CaBP (Schachter and Kowarski, 1980).

Finally, several other proteins with Ca-binding characteristics have been described; thus, Wilson and Lawson (1977) found two proteins of molecular weight 45,000 and 86,000, which appeared in the intestinal mucosa with a time course following the administration of vitamin D and just preceding an increase in Ca transport. On the basis of this temporal association, this protein, which localized in the brush border membrane, was thought to be a factor that increased the permeability of the mucosal cells to Ca. Finally, Miller *et al.* (1979) identified a vitamin D-dependent, Ca-binding protein that localized to the brush border membrane. Further studies with these proteins will be needed to clarify their role in Ca transport.

E. Intestinal ATPase, Alkaline Phosphatases, and Other Proteins

It has also been found that several other intestinal mucosal enzymes, primarily adenosine triphosphatase (ATPase) and alkaline phosphatase, may participate in Ca absorption, particularly that which is stimulated by vitamin D. Thus, Martin *et al.* (1969) and Melancon and DeLuca (1970) identified a vitamin D-stimulated, calcium-dependent ATPase, which was localized in the brush border of both rat and chick and which showed a correlation with Ca transport. Norman *et al.* (1970) suggested that the alkaline phosphatase present in the brush border may participate in Ca absorption. They found that the levels of both alkaline phosphate and calcium-activated ATPase in the brush border were increased by vitamin D, and that the time courses for the appearances of increased enzyme activities and increases in intestinal Ca absorption were similar. Haussler *et al.* (1970) reported a similarity between the alkaline phosphatase and Ca-activated ATPase, and suggested that brush border alkaline phosphatase was directly involved in Ca transport. By coincidence, the K_m for ATPase is very close to the previously determined K_t for Ca absorption by rat duodenum (Walling and Rothman, 1969; 1970); also, Mircheff *et al.* (1977) showed a strong correlation between Ca activated ATPase and Ca absorption by the rat duodenum and ileum. They compared the localization of ATPase in brush border membrane with that in basolateral membrane; the activity of Ca-activated ATPase was greater in the basolateral membrane than in the brush border membrane, while the reverse was true for alkaline phosphatase. Treatment with $1,25(OH)_2D_3$ increased Ca-activated ATPase two-fold and alkaline phosphatase was increased to a similar degree; nonetheless, the differential distribution of the enzymes in the basolateral and brush-border membranes was preserved. Such differences in distribution of alkaline phosphatase and Ca-activated ATPase between the brush border membrane and the basolateral membrane suggest that the activities of the two enzymes do not entirely reside in the same molecule. In the study by Mircheff *et al.* (1977), the degree of stimulation of Ca-activated ATPase was more than 100-fold greater than was the rate of net Ca absorption. The reason for this apparent discrepancy in rate of Ca transport compared to the change in enzymatic activity is unknown; it might relate to the Ca activity utilized in the assay of ATPase. On the other hand, Holdsworth (1970) presented evidence that alkaline phosphatase may not function in Ca transport. He demonstrated that vitamin D caused an equal increase in the activities of Ca-activated ATPase, *P*-nitrophenylphenol phosphatase, and pyrophosphatase activity in the brush border of chick intestine; however, the addition of a specific inhibitor of alkaline phosphatase inhibited all three activities, but had no effect on intestinal Ca transport.

The role of calcium-stimulated ATPase in Ca transport is also unclear. Clearly, this enzyme is not totally vitamin D-dependent and it can be present in the intestine of vitamin D-deficient animals (Martin *et al.*, 1969; Melancon and DeLuca, 1970; Norman *et al.*, 1970; Holdsworth, 1970; Haussler *et al.*, 1970; Mircheff *et al.*, 1977). Moreover, its activity may be stimulated by parathyroid hormone (Birge and Gilbert, 1974). The activity but not necessarily the synthesis of this enzyme might be stimulated by vitamin D in a manner that parallels changes in active Ca absorption. Further clarification of the role of these enzymes in Ca transport is needed.

Other proteins and molecular alterations in the intestine appear in response to vitamin D, the major stimulus to Ca absorption: they include a 42,000 molecular weight brush-border protein, which is similar to actin (Wilson and Lawson, 1978); increased activity of cAMP (Corradino, 1974; Wasserman *et al.*, 1977); increases in the activity of adenylate-cyclase (Corradino, 1974; Neville and Holdsworth, 1969); and an alteration in certain phospholipid components (Max *et al.*, 1978).

F. Effect of Other Ions

1. *Sodium*

One factor studied in relationship to Ca transport across the intestinal epithelium has been the role of sodium. Initial studies by Schachter *et al.* (1960a), Wasserman and Taylor (1963), and Harrison and Harrison (1963), which utilized the gut sac uptake technique in the duodenum, suggested that sodium was not required for Ca uptake. However, subsequent studies by Martin and DeLuca (1969b) indicated a dependence of Ca uptake upon the presence of sodium. The apparent discrepancy is related to the buffer used, with potassium phosphate employed in the earlier studies, while Martin and DeLuca used choline chloride buffer. Moreover, Martin and DeLuca found no sodium dependence when they employed a potassium phosphate buffer.

The mechanism whereby sodium may influence Ca transport is uncertain. Studies of cellular uptake of Ca have shown that the substitution of mannitol for sodium led to a substantial increase in Ca uptake (Barry and Eggenton, 1972). However, this procedure results in a decrease in intracellular potential difference and Ca uptake was not increased when choline chloride was substituted. Thus, the initial entry of Ca into the cell was not directly affected by sodium, and Martin and DeLuca (1969b) concluded that sodium is required for the transfer of Ca into the blood across the basolateral membrane of the cell. The inhibition of sodium transport by ethacrynic acid was found to inhibit Ca transport as well; on the other hand, inhibition of Na transport with ouabain had no effect on Ca (Birge *et al.*, 1972). With studies carried out using the Ussing system, Nellans and Kimberg (1978) evaluated fluxes of ^{45}Ca in the total absence of sodium using choline chloride or other sodium-free buffers as a replacement. Their data suggested that both the M–S and S–M fluxes had components that were inhibited by sodium removal. Voltage clamp analysis indicated that the fluxes independent of voltage change, i.e., the transcellular fluxes, were inhibited by the removal of sodium. On the other hand, the fluxes considered to be paracellular were increased concomitant with the marked decrease in conductance. Thus, available data provide evidence for a component of Ca transport, probably involving Ca extrusion from the cell, which is dependent upon sodium; whether situations ever exist *in vivo* where sodium fluxes are ever reduced to a degree that Ca transport may be inhibited is unknown.

2. *Magnesium*

A number of studies in man and several animal species suggest that Ca and magnesium (Mg) may compete for a common absorptive mechanism, and changes in the Mg content of the diet may affect Ca absorption. Utilizing balance techniques, Alcock and MacIntyre (1962, 1964) found that feeding a diet low in Mg to rats caused Ca absorption to increase; also, refeeding magnesium-depleted rats with a normal dietary Mg led to a decrease in Ca absorption. *In vitro* studies also suggest an interaction between the transport of Ca and that of Mg; thus, Schachter and Rosen (1959), Hendrix *et al.* (1963), and O'Donnell and Smith (1973b) found that Mg inhibited the uptake or transport of Ca by the duodenum of rats. Moreover, Brannan *et al.* (1976) found a decrease in Ca absorption, measured *in situ,* by the jejunum of humans when they increased the Mg concentration.

In contrast to these data, other observations are inconsistent with a competitive mechanism for the absorption of Ca and Mg. Thus, metabolic balance studies of Clark (1968), Miller *et al.* (1965), and Heaton and Parsons (1961) revealed that an increase in dietary Mg was associated with either augmented or unchanged Ca absorption in studies in rats, pigs, and man. In recent studies, Levine *et al.* (1980) studied the effect of varying Mg intake in vitamin D-deficient rats, and found marked inhibition of Ca absorption when dietary Mg intake was increased.

However, the administration of $1,25(OH)_2D_3$ led to nearly equal increments in Ca absorption independent of the dietary Mg content. They suggested that a high Mg intake can affect a Ca transport process that was independent of vitamin D, perhaps occurring via the paracellular pathway. The vitamin D-dependent transport of Ca, occurring primarily transcellularly, was little affected by changes in dietary Mg.

The effect of Mg-deficiency, per se, on intestinal Ca absorption has received attention primarily because of the marked hypocalcemia that occurs during Mg-depletion. The data of Morehead and Kessner (1969) and Walling *et al.* (1975) in the rat and studies by Reddy *et al.* (1973) in the chick provide evidence for enhanced intestinal transport of Ca during Mg-depletion. In the studies carried out in rats, the effect of low Mg diet on Ca transport was abolished by parathyroidectomy (Morehead and Kessner, 1969; Walling *et al.*, 1975); this finding is of interest since in many species other than the rat, Mg depletion leads to inhibition of PTH release. Preliminary data on vitamin D metabolism failed to provide evidence for altered vitamin D metabolism during Mg depletion (Coburn *et al.*, 1973c).

3. *Phosphate*

The specific interactions between the intestinal transport of Ca and that of phosphate are considered elsewhere (Chapter 1, this volume). The active trans-

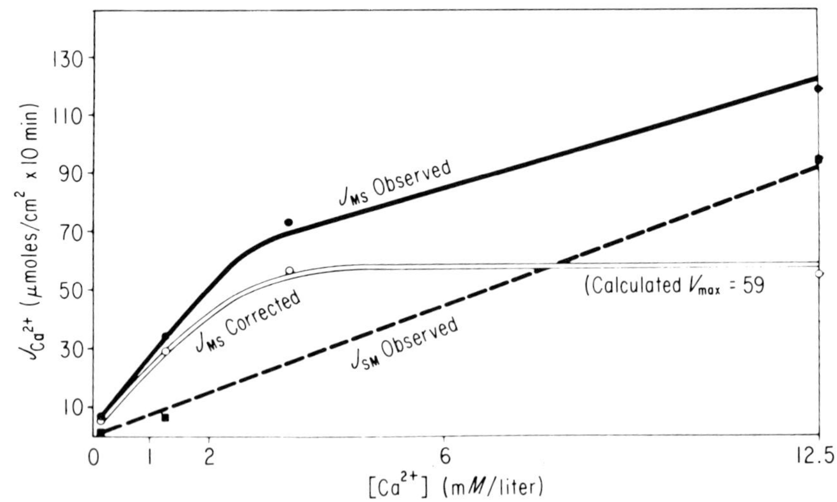

Fig. 7. Relationship between mucosal-to-serosal (MS) and serosal-to-mucosal (SM) fluxes of Ca (J_{Ca}) and the Ca concentration in the bathing media which was free of phosphate. The data demonstrate saturation of the J_{MS} for Ca in animals fed a low Ca diet. The V_{max} was calculated using a Lineweaver-Burke plot. The MS Ca flux was corrected for diffusion by subtracting $0.68 \times J_{SM}$ at each Ca concentration. (Reproduced from Walling and Rothman, 1969, with permission of *Am. J. Physiol.*)

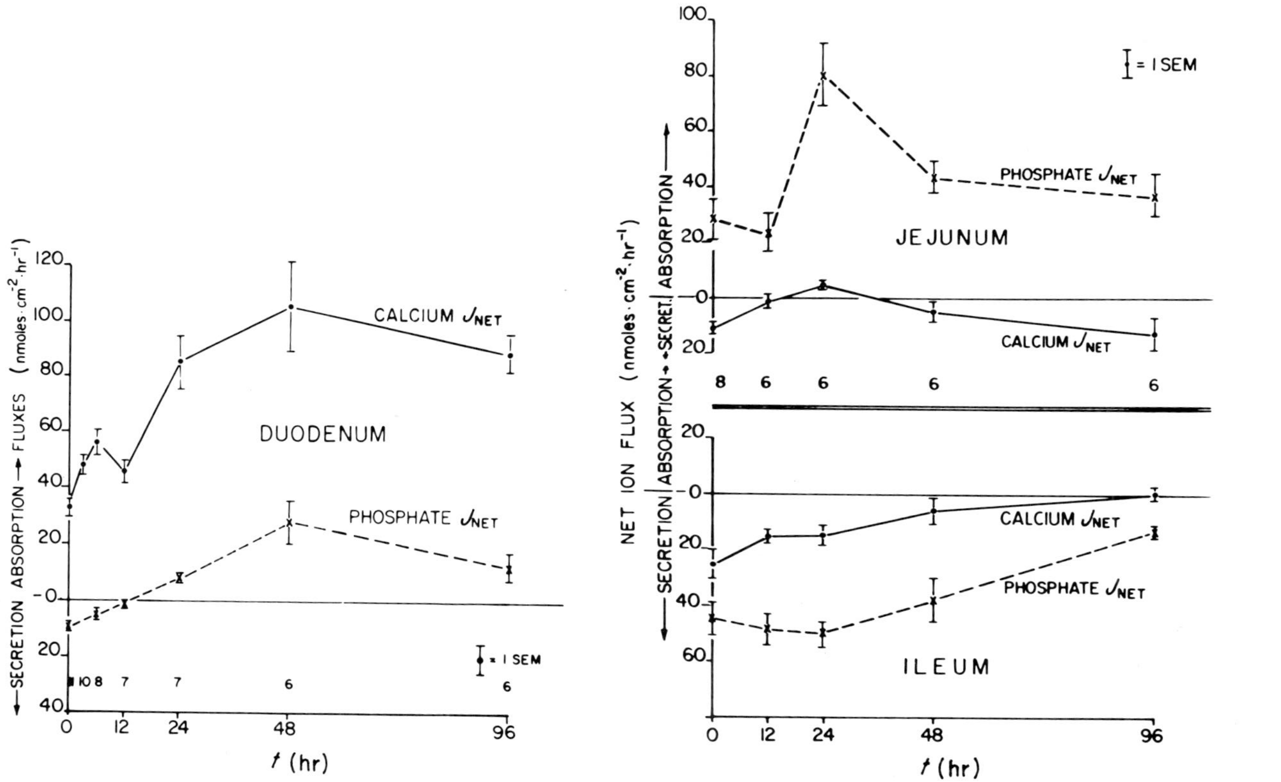

Fig. 8. The time course of the effects of a single dose of $1,25(OH)_2D_3$, 405 ng on the active transport of Ca and phosphate across various segments of the small intestine from a vitamin D-deficient rat; see text. The animals were vitamin D-deficient and the time is that between *in vivo* dosing and the measure of Ca transport. (Adapted from Walling, 1977a, with permission of *Arch. Biochem. Biophys.*)

port of both Ca and phosphate are stimulated by vitamin D, and it was suggested that the two may be absorbed by a co-transport process, with phosphate transport primary and that for Ca secondary (Helbock *et al.*, 1966). Birge and Miller (1977) suggested that 1,25$(OH)_2D_3$ may act to enhance the transport of phosphate, which in turn leads to increased in Ca absorption. Other data provide strong evidence that Ca and phosphate transport occur independent of each other. Thus, the removal of sodium from the incubation media causes substantial inhibition of phosphate transport without any effect on Ca (Harrison and Harrison, 1963). Walling and Rothman (1968, 1969) provided evidence for active Ca transport by the duodenum when phosphate is absent (Fig. 7). It has also been shown that different segments of the intestine have a predominance of transport of either Ca or phosphate; phosphate transport is greater in the jejunum, while Ca transport is greater in the duodenum and ileum (Fig. 8). Ferraro *et al.* (1976), using the ligated loop technique, showed a clear separation between the absorption of Ca and phosphate, providing further evidence that the intestinal transport of Ca and phosphate occurs via different mechanisms. Studies in the ascending colon indicate the existence of active transport for Ca that is stimulated by vitamin D, while there is no effect on phosphate transport (Lee *et al.*, 1980). The mechanisms whereby vitamin D acts independently to stimulate the transport of Ca and phosphate is uncertain. It was suggested (Walling, 1977b; Walling and Lee, 1979) that certain epithelial cells predominantly act to transport Ca, while others act predominantly to transport phosphate; the mechanisms whereby this may occur are unknown.

The effect of dietary phosphate restriction and phosphate depletion on intestinal Ca absorption have been subjects of considerable interest. There may be effects on Ca absorption that are due to changes in vitamin D metabolism (Tanaka and DeLuca, 1973), and there may be specific effects of phosphate depletion, per se; these are considered in detail elsewhere (Chapter 7, this volume; Chapter 6, Vol. III).

IV. HORMONAL EFFECTS ON CALCIUM ABSORPTION

A. Vitamin D

A review of the metabolism of vitamin D and its actions on various target tissues are presented in Chapter 7, this volume; however, a brief consideration of vitamin D is needed for the consideration of intestinal Ca absorption and disorders related to abnormal Ca absorption. There is overwhelming evidence that 1,25$(OH)_2D_3$, the natural hormonal form of vitamin D, is the most potent stimulus to intestinal Ca absorption. Also, there is evidence that adaptive processes for increasing Ca absorption involve enhanced bioconversion of vitamin

D_3 to its more active forms. In Chapter 7 there is a detailed discussion of the metabolism and mode of action of vitamin D. This chapter will review the mechanism whereby vitamin D enhances Ca transport across the intestine.

The evidence that vitamin D enhances intestinal Ca absorption is extensive: Nicolaysen (1937a,b) showed that net intestinal absorption of Ca by isolated small intestinal loops was enhanced by vitamin D. Furthermore, Liu *et al.* (1940) reported enhanced net absorption of Ca in humans given vitamin D. Subsequently, Schachter and Rosen (1959) and Harrison and Harrison (1960) provided evidence that the Ca transport stimulated by vitamin D is an active, carrier-mediated process. Thus, Schachter and Rosen (1959) showed that the vitamin D-stimulated uptake of ^{45}Ca by the everted gut sac resulted in an S/M ratio greater than 1.0, an observation suggesting active transport.

Studies in several species have provided data localizing the effect of vitamin D and $1,25(OH)_2D_3$ on various segments of the intestine. In the rat, hamster, rabbit, and guinea pig, vitamin D stimulates active Ca absorption to the greatest degree in the duodenum (Schacter and Rosen, 1959; Schacter *et al.*, 1960a, 1961; Harrison and Harrison, 1965). On the other hand, the vitamin D stimulation of phosphate absorption was greatest in the jejunum of rats and chicks (Freedman *et al.*, 1977). Favus *et al.* (1980) have shown that $1,25(OH)_2D_3$ can enhance active Ca absorption across descending colon by increasing mucosal to serosal flux. Studies evaluating the dose-response of different intestinal segments to $1,25(OH)_2D_3$ disclosed that the duodenum was the most responsive with the ileum the next most sensitive; the colon responded next after the ileum, and the jejunum was the most resistant (Lee *et al.*, 1980). Thus, it was suggested that the increased net Ca absorption produced by progressively larger quantities of $1,25(OH)_2D_3$ may occur via "recruiting" additional segments of the intestine rather than by increasing Ca absorption in a dose-dependent way throughout the gut (Lee *et al.*, 1980).

The mechanisms whereby vitamin D stimulates intestinal Ca absorption has been a subject of considerable interest. It has been shown that vitamin D can stimulate the oxygen-dependent component of Ca transport, and Sallis and Holdsworth (1962) showed that vitamin D can stimulate glycolysis in the chick. Evidence that vitamin D acts by inducing the synthesis of several proteins is reviewed in Chapter 4. As already discussed, the intestinal mucosal proteins that are stimulated by vitamin D include one or more Ca binding proteins, alkaline phosphatase, a Ca-activated ATPase, and a large molecular weight complex present in the brush border (Schachter and Kowarski, 1980). There may be two mechanisms whereby vitamin D stimulates Ca transport, one involving synthesis of new proteins and the other may involve a membrane effect of $1,25(OH)_2D_3$ to alter cell permeability.

Considerable data suggest that vitamin D acts to stimulate Ca entry into the cell. This possible mode of action of vitamin D has been strengthened by the

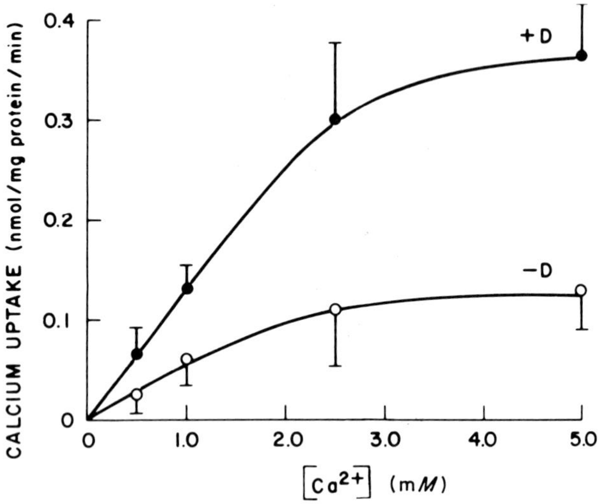

Fig. 9. Uptake of radiocalcium by brush-border membrane vesicles prepared from the duodenum of vitamin D-deficient chicks, which received 1α-hydroxyvitamin D_3, 1 μg (+D) or vehicle (−D) 6–18 hr before preparing the vesicles. (Reproduced from Rasmussen *et al.*, 1979, with permission from *J. Biol. Chem.*)

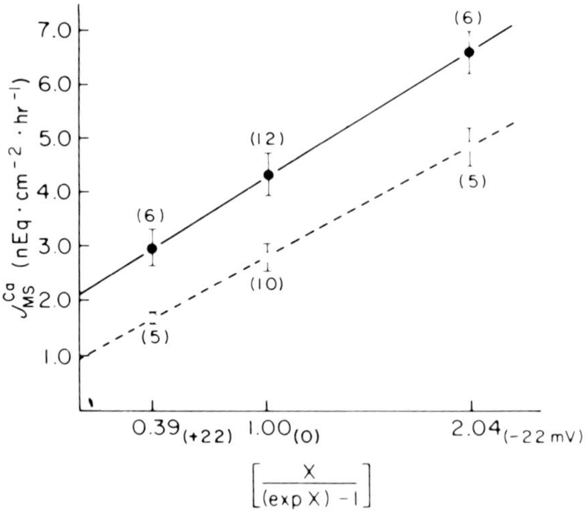

Fig. 10. The relationship between ileal Ca flux from mucosa to serosa of the rat ileum, J_{MS}^{Ca}, and potential difference, indicated by the expression $[\chi/(\exp \chi) - 1]$, where χ = ZF $(\Delta\Psi_{ms})$/RT. The lines are mean values of least-squares fit to individual experiments. The number of tissues studied is indicated in parentheses with mean ± SE at each point for rats fed a low calcium diet (●) or high calcium diet (○). Treating the animals with the low Ca diet raised the intercept, or the voltage-independent component of Ca transport, with no effect on slope or the voltage-dependent portion of Ca flux. The voltage-independent component of Ca transport is thought to represent primarily transcellular movement of Ca. See text for details. (Reproduced from Nellans and Kimberg, 1979b, with permission of *Am. J. Physiol.*)

observation of Rasmussen *et al.* (1979) that 1α-hydroxyvitamin D_3 produced a 2.5- to 5.3-fold increase in Ca accumulation by vesicles prepared from intestinal brush border membranes (Fig. 9). Also, pretreatment of these chicks with cycloheximide, an inhibitor of protein synthesis, did not block the Ca uptake stimulated by $1,25(OH)_2D_3$. Moreover, in intestinal brush border membranes from vitamin D-deficient chicks, two other compounds, the lipophilic polyene antibiotic, filipin, and a Ca ionophore, were both reported to stimulate Ca uptake.

The possibility that vitamin D may act on the diffusional or paracellular pathway of Ca absorption has also received consideration. Studies by Harrison

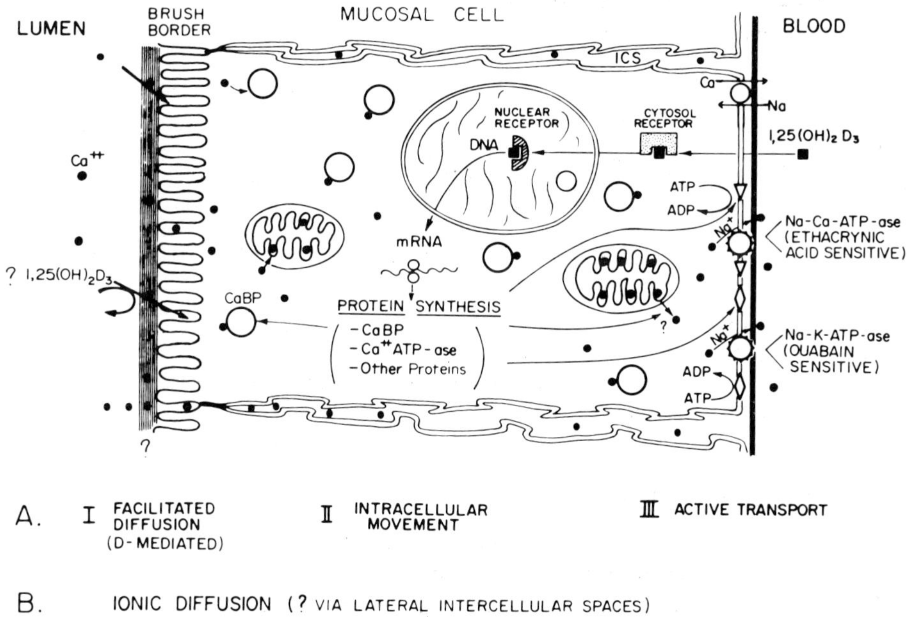

Fig. 11. A schematic model of proposed events believed to occur with vitamin D-stimulated transport of calcium across the intestinal epithelium. After it is transported from the blood, $1,25(OH)_2D_3$ is bound to a specific cytosolic receptor; the receptor-$1,25(OH)_2D_3$ complex is then transferred to a nuclear receptor, and there is increased formation of messenger RNA (mRNA). Synthesis of new proteins then occurs, including a specific vitamin D-dependent calcium-binding protein (CaBP), a calcium-activated ATPase, and perhaps others. Most data suggest that $1,25(OH)_2D_3$ stimulates the entry of calcium into the cell at the mucosal surface, probably through a carrier-mediated process although the carrier has not been identified. Other data suggest that $1,25(OH)_2D_3$ may have a direct effect on the brush border membrane to enhance the permeability. Once calcium enters the cell, its transcellular movement may involve binding to CaBP or being taken up by mitochondria. At the basolateral surface, calcium is actively extruded from the cell, probably via one or more ATPases. When there is a high luminal content of calcium, there also may be transport due to simple diffusion or by solvent drag via the lateral intercellular spaces. (Modified from Coburn *et al.*, 1977.)

and Harrison (1965) and by Wasserman and Kallfelz (1962) suggested that vitamin D increases the overall mucosal permeability to Ca. Subsequent data (M.W. Walling, unpublished) showed an increase in the conductance and short circuit current of the intestine of chicks given a supraphysiologic dose of 1,25$(OH)_2D_3$; however, no such effect could be identified in the rat, suggesting there may be a species difference. Moreover, the effect of 1,25$(OH)_2D_3$ on the rat intestine is due entirely to an increase the M–S flux with no effect on S–M movement. Younoszai *et al.* (1973) concluded that vitamin D increased only the lumen-to-plasma flux of Ca, while the plasma-to-lumen flux was unaffected. Moreover, Nellans and Kimberg (1978) studied the effect of a low Ca diet which presumably increases the synthesis of 1,25$(OH)_2D_3$, on voltage-dependent and -independent Ca flux across the ileum; the voltage-independent, or transcellular, Ca flux rather than voltage-dependent, or paracellular, flux was enhanced by the low Ca diet (Fig. 10). The details of these studies are reviewed above in the section on carrier-mediated transport processes.

Thus, available data indicate that vitamin D, or more appropriately 1,25$(OH)_2D_3$, is the most potent known hormone to enhance intestinal Ca absorption; it acts to increase an active component of Ca transport and probably does this by enhancing Ca entry into the cell. Whether it does this entirely by increasing the synthesis of new proteins or also by acting directly on the mucosal membrane to increase permeability or both has not been resolved. A schematic representation of the mechanisms whereby vitamin D might stimulate Ca transport is shown in Fig. 11.

B. Parathyroid Hormone

One of the most controversial peptide hormones with regard to having an effect on the intestine is parathyroid hormone (PTH). There are numerous reports showing increased Ca absorption in hyperparathyroid states and diminished absorption following parathyroidectomy (Rasmussen, 1959; Sammon *et al.*, 1970; Peacock, 1975). However, very few studies have shown a direct effect of PTH on intestinal epithelial cells. Thus, PTH has a potent effect to stimulate adenylate cyclase in the kidney with enhanced production of cyclic AMP; however, it does not appear to affect either parameter in the gut (Kimberg *et al.*, 1971; Walling 1978). Thus, the only direct action of PTH on intestinal epithelial cells has been to increase the activity of lysozymal enzymes (Nemere, 1979). All other changes in intestinal Ca and phosphate absorption that occur in relationship to changes in PTH may be related to altered generation of 1,25$(OH)_2D_3$, as discussed in Chapter 7.

The occasional results of an apparent increase in intestinal Ca absorption following the administration of PTH could arise due to the animals' being in a state of only partial vitamin D deficiency. Thus, some residual vitamin D might undergo conversion of 1,25$(OH)_2D_3$ (Toverud, 1964).

C. Thyroid Hormones

Clinical observations of a high incidence of skeletal disease (Golden and Abbot, 1933) and augmented fecal losses of Ca in patients with hyperthyroidism (Krane *et al.*, 1956; Gennari, 1964) prompted studies regarding the effect of thyroid hormone on intestinal absorption of Ca. In animals, Noble and Matty (1967) found that the administration of large doses of thyroxin to 200-gm rats caused a depression in the M–S flux of Ca and P in the duodenum; however, there was no overall effect on the mucosal uptake of Ca. Utilizing intragastric administration of ^{45}Ca, Williams *et al.* (1967) found decreased net and "true" absorption of ^{47}Ca in animals treated with triiodothyronine compared to controls. Moreover, Friedland *et al.* (1965) gave either triiodothyronine or thyrotropin for 7, 14, and 28 days to weanling rats; they found diminished S–M uptake of ^{45}Ca by the duodenum after treatment with either hormone regardless of the duration of treatment. In contrast to these findings, Krawitt (1967b) found that thyroxin had no effect on Ca absorption in intestinal loops perfused *in vivo;* however, these studies were in adult rats, with lower active transport than may have existed in the previously described studies utilizing young rats. It is not known whether the effect of thyroxin on intestinal Ca absorption is direct or indirect through altered vitamin D metabolism.

D. Pituitary Hormones

The absence or excess of several pituitary hormones may alter Ca absorption (see Chapter 9, this volume). Certain of these hormones may affect intestinal Ca absorption indirectly via an effect on the conversion of vitamin D to its hormonally active form or they could have a direct effect. It is known that prior hypophysectomy causes a reduction in the Ca transport by everted gut sacs from the rat duodenum (Finkelstein and Schacter, 1962; Kimberg *et al.*, 1961). Moreover, this inhibition of Ca transport can be partially corrected by treatment with either growth hormone or prolactin (Kimberg *et al.*, 1961; Spanos *et al.*, 1978). On the other hand, other pituitary hormones, including follicle-stimulating hormone, luteinizing hormone, adrenocorticotropic hormone, and thyrotropin had no effect. Subsequently, it has been shown that both growth hormone and prolactin can increase the plasma level of $1,25(OH)_2D$ (Spanos *et al.*, 1978; Spencer and Tobiassen, 1977), which may account for the increase in Ca absorption. It should be noted that hypophysectomy did not interfere with the adaptation to a low Ca diet (Kimberg *et al.*, 1961), an observation indicating that the absence of growth hormone or prolactin may not completely inhibit the adaptive change in vitamin D metabolism. Others (Krawitt *et al.*, 1977) could find no effect of hypophysectomy on intestinal Ca absorption, and it was suggested that the effects observed by others may have been due to changes in the mucosal weight of the intestine after hypophysectomy. On the other hand, Krawitt *et al.* fed their animals a high Ca diet, a factor which could have suppressed intestinal Ca absorption in hypophysectomized and control animals.

It has been shown that prolactin can stimulate the generation of $1,25(OH)_2D$, which could account for increased Ca absorption during lactation (Kumar *et al.*, 1979b).

E. Calcitonin (Thyrocalcitonin)

Initial studies in rats (Bronner *et al.*, 1967; Krawitt 1967a; Cramer *et al.*, 1969; Cramer, 1973) showed no effect of various preparations of calcitonin on the intestinal absorption of Ca. Subsequently, studies by Gray *et al.* (1973) showed a major effect of calcitonin to enhance the permeability of the jejunum, causing increased secretion of sodium and other electrolytes in normal man; however, there was no effect on Ca absorption. Olson *et al.* (1972) reported that low doses of calcitonin decreased luminal-to-plasma movement of ^{45}Ca in the *in situ* perfused intestine of vitamin D-replete rats, while high doses increased the flux of ^{45}Ca. They did not determine whether this was related to a change in permeability or an overall change in active sodium transport. Subsequently, *in vitro* studies carried out in the rat ileum demonstrated that calcitonin decreased the absorption of sodium while net chloride secretion occurred and short circuit current rose (Walling *et al.*, 1977b). There was an increase in the bidirectional flux of Ca, but net Ca movement did not occur. These effects on the intestinal mucosa were similar to those occurring with activation of adenylate cyclase; however, intestinal cyclic AMP did not change. Subsequent studies in human jejunum (Juan *et al.*, 1976) not only demonstrated the previously reported net secretory effect of calcitonin but also showed reduced absorption of Ca and phosphate. The discrepancy between the results of this study and the earlier experiment in humans may have arisen because the Ca concentration in the perfusate was 1.25 m*M* compared to 5 m*M* in the earlier study (Gray *et al.*, 1973). Thus, available data suggest that calcitonin may have considerable affect on overall electrolyte transport; if there is a specific effect on net Ca transport it is probably small. It should be noted that Nakhlal and Latif (1978) reported that calcitonin causes the local release of 5-hydroxytryptamine; indeed various effects of calcitonin may well occur indirectly.

F. Glucocorticoids

It is well established that adrenal glucocorticoids given in supraphysiologic doses can reduce the intestinal absorption of Ca (Harrison and Harrison, 1960; Sallis and Holdsworth, 1962; Collins *et al.*, 1962; Williams *et al.*, 1961). Inhibition of Ca absorption appears to arise primarily through a decrease in active Ca transport (Kimberg *et al.*, 1961). Moreover, adrenalectomy can produce enhanced *in vitro* Ca transport in gut sacs from rats eating a low Ca diet (Kimberg *et al.*, 1961). Ferraro *et al.* (1976) using the ligated loop technique, showed that glucocorticoids produce a significant inhibition of phosphate as well as Ca absorption in the rat. Studies evaluating the effects of glucocorticoids on intestinal absorption in humans reveal different results depending upon the dosage employed (Fig. 12). Thus, Lekkerkerker *et al.* (1972) found no effect of prednisolone, 15 mg/day, on intestinal Ca absorption, measured from the plasma appearance of radiocalcium following its oral ingestion. Observations of humans with Cushing syndrome have indicated variable results; there have been reports of increased intestinal absorption of Ca in some patients, while others have normal net Ca absorption (Bassett *et al.*, 1960; Wajchenberg *et al.*, 1969; Sjöberg, 1970). The relationship between Ca absorption and daily doses of prednisone in renal transplant recipients is shown in Fig. 13 (Coburn *et al.*, 1973a).

An unresolved question is whether glucocorticoids exert their effect on Ca transport by alterating vitamin D metabolism, or intestinal transport per se. Kimberg *et al.* (1961) showed that the effect of cortisone on active Ca transport could not be corrected by large doses of vitamin D. Favus *et al.* (1973a) demonstrated that cortisone did not change the rate of conversion of 25(OH)D to

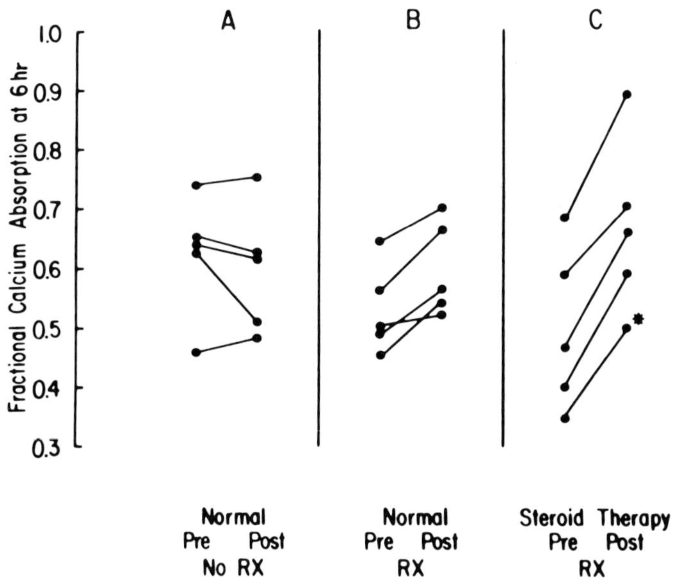

Fig. 12. Fraction of radiocalcium absorbed by normal individuals and patients receiving "high-dose" glucocorticoid therapy before and after treatment with $1,25(OH)_2D_3$, 0.4 μg/day, for 7 days. With steroid therapy there was correction of intestinal Ca absorption toward normal. (Reproduced from Klein *et al.*, 1977, with permission of *J. Clin. Invest.)*

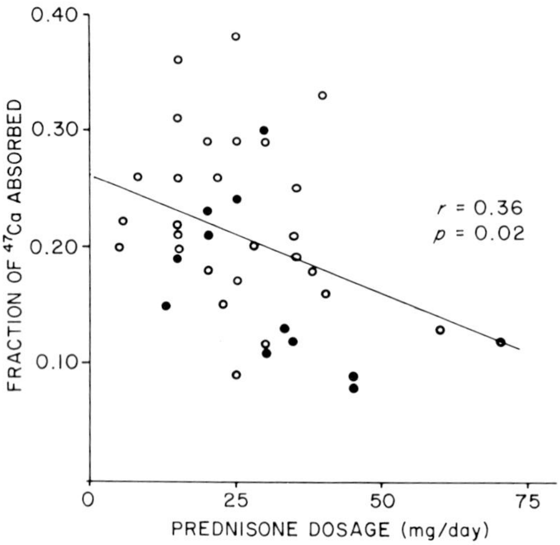

Fig. 13. The relationship between the fractional absorption of Ca in renal transplant recipients and the daily dosage of prednisone; the Ca absorption was measured utilizing a double isotope method; males (○), females (●). (Adapted from Coburn *et al.*, 1973a.)

$1,25(OH)_2D$ nor did it affect the localization of $1,25(OH)_2D_3$ in the intestine. It was suggested that the antivitamin D-like actions of glucocorticoids in the intestine were due to influences on biochemical processes responsible for Ca transport; the events were thought to occur independent of a direct interaction with vitamin D_3 or its active metabolite. In subsequent studies evaluating the biologic response to $1,25(OH)_2D_3$ in cortisone-treated rats, Favus *et al.* (1973b) showed a diminished rate of Ca flux, in vitamin D-deficient, cortisone-treated animals; M–S flux was decreased as was net absorptive flux in the vitamin D-deficient state. The administration of $1,25(OH)_2D_3$ improved but failed to correct completely either M–S or net flux of Ca. Younoszai and Ghishan (1978) perfused the jejunum and ileum of suckling, weanling, and "adolescent" rats; they found that pharmacologic doses of corticosteroids caused an inhibition of Ca transport in the suckling rats, while there was no effect in older rats. Also, they found that both the lumen-to-mucosa and mucosa-to-lumen fluxes of Ca were lower than in control rats; they suggested that the effect of pharmacologic doses of glucocorticoids was to change the permeability of the mucosa. Thus, glucocorticoids had an effect on a passive process for Ca absorption rather than on a vitamin D-dependent mechanism. Studies measuring intestinal enzymes also suggest that cortisone may directly affect the intestinal mucosa; thus, decreases in alkaline phosphatase, maltase, and total protein content of the intestine have been reported (Krawitt, 1972; Lafont and Pilon, 1975). Also, reduced CaBP has been reported in the intestine of cortisol-treated chicks (Fehar and Wasserman, 1979).

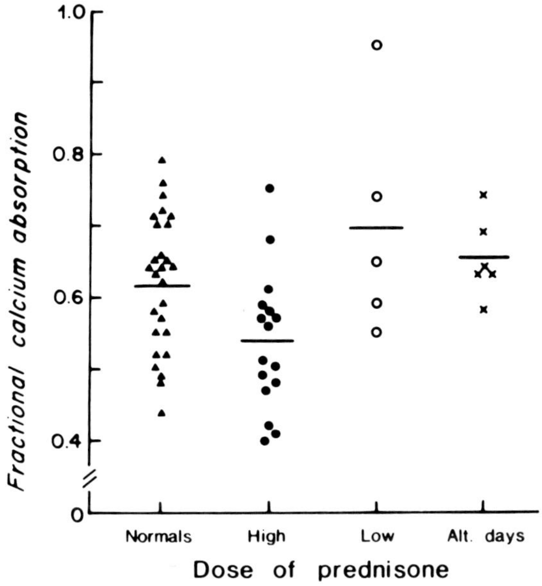

Fig. 14. Individual values of fractional intestinal absorption of Ca at 6 hr after ingestion of radiocalcium; the high dose glucocorticoids are those receiving more than 30 mg/day of prednisone. The mean value for Ca absorption in the "high-dose" group is significantly lower than that in normals. (From Klein *et al.,* 1977, with permission of *J. Clin. Invest.)*

Other studies provided strong evidence that cortisone exerts an effect on vitamin D metabolism. Thus, the turnover of radiolabeled vitamin D was increased during prednisone therapy (Avioli *et al.*, 1968), and it was shown that small doses of $1,25(OH)_2D_3$ could restore intestinal Ca absorption to normal in humans receiving more than 30 mg/day of cortisone, as is shown in Fig. 14 (Klein *et al.*, 1977). Moreover, reduced plasma levels of $1,25(OH)_2D$ have been reported in patients receiving large doses of corticosteroids (Chesney *et al.*, 1978).

Thus, there is an important effect of large doses of corticosteriods in inhibiting intestinal Ca transport; in part, this may be mediated by alterations in vitamin D metabolism; on the other hand, there is strong evidence that corticosteroids also may have significant actions beyond a possible effect on vitamin D metabolism.

G. Somatostatin

Interest has focused on possible effects of somatostatin on intestinal absorption of Ca. This hormone has been detected in the gastrointestinal tract as well as the hypothalamus. It has a number of effects on intestinal motility and blood flow as well as effects on various intestinal hormones. Recently, data from studies in man have provided evidence that an acute infusion of somatostatin decreases the intestinal absorption of Ca. This effect may occur via the inhibition of the secretion of other hormones; however, this seems unlikely as the effect is very rapid, occurring within 30 min (Evensen *et al.*, 1978; Scholz and Schwille, 1978). Moreover, studies utilizing everted gut sacs (Wagner *et al.*, 1978) indicate that somatostatin can directly augment the absorption of galactose, providing other evidence for an intestinal effect.

There is considerable evidence that somatostatin can decrease the influx of Ca into cells from tissues such as the pancreas; perhaps somatostatin could exert a similar effect on the influx of Ca into the intestinal mucosal cells.

V. PHYSIOLOGIC, DIETARY, AND LOCAL FACTORS AFFECTING CALCIUM ABSORPTION

There are a number of physiologic and nutritional factors that may have significant effects on Ca absorption. With newer insight into active Ca absorption and the important action of vitamin D, the study of certain of these factors has not received recent attention; however, some of these factors may have important effects on Ca absorption; others are probably mediated through vitamin D metabolism.

A. Adaptation to Low Dietary Calcium Intake

Observations made many years ago showed that feeding animals a low Ca diet led to an increased intestinal absorption of Ca (Nicolaysen, 1943). Moreover, it was shown that this adaptation to a low Ca diet required the presence of vitamin D (Nicolaysen *et al.*, 1953), observations confirmed subsequently in a series of studies by Schachter and colleagues (Dowdle *et al.*, 1960; Kimberg *et al.*, 1961). They found that the ability of rats to increase intestinal Ca transport in response to a low Ca diet was impaired following adrenalectomy, hypophysectomy, and thyroparathyroidectomy. The understanding of how intestinal Ca transport increases in response to a low Ca intake was greatly advanced when it was found that feeding a low Ca diet enhanced the conversion of $25(OH)D_3$ to $1,25(OH)_2D_3$ (Boyle *et al.*, 1971). Moreover, it was shown that the administration of exogenous $1,25(OH)_2D_3$ could abolish any further effect of a low Ca diet to enhance the intestinal absorption of Ca (Ribovich and DeLuca, 1975). Details of factors regulating vitamin D metabolism are reviewed in detail in Chapter 7, this volume; nonetheless, this important aspect related to Ca absorption will be reviewed briefly: The usual pathway for the adaptation to a low Ca diet is believed to involve increased PTH secretion in response to a slight fall in serum Ca; the PTH leads to increased generation of $1,25(OH)_2D_3$, which then stimulates intestinal Ca absorption (Hughes *et al.*, 1975; Rader *et al.*, 1979). On the other hand, there are numerous reports suggesting that feeding of a low Ca diet, itself, can stimulate the production and/or intestinal localization of $1,25(OH)_2D_3$ (Larkins *et al.*, 1973; Favus *et al.*, 1974). Moreover, a number of reports provide evidence that intestinal Ca absorption can increase in animals following removal of their parathyroid glands (Kimberg *et al.*, 1961; Sammon *et al.*, 1970; Favus *et al.*, 1974; Kemm, 1976; Pento *et al.*, 1977). In studies utilizing the Thiry-vella jejunal loops in pigs, Fox *et al.* (1977) found that prior feeding with a low Ca diet enhanced the Ca absorption through this loop, although an increased content of CaBP could not be detected. Gran (1960) and Benson *et al.* (1969) also found that the presence of PTH was not essential for adaptation to a low Ca diet. It should be mentioned that others, including Shah and Draper (1966), Winter *et al.* (1972), and Kenny (1975), reported that parathyroidectomy abolished the adaptation to a low Ca diet. It was even suggested that the adaptation might occur on certain occasions because of accessory tissue that produces PTH (Pento *et al.*, 1977). This possibility seems unlikely; thus, one would need to postulate that the amount of PTH produced would be inadequate to restore serum Ca and phosphorus to normal in the parathyroidectomized animals while it could restore the activity of the 25-hydroxyvitamin D_3-1α-hydroxylase.

Another point of controversy relates to whether or not adaptation to a low Ca diet occurs as readily in older as in younger animals. Initially, Nicolaysen (1943) did not find the Ca absorption to be as prominent in older rats receiving a low Ca diet. Subsequently Nicolaysen (1956) reported that old rats could maintain a Ca balance on a very low Ca intake, providing evidence for the presence of adaptation.

Henry *et al.* (1960) reported that rats, varying in age from 3 to 9 months, adapted to a low Ca diet within 2 to 6 months of the change in diet. There was a suggestion, however, that the older rats achieved this adaptation more slowly than did younger rats. Other studies suggest that adaptation can begin to occur within 6 to 8 days following initiation of a low Ca diet.

Whether a change in dietary Ca content can affect either endogenous Ca secretion or the S–M flux of Ca remains uncertain. Data of Walling and Kimberg (1974) suggest that the change from absorption to secretion of Ca by the rat ileum is dependent upon changes in dietary Ca intake and arises entirely from changes in the M–S flux. On the other hand, Kemm (1973), who measured endogenous secretion with the aid of isotope during metabolic balance studies, found greater endogenous fecal Ca in rats fed a high as opposed to a low Ca diet. Cohn *et al.* (1968) also presented evidence for enhanced endogenous fecal Ca as dietary Ca intake was increased.

Adaptation to changes in dietary Ca intake has clearly been shown to exist in man; thus Malm (1958), in metabolic balance studies, showed that most young adults could reduce their fecal Ca to achieve a net balance when their dietary Ca was reduced to 400–500 mg/day; moreover, Spencer *et al.* (1969), who utilized radioisotopic methods, found a mean improvement in intestinal Ca absorption from 30.5 to 63.6% as patients changed from a high to low Ca intake. Also, Begum and Pereira (1969) provided evidence that most children who were eating a dietary Ca intake of 200 mg/day were in positive balance for Ca with absorption at 50% of their intake. Interestingly, with this relatively low Ca diet there was a greater absorption and retention of Ca with an increase in dietary Ca to 280 mg/day. The relationship between habitual dietary Ca intake and the fraction of Ca absorbed in adults is shown in Fig. 15.

Studies by Krawitt *et al.* (1973) are of interest; utilizing an *in vitro* gut sac technique, they found increased Ca uptake by duodenum, jejunum, and terminal ileum from animals receiving a low Ca intake, however, there was increased alkaline phosphatase activity only in the duodenum. Thus, if alkaline phosphatase plays a role in Ca transport, its effect may be limited to the duodenum. Finally, Favus *et al.* (1980) found increased Ca uptake by everted sacs prepared from ascending and descending colon of rat placed on a low Ca diet.

Although total intake of Ca is the usual parameter evaluated is assessing the adequacy of dietary Ca, there is evidence that the manner of its administration,

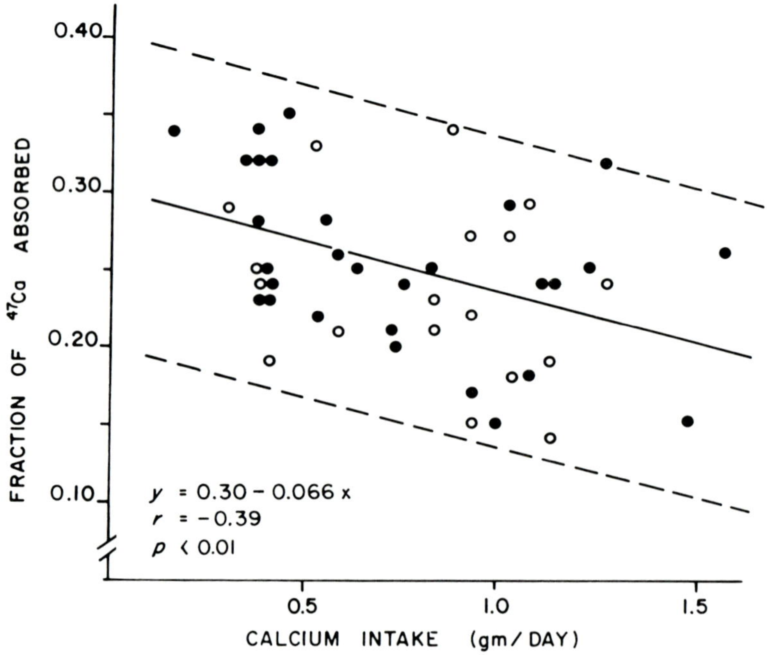

Fig. 15. Relationship between the fraction of ^{47}Ca absorbed measured by a double isotope technique and the habitual dietary intake of Ca in adult normal subjects; males are indicated by (○) and females by (●). (From Coburn *et al.*, 1973a, with permission of *Kidney Int.)*

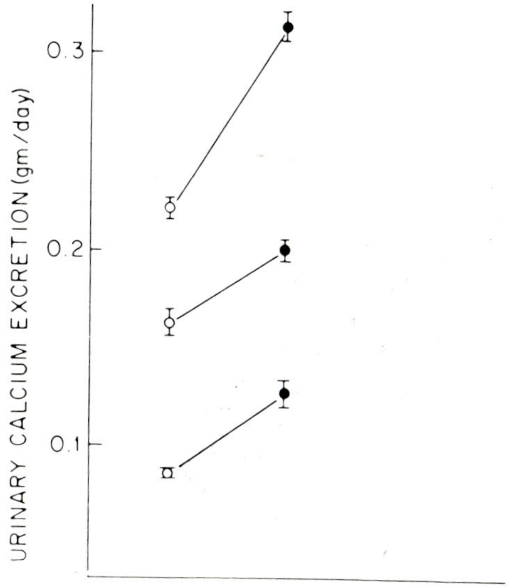

Fig. 16. A comparison of urinary calcium excretion in three normal subjects consuming a constant diet with one pint (408 ml) of milk given either as a single dose (○) or in six divided doses (●); values are mean ± SE for several 24-hr collections. (From Phang *et al.*, 1968, with permission of *Lancet*.)

i.e. whether it is taken in a single dose or as multiple divided doses, can significantly affect Ca absorption. Thus, Phang *et al.* (1968) administered two diets, each providing Ca (1000 mg with 700 mg provided as milk) to subjects studied on a metabolic ward; this resulted in widely different rates of urinary Ca excretion depending upon whether the milk was taken as a single dose or in six divided doses each day. Thus, urinary Ca excretion was 20–50% higher when the Ca was taken in the divided doses (Fig. 16). This provides confirmatory evidence that the mechanism for Ca transport involves a carrier-mediated mechanism that is not completely saturated. When the moderately large single dose of Ca is taken, the absorptive mechanism is "saturated"; on the other hand, when the same total amount of Ca is taken in frequent divided feedings, there is greater fractional absorption of Ca leading to higher urinary Ca. Therefore, studies which evaluate the effect of varying the intake of Ca must take into consideration not only the total quantity of Ca taken but the manner in which Ca is provided throughout the day.

B. Effect of Age

Results of studies that use radiocalcium techniques (Bronner *et al.*, 1963; Avioli *et al.*, 1965b; Bullamore *et al.*, 1970; Alevizaki *et al.*, 1973) or metabolic balance methods (Nordin *et al.*, 1976) indicate that there is a progressive decrease in intestinal Ca absorption with advanced age, particularly over age 70. Moreover, data in animals indicate that the active component of Ca transport decreases with age (Fig. 17). Bullamore *et al.* (1970), who measured intestinal absorption from the plasma appearance of radiocalcium following its oral ingestion, found significant malabsorption in all subjects over 80 years of age. This consideration is of particular importance regarding the decrease in bone mineral content with age. With a single exception (Avioli *et al.*, 1965b), osteoporotic patients have been found to have lower Ca absorption than do their age-matched controls (Bronner *et al.*, 1963; Syzmendera *et al.*, 1972; Gallagher *et al.*, 1973). A more detailed discussion of osteoporosis can be found in Chapter 2, Vol. III.

The mechanism for the decrease in intestinal Ca absorption with age is subject to speculation. Observations by Gallagher *et al.* (1979) indicate a progressive decrease in intestinal Ca absorption with age. Also, they reported that the plasma levels of $1,25(OH)_2D$ decrease after age 65 (Fig. 18), with a positive correlation between serum levels of $1,25(OH)_2D$ and fractional Ca absorption as measured with a double isotope technique. Data in humans suggest there is normal responsiveness of the intestine to exogenous $1,25(OH)_2D_3$ (Gallagher *et al.*, 1979); some data in rats suggest otherwise (Horst *et al.*, 1978), but Lee *et al.* (1980) have reported that mature rats respond promptly to very low doses of $1,25(OH)_2D_3$, resembling vitamin D-deficient weanling rats in their responsivity. Such observations suggest that the changes in Ca absorption with age may be

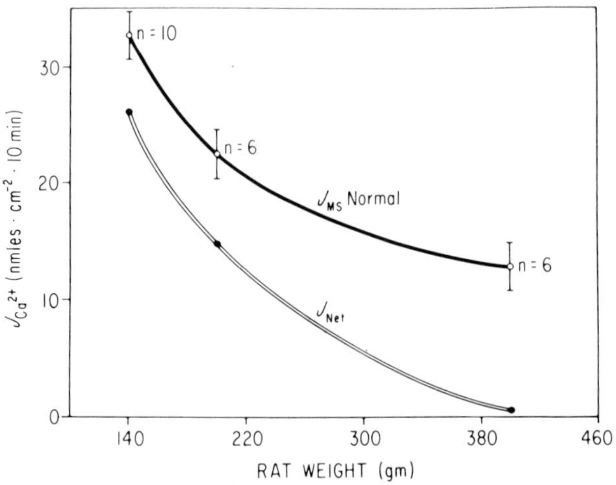

Fig. 17. Steady-state rates of Ca flux across the duodenum of rats of different ages. Data are shown as mean ± SE; $J_{net} = J_{MS} - J_{SM}$. There is a progressive decrease in net flux and J_{MS} with advancing age. (From Walling and Rothman, 1970, with permission of *J. Biol. Chem.*)

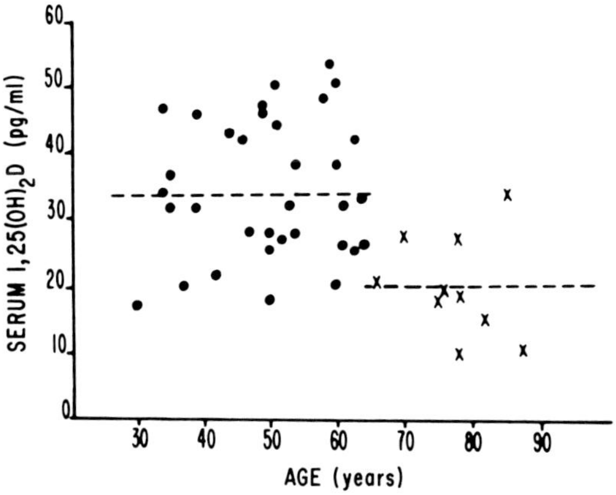

Fig. 18. Serum levels of 1,25(OH)$_2$D in relation to age. Normal subjects below age 64 years are indicated by (●) and patients aged 65 or over are indicated by (X). Mean serum 1,25(OH)$_2$D, indicated by the dashed lines, are significantly lower in the elderly than in the non-elderly subjects ($p < 0.001$). (From Gallagher *et al.*, 1979, with permission of *J. Clin. Invest.)*

associated with a decrease in the ability to generate 1,25(OH)$_2$D$_3$. Epstein *et al.* (1973) evaluated the change in serum Ca after a single large oral Ca load, which provided 4 gm of elemental Ca. Certain elderly subjects failed to show an increase in serum Ca equal to that observed in young subjects. On the other hand, pretreatment of the elderly subjects for 1 week with vitamin D$_2$, 5000 IU/day, increased the calcemic response to that observed in younger subjects. They suggested that certain elderly subjects may exhibit "sub-clinical" vitamin D-deficiency.

C. Form of Calcium in the Diet

There is evidence that certain soluble salts of Ca are more readily absorbed than are others, with calcium chloride > calcium gluconate or calcium lactate > calcium carbonate (Mautalen *et al.*, 1969; DeGrazia and Rich, 1964). Certain other salts of calcium, such as calcium oxalate and CaHPO$_4$, are highly insoluble. Despite the fact that substantial amount of Ca may be complexed or precipitated with phosphate or oxalate within the intestine, freely diffusible ionized Ca is also present. In rats on a very low Ca diet, Sernka and Borle (1969) found that the free Ca activity fell to as low as 0.09–0.31 m*M* on a Ca-free diet, while the level increased to 0.19–1.08 m*M* with a 0.15% Ca diet in samples taken from the duodenum, jejunum, and ileum. These studies provide evidence for the remarkable ability of the body to remove Ca from the intestinal contents.

There is some reason to believe that a greater fraction of Ca in intestinal fluid is in a precipitated form as a meal moves down the small bowel, since $CaHPO_4$ precipitates at a pH above 6.1, and the pH increases as a meal moves distally. (Fordtran and Locklear, 1966).

In studies carried out in the chick and hen, Hurwitz and Bar (1969) measured Ca activity as they varied dietary Ca from 0.31% to 3.94%. With the higher Ca diets the intestinal Ca activity reached 3–6 m*M* and the concentration decreased in the more distal small intestine; thus, with the high Ca diet there was evidence that Ca could be absorbed into the plasma down its chemical gradient. In man, Fordtran and Locklear (1966) showed a substantial variation in Ca content depending on the type of meal ingested. After a steak meal, the duodenal Ca content was below 2–4 m*M*, while after a meal consisting of milk and a doughnut the levels were 20–30 m*M* in the stomach; the Ca levels fell progressively to less than 1–3 m*M* in the distal small intestine.

D. Lactose and Other Carbohydrates

It has long been known that the addition of lactose to the diet could enhance the absorption of Ca; subsequently, it was shown that a number of other sugars, including mannose, raffinose, zylose, and various polyalcohols, such as mannitol and sorbitol, could also enhance net Ca absorption in rats (Wasserman and Comar, 1959; Wasserman and Taylor, 1969). Certain sugars, such as D-glucose, sucrose, and fructose, were ineffective; these sugars are rapidly absorbed in proximal intestine and fail to reach the ileum, where lactose exerts its major effect. It was shown by Kimberg *et al.* (1961) that this effect of lactose was most effective in enhancing ^{45}Ca absorption by the ileum of a normal rat, while lactose decreased Ca absorption in a rat having been fed a Ca-deficient diet. Also, vitamin D is not required for lactose to enhance Ca absorption (Dupuis and Fournier, 1963). The mechanism whereby lactose can enhance Ca absorption is not clear. It was suggested that lactose acts on the ileum to allow enhanced entry of Ca into the intestinal cells that are not adapted to high rates of Ca absorption. Thus, it was postulated that somehow lactose could act as a metabolic inhibitor and reduce an energy-dependent reaction that normally prevents the entry of Ca into the cell (Wasserman and Taylor, 1969). Other studies that evaluated the effect of long-term feeding of lactose on duodenal Ca absorption, measured *in situ,* and duodenal CaBP demonstrated a progressive decrease in Ca absorption and CaBP (Pansu *et al.*, 1979); it was suggested that the effect of lactose ingestion on the duodenum was similar to that from continued high Ca intake, i.e., causing a decrease in the efficiency of Ca absorption with reduced CaBP. In a subsequent study (Pansu *et al.*, 1981) the addition of lactose to the diet caused a significant depression in the saturable component of Ca absorption, measured in the duodenum *in situ;* there was a depression of the J_{MS} and the K_t and an associated decrease in CaBP. These studies were carried out in the duodenum and not the site of the intestine where lactose exerts its effect to enhance Ca absorption.

E. Amino Acids

Addition of certain amino acids to the diet may enhance the intestinal absorption of Ca (Wasserman *et al.*, 1956). Of various amino acids tested, lysine and arginine were particularly effective. Although it was suggested that these amino acids may enhance the solubility of certain Ca phosphate complexes, the mechanism of their action on Ca absorption is still uncertain.

F. Bile and Bile Salts

It has been known for some time that the normal secretion of bile is necessary for optimal absorption of vitamin D; however, it has also been shown that bile may directly enhance Ca absorption, as evaluated in the chick ileum (Webling and Holdsworth, 1965, 1966). The observation that bile can increase the absorption of an insoluble Ca salt, $CaHPO_4$, suggests that the action of bile may be primarily to increase the solubility of such salts (Wasserman and Taylor, 1969). Moreover, considerable Ca is secreted into the bile, and it has been suggested that biliary Ca may be more readily reabsorbed than are other sources of endogenous fecal Ca (Briscoe and Ragan, 1965).

G. Zinc

Zinc and copper are thought to inhibit the absorption of Ca (Van Campen and Scaife, 1970; Murphy *et al.*, 1974). In a study carried out in adolescent females, Greger *et al.* (1978) found that an alteration in the levels of dietary zinc had no effect on net Ca absorption measured during metabolic balance studies. Thus, the effects of zinc described in experimental animals may not be applicable to man.

H. Changes in Dietary Protein

Metabolic balance studies in animals have shown that increments in dietary protein intake lead to either an increase or no change in net Ca absorption (Engström and DeLuca, 1963; Bell *et al.*, 1975; Shenolikar and Rao, 1968). Utilizing *in situ* perfusion, Moyer *et al.* (1978) evaluated Ca transport in rats receiving varying protein intakes. Ca absorption, expressed per weight of mucosa, was unchanged in all diet groups. However, because of greater mucosal weight per unit intestinal length in animals that had received the higher protein diets, there was a greater Ca absorption per unit length of intestine. These observations suggest that the mass of absorptive cells may determine intestinal Ca absorption.

Increased urinary Ca excretion is commonly observed with increased protein intake (Johnson *et al.*, 1970; Walker and Linkswiler, 1972; Schwartz *et al.*, 1973); this has been attributed to the acid-load produced by such diets. It is possible that increased losses of urinary Ca may be important in leading to increased Ca absorption under these maneuvers.

I. Diphosphonates

Ethane-1-hydroxy-1,1-disphosphonate (EHDP), which has been found to retard both the formation and dissolution of bone crystals *in vitro,* has been utilized for the management of myositis ossificans progressiva and other forms of ectopic calcification. It has been found that EHDP can impair the conversion of vitamin D to 1,25$(OH)_2D_3$ (Hill *et al.*, 1973) and reduce the intestinal absorption of Ca in rats (Bonjour *et al.*, 1973). Uttley *et al.* (1975) performed balance studies in three children undergoing therapy with EHDP for extraskeletal calcification. All patients showed an overall reduction in Ca balance due to an increase in fecal excretion of Ca. It was suggested that diphosphonate, as employed clinically, decreased the intestinal absorption of Ca. Although not studied in these patients, it is likely that this effect arose through the action of EHDP on the metabolism of vitamin D.

J. Alterations in Dietary Fat

The observations that an increase in dietary fat increases the degree of steatorrhea and enhances the fecal loss of Ca is well known (Bassett *et al.*, 1939). Studying the effects of fats on Ca absorption, Agnew and Holdsworth (1971) compared the effects of a long-chain triglyceride with that of medium-chain triglyceride in both normal subjects and patients with certain intestinal disorders. They found a significant inhibition of intestinal Ca absorption by the long-chain triglyceride compared to baseline and the medium-chain triglyceride. Also it has been shown that medium-chain triglycerides can stimulate Ca absorption in normal rats and rats with bile-duct ligation (Kehayoglou *et al.*, 1968).

Premature infants fail to absorb both Ca and fat normally, with positive correlations between retention of Ca and fat absorption (Williams *et al.*, 1970; Hanna *et al.*, 1970). Tantibhedhyangkul and Hashim (1978) evaluated the effect on Ca absorption of medium-chain triglycerides, which are well absorbed by premature infants. The addition of medium-chain triglycerides to three different types of formulae fed to premature infants led to a significantly greater absorption of Ca with each diet. Such observations provide support for the view that the binding of

Ca by fat within the intestinal lumen can reduce intestinal Ca absorption under some circumstances.

K. Oxalic Acid and Phytic Acid

The chelation of Ca by either oxalic acid or phytic acid to form insoluble salts within the intestinal lumen can interfere with intestinal absorption of Ca (Recommended Dietary Allowances, 1974; Hegstead, 1973; Wills, 1973). As is discussed below, the presence of large quantities of phytates in the chapatti flour used for unleavened bread has been implicated as a contributory factor for osteomalacia observed in Asian and Middle-Eastern individuals (Berlyne *et al.*, 1973). Because of its effectiveness in binding Ca and rendering Ca nonabsorbable, sodium phytate has been employed for the management of recurrent nephrolothiaisis arising from the hyperabsorption of Ca (Pak *et al.*, 1974a). Studies to date have shown no detrimental effects from the use of such phytates on overall mineral metabolism (Pak, 1973).

L. Miscellaneous Factors

There are a number of studies (Wasserman and Lengemann, 1960; Heggeness, 1959) suggesting that there are certain antibiotics, including penicillin, chloramphenicol, and neomycin, that enhance the absorption of radiocalcium. Their mechanism of action is unknown; however, it has been suggested that they may act in a manner similar to lactose (Wasserman and Taylor, 1969).

The overall importance of some of these above-noted agents to modify Ca absorption is not entirely clear; they have been used under certain circumstances to modify or decrease hypocalcemia present in animals receiving a rachitogenic diet. Many of these substances or factors may have less effect on Ca absorption in a vitamin D-replete animal or an animal in which active Ca transport is stimulated.

VI. CONDITIONS WITH REDUCED CALCIUM ABSORPTION

A. Reduced Dietary Calcium Intake

One mechanism whereby the net absorption of Ca can be decreased is via a reduction in dietary Ca intake. Thus, the net absorption of Ca is reduced despite the substantial increase in the efficiency of its absorption. The consequences of a markedly reduced Ca intake remain somewhat unclear. Thus, Malm (1958) showed in long-term balance studies in man that only 3 of 25 subjects remained in negative balance when the dietary Ca intake was reduced from 940 to 450 mg/day; 19 had regained Ca equilibrium after a period of 1–8 months. In rats, there is evidence that the quantity of bone Ca is reduced when the animals are placed on low Ca diet, indicating that there is negative balance even though adaptation occurs with increased efficiency of absorption (Kemm, 1973). The question of whether a low Ca diet can lead to osteoporosis is of some concern; it has been suggested that the intake of adequate dietary Ca may prevent osteoporosis, and this subject is reviewed extensively in Chapter 2, Vol. III.

A bone disease that resembles "rickets" and is believed to be due to Ca deficiency has been described in children (Kooh *et al.*, 1977). The possibility has been raised that the radiographic skeletal lesions of Ca deficiency may be due to secondary hyperparathyroidism rather than rickets (Ritz and Mehls, 1978). Thus, although adaptation of the efficiency of Ca absorption may be pronounced, there is growing evidence that the intake of very low dietary Ca may be detrimental to man.

The overall needs of Ca in the diet of man have been the subject of much interest (McBean and Speckmann, 1974). For an adult, the Recommended Dietary Allowance (RDA) for Ca of 800 mg/day has remained unchanged from that formulated in 1963 and 1968. Data related to this are reviewed by McBean and Speckman (1974). Heaney *et al.* (1977) studied Ca in women aged 35–50 utilizing Ca balance techniques and measuring Ca kinetics with radiocalcium. They predicted that the dietary Ca intake required to produce an average neutral balance was 1250 mg/day. This quantity is significantly in excess of the RDA, and Heany *et al.* have suggested that dietary Ca intake be increased in peri- and postmenopausal women.

One method employed for management of morbid obesity has been the application of total starvation, a situation where obviously there is no Ca intake. Marked catabolism and loss of body weight occur, associated with negative balances for Ca as well as nitrogen, phosphorus, sodium, and water. Substantial hypercalciuria is also seen; this parallels the degree of ketoacidosis. When these patients receive a diet providing 600 kcal/day, there is prompt increase in anabolism with retention of Ca as well as nitrogen, phosphate, potassium, and sodium (Spencer *et al.*, 1966).

Another situation characterized by reduced or absent dietary Ca intake is the long-term treatment of patients with severe gastrointestinal disease with total parenteral nutrition. With this treatment, all nutrients are supplied intravenously; the source of calories is largely dextrose and the sources of protein are essential amino acids or casein hydrolysate (Byrne *et al.*, 1979). Despite the supply of adequate quantities of intravenous Ca, phosphate, and vitamin D_2, an unusual metabolic bone disease has been described (Targoff *et al.*, 1979; Klein *et al.*, 1980; Shike *et al.*, 1980). This bone disease is characterized by decreased bone turnover and patchy osteomalacia; the levels of serum Ca are normal or slightly increased, serum phosphorus levels are normal, and serum PTH levels are normal or reduced (Shike *et al.*, 1980; Klein *et al.*, 1980). The pathogenesis of this skeletal disease is uncertain, although adequate quantities of Ca are supplied parenterally, and no Ca absorption occurs. It is conveivable that alterations related to changes in gastrointestinal hormones or the lack of Ca supplied through the enteral route into the portal circulation could contribute to the bone disease; however these suggestions are speculative.

B. Vitamin D Deficiency

As would be predicted, reduced Ca absorption has been shown to exist in humans with vitamin D deficiency: Liu *et al.* (1940) found a high fecal excretion of Ca in pregnant women with osteomalacia prior to the administration of vitamin D. Following treatment with vitamin D, fecal Ca fell and the balance for Ca became substantially positive. Also, Ca retention significantly increased in infants receiving milk from the lactating, vitamin D-treated mothers. Subsequent studies showed that the metabolic balance for Ca was frequently negative in patients with nutritional osteomalacia prior to vitamin D treatment; in instances when a Ca balance was not negative, small amounts of vitamin D may have been provided in the diet. Moreover, the administration of only 50 μg/day (2000 IU) of vitamin D caused a marked reduction of fecal Ca and strikingly positive Ca balance (Dent and Smith, 1969). In a study of radiocalcium kinetics, Harris *et al.* (1965a,b) found that $33 \pm 4\%$ of Ca was absorbed in eight children and infants with active rickets; with vitamin D treatment or during spontaneous healing, the percentage of dietary Ca absorption was increased to $55 \pm 6\%$. Of interest, these children, with dietary Ca intakes between 900 and 2600 mg/day, exhibited positive balances for Ca prior to receiving vitamin D. These data confirm observations in animals that the high fecal Ca arises from unabsorbed dietary Ca and that the action of vitamin D on the intestine is primarily to improve the absorption of both dietary Ca and digestive juice Ca (Harris *et al.*, 1965b).

C. Malabsorption Syndromes

Abnormalities of Ca absorption occur frequently in patients with various malabsorption syndromes (Alpers, 1974). Although not all patients with the malabsorption syndrome and steatorrhea exhibit impaired absorption of Ca (Milhaud and Vesin, 1961), the excessive fecal loss of Ca may be remarkable and the quantities of Ca found in the stool may exceed the dietary Ca intake. Other manifestations of the intestinal disease often predominates, but the severity of Ca malabsorption and the attendant osteomalacia and secondary hyperparathyroidism often lead to profound hypocalcemia and skeletal symptoms (Hajjar *et al.*, 1974).

The mechanism responsible for impaired intestinal Ca absorption may differ from one patient to another: Thus, there may be a failure of intestinal absorption of vitamin D, rendering such individuals vitamin D-deficient; there may be alterations of the intestinal mucosa making it unresponsive to vitamin D; or a combination of both factors may exist. The presence of excessive nonabsorbed fat in the intestinal lumen can bind Ca and thereby render it nonabsorbable. Certain intestinal diseases, with altered absorption of sodium and water leading to rapid transit and a tendency towards diarrhea, may also impair Ca absorption.

The mechanism for impaired Ca absorption with the malabsorption syndrome can be assessed indirectly from sensitivity of such patients to vitamin D treatment. The results of such studies are somewhat conflicting; thus, Fourman and Spray (1948) found no improvement in Ca malabsorption after the oral administration of vitamin D, 1200 IU/day; however, the balance for Ca became positive when vitamin D was given intramuscularly. Subsequently, Badenoch and Fourman (1954) concluded from metabolic studies in two patients with steatorrhea that vitamin D absorption was reduced but that the defect could be overcome by giving the vitamin D either parenterally or by mouth in large doses. In patients with gluten-sensitive steatorrhea, Nassim *et al.* (1959) showed that a gluten-free diet led to clinical improvement and a markedly positive balance for Ca. When gluten was added to the diet, there was a clinical and biochemical relapse, with decreased Ca absorption; however there was no response to vitamin D, given orally or parenterally. In more recent studies, Bordier *et al.* (1974) found that oral treatment with 1α-hydroxyvitamin D_3, 2.5 μg/day, improved the Ca balance in two patients with idiopathic steatorrhea and two others with the blind-loop syndrome; the latter observations suggested that the intestine could respond to an active form of vitamin D. Thus, such data suggest that some patients may respond to vitamin D with improved Ca absorption; while in others, the intestine may be totally unresponsive, implying an intrinsic defect in the intestinal epithelium.

Other studies have evaluated the absorption of vitamin D utilizing radiolabeled vitamin D; they indicate that there is decreased absorption of the sterol with the degree of malabsorption related to the total losses of fat in the feces (Thompson *et al.*, 1966). Krawitt *et al.* (1979) found impaired intestinal absorption of both vitamin D_3 and 25(OH)D_3 in the malabsorption syndrome, although the net absorption of 25(OH)D_3 was somewhat greater than that of vitamin D_3. Nevertheless, the quantities of vitamin D_3 and 25(OH)D_3 absorbed, even with profound steatorrhea, were large enough to suggest that treatment with modest oral doses of vitamin D would be effective. Others (Arnaud *et al.*, 1979) found levels of 25(OH)D to be substantially subnormal in plasma from patients with nontropical sprue; moreover, the 25(OH)D was almost entirely in the vitamin D_3 rather than the vitamin D_2 form, suggesting that most had been generated in the skin. Hollander *et al.* (1978), studying vitamin D absorption in animals, found that the absorption of vitamin D, a passive process, was impaired by the presence of various fatty acids; such studies suggest that malabsorption of vitamin D may contribute to reduced Ca absorption in patients with the malabsorption syndromes.

Hypocalcemia and metabolic bone disease have been reported following jejuno-ileal bypass surgery for patients with morbid obesity (Johnson and Bynum, 1976); Teitelbaum *et al.* (1977) found reduced plasma levels of 25(OH)D and postulated that reduced absorption of vitamin D may be related to fat malabsorption. Treatment of such patients with supplemental Ca may not result in improvement. Magnesium deficiency and hypomagnesemia may contribute to the development of hypocalcemia in certain patients.

D. Gastrectomy

Following subtotal gastrectomy, there is evidence for impaired intestinal absorption of Ca, a factor that may contribute to the high incidence of osteomalacia, osteoporosis, and fractures following gastric surgery (Morgan *et al.*, 1970). Metabolic balance studies showed increased losses of fecal Ca (Caniggia *et al.*, 1964) and other observations showed reduced absorption of radiocalcium (Deller, 1966). Studies of bone density suggest that Ca loss from bone is more common following a gastrojejunostomy. Other observations indicate that the decrease in net absorption of Ca arose because of higher endogenous fecal secretion of Ca (Wortsman *et al.*, 1972). It should be noted, however, that the latter case had marked secondary hyperparathyroidism, which might have led to an increase in net Ca absorption. Results of yet another study (Agnew and Holdsworth, 1971) provided evidence for augmented absorption of radiocalcium in patients following a Billroth I gastroduodenostomy.

The mechanism for impaired intestinal Ca absorption following gastrectomy is not clear; the observation that it is more likely to occur following gastrojejunostomy raises the possibility that the lack of absorption of Ca in the duodenum and early jejunum may be a factor. Thus, the extent of the duodenum remaining intact could contribute to the role of gastrectomy in causing malabsorption of Ca and could explain differences in results from various reports. The association of abnormal Ca metabolism with the presence of steatorrhea has raised the possibility that the increased fat content of the gut contributes. The prompt response to dihydrotachysterol (Wortsman *et al.*, 1972) or pharmacologic doses of vitamin D (Morgan *et al.*, 1970) raises the possibility that there may be altered vitamin D metabolism. Levels of 25(OH)D have been low in some but not all patients following subtotal gastrectomy (Zansi *et al.*, 1977). Further studies are required to define the pathogenesis of altered Ca absorption under this condition.

E. Anticonvulsant Therapy

During the past decade, it has been recognized that osteomalacia is frequent in patients receiving the anticonvulsants phenobarbital and diphenylhydantoin. It has been shown by Shafer and Nuttal (1975) that Ca absorption was below normal in 25% of patients receiving both drugs.

There are data suggesting that anticonvulsants may have a direct effect on the intestine. Corradino (1976) observed that diphenylhydantoin caused a direct inhibition of vitamin D_3-stimulated Ca absorption in the duodenum of the chick embryo, as evaluated in organ culture. This observation makes it unlikely that these effects are mediated via a direct alteration in vitamin D metabolism. Also, de Wolff (1975) reported that diphenylhydantoin had a direct effect *in vitro* on Ca-ATPase in isolated brush borders from the rat jejunum; surprisingly, there was stimulation of intestinal Ca absorption, evaluated *in vivo*.

There is other evidence that a major effect of these agents is to alter the metabolism of vitamin D (Silver, 1977; Hahn and Avioli, 1975). Thus, the anticonvulsants can lead to a decrease in the plasma levels of 25(OH)D, while the levels of $1,25(OH)_2D$ remain normal (Jubiz *et al.*, 1977). The mechanism whereby this leads to abnormal intestinal Ca transport remains unexplained. These aspects are discussed in Chapter 7.

F. Thyroid Disorders

Disturbances of Ca metabolism are known to occur in hyperthyroidism, and a negative Ca balance with excessive fecal Ca loss is commonly recognized. In a study carried out in thyroidectomized patients, some of whom were receiving treatment with dihydrotachysterol for concomitant hyperparathyroidism, Lekkerkerker and Doorenbos (1973) found that the administration of thyroxin, with restitution of a euthyroid state, caused a substantial decrease in intestinal Ca absorption measured with a double isotope technique. Moreover, other studies in thyroidectomized patients showed an increase in serum Ca within two weeks after they discontinued therapy with triiodothyronine and treatment of hypoparathyroid patients with triiodothyronine reduced both serum and urinary Ca. These data provide additional evidence that thyroid hormone can modify Ca absorption.

On the other hand, Singhelakis *et al.* (1974) found that intestinal Ca absorption, measured utilizing a double isotope technique, was significantly below normal in patients with untreated hypothyroidism compared to both controls and patients with previous hypothyroidism who are clinically euthyroid after appropriate treatment for two or more months. The observations in patients who are hypoparathyroid and receiving constant doses of dihydrotachysterol suggest that alterations in vitamin D metabolism are not responsible. Also, these observations suggest that alterations in the secretion of PTH does not play a role in modifying Ca absorption in relation to thyroid hormone treatment. Plasma levels of 25(OH)D have been reported to be low in patients with hyperthyroidism (Valentzas *et al.*, 1977), suggesting that there may be an alteration in vitamin D metabolism.

G. Liver Disease and Alcoholism

There has been clinical evidence for a higher incidence and a greater severity of skeletal rarefaction in patients with advanced liver disease than in age-matched controls. This is particularly evident in patients with cholestatic liver disease or primary biliary cirrhosis. A substantial number of these patients show histologic evidence of osteomalacia (Atkinson *et al.*, 1956; Long *et al.*, 1978; Osk-Upmark, 1939) and Ca absorption is frequently depressed in patients with liver disease (Whelton *et al.*, 1971).

The liver plays a central role in the metabolism of vitamin D_3, and it has been thought that the alteration in Ca metabolism in liver disease arises from a failure of hepatic 25-hydroxylation of vitamin D to 25(OH)D. Indeed, plasma levels of 25(OH)D have been found to be low in some patients with liver disease (Long *et al.*, 1976). The possible role of vitamin D metabolism in liver disease is reviewed in Chapter 7.

Other evidence suggests that factors other than alterations in vitamin D metabolism may affect Ca absorption in patients with liver disease (Avioli, 1980). Measuring intestinal Ca absorption, Varghese *et al.* (1979) found reduced Ca absorption in patients with primary biliary cirrhosis, while there was improved absorption following treatment with either $1,25(OH)_2D_3$ or $1\alpha(OH)D_3$; however, the patients with biliary cirrhosis did require somewhat large doses of 1-$\alpha(OH)D_3$. Nonetheless, the data suggest that adequate 25-hydroxylation could occur. In another study, Kehayoglou *et al.* (1973) measured Ca absorption using the whole body counter. Ca absorption was less in patients with biliary cirrhosis than that in controls; there was good correlation between impaired Ca absorption and increased excretion of fecal fat. Treatment with medium-chain triglycerides restored Ca absorption to normal in seven of eight patients and there was decreased steatorrhea. These observations suggest that the fats which are more readily absorbed enhance the absorption of Ca and/or that of vitamin D. Farrington *et al.* (1979) measured Ca and phosphate absorption in patients with primary biliary cirrhosis before and after treatment with $1,25(OH)_2D_3$, 0.5 μg/day; there was marked improvement in the fractional absorption of both Ca and phosphate, implying that there was no end-organ-unresponsiveness of the intestine to the active vitamin D sterol level. In a prospective study evaluating 32 patients with cholestatic liver disease, Compston *et al.* (1980) found histologic evidence of osteomalcia in only four; half of the total group had been receiving parenteral therapy with vitamin D; those receiving vitamin D had normal levels of plasma 25(OH)D, and serum Ca was significantly higher than in the non-treated group. It was suggested that osteomalacia may be somewhat rare in cholestatic liver disease despite the abnormalities in vitamin D bioconversion and Ca absorption noted above.

The status of Ca metabolism in patients with chronic alcoholism, alcoholic liver disease, and Laennec's cirrhosis is unclear. An increased incidence of fractures and a decrease in bone density have been described (Dalen and Lamke, 1976); however, there is disagreement concerning the alterations in Ca homeostasis. Garcia-Pascual *et al.* (1977) reported depressed intestinal Ca absorption, low plasma levels of 25(OH)D, and reduced bone mineral content in patients with chronic alcoholism, with or without cirrhosis. Moreover, Hepner *et al.* (1976) showed that cirrhosis was associated with reduced serum levels of 25(OH)D, and they suggested that there was altered hepatic bioconversion of vitamin D. On the other hand, Skinner *et al.* (1977) and Sorensen *et al.* (1979) found low levels of 25(OH)D, but the plasma levels of 25(OH)D responded normally to treatment with vitamin D_3. It was suggested that dietary or environmental lack of vitamin D rather than an alteration of hepatic-hydroxylation of vitamin D was responsible for altered Ca metabolism.

It should be noted that alcohol can suppress duodenal Ca transport in experimental animals (Krawitt *et al.*, 1975). This abnormality of Ca transport was not reversed by treatment with $1,25(OH)_2D_3$; there were abnormalities in the mitochondria and other subcellular organelles of intestinal epithelial cells, suggesting that the inhibition of Ca transport was mediated at the intestinal level by mechanisms that are probably independent of vitamin D.

It is obvious that other nutritional problems often coexist in patients with alcoholism and alcoholic liver disease; these may play an important role in the malabsorption of Ca. It seems likely that a minor abnormality of hepatic 25-hydroxylation of vitamin D may place patients with biliary cirrhosis at greater risk for having reduced absorption of Ca with a likelihood of developing osteomalacia.

H. Renal Failure

Considerable data indicate that intestinal absorption of Ca is reduced in patients with renal failure. Results from studies employing classic metabolic balance methods often show that fecal Ca equals or even exceeds dietary Ca (Liu and Chu, 1943; McDonald *et al.*, 1964; Dent *et al.*, 1961; Kopple and Coburn, 1973). Other studies which have utilized various radiocalcium techniques invariably reveal subnormal intestinal Ca absorption in groups of uremic patients (Kaye and Silverman, 1965; Coburn *et al.*, 1973a; Ogg, 1968; Messner *et al.*, 1969; Recker and Saville, 1971). There is evidence from the timed evaluation of ^{47}Ca absorption in uremic patients that the abnormality of Ca absorption occurs primarily in the proximal small intestine (Brickman *et al.*, 1974a).

Considerable overlap exists between results obtained in patients with chronic renal failure and those found in normal individuals (Coburn *et al.*, 1973b). This may mean that a defect of absorption may not occur in all patients with renal disease. The quantity of Ca consumed by uremic patients is usually lower than normal; in one large group of patients with chronic renal failure, the average dietary Ca intake averaged only 300 mg/day, whereas patients undergoing regular dialysis consumed 400–500 mg Ca/day and normal adults of comparable age and sex ingested 800 mg/day (Coburn *et al.*, 1973b).

A decrease in the generation of $1,25(OH)_2D_3$ is probably a major factor leading to both decreased Ca absorption and secondary hyperparathyroidism in uremia (Coburn *et al.*, 1976). Thus, the serum levels of $1,25(OH)_2D$ have been uniformly low or undetectable in patients with advanced renal failure (Brumbaugh *et al.*, 1974; Eisman *et al.*, 1976). Moreover, treatment with small and presumably physiologic amounts of $1,25(OH)_2D_3$ increases intestinal absorption of Ca to normal in such patients (Brickman *et al.*, 1972, 1974b; Henderson *et al.*, 1974). Such data provide convincing evidence that the reduction in the generation of $1,25(OH)_2D$ plays a major role in causing decreased Ca absorption. When, in the course of renal insufficiency, vitamin D metabolism becomes abnormal and Ca absorption is reduced is not known. The fractional absorption of Ca has been found to be normal in patients with mild-to-moderate renal insufficiency, i.e., with serum creatinine levels <2.5 mg/dl (Coburn *et al.*, 1973b). Other studies also indicate that Ca absorption is normal in most patients with creatinine clearance above 60 ml/min (Malluche *et al.*, 1978). Preliminary observations indicate that the plasma levels of $1,25(OH)_2D$ are normal in patients with creatinine clearances above 30 ml/min (Slatopolsky *et al.*, 1978). These observations are inconsistent with the possibility that Ca malabsorption occurs early in the course of renal insufficiency and contributes to the early pathogenesis of secondary hyperparathyroidism. However, it should be noted that plasma levels of $1,25(OH)_2D$ are increased in patients with primary hyperparathyroidism (Haussler *et al.*, 1976) and they commonly exhibit hyperabsorption of Ca. Thus, the Ca absorption noted in patients with mild renal failure may be lower than expected.

Some data indicate that abnormal Ca absorption in uremia may be due, at least in part, to factors other than altered vitamin D metabolism. Thus, uremia, per se, may reduce the response of the intestine to $1,25(OH)_2D_3$ or adversely affect Ca transport via a mechanism not dependent upon vitamin D as shown in Fig. 19 (Wong *et al.*, 1972). Some degree of improvement in intestinal Ca absorption has been reported in uremic patients following the initiation of hemodialysis (Coburn *et al.*, 1973a; Chanard *et al.*, 1974; Juttmann *et al.*, 1979). It has been suggested that defective oxidative phosphorylation, which may occur in uremia, could alter mitochondrial binding of Ca in intestinal cells, reduce its transcellular movement, and thereby reduce absorption (Avioli, 1972). Russell and Avioli (1974) found reduced uptake and release of radiocalcium by the mitochondria from the intestine of chronically uremic rats. Thus, it is possible that Ca absorp-

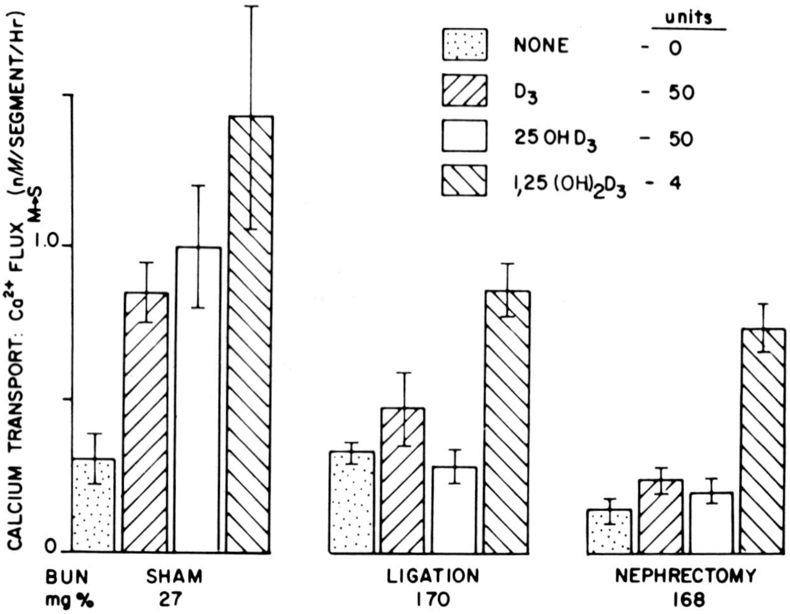

Fig. 19. Calcium transport, measured as *in vitro* Ca flux from mucosal-to-serosal surface of duodenal segments from vitamin D-deficient rats given the vitamin D sterol indicated. Treatment with $1,25(OH)_2D_3$ stimulated Ca transport in rats with urethral ligation or bilateral nephrectomy, but there was decreased Ca transport in uremic, vitamin D-deficient rats. These data suggest that uremia, per se, may impair Ca transport. (From Wong *et al.*, 1972, with permission of *J. Clin. Invest.*)

tion may be altered independent of the abnormality of vitamin D metabolism in renal disease. This is discussed elsewhere (Chapter 4, Vol. III and Chapter 7, Vol. II).

I. Chapatti Diets

An increased incidence of rickets or osteomalacia has been found among Asian immigrants to Western Europe and the United Kingdom; there has been the suggestion that this is related to diminished dietary intake of vitamin D as most Asian families continue to follow traditional diets in their new environments (Goel *et al.*, 1976). One characteristic of this diet is consumption of much chapatti flour, which contains large quantities of phytate. There is evidence that short-term consumption of chapatti flour can lower intestinal Ca absorption perhaps by binding Ca and making it unavailable (Reinhold *et al.*, 1976). Despite the incrimination of the chapatti diet per se, others (Dent *et al.*, 1973) reported that treatment with ultraviolet light could ameliorate the manifestations

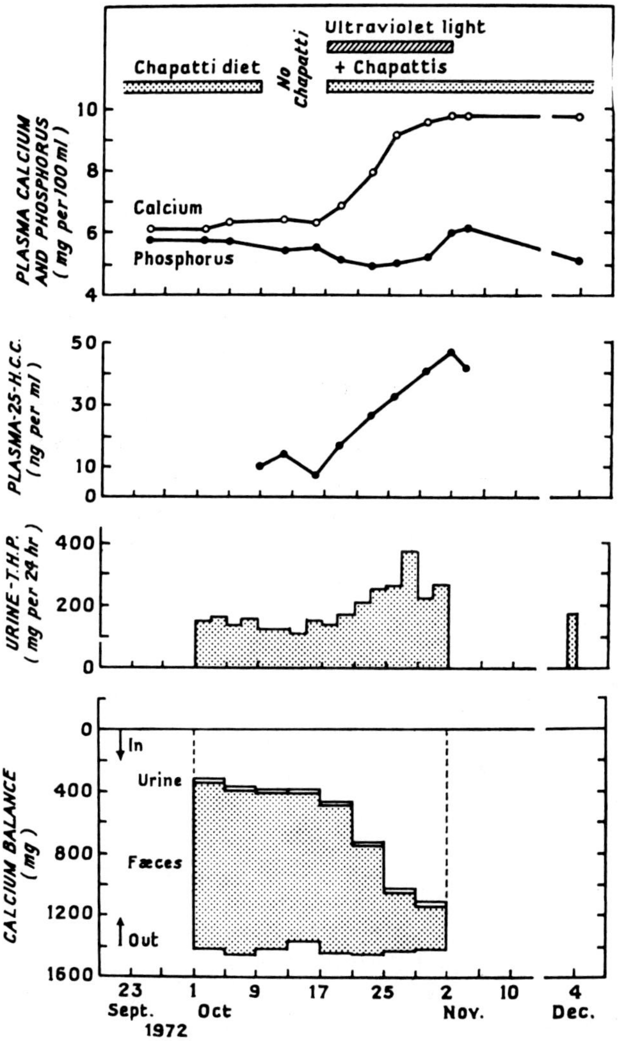

Fig. 20. Metabolic balance study in an Asian patient eating a chappati diet. He first received a vitamin D-free chappati diet, then a low phytate diet, followed by the chappati diet while he had ultraviolet light treatment. There was a marked increase in net Ca absorption during treatment with ultraviolet light. The abbreviations are 25-HCC, 25-hydroxyvitamin D_3, and THP, total hydroxyproline. The lower panel shows Ca balance; the stippled area represents fecal Ca and the open bars, urinary Ca; the area under the zero line represents positive calcium balance. (From Dent *et al.*, 1973, with permission of *Lancet.)*

of vitamin D deficiency despite continued ingestion of the chapatti diet (Fig. 20). Dunnigan and colleagues (1976) calculated that the sunlight exposure of Asian children was similar to that of other children in the United Kingdom who are not prone to rickets. However, they found a good correlation between the quantity of chapatti flour, the amounts of phosphorus and phytate, total dietary phosphate intake, and the degree of elevation of serum alkaline phosphatase levels in these patients. They admitted that the component of the chapatti flour which contributed to rickets was unidentified; the presence of excess quantities of phytate-derived polyphosphate esters or dietary phosphate itself could possibly also be incriminated in reducing Ca absorption. Thus, the mechanism for the decreased absorption of Ca in patients ingesting bread made from chapatti flour remains uncertain at this time. It is possible that the limited exposure to sunlight in the United Kingdom combined with the decreased availability of dietary Ca for absorption when taken with the chapatti flour act together to increase the risk for the development of osteomalacia.

J. Diabetes Mellitus

Interest has focused on the high prevalence of altered Ca absorption and Ca metabolism in patients with diabetes mellitus. Thus, Albright and Reifenstein (1948) noted the presence of osteoporosis in patients with long standing and poorly controlled diabetes. Subsequently, Berney (1952) reemphasized the coexistence of diabetes and osteoporosis and Menczel *et al.* (1972) reported a very high incidence of hip fractures in diabetic patients. Levin *et al.* (1976) measured the skeletal mass of the forearm with photoabsorptometry and noted a significant reduction in bone mass in both juvenile and adult-onset diabetics compared to age- and sex-matched controls. The finding of bone loss in those with juvenile diabetes even of brief duration suggested the possibility that Ca metabolism may be altered even before the appearance of overt diabetes. Measurements of intestinal Ca absorption have not been reported to date.

Supporting the possibility that vitamin D metabolism may be altered in diabetes are numerous studies showing a reduction in both intestinal Ca transport and intestinal CaBP in rats with diabetes produced with either alloxan or streptozocin (Schneider *et al.,* 1974, 1976; Schneider and Schedl, 1977; Schedl, 1979). Treatment of these animals with insulin restored intestinal Ca absorption and intestinal CaBP to normal. Treatment with various vitamin D metabolites, including vitamin D_3, 25(OH)D_3, 1,25$(OH)_2D_3$, 1α(OH)D_3 and an extract of *Solanum malacoxylon,* indicate that only 1,25$(OH)_2D_3$, 1α(OH)D_3 and the extract of *Solanum malocoxylon* could restore CaBP and intestinal Ca absorption to normal. Moreover, observations of low plasma levels of 1,25$(OH)_2$D confirmed the existence of altered vitamin D metabolism in these animals; however, its relationship to human diabetes has not been firmly established.

K. Osteoporosis

The etiology of osteoporosis is multifactorial and remains unknown. This disorder is considered in detail in Chapter 2, Vol. III. Nonetheless, a consideration of disorders related to reduced Ca absorption would not be complete without some mention of this complex disorder. Most observers have come to the opinion that decreased intestinal Ca absorption and Ca deficiency play a pathogenic role. Caniggia *et al.* (1963), measuring plasma radioactivity after an oral dose of ^{45}Ca, Bronner *et al.* (1963), using Ca balance and kinetic modeling, and Szymendera *et al.* (1972) and Gallagher *et al.* (1973), utilizing double isotope methods, have provided evidence that intestinal Ca absorption was reduced in patients with osteoporosis. Moreover, several investigators have reported that treatment with oral Ca supplements can increase Ca retention as measured by metabolic balance studies (Spencer *et al.*, 1964; Schwartz *et al.*, 1965). However, it has also been found that increased Ca retention does not persist and even disappears when a high Ca intake is maintained for a prolonged period (Harrison *et al.*, 1961; Schwartz *et al.*, 1965). It has been suggested that a high Ca intake can reduce the rate of bone turnover (Schwartz *et al.*, 1965; Sammon *et al.*, 1970; Riggs *et al.*, 1976). Other studies, particularly in patients with juvenile osteoporosis, suggest that oral Ca supplements combined with large doses of vitamin D can lead to favorable Ca retention (Munck, 1964). Studies by Gallagher *et al.* (1979) showed that the normal decline in intestinal Ca absorption that occurs with aging is accelerated with osteoporosis. Moreover, the patients with osteoporosis have slightly reduced serum levels of $1,25(OH)_2D$ compared to normal individuals,

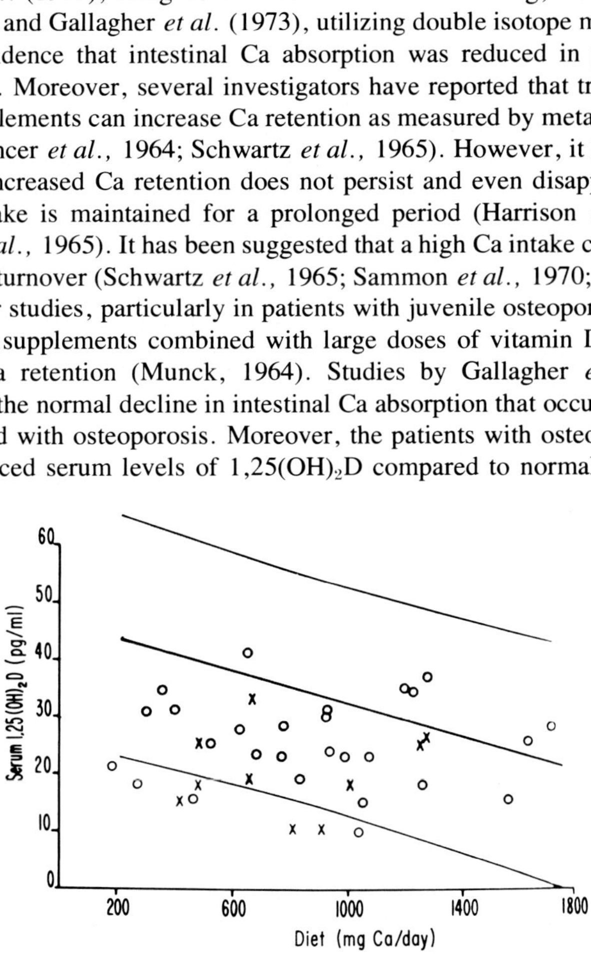

Fig. 21. The relationship between dietary Ca intake and serum level of $1,25(OH)_2D$ in patients with osteoporosis (○) and normal elderly subjects (X). The regression line and confidence limits for normal subjects are also shown. (From Gallagher *et al.*, 1979, with permission of *J. Clin. Invest.*)

particularly in relation to the dietary Ca intake (Fig. 21). The oral administration of $1,25(OH)_2D_3$ produced a significant increase in Ca absorption in patients with osteoporosis and in elderly individuals. Thus, there is evidence that intestinal Ca absorption is reduced in patients with osteoporosis and some data suggest that the serum levels of $1,25(OH)_2D$ are slightly lower in these patients than in elderly controls; the factors responsible for these abnormalities are still uncertain (Gallagher *et al.*, 1979).

L. Nephrotic Syndrome

The nephrotic syndrome is characterized by the excretion of large quantities of albumin in the urine, hypoalbuminemia, and hyperlipidemia. Abnormalities of Ca metabolism have been observed, even in patients with normal rates of glomerular filtration. Thus, decreased levels of total serum Ca, generally attributed to the presence of hypoalbuminemia, were found to be associated with low serum levels of ionized Ca (Lim *et al.*, 1977; Goldstein *et al.*, 1977). Moreover, reduced intestinal absorption of Ca has also been reported (Jones *et al.*, 1967; Emerson and Beckman, 1945). It has been suggested that there is an abnormality of vitamin D metabolism in patients with the nephrotic syndrome; this is believed to arise from excessive losses of 25(OH)D in the urine (Schmidt-Gayk *et al.*, 1977; Barragry *et al.*, 1977; Goldstein *et al.*, 1977). It has been suggested that such losses are believed to arise because of increased urinary excretion of serum vitamin D-binding protein (Massry and Goldstein, 1978). It should be noted that Mountokalakis *et al.* (1977), who measured Ca absorption using a double isotope technique, could find no abnormalities of Ca absorption in patients with nephrotic syndrome and normal renal function; abnormal Ca absorption was present only when renal insufficiency was present.

Thus, there is evidence for increased renal losses of 25(OH)D in patients with the nephrotic syndrome; this may contribute to decreased Ca absorption, and, in some cases this may lead to mild osteomalacia (Malluche *et al.*, 1979). However, it is not clear that this leads to an increased predilection for clinically significant skeletal disease as renal insufficiency progresses (Coburn *et al.*, 1977).

M. Hypoparathyroidism and Pseudohypoparathyroidism

Metabolic balance studies have shown that net absorption of Ca is reduced in the hypoparathyroid patient; and the absorption of Ca is decreased in the presence of marked hypocalcemia (Aub *et al.*, 1932). The identification of the role of PTH to stimulate the bioconversion of vitamin D_3 to its active form, $1,25(OH)_2D_3$, and the finding of reduced plasma levels of $1,25(OH)_2D$ in patients with hypoparathyroidism have provided the apparent mechanism for reduced Ca absorption. Moreover, the administration of 1,25$(OH)_2D_3$ in relatively small doses can lead to a correction of hypocalcemia and reduction in fecal Ca (Coburn *et al.,* 1974; Russell *et al.,* 1974). Moreover, treatment with 1,25$(OH)_2D_3$ or 1$\alpha$$(OH)D_3$ can restore serum Ca to normal in association with little change in the renal clearance of Ca and no change in hydroxyproline excretion (Neer *et al.,* 1975); thus, it was suggested that correction of hypocalcemia primarily involves stimulation of intestinal Ca absorption rather than an augmentation of bone resorption.

Pseudohypoparathyroidism is characterized by hypocalcemia, hyperphosphatemia, and defective phosphaturic and calcemic responses to exogenous PTH. The plasma levels of 1,25$(OH)_2D_3$ are also reduced in this condition (Drezner *et al.,* 1976). Metabolic balance studies indicate that there is impaired net intestinal absorption of Ca, with a marked increase in intestinal Ca absorption upon treatment with 1,25$(OH)_2D_3$ (Sinha and Bell, 1976).

Thus, there is evidence that the hypoabsorption of Ca seen in both hypoparathyroidism and pseudohypoparathyroidism arises, in large part, due to decreased renal generation of 1,25$(OH)_2D_3$ (Brickman *et al.,* 1978).

VII. CONDITIONS WITH INCREASED CALCIUM TRANSPORT

A. Milk Alkali Syndrome

The ''milk alkali'' syndrome is characterized by hypercalcemia, decreased renal function, and alkalosis. It arises in association with the ingestion of large quantities of milk and/or calcium carbonate. Its pathogenesis is unclear but the disorder probably arises from increased intestinal absorption of Ca. In a prospective study, McMillan and Freeman (1975) found that most patients given frequent oral doses of milk and calcium carbonate develop only modest degrees of hypercalciuria, probably due to increased net absorption of Ca; however, an occasional patient developed hypercalcemia and a decrease in renal function. The quantities of Ca administered were quite high, i.e., 13–14 gm/day; under such circumstances, it is almost certain that the increase in net Ca absorption occurs by a passive absorptive mechanism. However, it is not clear why only certain patients, given such massive loads of oral Ca, develop marked hypercalcemia. With continued administration of Ca, nephrocalcinosis and decreased renal function may occur. Studies utilizing radiocalcium are not available to indicate whether patients who have a propensity to develop this disorder absorb a greater fraction of Ca than would occur under normal circumstances. Serum levels of various vitamin D sterols have, as yet, not been reported in this syndrome.

B. Hyperparathyroidism

Metabolic balance studies and studies using radioactive Ca indicate that Ca absorption is often increased in patients with primary hyperparathyroidism (Sjöberg, 1970). However, this does not invariably occur; thus, Peacock (1975) found that patients with hyperparathyroidism and a history of renal stones almost always exhibited hyperabsorption of Ca, while it was less consistent in patients with other presenting features of hyperparathyroidism. The hyperabsorption of Ca that occurs in patients with nephrolithiasis and hyperparathyroidism is probably a consequence of increased plasma levels of $1,25(OH)_2D$. Thus, Broadus *et al.* (1980) found a strong correlation between the intestinal absorption of Ca, measured by changes in urinary Ca excretion in response to an acute load of Ca, and the plasma level of $1,25(OH)_2D$ in such patients.

C. Idiopathic Hypercalciuria and Calcium-Stone Formers

Idiopathic hypercalciuria is a syndrome that is usually detected after the finding of calcium-containing kidney stones. Intestinal absorption of Ca is generally increased when measured either by metabolic balance techniques (Edwards and Hodgkinson, 1965; Lemann, 1980) or radioisotopic methods (Pak *et al.*, 1972; Wills *et al.*, 1970). Recent studies have shown a direct correlation between intestinal absorption of Ca and the plasma levels of $1,25(OH)_2D$ (Kaplan *et al.*, 1977; Wilz *et al.*, 1979; Lemann, 1980). The cause for the increase in serum levels of $1,25(OH)_2D$ is uncertain and may differ from patient to patient. Thus, Shen *et al.* (1977) suggested that a renal "leak" of phosphate with consequent hypophosphatemia might stimulate the renal generation of $1,25(OH)_2D_3$. However, Kaplan *et al.* (1977) found normal levels of serum phosphate and concluded that a renal "leak" of phosphate was not responsible for the increased levels of $1,25(OH)_2D$. Another cause of hypercalciuria could be a primary renal "leak" of Ca, which would lead to mild hypocalcemia, stimulating the secretion of PTH and thereby increase the generation of $1,25(OH)_2D_3$. Such an increase in the levels of $1,25(OH)_2D$ could lead to secondary hyperabsorption of Ca (Bordier *et al.*, 1977). Serum immunoreactive parathyroid hormone (iPTH) levels have been shown to be increased in patients with hypercalciuria due to a renal Ca "leak" (Coe *et al.*, 1973; Coe, 1977), while the levels should be decreased when there is primary hyperabsorption of Ca. Thus, the serum levels of $1,25(OH)_2D$ and hyperabsorption of Ca could occur with hypercalciuria of any cause.

It should be noted that only 30–40% of patients with hypercalciuria studied have increased serum levels of $1,25(OH)_2D$ (Shen *et al.*, 1977; Gray *et al.*, 1977; Kaplan *et al.*, 1977); the cause of the increased intestinal absorption of Ca in the remaining patients is unknown. One could speculate that a subgroup of patients may have enhanced intestinal sensitivity to the action of $1,25(OH)_2D_3$ or might have an unrecognized alteration of vitamin D metabolism. Further studies will be useful in defining various subgroups of patients with the syndrome, idiopathic hypercalciuria.

D. Sarcoidosis

Sarcoidosis is a noninfectious, idiopathic, granulomatous disorder that is often associated with increased intestinal absorption of Ca, increased urinary Ca, and, less commonly, hypercalcemia (Anderson *et al.*, 1954). It has been shown that small quantities of vitamin D, which produce little or no effect in normal individuals, can cause increased intestinal absorption of Ca in these patients (Bell *et al.*, 1964). Moreover, the removal of vitamin D from the diet can lead to resolution of the hypercalciuria and hyperabsorption of Ca (Hendrix, 1966). Thus, there is evidence for increased sensitivity to vitamin D in patients with sarcoidosis and hypercalciuria. Serum levels of 25(OH)D have been normal (Belsey *et al.*, 1974), while the plasma levels of $1,25(OH)_2D$ have been increased (Papapoulous *et al.*, 1979; Stern *et al.*, 1980). Preliminary observations suggest that the administration of a modest dose of vitamin D to patients with sarcoidosis who lack evidence of altered Ca homeostasis leads to a greater increase in urinary Ca and serum $1,25(OH)_2D$ than occurs in normals. The source of the increased generation of $1,25(OH)_2D_3$ is uncertain; the persistence of hypercalcemia with increased serum levels of $1,25(OH)_2D$ following bilateral nephrectomy in a patient with sarcoidosis suggests that a tissue other than the kidney is responsible (Barbour *et al.*, 1980). Present data suggest that the increase in intestinal Ca absorption and most of the abnormalties of Ca metabolism seen in sarcoidosis may arise from the increased generation of $1,25(OH)_2D_3$.

E. Pituitary Disorders

Naturally occurring alterations in the secretion of pituitary hormones may lead to altered Ca absorption. Thus, Sjöberg (1969) has shown that patients with acromegaly had increased retention of ingested ^{47}Ca. This could have arisen from increased generation of $1,25(OH)_2D_3$, and the plasma levels of this sterol have been reported to be increased in patients with acromegaly or hyperprolactinemia (Brown *et al.*, 1979; Lund *et al.*, 1979). Moreover treatment with bromocriptine led to a significant fall in elevated plasma levels. On the other hand, Kumar *et al.* (1979a) failed to find elevated plasma levels of $1,25(OH)_2D$ in patients with either dwarfism or acromegaly.

F. Pregnancy

The skeleton of a newborn infant contains approximately 25 gm of Ca, and there is obviously an increased need for Ca during pregnancy. Heaney and

Skillman (1971) evaluated Ca metabolism in pregnant women, who were studied with metabolic balance techniques and Ca kinetics with ^{48}Ca, a stable radioisotope. In these women, intestinal Ca absorption was increased to twice the usual level at 20–24 weeks of gestation, the earliest time studied. These rates persisted throughout pregnancy but reverted to the normal "non-pregnant" levels by three months following delivery. The observation of Kumar *et al.* (1979b) of increased plasma levels of $1,25(OH)_2D$ make it likely that changes in vitamin D metabolism account, in part, for the increased Ca absorption. Heaney and Skillman found that high doses of both estrogen and progesterone given to a normal woman for seven weeks failed to produce the changes observed during pregnancy. Therefore, the hormonal mechanisms that stimulate the increased generation of $1,25(OH)_2D_3$ and augment Ca absorption remain unclear.

ACKNOWLEDGMENTS

We acknowledge the secretarial assistance provided by Carolyn Schaefer, Ella Manning, Elizabeth Atwell, Sally Shupien, and Michael Greene.

This study was supported in part by research funds from the Veterans Administration, USPHS Grants AM 14750 and AM 20919.

REFERENCES

Adams, T. H., and Norman, A. W. (1970). Studies on the mechanism of action of calciferol. *J. Biol. Chem.* **245,** 4421–4431.

Adams, T. H., Wong, R. G., and Norman, A. W. (1970). Studies on the mechanism of action of calciferol. II. Effects of the polyene antibiotic, filipin, on vitamin D-mediated calcium transport. *J. Biol. Chem.* **245,** 4432–4442.

Agnew, J. E., and Holdsworth, C. D. (1971). The effect of fat on calcium absorption from a mixed meal in normal subjects, patients with malabsorptive disease, and patients with a partial gastrectomy. *Gut* **12,** 973–877.

Albright, F., and Reifenstein, E. C. (1948). "Parathyroid Glands and Metabolic Bone Disease; Selected Studies," p. 150. Williams & Wilkins, Baltimore, Maryland.

Alcock, N., and MacIntyre, I. (1962). Interrelation of calcium and magnesium absorption. *Clin. Sci.* **22,** 185–193.

Alcock, N., and MacIntyre, I. (1964). Some effects of magnesium repletion on calcium metabolism in the rat. *Clin. Sci.* **26,** 219–225.

Alevizaki, C. C., Ikkos, D. C., and Singhelakis, P. (1973). Progressive decrease of true intestinal calcium absorption with age in normal man. *J. Nucl. Med.* **14,** 760–762.

Alpers, D. H. (1974). Calcium absorption and malabsorption. *Viewpoints Dig. Dis.* **6,** 1–4.

Anderson, J., Dent, C. E., Harper, C., and Philpot, G. R. (1954). Effect of cortisone on calcium metabolism in sarcoidoisis with hypercalcemia, possibly analogous actions on cortisone to vitamin D. *Lancet* **2,** 720–724.

Arnaud, S. B., Newcomer, A. D., Offord, K. P., and Go, V. L. W. (1979). 25-hydroxyvitamin D (25-OH-D) metabolism in nontropical sprue (NTS). Vitamin D: Basic Research and its Clinical

Application'' (A. W. Norman, K. Schaefer, D. von Herrath, H.-G. Grigoleit, J. W. Coburn, H. F. DeLuca, E. B. Mawer, and T. Suda, eds.), pp. 1023–1026. Gruyter, Berlin.

Arnold, B. M., Kovacks, K., and Murray, T. M. (1976). Cellular localization of intestinal calcium binding protein in pig duodenum. *Digestion* **14,** 77.

Asano, T. (1960). Transport of calcium and inorganic phosphate across the intestinal wall of the rat. *Seitai no Kagaku* **11,** 55–58.

Atkinson, M., Nordin, B. E. C., and Sherlock, S. (1956). Malabsorption and bone disease in prolonged obstructive jaundice. *Q. J. Med.* **25,** 299–304.

Aub, J. C., Albright, F., Bauer, W., and Rossmeisl, E. (1932). Studies of calcium and phosphorus metabolism. VI. In hypoparathyroidism and chronic steatorrhea with tetany with special consideration of the therapeutic effect of thyroid. *J. Clin. Invest.* **11,** 211–234.

Aubert, J. P., Cherian, A. G., Moukhtan, M. S., and Milhaud, G. (1964). Etude du metabolisme du calcium chez le rat à l'aide de calcium 45. V-LA thyroparathyroidectomie et l'effet de la thyroxine et de la parathormone. *Biochem. Pharmacol.* **13,** 31–44.

Avioli, L. V. (1972). Intestinal absorption of calcium. *Arch. Intern. Med.* **129,** 345–355.

Avioli, L. V. (1980). Mineral metabolism in chronic hepatic failure. *In* ''Pediatric Diseases Related to Calcium'' (H. F. DeLuca and C. S. Anast, eds.), pp. 433–441. Am. Elsevier, New York.

Avioli, L. V., McDonald, J. E., Singer, R. A., and Henneman, P. H. (1965a). A new oral isotopic test of calcium absorption. *J. Clin. Invest.* **44,** 128–139.

Avioli, L. V., McDonald, J. E., and Lee, S. W. (1965b). The influence of age on the intestinal absorption of ^{45}Ca in women and its relation to ^{45}Ca absorption in post-menopausal osteoporosis. *J. Clin. Invest.* **44,** 1960–1967.

Avioli, L. V., Birge, S. J., and Lee, S. W. (1968). Effects of Prednisone on vitamin D metabolism in man. *J. Clin. Endocrinol. Metab.* **28,** 1341–1346.

Badenoch, J., and Fourman, P. (1954). Osteomalacia in steatorrhoea. *Q. J. Med.* **23,** 165–176.

Bar, A., Cohen, A., Eisner, U., Resenfeld, G., and Hurwitz, S. (1978). Differential response of calcium transport systems in laying hens to exogenous and endogenous changes in vitamin D status. *J. Nutr.* **108,** 1322–1328.

Barbour, G. L., Coburn, J. W., Norman, A. W., and Slatopolsky, E. (1980). Non-renal hypercalcemia in Sarcoidosis. *Clin. Res.* **28,** 46A (abstr.).

Barragry, J. M., France, M. W., Crter, N. D., Auton, J. A., Beer, M., Boucher, B. J., and Cohen, R. D. (1977). Vitamin D metabolism in nephrotic syndrome. *Lancet* **2,** 626–629.

Barry, R. J. C., and Eggenton, J. (1972). Ionic basis of membrane potentials of epithelial cells in rat small intestine. *J. Physiol. (London)* **227,** 217–231.

Bassett, S. H., Keutmann, E. H., and van Hyde, Z. H. (1939). Metabolism in idiopathic steatorrhea: I. The influence of dietary and other factors on lipid and mineral balance. *J. Clin. Invest.* **18,** 101–120.

Bassett, S. H., Figueroa, W. G., Tuttle, S. G., and Jordan, T. (1960). Metabolic studies in Cushing's syndrome. The effect of steriod withdrawal, androgen and vitamin D on calcium, phosphorus and nitrogen balance. *Clin. Orthop.* **17,** 304.

Begum, A., and Pereira, S. (1969). Calcium balance studies on children accustomed to low calcium intakes. *Br. J. Nutr.* **23,** 905–911.

Behar, J., and Kerstein, M. D. (1976). Intestinal calcium absorption: Differences in transport between duodenum and ileum. *Am. J. Physiol.* **230,** 1255–1260.

Bell, N. H., Gill, J. R., and Bartter, F. C. (1964). On the abnormal calcium absorption in sarcoidosis. Evidence for increased sensitivity to vitamin D. *Am. J. Med.* **36,** 500–513.

Bell, R. R., Engelmann, D. T., Sie, T.-L., and Draper, H. H. (1975). Effect of high protein intake on calcium metabolism in the rat. *J. Nutr.* **105,** 475–483.

Belsey, R. E., DeLuca, H. F., and Potts, J. T., Jr. (1974). A rapid assay for 25-OH-vitamin D_3 without preparative chromatography. *J. Clin. Endocrinol. Metab.* **38,** 1046–1051.

Benson, J. D., Emery, R. S., and Thomas, J. W. (1969). Effects of previous calcium intakes on adaptation to low and high calcium diets in rats. *J. Nutr.* **97,** 53–60.

Berlyne, G. M., Ari, J. B., Nord, E., and Shainkin, R. (1973). Bedouin osteomalacia due to calcium deprivation caused by high phytic acid content of unleavened bread. *Am. J. Clin. Nutr.* **26,** 910–911.

Berney, P. W. (1952). Osteoporosis and diabetes mellitus. *J. Iowa Med. Soc.* **42,** 10–12.

Bhandarkar, S. D., Bluhm, M. M., MacGregor, J., and Nordin, B. E. C. (1961). Visceral scleroderma without skin involvement. *Br. Med. J.,* 1539–1541.

Bikle, D. B., Zolock, D. T., Morrissey, R. L., and Herman, R. H. (1978). Independence of 1,25-dihydroxyvitamin D_3-mediated calcium transport from de novo RNA and protein synthesis. *J. Biol. Chem.* **253,** 484–488.

Bikle, D. B., Morrissey, R. L., and Zolock, D. T. (1979). The mechanism of action of vitamin D in the intestine. *Am. J. Clin. Nutr.* **32,** 2322–2338.

Birge, S. J., and Gilbert, H. R. (1974). Identification of an intestinal sodium and calcium-dependent phosphatase stimulated by parathyroid hormone. *J. Clin. Invest.* **54,** 710–717.

Birge, S. J., and Miller, R. (1977). The role of phosphate in the action of vitamin D on the intestine. *J. Clin. Invest.* **60,** 980–988.

Birge, S. J., Peck, W. A., Berman, M., and Whendon, G. D. (1969). Study of calcium absorption in man: A kinetic analysis and physiologic model. *J. Clin. Invest.* **48,** 1705–1713.

Birge, S. J., Gilbert, H. R., and Avioli, L. V. (1972). Intestinal calcium transport: The role of sodium. *Science* **176,** 168–170.

Blau, M., Spencer, H., Swernov, J., and Laszlo, D. (1954). Utilization and intestinal excretion of calcium in man. *Science* **120,** 1029–1031.

Bonjour, J. P., Russell, R. G. G., Morgan, D. B., and Fleisch, H. A. (1973). Intestinal calcium absorption, Ca-binding protein, and Ca-ATPase in diphosphonate-treated rats. *Am. J. Physiol.* **224,** 1011–1017.

Bordier, P., Pechet, M. M., Hesse, R., Marie, P., and Rasmussen, H. (1974). Response of adult patients with osteomalacia to treatment with crystalline 1α-hydroxy vitamin D_3. *N. Engl. J. Med.* **291,** 866–871.

Bordier, P., Ryckewart, A., Gueris, J., and Rasmussen, H. (1977). On the pathogenesis of so called idiopathic hypercalciuria. *Am. J. Med.* **63,** 398–409.

Boyle, I. T., Gray, R. W., and DeLuca, H. F. (1971). Regulation by calcium of *in vivo* synthesis of 1,25-dihydroxycholecalciferol and 21,25-dihydroxycholecalciferol. *Proc. Natl. Acad. Sci. U.S.A.* **68,** 2131–2134.

Brannan, P. G., Vergne-Marini, P., Paks, C. Y. C., Hull, A. R., and Fordtran, J. S. (1976). Magnesium absorption in the human small intestine: Results in normal subjects, patients with absorptive hypercalciuria. *J. Clin. Invest.* **57,** 1412–1418.

Bredderman, P. J., and Wasserman, R. H. (1974). Chemical composition affinity for calcium and some related properties of the vitamin D-dependent calcium binding protein. *Biochemistry* **13,** 1687–1694.

Brickman, A. S., Coburn, J. W., and Norman, A. W. (1972). Action of 1,25-dihydroxycholecalciferol, a potent, kidney-produced metabolite of vitamin D_3, in uremic man. *N. Engl. J. Med.* **287,** 891–895.

Brickman, A. S., Coburn, J. W., Rowe, P. H., Massry, S. G., and Norman, A. W. (1974a). Impaired calcium absorption in uremic man: Evidence for defective absorption in the proximal intestine. *J. Lab. Clin. Med.* **84,** 791–801.

Brickman, A. S., Coburn, J. W., Massry, S. G., and Norman, A. W. (1974b). 1,25-dihydroxy-vitamin D_3 in normal man and patients with renal failure. *Ann. Intern. Med.* **80,** 161–168.

Brickman, A. S., Coburn, J. W., and Norman, A. W. (1978). Relative resistance to 1α-hydroxyvitamin D in hypo- and pseudohypoparathyroidism. *Clin. Res.* **26,** 158.

Briscoe, A. M., and Ragan, C. (1965). Bile and endogenous fecal calcium in man. *Am. J. Clin. Nutr.* **16,** 281–286.

Broadus, A. E., Dominguez, M., and Bartter, F. C. (1978). Pathophysiologic studies in idiopathic hypercalciuria: Use of an oral calcium tolerance test to characterize distinctive hypercalciuria subgroups. *J. Clin. Endocrinol. Metab.* **47,** 751–760.

Broadus, A. E., Horst, R. L., Lang, R., Littledike, E. T., and Rasmussen H. (1980). The importance of circulating 1,25-dihydroxyvitamin D in the pathogenesis of hypercalciuria and renalstone formation in primary hyperparathyroidism. *N. Engl. J. Med.* **302,** 421–426.

Bronner, F., Richelle, L. J., Saville, P. D., Nicholas, J. A., and Cobb, J. R. (1963). Quantitation of calcium metabolism in postmenopausal osteoporosis and in scoliosis. *J. Clin. Invest.* **42,** 898–905.

Bronner, F. (1962). Experimental studies of calcium absorption in man. *Bibl. "Nutr. Dieta"* **3,** 22.

Bronner, F., Sammon, P. J., Stacy, R. E., and Shah, B. G. (1967). Role of thyrocalcitonin in the regulation of the blood calcium level. *Biochem. Med.* **1,** 261–279.

Bronner, F., Charnot, Y., Globub, E. E., and Freund, T. (1976). Calcium binding protein and regulation of calcium transport. *Calcif. Tissue Res.* **21,** Suppl., 27–38.

Brown, D. J., Spanos, E., Raptis, P., and MacIntyre, I. (1979). Effect of pregnancy, acromegaly, primary hyperparathyroidism and prolactinoma on 1,25-dihydroxyvitamin D in man. *In* "Vitamin D: Basic Research and Its Clinical Application" (A. W. Norman, K. Schaefer, D. von Herrath, H.-G. Grigoleit, J. W. Coburn, H. F. DeLuca, E. B. Mawer, and T. Suda, eds.), pp. 625–635. de Gruyter, Berlin.

Brumbaugh, P. F., Haussler, D. H., Bressler, R., and Haussler, M. R. (1974). Radio-receptor assay for 1α,25-dihydroxy-vitamin D_3. *Science* **183,** 1080–1091.

Bullamore, J. R., Gallagher, J. C., Wilkson, R., and Nordin,B. E. C. (1970). Effect of age on calcium absorption. *Lancet* **2,** 535–537.

Byrne, W. J., Ament, M. E., Burke, M., and Fonkalsrud, E. (1979). Home parenteral nutrition. *Surg., Gynecol. Obstet.* **149,** 593–599.

Caniggia, A., Gennari, C., Bianchi, V., and Guideri, R. (1963). Intestinal absorption of ^{45}Ca in senile osteoporosis. *Acta Med. Scand.* **173,** 613–617.

Caniggia, A., Gennari, G., and Cesari, L. (1964). Intestinal absorption of ^{45}Ca and dynamics of ^{45}Ca in gastrectomy osteoporosis. *Acta Med. Scand.* **176,** 599–605.

Chanard, J., Jacques, A., Cyrille, B., and Funch-Brentano, J. L. (1974). A rapid method for measurement of fractional intestinal absorption of calcium. *J. Nucl. Med.* **15,** 588–592.

Cherney, R. W., Mazess, I., Hamstra, R. B., DeLuca, H. F., and O'Reagan, S. (1978). Reduction of serum 1,25-dihydroxyvitamin D in children receiving glucocorticoids. *Lancet* **2,** 1123–1125.

Clark, I. (1968). Effects of magnesium ions on calcium and phosphorus metabolism. *Am. J. Physiol.* **214,** 348–356.

Coburn, J. W., Koppel, M. H., Brickman, A. S., and Massry, S. G. (1973a). Study of intestinal absorption of calcium in patients with renal failure. *Kidney Int.* **3,** 264–272.

Coburn, J. W., Hartenbower, D. L., and Massry, S. G. (1973b). Intestinal absorption of calcium and the effect of renal insufficiency. *Kidney Int.* **4,** 96–104.

Coburn, J. W., Reddy, C. R., Brickman, A. S., Hartenbower, D. L., Friedler, R. M., and Norman, A. W. (1973c). Vitamin D metabolism in magnesium deficiency. *Fed. Proc., Fed. Am. Soc. Exp. Biol.* **62,** 3933.

Coburn, J. W., Brickman, A. S., Kurokawa, K., Massry, S. G., Bethune, J. E., Harrison, H. E., and Norman, A. W. (1974). Action of 1,25-dihydroxycholecalciferol in normal man and patients with hypophosphatemic resistant rickets, pseudohypoparathyroidism, and uremia. *Endocrinol., Proc. Int. Symp., 4th,* pp. 385–392.

Coburn, J. W., Hartenbower, D. L., and Brickman, A. S. (1976). Advances in vitamin D metabolism as they pertain to chronic renal disease. *Am. J. Clin. Nutr.* **29,** 1283–1299.

Coburn, J. W., Hartenbower, D. L., Brickman, A. S., Massry, S. G., and Kopple, J. D. (1977). Intestinal absorption of calcium, magnesium and phosphorus in chronic renal insufficiency. *In* "Calcium Metabolism in Renal Failure and Nephrolithiasis" (D. S. David, ed.), pp. 77–109. Wiley, New York.

Coe, F. L. (1977). Treated and untreated recurrent calcium nephrolithiasis in patients with idiopathic hypercalciuria, hyperurocosuria or no metabolic disorder. *Ann. Intern. med.* **87,** 404–410.

Coe, F. L., Canterbury, J. M., Firpo, J. J., and Reiss, E. (1973). Evidence for secondary hyperparathyroidism in idiopathic hypercalciuria. *Clin. Invest.* **52,** 134–142.

Cohn, S. H., Teree, T. M., and Gusmano, E. A. (1968). Effect of varying calcium intake on the parameters of calcium metabolism in the rat. *J. Nutr.* **94,** 261–267.

Collins, E. J., Garrett, E. R., and Johnson, R. L. (1962). Effects of adrenal steroids on radiocalcium metabolism in dogs. *Metab., Clin. Exp.* **11,** 716–726.

Compston, J. E., Crow, J. P., Wells, I. P., Horton L. W. L., Hirst, D., Merrett, A. L., Woodhead, J. S., and Williams, R. (1980). Vitamin D prophylaxis and osteomalacia in chronic cholestatic liver disease. *Digest. Dis. Sci.* **25,** 28–32.

Corradino, R. A. (1974). Embryonic chick intestine in organ culture: Interaction of adenylate cyclase system and vitamin D_3 mediated calcium absorptive mechanism. *Endocrinology* **94,** 1607–1614.

Corradino, R. A. (1976). Diphenylhydantoin: Direct inhibition of the vitamin D_3-mediated calcium absorptive mechanism in organ-cultured duodenum. *Biochem. Pharmacol.* **25,** 863–864.

Corradino, R. A. (1977). Cyclic AMP regulation of the $1,25(OH)_2D_3$ mediated intestinal calcium absorptive mechanics. *In* "Vitamin D: Biochemical, Chemical and Clinical Aspects Related to Calcium Metabolism" (A. W. Norman, K. Schaefer, J. W. Coburn, H. F. DeLuca, D. Fraser, H.-G. Grigoleit, and D. von Herrath, eds.), pp. 231–230. de Gruyter, Berlin.

Corradino, R. A., Ebel, J. G., Craig, P. H., Taylor, A. N., and Wasserman, R. H. (1971). Calcium absorption and the vitamin D_3-dependent calcium-binding protein. I. Inhibition by dietary strontium. *Calcif. Tissue Res.* **7,** 81–92.

Cramer, C. F. (1973). Effect of salmon calcitonin on in vivo calcium absorption in rats. *Calcif. Tissue Res.* **13,** 169–172.

Cramer, C. F., and Dueck, J. (1962). In vivo transport of calcium from healed thirty-vella fistulas in dogs. *Am. J. Physiol.* **202,** 161–614.

Cramer, C. F., Parkes, C. O., and Copp, D. H. (1969). The effect of chicken and hog calcitonin on some parameters of Ca, P, and Mg metabolism in dogs. *Can. J. Physiol. Pharmacol.* **47,** 181–184.

Curtis, F. K., Fellows, H., and Rich, C. (1967). Estimation of human calcium absorption of external radiosotope counting. *J. Lab. Clin. Med.* **69,** 1036–1041.

Dalen, N., and Lamke, B. (1976). Bone mineral loses in alcoholics. *Acta Orthop. Scand.* **47,** 469–471.

Davis, W. L., Jones, R. G., and Hagler, H. K. (1979). Calcium containing lysosomes in the normal chick duodenum: A histochemical and analytical electron microscopic study. *Tissue Cell* **11,** 127.

DeGrazia, J. A., and Rich, C. (1964). Intestinal absorption of calcium^{45} in man. *Metab., Clin. Exp.* **13,** 650–660.

DeGrazia, J. A., Ivanovich, P., Fellows, H., and Rich, C. (1965). A double isotope method for measurement of intestinal absorption of calcium in man. *J. Lab. Clin. Med.* **66,** 822–829.

Deller, D. J. (1966). Radiocalcium absorption after partial gastrectomy. *Am. J. Dig. Dis.* **11,** 10–19.

Deller, D. J., Worthley, B. W., and Martin H. (1965). Measurement of calcium^{47} absorption by whole body gamma spectrometry. *Australas. Ann. Med.* **14,** 223–231.

Demel, R. A., and van Deenen, L. L. M. (1965). Penetration of lipid monolayers by polyene antibiotics. Correlation with selective toxicity and mode of action. *J. Biol. Chem.* **240,** 2749+.

Dent, C. E., and Smith, R. (1969). Nutritional osteomalacia. *Q. J. Med.* **38,** 195–209.

Dent, C. E., Harper, C. N., and Philpot, G. R. (1961). Treatment of renal-glomerular osteodystrophy. *Q. J. Med.* **30,** 1–31.

Dent, C. E., Rowe, D. J. E., Round, J. M., and Stamp, T. C. (1973). Effect of Chapattis and ultraviolet irradiation on nutritional rickets in an Indian immigrant. *Lancet* **1,** 1282–1284.

de Wolff, F. A. (1975). Stimulation of vitamin D-dependent Ca-ATPase and of intestinal calcium absorption by diphenyhydantoin. *Eu. J. Pharmacol.* **33,** 71–79.

Dorrington, K. J., Hui, A., Hofman, T., Hitchman, A. J. W., and Harrison, J. E. (1974). Spectroscopic studies on the binding of divalent cations to procine intestinal calcium-binding protein. Molecular properties and the effect of binding calcium ions. *J. Biol. Chem.* **249,** 199–204.

Dorrington, K. J., Kells, D. I. C., Hitchman, A. J. W., Harrison, J. E., and Hofmann, T. (1978). Spectroscopic studies on the binding of divalent cations to porcine intestinal calcium-binding protein. *Can. J. Biochem.* **56,** 492–499.

Dowdle, E. B., Schachter, D., and Schenker, H. (1960). Requirement for vitamin D for the active transport of calcium by the intestine. *Am. J. Physiol.* **198,** 269–274.

Drezner, M. K., Neelon, F. A., Haussler, M., McPherson, H. T., and Lebovitz, H. E. (1976). 1,25-dihydroxycholecalciferol deficiency: The probable cause of hypocalcemia and metabolic bone disease in pseudohypoparathyroidism. *J. Clin. Endocrinol. Metab.* **42,** 621–628.

Dumont, P. A., Curran, P. F., and Solomon, A. K. (1960). Calcium and strontium in rat small intestine, their fluxes and their effect on Na flux. *J. Gen. Physiol.* **43,** 1119–1135.

Dunnigan, M. G., McIntosh, W. B., and Ford, J. A. (1976). Rickets in Asian immigrants. *Lancet* **1,** 1346.

Dupuis, Y., and Fournier, P. (1963). Lactose and the absorption of calcium and strontium. *In* "The Transfer of Calcium and Strontium Across Biological Membranes" (R. H. Wasserman, ed.), pp. 277–293. Academic Press, New York.

Edwards, W. A., and Hodgkinson, A. (1965). Metabolic studies in patients with idiopathic hypercalciuria. *Clin. Sci.* **29,** 143–157.

Eisman, J. A., Hamstra, A. J., Kream, B. E., and DeLuca, H. F. (1976). 1,25-dihydroxyvitamin D in biological fluids: A simplified and sensitive assay. *Science* **193,** 1021–1023.

Emerson, K., and Beckman, W. W. (1945). Calcium metabolism in nephrosis. I. A description of an abnormality in calcium metabolism in children with nephrosis. *J. Clin. Invest.* **24,** 564–572.

Engström, G. W., and DeLuca, H. F. (1963). Effect of egg white diets on calcium metabolism in the rat. *J. Nutr.* **81,** 218–222.

Epstein, S., Van Mieghem, W., Sagel, J., and Jackson, W. P. U. (1973). Effect of single large doses of oral calcium on serum calcium levels in the young and the elderly. *Metab., Clin. Exp.* **22,** 1163–1173.

Evensen, D., Hanssen, K. F., and Berstad, A. (1978). Inhibition of intestinal calcium absorption by somatostatin in man. *Metab., Clin. Exp.* **27,** 1345–1347.

Farrington, K., Epstein, O., Varghese, Z., Newman, S. P., Moorhead, J. F., and Sherlock, S. (1979). Effect of oral 1,25-dihydroxycholecalciferol on calcium and phosphate malabsorption in primary biliary cirrhosis. *Gut* **20,** 616–619.

Favus, M. J., Kimberg, D. V., Millar, G. N., and Gershon, E. (1973a). Effects of cortisone administration on the metabolism and localization of 25-hydroxycholecalciferol in the rat. *J. Clin. Invest.* **52,** 1328–1335.

Favus, M. J., Walling, M. W., and Kimberg, D. V. (1973b). Effects of 1,25-dihydroxycholecalciferol on intestinal calcium transport in cortisone-treated rats. *J. Clin. Invest.* **52,** 1680–1685.

Favus, M. J., Walling, M. W., and Kimberg, D. V. (1974). Effects of dietary calcium restriction and chronic thyroparathyroidectomy on the metabolism of [^{3}H]25-hydroxyvitamin D_3 and the active transport of calcium by rat intestine. *J. Clin. Invest.* **53,** 1139–1148.

Favus, M. J., Kathpalia, S. C., Coe, F. L., and Monod, A. E. (1980). Effects of diet calcium and 1,25-dihydroxyvitamin D_3 on colon calcium active transport. *Am. J. Physiol.* **238,** G75–G78.

Feher, J. J., and Wasserman, R. H. (1979). Calcium binding protein, alkaline phosphatase and calcium absorption in cortisol-treated chicks. *Endocrinology* **104,** 547–551.

Ferraro, C., Ladizesky, M., Cabrejas, M., Montoreano, R., and Mautalen, C. (1976). Intestinal absorption of phosphate: Action of protein synthesis inhibitors and glucocorticoids in rat. *J. Nutr.* **106,** 1752–1756.

Finkelstein, J. D., and Schachter, D. (1962). Active transport of calcium by intestine: Effects of hypophysectomy and growth hormone. *Am. J. Physiol.* **103,** 873–880.

Fordtran, J. S., and Locklear, T. W. (1966). Ionic constituents and osmolality of gastric and small-intestinal fluids after eating. *Am. J. Dig. Dis.* **11,** 503–521.

Fourman, L. P. R., and Spray, G. H. (1948). Absorption of vitamin D in Steatorrhoea. *Br. Med. J.* **1,** 142–144.

Fox, J. Swaminathan, R., Murray, T. M., and Care, A. D. (1977). Role of the parathyroid glands in the enhancement of intestinal calcium absorption in response to a low calcium diet. *J. Endocrinol.* **74,** 345–354.

Freedman, R. A., Weiser, M. M., and Isselbacher, K. J. (1977). Calcium translocation by Golgi and lateral-basal membrane vesicles from rat intestine: Decrease in vitamin D-deficient rats. *Proc. Natl. Acad. Sci. U.S.A.* **74,** 3612–3616.

Freund, T. S., and Bronner, F. (1975). Stimulation in vitro by 1,25-dihydroxyvitamin D_3 of intestinal cell calcium uptake and calcium-binding protein. *Science* **190,** 1300–1302.

Friedland, J. A., Williams, G. A., Bowser, E. N., Henderson, W. J., and Hoffeins, E. (1965). Effect of hyperthyroidism on intestinal absorption of calcium in rat. *Proc. Soc. Exp. Biol. Med.* **120,** 20–23.

Frizzell, R. A., and Schultz, S. G. (1972). Ionic conductance of extracellular shunt pathway in rabbit ileum. *J. Gen. Physiol.* **59,** 318–346.

Fullmer, C. S., and Wasserman, R. H. (1973). Bovine intestinal calcium-binding: Purification and some properties. *Biochim. Biophys. Acta* **317,** 172–186.

Fullmer, C. S., Wasser, R. H., Cohn, D. V., and Hamilton, J. W. (1977). Chemical studies on bovine intestinal calcium binding protein and related peptides minor A and minor B. *In* "Vitamin D: Biochemical, Chemical and Clinical Aspects Related to Calcium Metabolism" (A. W. Norman, K. Schaefer, J. W. Coburn, H. F. DeLuca, D. Fraser, H.-G. Grigoleit, and D. von Herrath, eds.), pp. 245–252. de Gruyter, Berlin.

Gallagher, J. C., Aaron, J., Horsman, A., Marshall, D. H., Wilkinson, R., and Nordin, B. E. C. (1973). The crush fracture syndrome in postmenopausal women. *Clin. Endocrinol. Metab.* **2,** 293.

Gallagher, J. C., Riggs, B. L., Eisman, J., Hamstra, A., Arnaud, S. B., and DeLuca, H. F. (1979). Intestinal calcium absorption and serum vitamin D metabolites in normal subjects and osteoporotic patients. *J. Clin. Invest.* **64,** 729–736.

Garcia-Pascual, B., Donath, A., and Courvoisier, B. (1979). Plasma 25-OH-D, bone mass densitometry and f^{47}Ca intestinal absorption deficiency in chronic alcoholism. *In* "Vitamin D: Basic Research and Its Clinical Application" (A. W. Norman, K. Schaefer, D. von Herrath, H.-G. Grigoleit, J. W. Coburn, H. F. DeLuca, E. B. Mawer, and T. Suda, eds.), pp. 819–821. de Gruyter, Berlin.

Gennari, C. (1964). Radiocalcium intestinal absorption in thyrotixic osteoporosis. *Boll. Soc. Ital. Biol. Sper.* **40,** 253–256.

Goel, K. M., Logan, R. W., Arnell, G. C., Sweet, E. M., Warren, J. M., and Shanks, R. A. (1976). Florid and subclinical tickets among immigrant children in Glasgow. *Lancet* **1,** 1141–1148.

Golden, R., and Abbot, H. (1933). Relation of thyroid, adrenals, and islands of Langerhans to malacic diseases of bone. *Am. J. Roentgenol. Radium Ther.* **30,** 641.

Goldman, D. E. (1943). Potential, impedance, and rectification in membranes. *J. Gen. Physiol.* **27,** 37–60.

Goldstein, D. A., Oda, Y., Kurokawa, K., and Massry, S. G. (1977). Blood levels of 25-hydroxyvitamin D in nephrotic syndrome. Studies in 26 patients. *Ann. Intern. Med.* **87,** 664–668.

Gran, F. C. (1960). Vitamin D and calcium absorption in parathyroidectomized rats. *Acta Physiol. Scand.* **49,** 211–215.

Gray, R. W., Wilz, D. L., Caldas, A. E., and Lemann, J., Jr. (1977). The importance of phosphate in regulating plasma 1,25$(OH)_2$-vitamin D levels in humans: Study in healthy subjects, in calcium-stone formers and in patients with primary hyperparathyroidism. *J. Clin. Endocrinol. Metab.* **45,** 299–306.

Gray, T. K., Bieberdorf, F. A., and Fordtran, J. S. (1973). Thyrocalcitonin and the jejunal absorption of calcium, water, and electrolytes in normal subjects. *J. Clin. Invest.* **52,** 3084–3088.

Greger, J. L., Baligar, P., Abernathy, R. P., Bennett, O. A., and Paterson, T. (1978). Calcium, magnesium, phosphorus, copper, and magnesium balance in adolescent females. *Am. J. Clin. Nutr.* **31,** 117–121.

Hahn, T. J., and Avioli, L. V. (1975). Anticonvulsant osteomalacia. *Arch. Intern. Med.* **135,** 997–1000.

Hajjar, E. T., Vincenti, F., and Salti, I. S. (1974). Gluten-induced enteropathy. *Arch. Intern. Med.* **134,** 565–566.

Hanna, F. M., Navarrette, D. A., and Hsu, F. A. (1970). Calcium-fatty acid absorption in term infants fed human milk and prepared formulas simulating human milk. *Pediatrics* **45,** 216–224.

Harris, F., Hoffenberg, R., and Black, E. (1965a). Calcium kinetics in vitamin D deficiency rickets. I. Plasma kinetic studies after intravenous and oral Ca^{47}. *Metab., Clin. Exp.* **14,** 1101–1111.

Harris, F., Hoffenberg, R., and Black, E. (1965b). Calcium kinetics in vitamin D deficiency rickets. II. Intestinal handling of calcium. *Metab., Clin. Exp.* **14,** 1112–1121.

Harris, J. L., and Innes, J. R. M. (1931). The mode of action of vitamin D. Studies on hypervitaminosis D. The influence of the calcium phosphate intake. *Biochem. J.* **25,** 367–390.

Harrison, H. E., and Harrison, H. C. (1960). Transfer of Ca^{45} across intestinal wall in vitro in relation to action of vitamin D and cortisol. *Am. J. Physiol.* **199,** 265–271.

Harrison, H. E., and Harrison, H. C. (1963). Sodium potassium, and intestinal transport of glucose, L-tyrosine, phosphate, and calcium. *Am. J. Physiol.* **205,** 107–111.

Harrison, H. E., and Harrison, H. C. (1965). Vitamin D and permeability of intestinal mucosa to calcium. *Am. J. Physiol.* **208,** 370–374.

Harrison, M., Fraser, R., and Mullan, B. (1961). Calcium metabolism in osteoporosis: Acute and long-term responses to increased calcium intake. *Lancet* **1,** 1015–1019.

Haussler, M. R., Nagode, L. A., and Rasmussen, H. (1970). Induction of intestinal brush border alkaline phosphatase by vitamin D and identity with Ca-ATPase. *Nature (London)* **228,** 1199–1200.

Haussler, M. R., Baylink, D. J., Hughes, M. R., Brumbaugh, P. F., Wergedal, J. E., Shen, F. H., Nielsen, R. L., Counts, S. J., Bursac, K. M., and McCain, T. A. (1976). The assay of 1-alpha, 25-dihydroxyvitamin D_3; Physiologic and pathologic modulation of circulating hormone levels. *Clin. Endocrinol. (Oxford)* **5,** 151s–165s.

Heaney, R. P., and Skillman, T. G. (1964). Secretion and excretion of calcium by the human gastrointestinal tract. *J. Lab. Clin. Med.* **64,** 29–41.

Heaney, R. P., and Skillman, T. G. (1971). Calcium metabolism in normal human pregnancy. *J. Clin. Endocrinol. Metab.* **33,** 661–670.

Heaney, R. P., and Whedon, G. D. (1958). Radiocalcium studies of bone formation rate in human metabolic bone disease. *J. Clin. Endocrinol. Metab.* **18,** 1246–1267.

Heaney, R. P., Saville, P. D., and Recker, R. R. (1975). Calcium absorption as a function of calcium intake. *J. Lab. Clin. Med.* **85,** 881–890.

Heaney, R. P., Recker, R. R., and Saville, P. D. (1977). Calcium balance and calcium requirements in middle-aged women. *Am. J. Clin. Nutr.* **30,** 1603–1611.

Heaton, F. W., and Parsons, F. M. (1961). The metabolic effect of high magnesium intake. *Clin. Sci.* **21,** 273–284.

Heggeness, F. W. (1959). Effect of antibiotics on the gastrointestinal absorption of calcium and magnesium in the rat. *J. Nutr.* **68,** 573–582.

Hegsted, D. M. (1973). Calcium and phosphorus. *In* "Modern Nutrition in Health and Disease" (R. S. Goodhart, and M. E. Shils, eds.), 5th ed., p. 268. Lea & Febiger, Philadelphia, Pennsylvania.

Helbock, H. J., Forte, J. G., and Saltman, P. (1966). The mechanism of calcium transport by rat intestine. *Biochim. Biophys. Acta* **126,** 81–93.

Henderson, R. G., Russell, G. G., Ledingham, J. G. G., Smith, R., Preston, C., Warner, G. T., and Norman, A. W. (1974). Effects of 1,25-dihydroxycholecalciferol on calcium absorption, muscle weakness, and bone disease in chronic renal failure. *Lancet* **1,** 379–384.

Hendrix, J. A., Alcock, N. W., and Archibald, R. M. (1963). Competition between calcium, strontium, and magnesium for absorption in the isolated rat intestine. *Clin. Chem. (Winston-Salem, N.C.)* **9,** 734–744.

Hendrix, J. Z. (1966). Abnormal skeletal mineral metabolism in sarcoidosis. *Ann. Intern. Med.* **64,** 797–805.

Henry, K. M., Kon, S. K., Todd, P. E. E., Toothil, J., and Tomlin, D. M. (1960). Calcium and phosphorus metabolism in the rat: Effect of age on rate of adaptation to a low calcium intake. *Acta Biochim. Pol.* **7,** 167–185.

Hepner, G. W., Roginsky, M., and Moo, H. F. (1976). Abnormal vitamin D metabolism in patients with cirrhosis. *Dig. Dis. Sci.* **21,** 527–532.

Hill, L. F., Lumb, G. A., Mawer, E. B., and Stanbury, S. W. (1973). Indirect inhibition of the biosynthesis of 1,25-dihydroxycholecalciferol in rats treated with diphosphonate. *Clin. Sci.* **44,** 335–347.

Hitchman, A. J. W., and Harrison, J. E. (1972). Calcium binding proteins in the duodenal mucosal of the chick, rat, pig and human. *Can. J. Biochem.* **50,** 758–765.

Holdsworth, E. S. (1970). The effect of vitamin D on enzyme activities in the mucosal cells of the chick small intestine. *J. Membr. Biol.* **3,** 43–53.

Hollander, D., Muradidhara, K. S., and Zimmerman, A. (1978). Vitamin D_3 intestinal absorption in vivo: Influence of fatty acids, bile salts and perfusate pH on absorption. *Gut* **19,** 267–272.

Horst, R. W., DeLuca, H. F., and Jorgenson, N. (1978). The effect of age on calcium absorption and accumulation of $1,25(OH)_2D_3$ in intestinal mucosa of rats. *Metab. Bone Dis. Relat. Res.* **1,** 29–33.

Hughes, M. R., Brumbaugh, P. F., Haussler, M. R., Wergedal, J. E., and Baylink, D. J. (1975). Regulation of serum 1α,25-dihydroxyvitamin D_3 by calcium and phosphate in the rat. *Science* **190,** 578–579.

Hurwitz, S., and Bar, A. (1969). Relation between the lumen-blood electrochemical potential difference of calcium, calcium absorption and calcium-binding protein in the intestine of the fowl. *J. Nutr.* **99,** 217–224.

Ireland, P., and Fordtran, J. S. (1973). Effect of dietary calcium and age on jejunal calcium absorption in humans studied by intestinal perfusion. *J. Clin. Invest.* **52,** 2672–2681.

Jaworski, Z. F., Brown, E. M., Federuk, S., and Seitz, H. (1963). A method for the study of calcium absorption by the human gut using a standard dose of calcium labelled with calcium^{47}. *N. Engl. J. Med.* **269,** 1103–1111.

Johnson, C. C., and Bynum, T. E. (1976). Hypocalcemia as a complication of jejunoileal bypass for morbid obesity. *South. Med. J.* **69,** 616–618.

Johnson, N. E., Alcantara, E. N., and Linkswiler, H. (1970). Effect of level of protein intake on urinary and fecal calcium and calcium retention of young adult males. *J. Nutr.* **100,** 1425–1430.

Jones, J. H., Peter, D. K., and Morgan, D. B. (1967). Observations on calcium metabolism in the nephrotic syndrome. *Q. J. Med.* **36,** 301–320.

Juan, D., Liptak, P., and Gray, T. K. (1976). Absorption of inorganic phosphate in the human jejunum and its inhibition by salmon calcitonin. *J. Clin. Endocrinol. Metab.* **43,** 517–522.

Jubiz, W., Haussler, M. R., McKain, T. A., and Tolman, K. O. (1977). Plasma 1,25-dihydroxyvitamin D levels in patients receiving anticonvulsant drugs. *J. Clin. Endocrinol. Metab.* **44,** 617–621.

Juttmann, J. R., Hagenouw-Taal, J. C. W., Lameyer, L. D. F., Ruis, A. M., and Birkenhager, J. C. (1979). A longitudinal study of bone-mineral content and intestinal calcium absorption in patients with chronic renal failure. *Metab., Clin. Exp.* **28,** 1114–1121.

Kapitola, J., Hrba J., and Vilimovska, D. (1979). A simplified method for the determination of intestinal calcium absorption. *Nucl. Med.* **18,** 151–153.

Kaplan, R. A., Haussler, M. R., Keftos, L. J., Bone, H., and Pak, C. Y. C. (1977). The role of 1α,25-dihydroxyvitamin D in the mediation of intestinal hyperabsorption of calcium in primary hyperparathyroidism and absorptive hypercalciuria. *J. Clin. Invest.* **59,** 756–760.

Kaye, M., and Silverman, M. (1965). Calcium metabolism in chronic renal failure. *J. Lab. Clin. Med.* **66,** 535.

Kehayoglou, C. K., Williams, H. S., Whimster, W. F., and Holdsworth, C. D. (1968). Calcium absorption in the normal, bile duct ligated and cirrhotic rat, with observations on the effect of long- and medium-chain triglycerides. *Gut* **9,** 597–603.

Kehayoglou, K., Hadziyannis, S. T., Kostamis, P., and Malamos, B. (1973). The effect of medium-chain triglyceride on ^{47}calcium absorption in patients with primary biliary cirrhosis. *Gut* **14,** 653–656.

Kemm, J. R. (1973). Effects of previous dietary history of calcium intake on the skeleton and calcium absorption in the rat. *J. Physiol. (London)* **230,** 643–658.

Kemm, J. R. (1976). The effect of parathyroidectomy and large doses of cholecalciferol on the ability of rats to adapt to changes in dietary intake of calcium. *J. Physiol. (London)* **256,** 103–115.

Kenny, A. D. (1975). Gastrointestinal absorption of alkaline earth ions. *In* "International Encyclopaedia of Pharmacology and Therapeutics" (W. Rummel and W. Forth, eds.), pp. 507–597. Pergamon, Oxford.

Kimberg, D. V., Schachter, D., and Schenker, H. (1961). Active transport of calcium by intestine: Effects of dietary calcium. *Am. J. Physiol.* **200,** 1256–1262.

Kimberg, D. V., Field, M., Johnson, J., Henderson, A., and Gershon, E. (1971). Stimulation of intestinal mucosal adenyl cyclase by cholera enterotoxin and prostaglandins. *J. Clin. Invest.* **50,** 1218–1230.

Klein, G. L., Ament, M. E., Bluestone, R., Norman, A. W., Targoff, C. M., Sherrard, D. J., Young, J. H., and Coburn, J. W. (1980). Bone disease associated with total parenteral nutrition. *Lancet* **2,** 1041–1044.

Klein, R. G., Arnaud, S. B., Gallagher, J. C., DeLuca, H. F., and Riggs, B. L. (1977). Intestinal calcium absorption in exogenous hypercortisonism. *J. Clin. Invest.* **60,** 253–259.

Kooh, S. W., Fraser, D., Reilly, J. R., Hamilton, J. R., Grant, D. G., and Bell, L. (1977). Rickets due to calcium deficiency. *N. Engl. J. Med.* **297,** 1264–1266.

Kopple, J. D., and Coburn, J. W. (1973). Metabolic studies of low protein diet in uremia. *Medicine (Baltimore)* **52,** 597–607.

Kowarski, S., and Schachter, D. (1975). Vitamin D-dependent, particulate calcium-binding activity and intestinal calcium transport. *Am. J. Physiol.* **229,** 1198–1204.

Krane, S. M., Brownell, G. L., Stanbury, J. B., and Corrigan, H. (1956). Effect of thyroid disease on calcium metabolism in man. *J. Clin. Invest.* **35,** 874–887.

Krawitt, E. L. (1967a). Duodenal calcium transport in hyperthyroidism. *Proc. Soc. Exp. Biol. Med.* **125,** 417–419.

Krawitt, E. L. (1967b). Effect of thyrocalcitonin on duodenal calcium transport. *Proc. Soc. Exp. Biol. Med.* **125,** 1084–1086.

Krawitt, E. L. (1972). The role of intestinal transport proteins in cortisone-mediated suppression of Ca^{2+} absorption. *Biochim. Biophys Acta* **274,** 179–188, 1972.

Krawitt, E. L., Stubbert, P. A., and Ennis, P. H. (1973). Calcium absorption and brush border phosphatases following dietary calcium restriction. *Am. J. Physiol.* **224,** 548–551.

Krawitt, E. L., Sampson, H. W., and Katagiri, C. (1975). Effect of 1,25-dihydroxycholecalciferol on ethanol mediated suppression of calcium absorption. *Calcif. Tissue Res.* **18,** 119–124.

Krawitt, E. L., Kunin, A. S., Sampson, H. W., and Bacon, B. J. F. (1977). Effect of hypophysectomy on calcium transport by rat duodenum. *Am. J. Physiol.* **232**(2), E229–E233.

Krawitt, E. L., Mawer, B., and Davies, M. (1979). Absorption of vitamin D and 25-OH vitamin D in patients with intestinal malabsorption. *In* "Vitamin D: Basic Research and Its Clinical Application" (A. W. Norman, K. Schaefer, D. von Herrath, H.-G. Grigoleit, J. W. Coburn, H. F. DeLuca, E. B. Mawer, and T. Suda, eds.), pp. 975–978. de Gruyter, Berlin.

Kumar, R., Merimee, T. J., Silva, P., and Epstein, F. H. (1979a). The effect of chronic excess or deficiency of growth hormone on plasma 1,25 dihydroxyvitamin D levels in man. *In* "Vitamin D: Basic Research and Its Clinical Application" (A. W. Norman, K. Schaefer, D. von Herrath, H.-G. Grigoleit, J. W. Coburn, H. F. DeLuca, E. B. Mawer, and T. Suda, eds.), pp. 1005–1009. de Gruyter, Berlin.

Kumar, R., Wayne, R. C., Silva, P., and Epstein, F. H. (1979b). Elevated, 1,25-dihydroxyvitamin D plasma levels in normal human pregnancy and lactation. *J. Clin. Invest.* **63,** 342–344.

Lafont, J., and Pilon, R. (1975). Influence of glucocorticoids on some morphological and biochemical aspects of rat small intestinal mucosa. *Biochim. Biophys. Acta* **392,** 288–298.

Larkins, R. G., Colston, K. W., Galante, L. S., MacAuley, S. J., Evans, I. M. A., and MacIntyre, I. (1973). Regulation of vitamin D metabolism without parathyroid hormone. *Lancet* **2,** 289–291.

Lee, D. B. N., Walling, M. W., Silis, V., and Coburn, J. W. (1980). Calcium and inorganic phosphate transport in rat colon: Dissociated response to 1,25-dihydroxyvitamin D_3. *J. Clin. Invest.* **65,** 1326–1331.

Lee, D. B. N., Walling, M. W., Levine, B. S., Gafter, V., Silas, V., Hodsman, A., and Coburn, J. W. (1981). Intestinal and metabolic effect of 1,25-dihydroxyvitamin D3 in the normal adult rat. *Am. J. Physiol.* **240,** G90–G96.

Lekkerkerker, J. F. F., and Doorenbos, H. (1973). The influence of thyroid hormone on calcium absorption from the gut in relation to urinary calcium excretion. *Acta Endocrinol. (Copenhagen)* **73,** 672–680.

Lekkerkerker, J. F. F., von Woudenberg, F., and Doorenbos, H. (1972). Influence of low dose of steriod therapy on calcium absorption. *Acta Endocrinol. (Copenhagen)* **69,** 488–496.

Lemann, J. (1980). Idiopathic hypercalciuria. *In* "Nephrolithiasis: Contemporary Issues in Nephrology" (B. M. Brenner and J. H. Stein, eds.), pp. 86–115. Churchill-Livingstone, New York. Edinburgh and London.

Levin, M. E., Boisseau, V. C., and Avioli, L. V. (1976). Effects of diabetes mellitus on bone mass in juvenile and adult-onset diabetes. *N. Engl. J. Med.* **294,** 241–245.

Levine, B. S., Brautbar, N., Walling, M. W., Lee, D. B. N., and Coburn, J. W. (1980). Effects of vitamin D and diet magnesium on magnesium metabolism. *Am. J. Physiol.* **239,** E515–E523.

Lim, P., Jacob, E., Tock, E. P. C., and Pwee, H. S. (1977). Calcium and phosphorus metabolism and nephrotic syndrome. *Q. J. Med.* **46,** 327–338.

Liu, S. H., and Chu, H. I. (1943). Studies of calcium and phosphorus metabolism with special reference to the pathogenesis and effect of dihydrotachysterol (AT-IO) and iron. *Medicine (Baltimore)* **22,** 103–161.

Liu, S. H., Chu, H. I., Su, C. C., Yu, T. F., and Cheng, T. Y. (1940). Calcium and phosphorus metabolism in osteomalacia. IX. Metabolic behavior of infants fed on breast milk from mothers showing various states of vitamin D Nutrition. *J. Clin. Invest.* **19,** 327–347.

Long, R. G., Wills, M. R., Skinner, R. K., and Sherlock, S. (1976). Serum-25-hydroxy-vitamin D in untreated parechymal and cholestatic liver disease. *Lancet* **2,** 650–652.

Long, R. G., Meinhard, E., Skinner, R. K., Varghese, Z., Wills, M. R., and Sherlock, S. (1978). Clinical, biochemical, and histological studies of osteomalacia, osteoporosis, and parathyroid function in chronic liver disease. *Gut* **19,** 85–90.

Lund, B. J., Eskildsen, P. C., Lund, B. I., Norman, A. W., Svendsen, P. A., and Sorensen, O. H. (1979). High serum $1,25(OH)_2D$ in acromegaly. Effect of bromocriptine treatment. *In* "Vitamin D: Basic Research and Its Clinical Application" (A. W. Norman, K. Schaefer, D. von Herrath, H.-G. Grigoleit, J. W. Coburn, H. F. DeLuca, E. B. Mawer, and T. Suda, eds.), pp. 1051–1055. de Gruyter, Berlin.

Lutwak, L. (1969). Tracer studies of intestinal calcium absorption in man. *Am. J. Clin. Nutr.* **22,** 771–785.

Lutwak, L., and Shapiro, J. R. (1964). Calcium absorption in man: Based on large volume liquid scintillation counter studies. *Science* **144,** 1155–1156.

McBean, L. D., and Speckmann, E. W. (1974). A recogniton of the interrelationship of calcium with various dietary components. *Am. J. Clin. Nutr.* **26,** 603–609.

McDonald, S. J., Clarkson, E. M., and DeWardener, H. E. (1964). The effect of a large intake of calcium citrate in normal subjects and patients with chronic renal failure. *Clin. Sci.* **26,** 27–39.

McMillan, D. D., and Freeman, R. B. (1965). The milk alkali syndrome: A study of the acute disorder with comments on the development of the chronic condition. *Medicine (Baltimore)* **44,** 485-501.

Malluche, H. H., Werner, E., and Ritz, E. (1978). Intestinal absorption of calcium and whole body retention in incipient and advanced renal failure. *Miner. Electrolyle Metab.* **1,** 263–270.

Malluche, H. H., Goldstein, D. A., and Massry, S. G. (1979). Osteomalacia and hyperparathyroid bone disease in patients with nephrotic syndrome. *J. Clin. Invest.* **63,** 494–500.

Malm, O. J. (1958). Calcium requirement and adaptation in adult men. *Scand. J. Clin. Lab. Invest.* **10,** 1–286.

Martin, D. L., and DeLuca, H. F. (1969a). Calcium transport and the role of vitamin D. *Arch. Biochem. Biophys.* **134,** 139–148.

Martin, D. L., and DeLuca, H. F. (1969b). Influence of sodium on calcium transport by the rat small intestine. *Am. J. Physiol.* **216,** 1351–1359.

Martin, D. L., Melancon, M. J., Jr., and DeLuca, H. F. (1969). Vitamin D stimulated, calcium-dependent adenosine triphosphatase from brush borders of small intestine. *Biochem. Biophys. Res. Commun.* **35,** 819–823.

Massry, S. G., and Goldstein, D. A. (1978). Calcium metabolism in patients with nephrotic syndrome. *Am. J. Clin. Nutr.* **31,** 1572–1580.

Mautalen, C. A., Cabrejas, M. L., and Soto, R. J. (1969). Isotopic determination of intestinal calcium absorption in normal subjects. *Metab., Clin. Exp.* **18,** 395–405.

Max, E. E., Goodman, D. B. P., and Rasmussen, H. (1978). Purification and characterization of chick intestine brush border membrane: Effects of $1\alpha(OH)$ vitamin D_3 treatment. *Biochim. Biophys. Acta* **511,** 224–239.

Melancon, M. J., Jr., and DeLuca, H. F. (1970). Vitamin D stimulation of calcium dependent adenosine triphosphatase in chick intestinal brush borders. *Biochemistry* **9,** 1658–1664.

Menczel, J., Makin, M., Robin, G., Jaye, I., and Naor, E. (1972). Prevalence of diabetes mellitus in Jerusalem: Its association with presenile osteoporosis. *Isr. J. Med. Sci.* **8,** 918–919.

Messner, R., Smith, H. T., Shapiro, F. L., and Gregory, D. H. (1969). The effect of hemodialysis, vitamin D, and renal homotransplantation on the calcium malabsorption of chronic renal failure. *J. Lab. Clin. Med.* **74,** 472–481.

Milhaud, G., and Vesin, P. (1961). Calcium metabolism in man with calcium^{45}: Malabsorption syndrome and exudative enteropathy. *Nature (London)* **191,** 872–874.

Miller, A., Ueng, T. H., and Bronner, F. (1979). Isolation of vitamin D-dependent, calcium-binding protein from brush borders of rat duodenal mucosa. *FEBS Lett.* **103,** 319–322.

Miller, E. R., Ullrey, D. E., Zutaut, C. L., Hoeter, J. A., and Luecke, R. W. (1965). Mineral balance studies with the baby pig: Effects of dietary magnesium level upon calcium, phosphorus and magnesium balance. *J. Nutr.* **86,** 209–212.

Mircheff, A. K., Walling, M. W., van Os, C. H., and Wright, E. M. (1977). Distribution of alkaline phosphatase and Ca-ATPase in intestinal epithelial cell plasma membranes: Differential response to $1,25(OH)_2D_3$. *In* "Vitamin D: Biochemical, Chemical and Aspects Related to Calcium Metabolism" (A. W. Norman, K. Schaefer, J. W. Coburn, H. F. DeLuca, D. Fraser, H.-G. Grigoleit, and D. von Herrath, eds.), pp. 281–283. de Gruyter, Berlin.

Morehead, R. M., Jr., and Kessner, D. M. (1969). Effects of Mg deficiency and parathyroidectomy on gastrointestinal Ca transport in the rat. *Am. J. Physiol.* **217,** 1608–1613.

Morgan, D. B., Hunt, G., and Paterson, C. R. (1970). The osteomalacia syndrome after stomach operations. *Q. J. Med.* **155,** 395–410.

Morrissey, R. L., and Wasserman, R. H. (1971). Calcium absorption and calcium-binding protein in chicks on differing calcium and phosphorus intakes. *Am. J. Physiol.* **220,** 1509–1515.

Morrissey, R. L., Empson, R. N., Jr., Zolock, D. T., Bikle, D. D., and Bucci, T. J. (1978a). Intestinal response to $1\alpha 25$-dihydroxycholecalciferol. II. A timed study of the intracellular localization of calcium binding protein. *Biochim. Biophys. Acta* **538,** 34.

Morrissey, R. L., Zolock, D. T., Bucci, T. J., and Bikle, D. D. (1978b). Immunoperoxidase localization of vitamin D-dependent calcium binding protein. *J. Histochem. Cytochem.* **26,** 628–634.

Mountokalakis, T., Virvidakis, C., Singhellakis, P., Alevizani, C., and Ikkos, D. (1977). Intestinal calcium absorptionin the nephrotic syndrome. *Ann. Intern. Med.* **86,** 746–747.

Moyer, G. L., Wilson, H. D., and Schedl, H. P. (1978). Effects of dietary protein on body weight, mucosal growth, and calcium absorption in the rat. *Dig. Dis. Sci.* **23,** 545–549.

Munck, O. (1964). Osteoporosis due to malabsorption of calcium responding favorably to large doses of vitamin D. *Q. J. Med.* **33,** 209–221.

Murphy, L., Klevay, L. M., and Petering, H. G. (1974). Interrelationships of zinc and copper nutriture in the rat. *J. Nutr.* **104,** 1458–1465.

Nakhla, A. M., and Latif, A. (1978). A possible role for 5-hydroxytryptamine as a mediator for calcitonin actions on the gastrointestinal tract and pancreas in rats. *Biochem. J.* **176,** 339–342.

Nassim, J. R., Saville, P. D., Cook, P. B., and Mulligan, L. (1959). The effects of vitamin D and given free net in idiopathic sicanrrhegh. *Q. J. Med.* **28,** 141–162.

Neer, R. M., Holick, M. F., DeLuca, H. F., and Potts, J. T., Jr. (1975). Effects of 1α-hydroxyvitamin D3 and 1,25-dihydroxyvitamin D3 on calcium and phosphorus metabolism in hypoparathyroidism. *Metab., Clin. Exp.* **24,** 1403–1413.

Nellans, H. N., and Kimberg, D. V. (1978). Cellular and paracellular calcium transport in rat ileum: Effects of dietary calcium. *Am. J. Physiol.* **236,** E726–E737.

Nellans, H. N., and Kimberg, D. V. (1979a). Intestinal calcium transport absorption, secretion, and vitamin D. *Int. Physiol.* **19,** 227–261.

Nellans, H. N., and Kimberg, D. V. (1979b). Anomalous secretion of calcium in rat ileum: Role of the paracellular pathway. *Am. J. Physiol.* **236,** E473–E481.

Nemere, I. M. (1979). Parathyroid hormone: Limited activation of lysosomes in isolated intestinal cells. *Program Abstr., 61st Annu. Meet. Endocr. Soc.* p. 85.

Neville, E., and Holdsworth, E. S. (1969). A "second messenger" for vitamin D. *FEBS Lett.* **2,** 313–316.

Nicolaysen, R. (1934). *Acta Physiol.* **69,** (1), 1–11.

Nicolaysen, R. (1937a). Studies upon mode of action of vitamin D; influence of vitamin D on faecal output of endogenous calcium and phosphorus in the rat. *Biochem. J.* **31,** 107–121.

Nicolaysen, R. (1937b). Studies upon the mode of action of vitamin D. III. The influence of vitamin D on absorption of calcium and phosphorus. *Biochem. J.* **31,** 122–129.

Nicolaysen, R. (1943). The absorption of calcium as a function of body saturation with calcium. *Acta Physiol. Scand.* **6,** 201–209.

Nicolaysen, R. (1956). Studies in calcium metabolism in rats; adaptation to low Ca intakes in old rats. *Acta Physiol. Scand.* **36,** 114–118.

Nicolaysen, R., Eeg-Larsen, N., and Malm, O. J. (1953). Physiology of calcium metabolism. *Physiol. Rev.* **33,** 424–444.

Noble, H. M., and Matty, A. J. (1967). The effect of thyroxiine on the movement of calcium and inorganic phosphate through the small intestine of the rat. *J. Endocrinol.* **37,** 111–117.

Nordin, B. E., Williams, C. R., Marhsall, D. H., Gallagher, J. C., Williams, A., and Peacock, M. (1976). Calcium absorption in the elderly. *Calcif. Tissue Res.* **215,** 422–451.

Nordin, B. E. C., Young, M. M., Oxby, C., and Bulusu, L. (1968). Calculation of calcium absorption rate from plasma radioactivity. *Clin. Sci.* **35,** 177–182.

Norman, A. W., Mircheff, A. K., Adams, T. H., and Spievogel, A. (1970). Studies on the mechanism of action of calciferol III. Vitamin D-mediated increase of intestinal brush border alkaline phosphate activity. *Biochim. Biophys. Acta* **215,** 348–359.

Norman, A. W., Demel, R. A., de Kruyff, B., and van Deenen, L. L. M. (1972). Studies on the biological properties of polyene antibiotics. Evidence for the direct interaction of filipin with cholesterol. *J. Biol. Chem.* **247,** 1918+.

O'Donnell, J. M., and Smith, M. W. (1973a). Influence of cholecalciferol (vitamin D_3) on the initial kinetics of the uptake of calcium by rat small-intestinal mucosa. *Biochem. J.* **134,** 667–669.

O'Donnell, J. M., and Smith, M. W. (1973b). Uptake of calcium and magnesium by rat duodenal mucosa analysed by means of competing metals. *J. Physiol. (London)* **229,** 733–749.

Ogg, C. S. (1968). The intestinal absorption of ^{47}Ca by patients in chronic renal failure. *Clin. Sci.* **34,** 467–471.

Okada, Y., Sato, T., and Inouye, A. (1975). Effects of potassium ions and sodium ions on membrane potential of epithelial cells in rat duodenum. *Biochim. Biophys. Acta* **413,** 104–115.

Olson, E. B., Jr., DeLuca, H. F., and Potts, J. T., Jr. (1972). Calcitonin inhibition of vitamin D-induced intestinal calcium absorption. *Endocrinology* **90,** 151–157.

Osk-Upmark, E. (1939). Osteomalacia hepatica. *Acta Med. Scand.* **99,** 204–208.

Pak, C. Y. C. (1973). Sodium cellulose phosphate: Mechanism of action and effect on mineral metabolism. *J. Clin. Pharmacol.* **13,** 15–27.

Pak, C. Y. C., East, D. A., Sanzenbacher, L. J., Delea, C. S., and Bartter, F. C. (1972). Gastrointestinal calcium absorption in nephrolithiasis. *J. Clin. Endocrinol. Metab.* **35,** 261–270.

Pak, C. Y. C., Delea, C. S., and Bartter, F. C. (1974a). Successful treatment of recurrent nephrolithiasis (Ca stones) with cellulose phospahte. *N. Engl. J. Med.* **290,** 175–180.

Pak, C. Y. C., Kaplan, R., Bone, H., Towsend, J., and Waters, O. (1975). A simple test for the diagnosis of absorptive, resorptive and renal hypercalciurias. *N. Engl. J. Med.* **292,** 497–500.

Pansu, D., Bellaton, C., and Bronner, F. (1979). Effect of lactose on duodenal calcium-binding protein and calcium absorption. *J. Nutr.* **109,** 508–512.

Pansu, D., Bellaton, C., and Bronner, F. (1981). The effect of calcium intake on the saturable and nonsaturable components of duodenal calcium transport. *Am. J. Physiol.* **240,** G32–G37.

Papapoulous, S. E., Fraher, L. J., Sandler, L. M., Clemens, T. L., Lewin, I. G., and O'Riordan, J. L. H. (1979). 1,25-dihydroxyvicholecalciferol in the pathogenesis of the hypercalcemia of sarcoidosis. *Lancet* **1,** 627–630.

Papworth, D. G., and Patrick, G. (1970). The kinetics of influx of calcium and strontium into rat intestine *in vitro*. *J. Physiol. (London)* **210,** 999–1020.

Parker, T. F., Vergne-Marini, P., Hull, A. R., Pak, C. Y. C., and Fordtran, J. S. (1974). Jejunal absorption and secretion of calcium in patients with chronic renal disease on hemodialysis. *J. Clin. Invest.* **54,** 358.

Parsons, V., Veall, N., and Butterfield, W. J. H. (1968). The clinical use of orally administered ^{45}Ca for the investigation of intestinal calcium absorption. *Calcif. Tissue Res.* **2,** 83–92.

Peacock, M. (1975). Renal stone disease and bone disease in primary hyperparathyroidism and their relationship to the action of parathyroid hormone on calcium absorption. *Parathyroid Conf., 5th, 1974* pp. 78–81.

Pento, J. T., Waite, L. C., Tracy, P. J., and Kenny, A. D. (1977). Adaptation to calcium deprivation in the rat: Effects of parathyroidectomy. *Am. J. Physiol.* **232,** E336–E342.

Phang, J. M., Kales, A. N., and Hahn, T. J. (1968). Effect of divided calcium intake on urinary calcium excretion. *Lancet* **2,** 84–85.

Rader, J. I., Baylink, D. J., Hughes, M. R., Safilian, E. F., and Haussler, M. R. (1979). Calcium and phosphorus deficiency in rats: Effects of PTH and 1,25-dihydroxyvitamin D_3. *Am. J. Physiol.* **236,** E118–E122.

Rasmussen, H. (1959). The influence of parathyroid function upon the transport of calcium in isolated sacs of rat small intestine. *Endocrinology* **65,** 517–519.

Rasmussen, H., Fontaine, O., Max, E. E., and Goodman, D. B. P. (1979). The effect of 1α-hydroxyvitamin D_3 administration on calcium transport in chick intestine brush border membrane vesicles. *J. Biol. Chem.* **254,** 2993–2999.

Recker, R. R., and Saville, P. D. (1971). Calcium absorption in renal failure: Its relationship to blood urea nitrogen, dietary calcium intake, time on dialysis, and other variables. *J. Lab. Clin. Med.* **78,** 380–388.

Recommended Dietary Allowances (1974). 8th rev. ed. *N.A.S.-N.R.C., Publ.* **2216.**

Reddy, C. R., Coburn, J. W., Hartenbower, D. L., Friedler, R. M., Brickman, A. S., Massry, S. G., and Jowsey, J. (1973). Studies on mechanisms of hypocalcemia of magnesium depletion. *J. Clin. Invest.* **52,** 3000–3010.

Reinhold, J. G., Faradji, B., Abadi, P., and Ismail-Beigi, F. (1976). Decreased absorption of calcium, magnesium, zinc and phosphorus by humans due to increased fiber and phosphorus consumption as wheat bread. *J. Nutr.* **106,** 493–503.

Ribovich, M. L., and DeLuca, H. F. (1975). The influence of dietary calcium and phosphorus on intestinal calcium transport in rats given vitamin D metabolites. *Arch. Biochem. Biophys.* **170,** 529–535.

Rich, C., and Ivanovich, P. (1964). Radioisotope tests of calcium absorption. *Northwest Med.* **63,** 792–796.

Riggs, B. L., Jowsey, J., Kelly, P. J., Hoffman, D. L., and Arnaud, C. D. (1976). Effects of oral therapy with calcium and vitamin D in primary osteoporosis. *J. Clin. Endocrinol. Metab.* **42,** 1139–1144.

Ritz, E., and Mehls, D. (1978). Rickets due to calcium deficiency. *N. Engl. J. Med.* **298,** 799 (lett.).

Russell, J. E., and Avioli, L. V. (1974). The effect of chronic uremia on intestinal mitochondrial activity. *J. Lab. Clin. Med.* **84,** 317.

Russell, R. G. G., Walton, R. J., Smith, R., Preston, C., Basson, R., Henderson, R. G., and Norman, A. W. (1974). 1,25-dihydroxycholecalciferol and 1α-hydroxycholecalciferol in hypoparathyroidism. *Lancet* **2,** 14–17.

Sakhaee, K., Peterson, R., Northcutt, C., and Pak, C. Y. C. (1979). Critical appraisal of oral calcium load test for indirect assessment of intestinal calcium absorption. *Urology* **14,** 251–255.

Sallis, J. D., and Holdsworth, E. S. (1962). Calcium metabolism in relation to vitamin D and adrenal function in the chick. *Am. J. Physiol.* **203,** 506–512.

Samachson, J. (1965). The detection of changes in the absorption of calcium and phosphorus. *Am. J. Clin. Nutr.* **16,** 292–298.

Sammon, P. J., Stacey, R. E., and Bronner, F. (1970). Role of parathyroid hormone in calcium homeostasis and metabolism. *Am. J. Physiol.* **218,** 479–485.

Sampson, H. W., Matthews, J. L., Martin, J. H., and Kunin, A. S. (1970). An electron microscopic localization of calcium in the small intestine of normal, rachitic and vitamin D-treated rats. *Calcif. Tissue Res.* **5,** 305.

Schachter, D., and Kowarski, S. (1980). Membrane components of the vitamin D dependent intestinal transport mechanism for calcium. *In* "Pediatric Diseases Related to Calcium" (H. F. DeLuca and C. S. Anast, eds.). Am. Elsevier, New York.

Schachter, D., and Rosen, S. M. (1959). Active transport of Ca^{45} by the small intestine and its dependence on vitamin D. *Am. J. Physiol.* **196,** 357.

Schachter, D., Dowdle, E. B., and Schenker, H. (1960a). Active transport of calcium by the small intestine of the rat. *Am. J. Physiol.* **198,** 263–268.

Schachter, D., Dowdle, E. B., and Schenker, T. T. (1960b). Accumulation of ^{45}Ca by slices of the small intestine. *Am. J. Physiol.* **198,** 275–279.

Schachter, D., Kimberg, D. V., and Schenker, H. (1961). Active transport of calcium by intestine: Action and bio-assay of vitamin D. *Am. J. Physiol.* **200,** 1263–1271.

Schedl, H. P. (1979). Effects of experimental diabetes in the rat on calcium transport and vitamin D metabolism. *In* "Vitamin D: Basic Research and Its Application" (A. W. Norman, K. Schaefer, D. von Herrath, H.-G. Grigoleit, J. W. Coburn, H. F. DeLuca, E. B. Mawer, and T. Suda, eds.), pp. 967–974. de Gruyter, Berlin.

Schedl, H. P., Osbaldiston, G. W., and Mills, I. H. (1968). Absorption, secretion, and precipitation of calcium in the small intestine of the dog. *Am. J. Physiol.* **214**(4), 814–819.

Schmidt-Gayk, H., Schmitt, W., Grawunder, C., Ritz, E., Tschoepe, W., Pietsch, V., Andrassy, K., and Bouillon, R. (1977). 25-hydroxyvitamin D in nephrotic syndrome. *Lancet* **2,** 105–108.

Schneider, L. E., and Schedl, H. P. (1977). Effects of Solanum malacoxylon on duodenal calcium binding protein in the diabetic rat. *Endocrinology* **100,** 928–933.

Schneider, L. E., Wilson, H. D., and Schedl, H. P. (1974). Effects of alloxan diabetes on duodenal calcium-binding protein in the rat. *Am. J. Physiol.* **227**(4), 832–838.

Schneider, L. E., Omdahl, J., and Schedl, H. P. (1976). Effects of vitamin D and its metabolites on calcium transport in the diabetic rat. *Endocrinology* **99,** 793–799.

Scholz, D., and Schwille, P. O. (1978). Somatostatin and intestinal calcium absorption in man. *Metab., Clin. Exp.* **27,** 1349–1352.

Schwartz, E., Panariello, A., and Saeli, J. (1965). Radioactive calcium kinetics during high calcium intake in osteoporosis. *J. Clin. Invest.* **44,** 1547–1560.

Schwartz, R., Woodcock, N. A., Blakely, J. D., and MacKeller, I. (1973). Metabolic responses of adolescent boys to two levels of dietary magnesium and protein. II. Effect of magnesium, and protein level on calcium balance. *Am. J. Clin. Nutr.* **26,** 519–523.

Sernka, T. J., and Borle, A. B. (1969). Calcium in the intestinal contents of rats on different calcium diets. *Proc. Soc. Exp. Biol. Med.* **131,** 1420–1423.

Shafer, R. B., and Nuttall, F. Q. (1975). Calcium and folic acid absorption in patients taking anticonvulsant drugs. *Metab., Clin. Exp.* **41,** 1125–1129.

Shah, B. G., and Draper, H. H. (1966). Depression of calcium absorption in parathyroidectomized rats. *Am. J. Physiol.* **211,** 963–966.

Shen, F. H., Baylink, D. J., Nielsen, R. L., Sherrard, D. J., Ivey, J. L., and Haussler, M. R. (1977). Increased serum 1,25-dihydroxyvitamin D in idiopathic hypercalciuria. *J. Lab. Clin. Med.* **90,** 955-962.

Shenolikar, I. S., and Rao, N. (1968). Influence of dietary protein on calcium metabolism in young rats. *Indian J. Med. Res.* **56,** 1412-1422.

Shike, M., Harrison, J. G., Sturtridge, W. T., Tam, C. S., Bobechko, P. E., Jones, G., Murray, T. M., and Jeejeebhoy, K. N. (1980). Metabolic bone disease in patients receiving long-term total parenteral nutrition. *Ann. Intern. Med.* **92,** 343-350.

Silver, J. (1977). Anticonvulsant osteomalacia - an overview. *In* "Vitamin D: Biochemical, Chemical and Clinical Aspects Related to Calcium Metabolism" (A. W. Norman, K. Schaefer, J. W. Coburn, H. F. DeLuca, D. Fraser, H.-G. Grigoleit, and D. von Herrath, eds.), pp. 781-783. de Gruyter, Berlin.

Singhelakis, P., Alevizaki, C. C., and Ikkos, D. G. (1974). Intestinal calcium absorption in hyperthyroidism. *Metab., Clin. Exp.* **23,** 311-321.

Sinha, T. K., and Bell, N. H. (1976). 1,25-dihydroxyvitamin D, and pseudohypoparathyroidism. *N. Engl. J. Med.* **294,** 612.

Sjöberg, H. E. (1969). Retention of oral ^{47}calcium in acromegaly. *Horm. Metab. Res.* **1,** 136-138.

Sjöberg, H. E. (1970). ^{47}Calcium administered orally in patients with primary hyperparathyroidism. *Horm. Metab. Res.* **2,** 32-34.

Skinner, R. K., Long, R. G., Sherlock, S., and Wills, M. R. (1977). 25-hydroxyvitamin D values in chronic liver disease and response to treatment with parenteral vitamin D. *In* "Vitamin D: Biochemical, Chemical and Clinical Aspects Related to Calcium Metabolism" (A. W. Norman, K. Schaefer, J. W. Coburn, H. F. DeLuca, D. Fraser, H. G. Grigbleit, and D. von Herrath, eds.), pp. 839-841. de Gruyter, Berlin.

Slatopolsky, E., Gray, R., Adams, N. D., Lewis, J., Hruska, K., Martin, K., Klahr, S., DeLuca, H., and Lemann, J. (1978). Low serum levels of $1,25(OH)_2D_3$ are not responsible for the development of secondary hyperparathyroidism in early renal failure. *Kidney Int.* **14,** 733 (abstr.).

Sorensen, O. H., Lund, B., Hilden, M., and Lund, B. (1979). 25-hydroxylation in chronic alcoholic liver disease. *In* "Vitamin D: Basic Research and Its Clinical Application" (A. W. Norman, K. Schaefer, D. von Herrath, H.-G. Grigoleit, J. W. Coburn, H. F. DeLuca, E. B. Mawer, and T. Suda, eds.), pp. 843-845. de Gruyter, Berlin.

Spanos, E., Barrett, D., MacIntyre, I., Pike, J. W., Safilian, E. F., and Haussler, M. R. (1978). Effect of growth hormone on vitamin D metabolism. *Nature (London)* **273,** 246-247.

Spencer, E. M., and Tobiassen, O. (1977). The effects of hypophysectomy on 25-hydroxyvitamin D_3 metabolism in the rat. *In* "Vitamin D: Biochemical, Chemical and Clinical Aspects Related to Calcium Metabolism" (A. W. Norman, K. Schaefer, J. W. Coburn, H. F. DeLuca, D. Fraser, H.-G. Grigoleit, and D. von Herrath, eds.), pp. 197-199. de Gruyter, Berlin.

Spencer, H., Menczel, J., Lewin, I., and Samachson, J. (1964). Absorption of calcium in osteoporosis. *Am. J. Med.* **37,** 223-234.

Spencer, H., Lewin, I., Samachson, J., and Laszlo, J. (1966). Changes in metabolism in obese persons during starvation. *Am. J. Med.* **40**(1), 27-37.

Spencer, H., Lewin, I., Fowler, J., and Samachson, J. (1969). Influence of dietary calcium intake in Ca^{47} absorption in man. *Am. J. Med.* **46,** 197-205.

Spencer, R., Charman, M., Wilson, P., and Lawson, E. (1976). Vitamin D-stimulated intestinal calcium absorption may not involve calcium-binding protein directly. *Nature (London)* **263,** 161-163.

Steggerda, T. J., and Mitchell, H. H. (1946). Effect of citrate ion on calcium metabolism of adult human subjects. *J. Nutr.* **31,** 423-438.

Stern, P. H., Olazabel, J. D., and Bell, N. H. (1980). Evidence for abnormal metabolism in patients with sarcoid and normal calcium metabolism. *Am. Soc. Bone Mineral. Res., 2nd Annu. Meet.* Abstract Book, p. 41A.

Szymendera, J., Heaney, R. P., and Saville, P. (1972). Intestinal calcium absorption: Concurrent use of oral and intravenous tracers and calculation by the inverse convolution method. *J. Lab. Clin. Med.* **79,** 570–578.

Tanaka, Y., and DeLuca, H. F. (1973). The control of 25-hydroxyvitamin D metabolism by inorganic phosphorus. *Arch. Biochem. Biophys.* **154,** 566–574.

Tantibhedhyangkul, P., and Hashim, S. A. (1978). Medium-chain triglyceride feeding in premature infants: Effects on calcium and magnesium absorption. *Pediatrics* **61,** 537–545.

Targoff, C. M., Coburn, J. W., Ament, M. E., Byrne, W. J., Miller, D. G., Sherrard, D. J., Brickman, A. S., and Bluestone, R. (1979). Bone disease associated with total parenteral nutrition, a new syndrome. *In* "Vitamin D: Basic Research and Its Clinical Application" (A. W. Norman, K. Schaefer, D. von Herrath, H.-G. Grigoleit, J. W. Coburn, H. F. DeLuca, E. B. Mawer, and T. Suda, eds.), pp. 1172–1176. de Gruyter, Berlin.

Taylor, A. N., and Wasserman, R. H. (1967). Vitamin D_3-induced calcium-binding protein: Partial pruification, electrophoretic visualization, and tissue distribution. *Arch. Biochem. Biophys.* **119,** 536–540.

Taylor, A. N., and Wasserman, R. H. (1970). Immunofluorescent localization of vitamin D-dependent CaBP. *J. Histochem. Cytochem.* **18,** 107–115.

Teitelbaum, S. L., Halverson, J. D., Bates, M., Wise, L., and Haddad, J. G. (1977). Abnormalities of circulating 25-hydroxyvitamin D after jejunal ileal by pass for obesity, evidence of an adaptive response. *Ann. Intern. Med.* **86,** 289–293.

Thomasset, M., Cuisinier-Gleizes, P., and Mathieu, H. (1976). Duodenal calcium-binding protein (CaBP) and phosphorus deprivation in growing rats. *Biomedicine* **25,** 333–337.

Thompson, G. R., Lewis, B., and Booth, C. C. (1966). Absorption of vitamin D_3-^3H in control subjects and patients with intestinal malabsorption. *J. Clin. Invest.* **43,** 94–102.

Tothill, P., Dellipiani, A. W., and Calbert, J. (1970). Plasma concentrations of radiocalcium after oral administration, and their relationship to absorption. *Clin. Sci.* **38,** 27–39.

Toverud, S. U. (1964). Parathyroid effect on intestinal absorption of calcium and on secretion of calcium with the digestive juices in vitamin D-deficient rats. *Acta Physiol. Scand.* **62,** 1–31.

Ueng, T.-H., Golub, E. E., and Bronner, F. (1979). The effect of age and 1,25-dihydroxyvitamin D_3 treatment on the intestinal calcium-binding protein of suckling rats. *Arch. Biochem. Biophys.* **196,** 624–630.

Ussing, H. H. (1949). The distinction by means of tracers between active transport and diffusion. *Acta Physiol. Scand.* **19,** 43–56.

Ussing, H. H., and Zerahn, K. (1951). Active transport of sodium as the source of electric current in the short circuited isolated frog skin. *Acta Physiol. Scand.* **23,** 110–127.

Uttley, W. S., Belton, N. R., Syme, J., and Sheppard, H. (1975). Calcium balance in children treated with diphosphonates. *Arch. Dis. Child.* **50,** 187–190.

Valentzas, C., Oreopoulos, D. G., From, G., Porrett, B., and Rapoport, A. (1977). Vitamin-D levels in thyrotoxicosis. *Lancet* **1,** 370–371.

Varghese, Z., Epstein, O., Farrington, K., Newman, S. P., Moorehead, J. F., and Sherlock, S. (1979). The effect of oral 1 alpha hydroxy vitamin D_3 and 1,25-$(OH)_2D_3$ on the intestinal absorption of calcium and phosphate in primary biliary cirrhosis. *In* "Vitamin D: Basic Research and Its Clinical Application" (A. W. Norman, K. Schaefer, D. von Herrath, H.-G. Grigoleit, J. W. Coburn, H. F. DeLuca, E. B. Mawer, and T. Suda, eds.), pp. 1045–1049. de Gruyter, Berlin.

Villareal, M., Gould, L. V., Wasserman, R. H., Bar, A., Chiroff, R. T., and Bergström, W. H. (1974). Diphenylhydantoin: Effects on calcium metabolism in the chick. *Science* **183,** 671–673.

Wagner, H., Hengst, K., Jansen, H., and Gerlach, U. (1978). Effects of somatostatin on absorption of mono-and disaccharides in small intestine in vivo and in vitro in man and rats. *Metab., Clin. Exp.* **27,** 1329–1332.

Wajchenberg, B. L., Pereira, V. G., Kieffer, J., and Ursic, S. (1969). Effect of dexamethasone on calcium metabolism and ^{47}Ca kinetics in normal subjects. *Acta Endocrinol. (Copenhagen)* **61,** 173–192.

Walker, R. M., and Linkswiler, H. M. (1972). Calcium retention in the adult human male as affected by protein intake. *J. Nutr.* **102,** 1297–1301.

Wallace, H. D., Shirley, R. L., and Davis, G. K. (1951). Excretion of Ca^{45} into gastrointestinal tract of young and mature rats. *J. Nutr.* **43,** 469–475.

Walling, M. W. (1977a). Intestinal Ca and phosphate transport: Differential responses to vitamin D_3 metabolites. *Am. J. Physiol.* **233,** E488–E494.

Walling, M. W. (1977b). Effects of 1α,25-dihydroxyvitamin D_3 on active intestinal inorganic phosphate absorption. *In* "Vitamin D: Biochemical, Chemical and Clinical Aspects Related to Calcium Metabolism" (A. W. Norman, K. Schaefer, J. W. Coburn, H. F. DeLuca, D. Fraser, H.-G. Grigoleit, and D. von Herrath, eds.), pp. 321–330. de Gruyter, Berlin.

Walling, M. W. (1978). Intestinal inorganic phosphate transport. *Adv. Exp. Med. Biol.* **103,** 131–147.

Walling, M. W., and Kimberg, D. V. (1973). Active secretion of calcium by adult rat ileum and jejunum in vitro. *Am. J. Physiol.* **225,** 415–422.

Walling, M. W., and Kimberg, D. V. (1974). Calcium absorption or secretion by rat ileum in vitro: Effects of dietary calicum intake. *Am. J. Physiol.* **226,** 1124–1130.

Walling, M. W., and Kimberg, D. V. (1975a). Calcium absorption by intestine stimulation in vitamin D-deficient nephrectomized rats by *Solanum glaucophyllum*. *Gastroenterology* **69,** 200.

Walling, M. W., and Kimberg, D. W. (1975b). Effects of 1α,25-Dihydroxyvitamin D_3 and *Solanum Glaucophyllum* on intestinal calcium and phosphate transport and on plasma Ca, Mg, and P levels in the rat. *Endocrinology* **97,** 1567–1576.

Walling, M. W. and Lee, D. B. N. (1979). Theories on the mechanism of action of $1,25(OH)_2D_3$ on active intestinal calcium and inorganic phosphate absorption: are the calcium and phosphate transport processes coupled, uncoupled, or both? *In* "Vitamin D: Basic Research and Its Clinical Applications" (A. W. Norman, K. Schaefer, D. von Herrath, H.-G. Grigoleit, E. B. Mawer, T. Suda, H. F. DeLuca, and J. W. Coburn, eds.), pp. 687–692. de Gruyter, Berlin.

Walling, M. W., and Rothman, S. S. (1968). Kinetic evidence for active carrier-mediated calcium transport across the small intestine. *Fed. Proc., Fed. Am. Soc. Exp. Biol.* **27,** 386.

Walling, M. W., and Rothman, S. S. (1969). Phosphate-independent, carrier-mediated transport of calcium by rat intestine. *Am. J. Physiol.* **217,** 1144.

Walling, M. W., and Rothman, S. S. (1970). Apparent increase in carrier affinity for intestinal calcium transport following dietary calcium restriction. *J. Biol. Chem.* **245,** 5007–5011.

Walling, M. W., and Rothman, S. S. (1973). Adaptive uptake of calcium at the duodenal brush border. *Am. J. Physiol.* **225,** 618–623.

Walling, M. W., Favus, M. J., and Kimberg, D. V. (1974). Effects of 25-hydroxyvitamin D_3 on rat duodenum, jejunum, and ileum. *J. Biol. Chem.* **249,** 1156–1161.

Walling, M. W., Favus, M. J., and Kimberg, D. V. (1975). Effects of magnesium deficiency and thyroparathyroidectomy on calcium active transport by rat duodenum. *Proc. Soc. Exp. Biol. Med.* **148,** 1038–1043.

Walling, M. W., Hartenbower, D. L., Coburn, J. W., and Norman, A. W. (1977). Effects of

1α,25-,24R,25-, and 1α,24R,25-hydroxylated metabolites of vitamin D_3 on calcium and phosphate absorption by duodenum from intact and nephrectomized rats. *Arch. Biochem. Biophys.*, **182,** 251-257.

Walling, M. W., Hartenbower, D. L., Coburn, J. W., and Norman, A. W. (1977a). Effects of 1α,25-, 24R,25- and 1α,24,25-hydroxylated metabolites of vitamin D_3 on calcium and phosphate absorption by duodenum from intact and nephrectomized rats. *Arch. Biochem. Biophys.* **182,** 251.

Walling, M. W., Brasitus, T. A., and Kimberg, D. V. (1977b). Effects of calcitonin and substance P on the transport of Ca Na and Cl across rat ileum in vitro. *Gastroenterology* **73,** 89-94.

Warner, R. R., and Coleman, J. R. (1975). Electron probe analysis of calcium transport by small intestine. *J. Cell Biol.* **64,** 54-74.

Wasserman, R. H. (1980). Molecular aspects of the intestinal absorption of calcium and phosphorus. *In* "Pediatric Diseases Related to Calcium" (H. F. DeLuca and C. S. Anast, eds.), pp. 107-132. Am. Elsevier, New York.

Wasserman, R. H., and Comar, C. L. (1959). Carbohydrates and gastrointestinal absorption of radiostrontium and radiocalcium in the rat. *Proc. Soc. Exp. Biol. Med.* **101,** 314-317.

Wasserman, R. H., and Kallfelz, F. A. (1962). Vitamin D_3 and unidirectional calcium fluxes across the rachitic chick duodenum. *Am. J. Physiol.* **203,** 221-224.

Wasserman, R. H., and Lengemann, F. W. (1960). Further observations on lactose stimulation of the gastrointestinal absorption of calcium and strontium in the rat. *J. Nutr.* **70,** 377-384.

Wasserman, R. H., and Taylor, A. N. (1963). The nonessentiality of sodium ions for intestinal calcium transport. *Proc. Soc. Exp. Biol. Med.* **114,** 479-482.

Wasserman, R. H., and Taylor, A. N. (1969). Some aspects of the intestinal absorption of calcium with special reference to vitamin D. *In* "Mineral Metabolism. An Advanced Treatise" (C. L. Comar and F. Bronner, eds.), Vol. 3, pp. 321-403. Academic Press, New York.

Wasserman, R. H., and Taylor, A. N. (1973). Intestinal absorption of phosphate in the chick: Effect of vitamin D_2 and other parameters. *J. Nutr.* **103,** 589-599.

Wasserman, R. H., Comar, C. L., and Noid, M. M. (1956). The influence of amino acids and other organic compounds on the gastrointestinal absorption of calcium 45 and strontium 89 in the rat. *J. Nutr.* **59,** 371-383.

Wasserman, R. H., Kallfelz, F. A., and Comar, C. L. (1961). Active transport of calcium by rat duodenum in vivo. *Science* **133,** 883-884.

Wasserman, R. H., Corradino, R. A., and Tafylor, A. N. (1968). Vitamin D-dependent calcium binding protein. Purification and some properties. *J. Biol. Chem.* **243,** 3978-3986.

Wasserman, R. H., Corradino, R. A., Feher, J., and Armbrecht, H. J. (1977). Temporal patterns of response of the intestinal calcium absorptive system and related parameters to 1,25-dihydroxycholecalciferol. *In* "Vitamin D: Biochemical and Clinical Aspects Related to Calcium Metabolism" (A. W. Norman, K. Schaefer, J. W. Coburn, H. F. DeLuca, D. Fraser, H.-G. Grigoleit, and D. von Herrath, eds.), pp. 331-340. de Gruyter, Berlin.

Webling, D. D'A., and H:oldsworth, E. S. (1965). The effect of bile, bile acids and detergents on calcium absorption in the chick. *Biochem. J.* **97,** 408-421.

Webling, D. D'A., and Holdsworth, E. W. (1966). Bile salts and calcium absorption. *Biochem. J.* **100,** 652-660.

Wensel, R. H., Rich, C., Brown, D. C., and Volwiler, W. (1969). Absorption of calcium measured by intubation and perfusion of the intact human small intestine. *J. Clin. Invest.* **48,** 1768-1775.

Whelton, M. J., Kehayoglou, A. K., Agnew, J. E., Turnberg, L. A., and Sherlock, S. (1971). ^{47}Calcium absorption in parenchymatous and biliary liver disease. *Gut* **12,** 978-983.

Whitby, L. G., and Lang, G. (1960). Experiences with the chromic oxide method of fecal marking in metabolic investigation on humans. *J. Clin. Invest.* **39,** 854-863.

Williams, G. A., Bowser, E. N., Henderson, W. J., and Uzgiries, V. (1961). Effects of vitamin D and cortisone on intestinal absorption of calcium in the rat. *Proc. Soc. Exp. Biol. Med.* **106,** 664.

Williams, G. A., Bowser, E. N., and Henderson, W. J. (1967). Calcium-^{47} absorption in rats with induced hyperthyroidism. *Isr. J. Med. Sci.* **3,** 639–642.

Williams, M. L., Rose, C. S., and Morrow, G., III (1970). Calcium and fat absorption in neonatal period. *Am. J. Clin. Nutr.* **23,** 1322–1330.

Wills, M. R. (1973). Intestinal absorption of calcium. *Lancet* **1,** 820–822.

Wills, M. R., Zisman, E., Wortsman, J., Evens, R. G., Pak, C. Y. C., and Bartter, F. C. (1970). The measurement of intestinal calcium absorption by external radiosotope counting: Application to study of nephrolithiasis. *Clin. Sci.* **39,** 95–108.

Wilson, P. W., and Lawson, D. E. M. (1977). 1,25-dihydroxyvitamin D stimulation of specific membrane proteins in chick intestine. *Biochim. Biophys. Acta* **497,** 805–811.

Wilson, P. W., and Lawson, D. E. M. (1978). Incorporation of (^{3}H) leucine into an actin-like protein in response to 1,25-dihydroxycholecalciferol in chick intestinal brush borders. *Biochem. J.* **173,** 527–631.

Wilson, T. H., and Wiseman, G. (1954). The use of sacs of everted small intestine for the study of the transference of substances from the mucosal to the serosal surface. *J. Physiol. (London)* **123,** 116–125.

Wilz, D. R., Gray, R. W., Dominguez, J. H., and Lemann, J., Jr. (1979). Plasma 1,25$(OH)_2$-vitamin D concentrations and net intestinal calcium, phosphate, and magnesium absorption in humans. *Am. J. Clin. Nutr.* **32,** 2052–2060.

Winter, M., Morava, E., Horvath, T., Simon, G., and Sos, J. (1972). Some findings on the mechanism of adaptation of the intestine to calcium deficiency. *Br. J. Nutr.* **28,** 105–111.

Wong, R. G., and Norman, A. W. (1975). Studies on the mechanism of action of calciferol. VIII. The effects of dietary vitamin D and the polyene antibiotic, filipin, in vitro, on the intestinal cellular uptake of calcium, *J. Biol. Chem.* **250,** 2411–2419.

Wong, R. G., Norman, A. W., Reddy, C. R., and Coburn, J. W. (1972). Biologic effects of 1,25-dihydroxycholecalciferol (a highly active vitamin D metabolite) in acutely uremic rats. *J. Clin. Invest.* **51,** 1287–1291.

Wortsman, J., Pak, C. Y. C., Bartter, F. C., Deftos, L., and Delea, C. (1972). Pathogenesis of osteomalacia in secondary hyperparathyroidism after gastrectomy. *Am. J. Med.* **52,** 556–564.

Younoszai, M. K., and Ghishan, F. K. (1978). In vivo intestinal calcium absorption in infant rats: Influence of methylprednisolone and vitamin D_1. *Proc. Soc. Exp. Biol. Med.* **158,** 174–178.

Younoszai, M. K., Urban, E., and Schedl, H. P. (1973). Vitamin D and intestinal calcium fluxes in vivo in the rat. *Am. J. Physiol.* **225,** 287–292.

Zansi, I., Schoen, M., Roginsky, M. S., Ellis, K. J., Holt, P., and Cohn, S. H. (1977). Skeletal mass and serum levels of 25-hydroxyvitamin D in postgastrectomy patients. *In* "Vitamin D: Biochemical, Chemical and Clinical Aspects Related to Calcium Metabolism" (A. W. Norman, K. Schaefer, J. W. Coburn, H. F. DeLuca, D. Fraser, H.-G. Grigoleit, and D. von Herrath, eds.), pp. 859–861. de Gruyter, Berlin.

Zornitzer, A. E., and Bronner, F. (1971). In situ studies of calcium absorption in rats. *Am. J. Physiol.* **220,** 1261–1266.

4

Renal Handling of Calcium

SHAUL G. MASSRY

I. INTRODUCTION

Total plasma calcium consists of two components: a protein-bound fraction ($40 \pm 5\%$) and a diffusible fraction ($60 \pm 5\%$) that passes the glomerular membrane and gains access to the tubular lumen. Indeed, micropuncture studies have confirmed that about 60% of total plasma calcium is filtered across the glomerulus (Harris *et al.*, 1974; LeGrimellec *et al.*, 1975). Harris *et al.* (1974) measured calcium concentration in the fluid obtained from Bowman's space and

Disorders of Mineral Metabolism, Vol. II

ISBN 0-12-135302-8

found that the ratio between it and plasma calcium averged 0.63 ± 0.02. In the average person, approximately 11,000 mg of calcium are lost from the blood into the glomerular filtrate each day. However, only less than 2% of filtered calcium appears in the urine; this indicates that most of the filtered calcium is reabsorbed by the tubules.

Since no evidence for secretion of calcium by the kidney exists, the renal handling of calcium must be controlled by glomerular filtration and tubular reabsorption. A multitude of hormonal and nonhormonal factors affect calcium transport along the various segments of the nephron (Massry and Coburn, 1973), but available data indicate that it is the distal nephron that exerts the major regulation of urinary calcium.

II. TUBULAR TRANSPORT OF CALCIUM

The concentration of calcium in the urine under diuretic conditions is lower than its concentration in the glomerular filtrate; this suggests active transport of calcium along the nephron. The nature, characteristics, and cellular processes responsible for calcium transport in the various segments of the nephron have not been fully elucidated. The reader is referred to the recent symposium report on renal handling of calcium (Sutton and Dirks, 1978), which is a detailed exposition of current news.

The proximal convoluted tubule is responsible for the reabsorption of 50–60% of filtered calcium. In this part of the nephron, the ratio between calcium concentration in the tubular fluid and plasma ultrafiltrate (TF/UF Ca) is slightly above 1.0 and ranges between 1.0–1.2 in most studies (Lassiter *et al.*, 1963; Duarte and Watson, 1967; Agus *et al.*, 1973; LeGrimellec *et al.*, 1973; Jamison *et al.*, 1974; LeGrimellec, 1975). This finding could be consistent with passive reabsorption of calcium secondary to transport of sodium and water, especially since a potential difference of +2 mV (lumen positive) has been measured across the renal tubular wall (Fromter and Gersner, 1974). This, however, does not rule out active transport of calcium. In fact, certain data support the latter possibility. Thus, values of TF/UF Ca slightly below 1.0 have been noted during saline or mannitol infusion (Lassiter *et al.*, 1963; Duarte and Watson, 1967). In addition, Murayama *et al.* (1972) have demonstrated a substantial back leak of calcium into the proximal tubule of the rat; such a process could prevent the fall in TF/UF Ca below 1.0. Finally, Ullrich *et al.* (1976) found that calcium is transported by both passive and active processes in the proximal tubule of the rat. These authors, utilizing a stop flow microperfusion technique with simultaneous perfusion of the peritubular capillaries, found that 20% of total calcium transport in the proximal tubule is active, while the bulk of calcium reabsorption is passive and related to sodium reabsorption. They demonstrated that the active component of calcium transport also is sodium-dependent, since the removal of sodium from the perfusate or the inhibition of sodium transport by ouabain almost abolished the active reabsorption of calcium.

Micropuncture data indicate that the calcium concentration in the tubular fluid rises slightly in the early part of the proximal tubule but remains unchanged throughout the rest of this segment of the nephron; this indicates that the transport of sodium and calcium in the proximal tubule parallel each other (Lassiter *et al.*, 1963; Duarte and Watson, 1967; Agus *et al.*, 1973; LeGrimellec, 1975). The data of Ullrich *et al.* (1976) provide further support for the interrelationships between the reabsorption of these two ions in the proximal tubule. Frick *et al.* (1965), utilizing micropuncture studies of the proximal tubule, found distinct similarities in the transport characteristics of calcium and sodium in this segment of the nephron; their results support the claim that a common transport mechanism for these two ions exists in the proximal tubule. However, direct evidence for such a common transport mechanism is not available. The interdependence between the transport of these two ions could be due to calcium reabsorption being largely passive following that of sodium and water, whereas active calcium transport would be coupled to that of sodium through a process of counter-transport at the antiluminal cell membrane.

Under certain experimental conditions, such as the infusion of calcium (Edwards *et al.*, 1974; LeGrimellec *et al.*, 1974), sulfate (Lechene *et al.*, 1975), or ferrocyanide (LeGrimellec *et al.*, 1974), TF/UF Ca in the proximal tubule rises. This is the result of a decrease in calcium reabsorption probably due to augmented complexing of calcium rendering it unabsorbable (sulfate or ferrocyanide) or due to a direct effect on calcium transport (hypercalcemia). In addition, very high TF/UF Ca ratios (1.5–1.6) have been reported in rats (Kuntziger *et al.*, 1974) or hamsters (Harris *et al.*, 1976) after acute thyroparathyroidectomy (TPTX); the administration of cyclic AMP to the TPTX rats or of parathyroid hormone to the TPTX hamsters produced a significant fall in TF/UF Ca. These observations suggest that calcium transport in the proximal tubule may be impaired immediately after the removal of the parathyroid glands. In contrast, other investigators found no change in TF/UF Ca in acutely TPTX dogs (Beck and Goldberg, 1973; Quamme *et al.*, 1975; Goldfarb *et al.*, 1977) or rats (Agus *et al.*, 1977c).

Data on calcium transport between the end of the proximal convoluted tubule and the ascending limb of the loop of Henle are limited, but available information indicates that 10% of filtered calcium is reabsorbed by this segment. Micropuncture studies in the psammomys (DeRouffignac *et al.*, 1973) and rats (Jamison *et al.*, 1974) have demonstrated that TF/UF Ca at the hairpin turn of the loop of Henle is significantly lower than the TF/P Na and that this difference is abolished by furosemide (Jamison *et al.*, 1974). These findings indicate a reversal of the situation prevailing in the proximal convoluted tubule and suggest that calcium is preferentially reabsorbed in this part of the nephron; however, addition of sodium by the pars recta or the descending limb of the loop of Henle would provide an alternative explanation. Results obtained from microperfusion of isolated segments of the nephron suggest that calcium reabosrption occurs in the pars recta (Rouse *et al.*, 1977; Almeida *et al.*, 1978) and not in the thin descending limb (Rocha *et al.*, 1977; Suki, 1979b). The rate of the net calcium efflux in the pars recta is in excess of that predicted from the rate of water reabsorption (Rouse and Suki, 1978) and calcium reabsorption in this segment is dependent upon an energy-producing metabolic process (Suki, 1979b).

There is no evidence for calcium transport in the thin ascending limb of the loop of Henle (Rocha *et al.*, 1977; Suki, 1979b). In contrast, about 20% of the filtered calcium is reabsorbed by the thick ascending limb, and TF/UF Ca and TF/P Na ratios in the early distal tubule are reduced in parallel to values of 0.5 or less (Lassiter *et al.*, 1963; Edwards *et al.*, 1973; Goldberg *et al.*, 1976). This suggests that calcium reabsorption occurs in the thick ascending limb of the loop of Henle and could be secondary to the electric potential gradient generated by chloride reabsorption in this segment of the nephron (Rocha and Kokko, 1973; Burg and Green, 1973).

Calcium transport in the medullary and cortical segments of the thick ascending limb of the loop of Henle has been studied by several investigators utilizing an *in vitro* perfusion of isolated segments of rabbit renal tubule (Rocha *et al.*, 1977; Imai, 1978; Shareghi and Stoner, 1978; Bourdeau and Burg, 1979a; Suki and Rouse, 1978). Although all agree that the thick ascending limb contributes significantly to calcium reabsorption by the nephron, their results differ regarding the nature of calcium transport in this segment of the nephron. The data of Shareghi and Stoner (1978) and of Bourdeau and Burg (1979a) indicate that calcium reabsorption in the cortical thick ascending limb of the loop of Henle is purely passive, while the results of Rocha *et al.* (1977), Imai (1978), and Suki and Rouse (1979) are consistent with active calcium transport in this segment of the nephron. Moreover, parathyroid hormone (PTH) stimulates calcium reabsorption in this segment (Suki and Rouse, 1979; Bourdeau and Burg, 1979a; Shareghi and Agus, 1979). Calcium reabsorption in the medullary part of the thick ascending limb of the loop of Henle appears to be passive and is not influenced by PTH (Suki and Rouse, 1979). Thus, it appears that the thick ascending limb of the loop of Henle is a heterogeneous structure with respect to its calcium reabsorption.

Both micropuncture studies of the distal nephron and evaluation of urine samples collected following transient ureteral occlusion (stop flow) demonstrated TF/UF Ca ratios well below unity (0.3–0.5) (Howard *et al.*, 1959; Samiy *et al.*, 1960; Lassiter *et al.*, 1963; Edwards *et al.*, 1973; Agus *et al.*, 1975; Goldberg *et al.*, (1975), even though an electrical potential difference across the tubule should have led to the appearance of greater concentration of calcium in urine than found in ultrafiltrate of plasma. These observations indicate that calcium is actively reabsorbed in the distal nephron. Indeed, Costanzo and Windhager (1978b) demonstrated active calcium reabsorption in this part of the nephron and the absorption of calcium was independent of sodium and of a potential difference. Shareghi and Stoner (1978) arrived at similar conclusions in studies utilizing perfusion of isolated segments of distal convoluted tubule. Calcium is also reabsorbed by the collecting tubule (Lassiter *et al.*, 1963; LeGrimellec *et al.*, 1975; Agus *et al.*, 1975). Shareghi and Stoner (1978) found that the granular segment of the collecting tubule exhibits significant calcium transport in the face of negative potential difference. About 10% of filtered calcium is reabsorbed between the early distal tubule and the terminal portion of the nephron.

Thus, the distal nephron and the collecting duct appear to be the fine modulators of urinary calcium excretion and most factors that influence the excretory rate of calcium exert their effects through alterations of calcium transport in these segments of the nephron (Sutton and Dirks, 1977; Agus, 1978). It should also be mentioned that although the reabsorption of calcium and sodium in the distal nephron may be parallel, their transport can be dissociated. Furthermore, differences in calcium reabsorption among deep and superficial nephron (nephron heterogenity) under the influence of various hormonal and non-hormonal factors could contribute to changes in urinary calcium excretion.

III. FACTORS AFFECTING URINARY EXCRETION OF CALCIUM

An increase in the urinary excretion of calcium could occur following a rise in filtered load of this ion, a decrease in its tubular reabsorption, or both.

A. Changes in Filtered Loads of Calcium

An augmentation in filtered loads of calcium could be produced either by raising the concentrations of calcium in blood or by increasing glomerular filtration rate (GFR). The effects of these procedures on urinary excretion of calcium are different.

Massry and Kleeman (1972) found that acute rises in GFR of 10–85% produced by protein feeding or intravenous administration of dexamethasone or dopamine are associated with only slight increments in urinary calcium or sodium excretion; this is in contrast to marked calciuresis noted during comparable rises in GFR produced during extracellular fluid volume expansion (ECVE) with saline infusion (Fig. 1); the later decreases tubular reabsorption of calcium (Walser, 1961a; Duarte and Watson, 1967; Massry *et al.*, 1967b; Blythe *et al.*, 1968). These observations are consistent with the following sequence of events: In the absence of ECVE, the fractional reabsorption of calcium and sodium in the

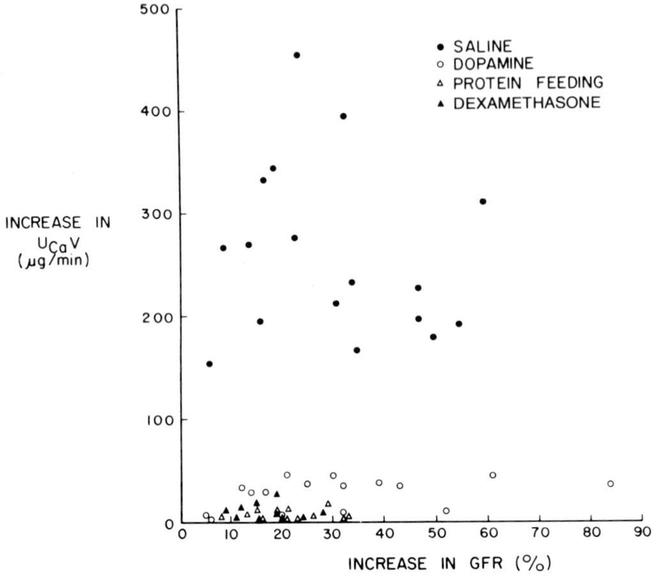

Fig. 1. Changes in urinary calcium ($U_{Ca}V$) in dogs following an acute augmentation in glomerular filtration rate (GFR). (Data adapted from Massry and Kleeman, 1972.)

proximal tubule remain unchanged. Therefore, a major portion of the increment in filtered loads of these ions due to increased GFR is reabsorbed at this site of the nephron, and the remainder is delivered to more distal sites. The increments in distal delivery are almost completely reabsorbed and, hence, there is little change in calcium and sodium excretion. It should be emphasized, however, that if the modest increments in the excretion of calcium observed during acute studies were to continue for a longer period of time, a considerable amount of calcium would be eliminated in the urine.

An increase in filtered loads of calcium secondary to acute or chronic elevation in the concentrations of serum calcium is associated with marked increments in urinary calcium. Both urinary excretion of calcium and the fraction of filtered calcium excreted increase during calcium infusion (Massry *et al.*, 1968b). Edwards *et al.* (1974) and LeGrimellec *et al.* (1974) found that TF/UF Ca in the proximal tubule is higher during calcium infusion and marked hypercalcemia, an observation consistent with a decrease in proximal calcium reabsorption. Indeed, others have found that although the absolute amount of calcium reabsorbed during hypercalcemia is greater than during normocalcemia, the fraction of filtered calcium reabsorbed is lower (Massry *et al.*, 1968b; Coburn *et al.*, 1970). Another factor that may contribute to the decrease in tubular calcium reabsorption during calcium infusion is the suppression of the parathyroid gland activity

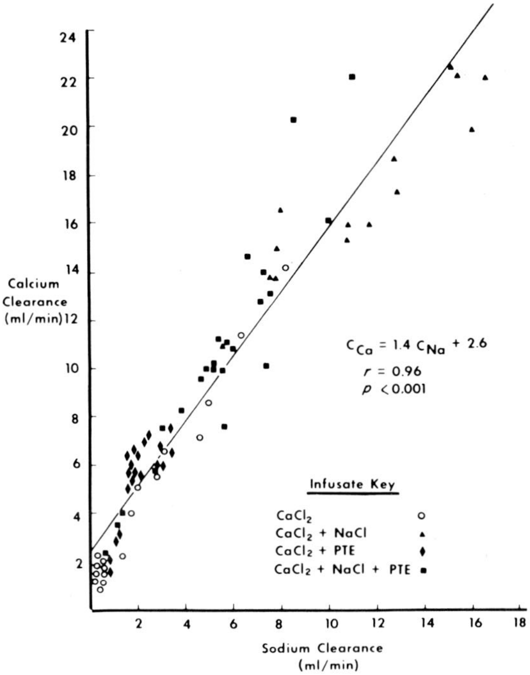

Fig. 2. Relationship between the clearances of calcium and of sodium in thyroparathyroidectomized dogs infused with calcium chloride with and without saline or parathyroid extract (PTE). (From Massry *et al.,* 1968b.)

by hypercalcemia (Sherwood *et al.,* 1966). Finally, if the anions of the calcium salts infused are not readily reabsorbable by the renal tubule, complexing of the calcium with these anions in the tubular fluid may hinder calcium reabsorption and contribute to the hypercalciuria.

Hypercalcemia is also associated with natriuresis (Massry *et al.,* 1968b). This is due to a decrease in tubular reabsorption of sodium along the nephron (Guttman and Gottschalk, 1966; Massry *et al.,* 1968b; Suki *et al.,* 1969; DiBona, 1971). The relationship between the clearances of calcium (C_{Ca}) and sodium (C_{Na}) during acute hypercalcemia differs from that seen during saline infusion in that C_{Ca} significantly exceeds C_{Na} for any degree of natriuresis (Massry *et al.,* 1968b). This altered relationship persists even when ECVE with saline is superimposed on the hypercalcemia (Fig. 2).

The urinary excretion of calcium in patients with hypercalcemic disorders is markedly increased. However, in patients with hypercalcemia due to excess parathyroid hormone, C_{Ca} for any given level of serum calcium is less than in those with other types of hypercalcemia (Kleeman *et al.,* 1961; Bernstein *et al.,*

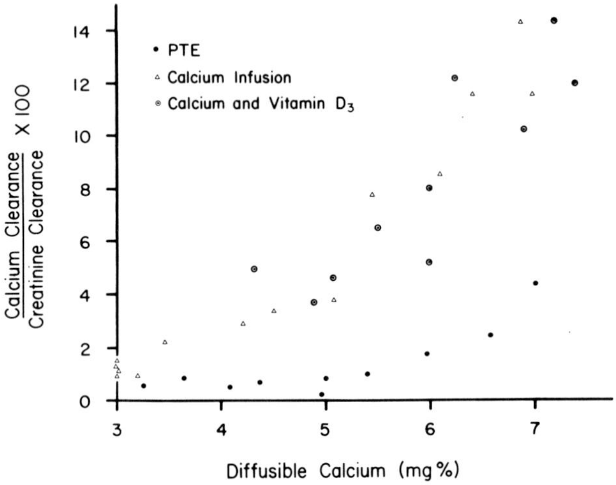

Fig. 3. The effect of calcium infusion, oral calcium and vitamin D_3, and parathyroid extract (PTE) on the renal clearance of diffusible calcium at increasing concentrations of plasma-diffusible calcium in a patient with hypoparathyroidism. Note that for any given level of plasma calcium the clearance is significantly lower while the patient is receiving parathyroid extract. (From Bernstein *et al.*, 1963.)

1963; Transbol *et al.*, 1970; Fig. 3). It should also be emphasized that hypercalciuria may be blunted or absent in hypercalcemic patients with impaired renal function. Therefore, in assessing urinary calcium excretion, renal function must have been evaluated, since even mild renal failure is associated with hypocalciuria (Better *et al.*, 1967; Friis *et al.*, 1968; Popovtzer *et al.*, 1970).

B. Changes in Tubular Reabsorption

Numerous hormonal and nonhormonal factors influence urinary excretion of calcium. These are listed in Table I and include the following.

1. *Extracellular Fluid Volume Expansion*

Expansion of extracellular fluid volume by saline infusion is associated with marked natriuresis and calciuresis (Walser, 1961a; Massry *et al.*, 1967b; Blythe *et al.*, 1968). Under these circumstances, the relationships between the C_{Ca} and C_{Na} is near unity over a wide range of C_{Na} (C_{Ca} = 0.85 to 0.95 C_{Na}). Clearance studies by Massry *et al.* (1967b) and Blythe *et al.* (1968) demonstrated that an increase in urinary calcium excretion occurs during ECVE even with marked reduction of filtered loads of calcium produced by acute lowering of glomerular filtration rate. Furthermore, the latter procedure did not affect the relationships between C_{Ca} and C_{Na} (Fig. 4). These observations indicate that ECVE reduces the tubular reabsorption of both calcium and sodium along the nephron. Indeed,

TABLE I

Factors Affecting Urinary Excretion of Calcium

1. Factors that increase urinary calcium excretion
Extracellular fluid volume expansion
Renal vasodilatation
Hypercalcemia
Hypermagnesemia
Osmotic diuresis
All diuretics except thiazides
Cardiac glycosides
Phosphate depletion
Acidosis
Carbohydrate ingestion
Alcohol ingestion
High sodium intake
Calcitonin[a]
Chronic Vitamin D administration and its metabolites
Growth hormone
Thyroid hormone
Chronic mineralocorticoid effect
2. Factors that decrease urinary calcium excretion
Chronic thiazide administration
Phosphate loading
Parathyroid hormone
Acute administration of Vitamin D and its metabolites

[a] In certain species.

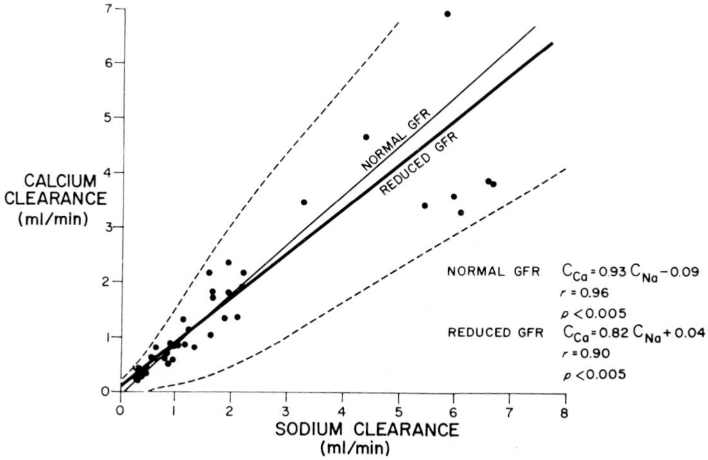

Fig. 4. The relationship between calcium clearance and sodium clearance in dogs receiving saline infusion before and during acute reduction in glomerular filtration rate (GFR). The data points during reduced GFR are superimposed upon the regression slope and 95% confidence limits of data obtained during normal GFR. (From Massry *et al.*, 1967b.)

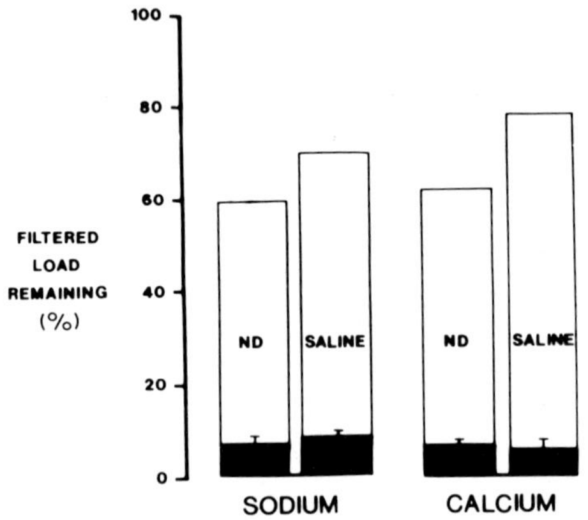

Fig. 5. Fraction of the filtered load of sodium and calcium remaining in the late proximal tubule in nondiuretic (ND) and saline-loaded intact rats. Delivery out of the proximal tubule is indicated by thin lines. Despite differences in delivery out of the proximal tubule, there were no differences in the amount of sodium and calcium remaining in the late distal tubule. These observations suggest that the calciuresis and natriuresis of saline infusion must be due to inhibition of their reabsorption in the terminal nephron. (From Agus, 1978.)

data from micropuncture experiments have shown that ECVE produced by saline infusion suppresses proximal tubular reabsorption of sodium (Dirks *et al.*, 1965) and calcium (Duarte and Watson, 1967).

A decrease in sodium reabsorption in the proximal tubule is not adequate to produce natriuresis (Howards *et al.*, 1968). ECVE with saline infusion inhibits sodium reabsorption both at proximal and distal sites of the nephron (Stein *et al.*,

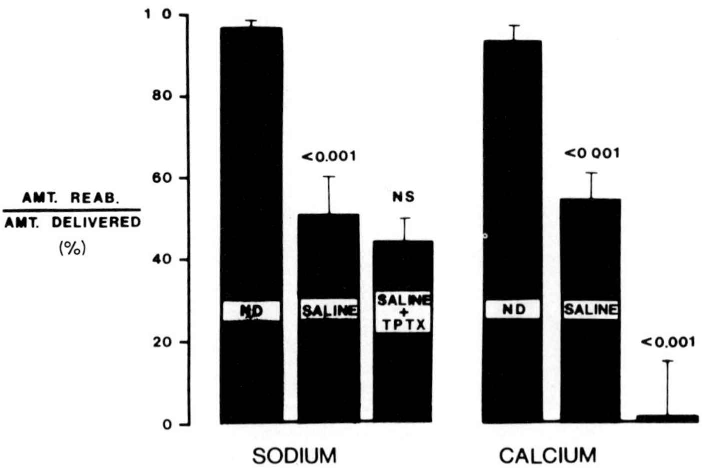

Fig. 6. Fraction of the sodium and calcium absorbed out of that delivered to the terminal nephron in nondiuretic (ND) saline loaded and TPTX-saline loaded rats. (From Agus, 1978.)

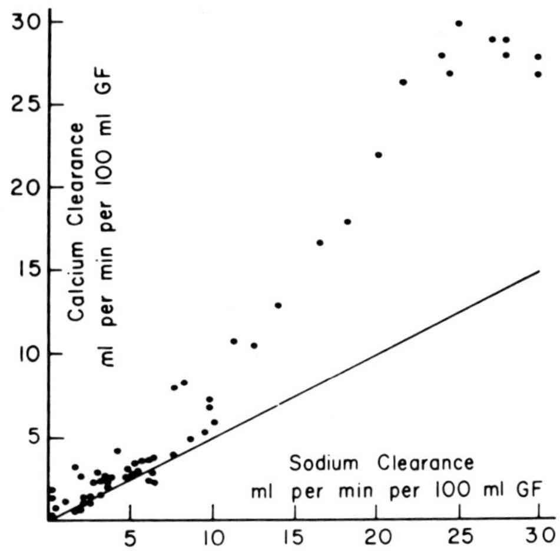

Fig. 7. The relationship between calcium clearance and sodium clearance during infusion of sodium sulphate (solid points) compared to the relationship during infusion of saline or osmotic diuresis (solid line). The clearance of calcium is expressed in terms of total serum calcium. GF = glomerular filtration. (From Walser, 1961a.)

1973), and it is the latter effect that is responsible for the increments in urinary sodium excretion. Since the renal excretions of sodium and calcium parallel each other during ECVE, one may assume that the calciuresis of ECVE is most probably due to inhibition of calcium transport in the distal nephron. The data of Agus (1978) provide support for this notion (Figs. 5 and 6).

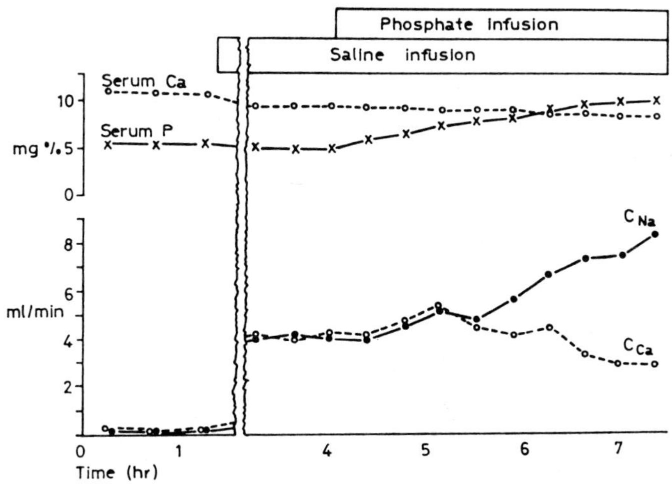

Fig. 8. The effect of phosphate infusion on the clearances of sodium (C_{Na}) and calcium (C_{Ca}) in dogs receiving saline infusion. (Data adapted from Coburn *et al.*, 1971.)

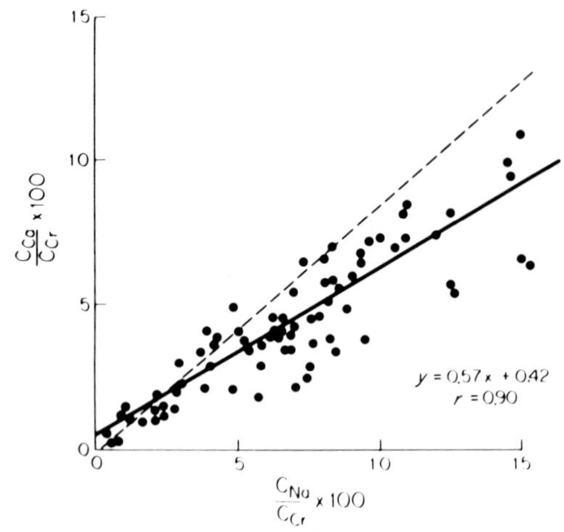

Fig. 9. Relationship between fraction of filtered calcium excreted ($C_{Ca}/C_{Cr} \times 100$) and that of sodium ($C_{Na}/C_{Cr} \times 100$) on days 8, 10, and 12 of daily repeated saline infusion in dogs being fed a low-calcium diet. Interrupted line is regression slope for days 1 and 3 of saline infusions. Each point represents a single clearance period. (From Brickman *et al.,* 1971.)

The close relationship between C_{Ca} and C_{Na} during ECVE may be modified by several factors, such as complexing of calcium by unabsorbable anions (Walser, 1961b; see Fig. 7), phosphate infusion (Coburn *et al.*, 1971;see Fig. 8), calcium deprivation and negative calcium balance (Brickman *et al.*, 1971; see Fig. 9), and duration of saline infusion (Antoniou *et al.*, 1969).

2. *Renal Vasodilatation*

Gonda *et al.* (1969), Ahumada and Massry (1971), and Thompson *et al.* (1971) demonstrated that renal vasodilatation produced by the infusion of acetylcholine or bradykinin into the renal artery, with and without the intravenous administration of angiotensin, augments the urinary excretion of calcium due to a decrease in its tubular reabsorption (Fig. 10). In these studies, the slope for the relationship between C_{Ca} and C_{Na} were 1.21, 1.08, and 1.00, respectively. These values are slightly greater than those usually observed during saline infusion. This small difference may be related to the inhibition of electrolyte transport in the loop of Henle (Massry and Ahumada, 1972), where calcium may be reabsorbed more avidly than sodium.

3. *Hypermagnesemia*

Hypermagnesemia produced by the infusion of magnesium salts is associated with natriuresis and calciuria (Massry *et al.*, 1970b; DiBona, 1971; Quamme and Dirks, 1978). Under these circumstances, the relationship between the renal

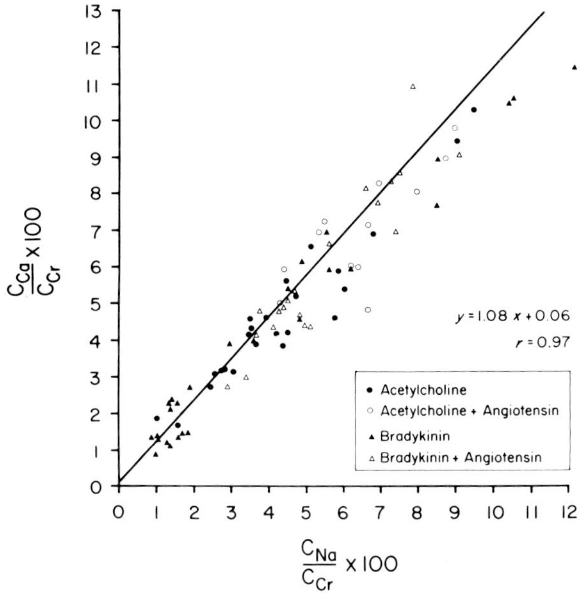

Fig. 10. The relationship between the fractional excretion of calcium ($C_{Na}/C_{Cr} \times 100$) and of sodium ($C_{Na}/C_{Cr} \times 100$) in dogs undergoing renal vasodilatation with and without the infusion of angiotensin. (From Ahumada and Massry, 1971.)

clearances of sodium and calcium differ from that found during ECVE (Massry *et al.*, 1968b). The increase in urinary excretion of calcium appears 2 to 3 hr earlier than the natriuresis and C_{Ca} is significantly greater than C_{Na} even during the periods of the highest sodium excretion (Massry *et al.*, 1970b). These differences may be related to at least two factors. First, hypermagnesemia inhibits sodium reabsorption in the proximal tubule (DiBona, 1971), but reduces calcium transport in the loop of Henle (Quamme and Dirks, 1978). Second, hypermagnesemia inhibits the activity of the parathyroid glands (Buckle *et al.*, 1968; Massry *et al.*, 1970a) and, therefore, is associated with greater excretion of calcium than sodium. Indeed, the administration of parathyroid extract during magnesium infusion causes a substantial decrease in C_{Ca} in relation to C_{Na}, but C_{Ca} remains significantly above C_{Na} (Massry *et al.*, 1970b). These data indicate that the preponderance of C_{Ca} over C_{Na} during magnesium infusion is not entirely related to suppression of the parathyroid gland activity.

4. *Diuretic Agents*

a. Osmotic Diuresis. Osmotic agents such as mannitol, glucose, and urea inhibit the tubular reabsorption of calcium and sodium and augment their urinary excretion (Wesson, 1962; Lassiter *et al.*, 1963; Duarte and Watson, 1967; Parfitt, 1969). In general, the relationship between C_{Ca} and C_{Na} during osmotic diuresis is similar to that seen during ECVE produced by saline infusion. The inhibition of the tubular reabsorption of calcium during osmotic diuresis could be explained by the decrease in its concentration in tubular fluid secondary to inhibition of water reabsorption along the nephron. Indeed, micropuncture studies have confirmed that mannitol inhibits water transport in the proximal tubule and in the loop of Henle (Seely and Dirks, 1969). Studies by Wong *et al.* (1978) have demonstrated that calcium reabsorption in the proximal tubule and the loop of Henle is inhibited during mannitol infusion.

b. Acetazolamide. Administration of acetazolamide produces either a fall or no change in calcium excretion in man and dogs (McIntosh and Seraglia, 1963; Massry *et al.*, 1968a; Beck and Goldberg, 1973). Micropuncture studies by Beck and Goldberg (1973) have shown that acetazolamide causes a parallel inhibition of calcium and sodium in the proximal tubule, without, however, leading to calciuria. These clearance and micropuncture studies indicate that the increased amount of calcium delivered from the proximal tubule during acetazolamide administration is completely reabsorbed at distal sites of the renal tubule. The drug, however, inhibits sodium reabsorption at the distal nephron, with the net effect being that natriuresis occurs without calciuria.

Because acetazolamide inhibits the Na^+–H^+ exchange, sodium reabsorption in the distal nephron, which is coupled with Na^+–H^+ exchange, cannot be linked to calcium transport. This conclusion is further supported by studies in which sodium diuresis was produced by the infusion of potassium salts. The latter inhibits Na^+–H^+ exchange secondary to intracellular alkalosis, yet, despite significant natriuresis, urinary calcium excretion did not rise (Massry *et al.*, 1968a).

c. Mercurial Diretics, Furosemide, and Ethacrynic Acids. All of these diuretics augment the urinary excretion of calcium and sodium with a greater increase in C_{Ca} than C_{Na} (Demartini *et al.*, 1967; Duarte, 1968; Sotornik *et al.*, 1969; Parfitt, 1969; Eknoyan *et al.*, 1970). Although these agents may have some action in the proximal tubule, they primarily inhibit tubular transport in the thick ascending limb of the loop of Henle (Seldin *et al.*, 1966). These data also suggest that the reabsorption of calcium and sodium are not parallel in this part of the nephron. Further support to this notion is provided by the studies of Rocha *et al.* (1977). However, it is also possible that the greater effect of these diuretics on calcium excretion than on that of sodium is due to a dissociation in their transport at sites distal to the early part of the distal tubule (Antoniou *et al.*, 1969; Edwards *et al.*, 1973).

The effect of furosemide in patients with nephrotic syndrome deserves comment since it may shed light on the genesis of the hypocalciuria frequently seen in

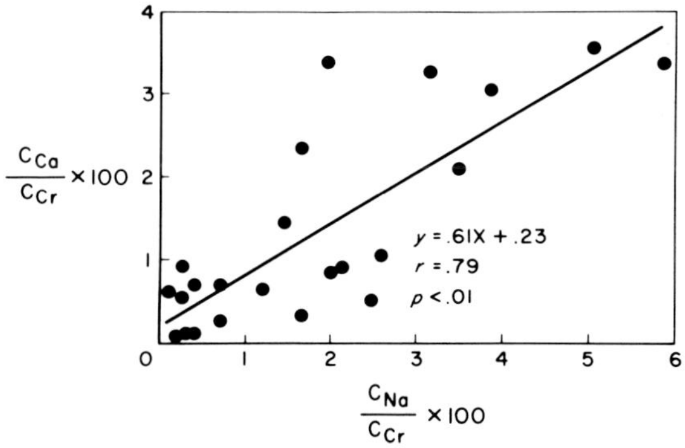

Fig. 11. The relation between the fractional excretion of calcium ($C_{Ca}/C_{Cr} \times 100$) and sodium ($C_{Na}/C_{Cr} \times 100$) in 24 patients with the nephrotic syndrome. Thirteen of these data points were obtained during administration of furosemide. (From Goldstein *et al.,* 1977.)

these patients (Scriver, 1928; Emerson and Beckman, 1945; Jones *et al.*, 1967; Goldstein *et al.*, 1977). Although the administration of furosemide to these patients produces natriuresis and calciuria, the slope for the relationships between the fractional excretions of sodium and calcium is 0.61 (Goldstein *et al.*, 1977; Fig. 11), this indicates that the diuretic had a greater effect on the urinary excretion of sodium than of calcium. This is contrary to the effect of furosemide in normal and thyroparathyroidectomized animals (Antoniu *et al.*, 1969; Eknoyan *et al.*, 1970). Further, the slope of 0.61 is similar to that of 0.57 observed for the relationship between the fractional excretion of sodium and calcium in calcium-deficient dogs undergoing ECVE with saline infusion (Brickman *et al.*, 1971). Also, the slope for the relationship between the fractional excretion of sodium and calcium in the nephrotics is significantly lower than that of 0.98 noted in patients with renal failure but without nephrosis (Popovtzer *et al.*, 1969). These observations suggest that patients with nephrotic syndrome may have strong calcium-retaining forces and that their hypocalciuria cannot be entirely explained by alterations in the renal handling of sodium in these patients.

d. Benzothiadiazine Diuretics. Although the acute administration of thiazide diuretics produces natriuresis and calciuria, the increment of C_{Ca} is smaller than that in C_{Na} (Duarte and Bland, 1965; Parfitt, 1969; Sotornik *et al.*, 1969; Eknoyan *et al.*, 1970; Costanzo and Weiner, 1974). This dissociation between the excretory rates of sodium and calcium is probably due to events that take place in the early distal tubule (Edwards *et al.*, 1973).

In contrast to other diuretics, the chronic administration of thiazides produces hypocalciuria (Lamberg and Kuhlback, 1959; Higgins *et al.*, 1964; Walser, 1961b; Brickman *et al.*, 1972; Parfitt, 1972), and this effect has made these drugs useful in the management of idiopathic hypercalciuria (Yendt *et al.*, 1966). The mechanisms responsible for the hypocalciuria of chronic thiazide administration are complex and not fully understood. Suki (1979a) has provided an interesting analysis of the available information on this issue.

Studies in man have shown that both a certain degree of extracellular volume depletion and intact parathyroid glands must be present before hypocalciuria develops (Brickman *et al.*, 1972; Parfitt, 1972; Fig. 12). Thus, if the sodium losses produced by thiazides are quantitatively replaced, the hypocalciuria fails to occur. Patients with hypoparathyroidism do not develop hypocalciuria during thiazide administration despite a similar degree of sodium losses and reduction in body weight. During depletion of extracellular fluid volume, the proximal reabsorption of both sodium and calcium are enhanced. This leads to a decrease in the delivery of these ions to the distal nephron, where thiazides primarily inhibit sodium reabsorption. The mechanisms by which parathyroid hormone (PTH) exerts its role in the hypocalciuria induced by chronic thiazide therapy are not clear. First, thiazide may potentiate the action of PTH on the kidney. There is

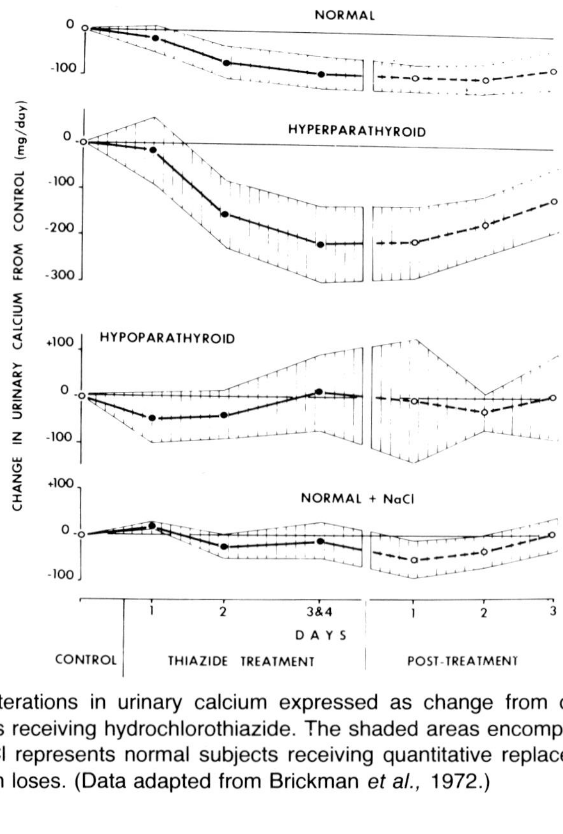

Fig. 12. Alterations in urinary calcium expressed as change from control values in human subjects receiving hydrochlorothiazide. The shaded areas encompass mean ± SE. Normal + NaCl represents normal subjects receiving quantitative replacement of diuretic induced sodium loses. (Data adapted from Brickman *et al.*, 1972.)

evidence that PTH exerts its renal action by stimulation of an adenylate cyclase-cyclic AMP system (Chase and Aurbach, 1967; Chase *et al.*, 1969). Certain data indicate that thiazides inhibit phosphodiesterase (Moore, 1968; Senft *et al.*, 1968), an enzyme that accelerates the degradation of cyclic AMP. It is possible, therefore, that in the presence of parathyroid hormone thiazides might lead to increased renal concentration of cyclic AMP, which would potentiate the action of the hormone, ultimately leading to enhanced calcium reabsorption. Second, Costanzo and Weiner (1974) found that the secretion of chlorothiazide by the renal tubule is defective in acutely TPTX dogs. They suggested that this defect may be responsible for the lack of the hypocalciuric effect of the diuretic in the absence of parathyroid hormone. Unfortunately, these authors did not provide data that demonstrate that such a defect in the renal handling of chlorothiazide exists in states of chronic hypoparathyroidism.

In contrast to the data of Brickman *et al.* (1972) and Parfitt (1972), other studies suggest that PTH is not necessary for the hypocalciuric action of thiazides. Porter *et al.* (1978) found that administration of these diuretics to patients with hypoparathyroidism receiving sodium-restricted diet is associated with a moderate fall in urinary calcium. Furthermore, thiazides produced a fall in urinary calcium excretion in hypoparathyroid rats (Jorgensen, 1971). Finally, Quamme *et al.* (1975), utilizing micropuncture techniques, found that PTH administration to hypoparathyroid dogs treated with thiazides did not alter the diuretic-induced dissociation between the renal handling of sodium and calcium.

Thiazides may also directly affect distal calcium reabsorption. The micropuncture data of Sutton *et al.* (1972) indicate that the diuretic inhibits distal sodium reabsorption without effect on calcium. During hydropenia, the mean value for the ratio TF/P Na was 0.34 and that for ultrafiltrable calcium was 0.31, with a highly significant correlation between them. During chlorothiazide administration, distal sodium reabsorption was inhibited, with TF/P Na rising from 0.26 to 0.54, while there was no effect on calcium transport. The net effect of chlorothiazide is, therefore, natriuresis without calciuria. In contrast, Costanzo and Windhager (1978b) demonstrated that thiazides directly enhance calcium transport in the distal tubule. This effect was demonstrated during conditions with increased distal delivery of calcium. The discrepancy between these data and those of Sutton *et al.* (1972) may be related to variations in distal calcium delivery in the two studies.

e. Cardiac Glycosides. The infusion of cardiac glycosides (ouabain, digoxin, or strophantin) into the renal artery produces natriuresis and calciuria (Walser and Trounce, 1961b; Kupfer and Kosovsky, 1965) with greater increments in C_{Ca} than C_{Na} (Kupfer and Kosovsky, 1965). The mechanism underlying this effect of cardiac glycosides is not understood, but it may be mediated by the inhibition of a sodium-potassium activated ATPase.

5. *Interrelation with Phosphate*

The state of body stores of phosphate has a significant effect on the renal handling of calcium. Phosphate loading decreases and phosphate depletion increases the urinary excretion of calcium.

a. Phosphate Loading. The oral or intravenous administration of phosphate is usually associated with a reduction in urinary calcium excretion (Albright *et al.*, 1932; Bernstein and Newton, 1966; Hebert *et al.*, 1966; Massry *et al.*, 1968c; Coburn *et al.*, 1971) and phosphate infusion can even blunt the potent calciuretic effect of ECVE (Coburn *et al.*, 1971). The hypocalciuric effect of phosphate loading is probably not due to a direct effect on the kidney since the infusion of phosphate into the renal artery does not reduce urinary calcium excretion (Hulley *et al.*, 1969). The effect of intravenous phosphate infusion on urinary calcium is not immediate and usually appears 90–120 min after the start of the infusion (Hulley *et al.*, 1969; Coburn *et al.*, 1971). These observations suggest that this action of phosphate loading, whether direct on the kidney or through an extrarenal mechanism, involves intermediate steps or reactions. Some studies with stop flow (Coburn *et al.*, 1971) and micropuncture (Goldfarb *et al.*, 1977) techniques suggest that the site of action of phosphate loading on tubular calcium reabsorption is the distal nephron.

Urinary calcium excretion may increase in dogs when enough phosphate is infused to raise serum phosphorus to high levels (Jahan and Pitts, 1948). These increments in urinary calcium may be related to the formation of soluble complexes of calcium phosphate (Greenwald *et al.*, 1940; Greenwald, 1945), to the natriuresis that may follow such phosphate administration, or to obligatory urinary cation losses that may occur secondary to phosphate acting as a nonabsorbable anion when filtered in high concentrations.

b. Phosphate Depletion. Marked hypercalciuria has been reported during phosphate depletion in humans (Lotz *et al.*, 1968), sheep (Young *et al.*, 1966), rats (Day and McCollum, 1939), dogs (Coburn and Massry, 1970), and rabbits (Ben-Isaac *et al.*, 1975). The increase in calcium excretion may occur within one day of dietary phosphate restriction (Kreusser *et al.*, 1978). Furthermore, clearance studies in phosphate-depleted dogs (Coburn and Massry, 1970) and rats (Kreusser *et al.*, 1978) demonstrated that the magnitude of the hypercalciuria is related to the severity of phosphate depletion and the degree of hypophosphatemia (Fig. 13).

Data from clearance studies in phosphate-depleted dogs indicate that the hypercalciuria is the result of a decrease in the tubular transport of calcium (Coburn and Massry, 1970) in the loop of Henle (Gold *et al.*, 1973). Indeed, micropuncture data have confirmed that the hypercalciuria in phosphate deple-

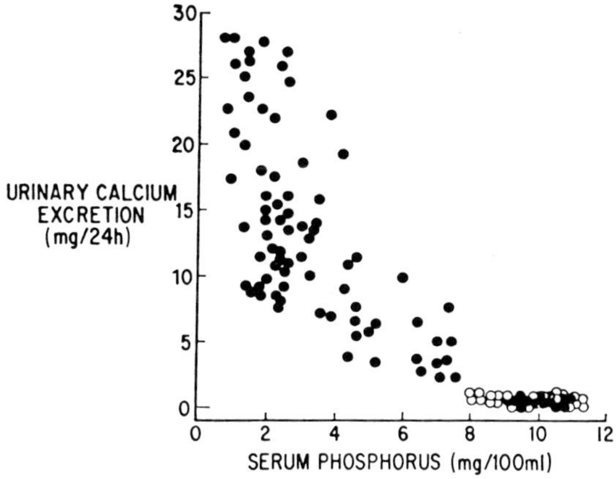

Fig. 13. The relationship between the concentration of serum phosphorus and urinary excretion of calcium in phosphate depleted (●) and pair-weighed (○) rats. (From Kreusser *et al.*, 1978.)

tion is due to suppression of calcium reabsorption at a site distal to the proximal tubule and prior to the distal sampling site (Quamme *et al.*, 1976; Goldfarb *et al.*, 1977), most probably at the ascending limb of the loop of Henle. Meyer *et al.* (1979) reported that thiazides blunt the hypercalciuria of phosphate depletion; their data are consistent with the notion that the defect in calcium transport during phosphate depletion is located at a site proximal to where these diuretics exert their action.

The mechanisms responsible for the increased urinary calcium excretion during phosphate depletion are not evident. Since phosphate depletion is associated with a state of hypoparathyroidism (Stoerk and Carnes, 1945; Dominguez *et al.*, 1976), it is possible that a deficiency in PTH is responsible for the hypercalciuria. Indeed, the administration of PTH to phosphate-depleted dogs produced a significant decrease in urinary calcium excretion, but did not abolish the hypercalciuria (Coburn and Massry, 1970); furthermore, parathyroidectomy of these dogs did not augment the hypercalciuria (Cuisinier-Gleizes *et al.*, 1976). Grabie *et al.* (1978) evaluated the role of PTH in the genesis of hypercalciuria in phosphate-depleted rats. They also found that repeated administration of PTH significantly lowered urinary calcium excretion but the rats remained hypercalciuric. Although these data suggest that a deficiency in PTH during phosphate depletion may contribute to the hypercalciuria, other factors must be operative. Studies carried out in our laboratory provided evidence that blood of phosphate-depleted rabbits contain a humoral factor capable of producing hypercalciuria in normal kidneys perfused *in vitro* with such blood (Ben-Isaac *et al.*, 1975).

6. *Acid-Base Balance*

Hypercalciuria is usually present during acute or chronic metabolic acidosis (Givens and Mendel, 1917; Farquharson *et al.*, 1931; Atchley *et al.*, 1933; Lemann *et al.*, 1967; Reidenberg, 1967; Lavan, 1969; Lennon and Piering, 1970; Sutton *et al.*, 1975b, 1979). Lemann *et al.* (1967) noted that the hypercalciuria of metabolic acidosis occurred in the face of falling filtered loads of calcium and that C_{Ca} was far greater than C_{Na}. They suggested that metabolic acidosis decreases tubular reabsorption of calcium and that this effect is not related to sodium transport. On the other hand, Walser (1971) found that C_{Ca} and C_{Na} correlated well during acute metabolic acidosis but calcium excretion correlated better with the sum of sodium and ammonium excretion. Since the latter parameter is a better estimate of distal sodium delivery than urinary sodium alone, metabolic acidosis may inhibit calcium and sodium transport in the proximal tubule. In that situation the relationship between C_{Ca} and C_{Na} is altered by enhanced ammonium addition. This reflects the Na^+–H^+ exchange process in the distal nephron.

Micropuncture studies have shown that acute metabolic acidosis inhibits sodium transport in the proximal and distal tubule (Stein *et al.*, 1968; Dubb *et al.*, 1977). Since the excretory rates of sodium and calcium correlate well during acute metabolic acidosis (Walser, 1971), it is plausible to suggest that calcium reabsorption is also inhibited. Sutton *et al.* (1979) found that chronic metabolic acidosis selectively inhibits calcium reabsorption in the distal sites of the nephron.

The data on the effect of metabolic alkalosis on urinary calcium excretion are inconsistent (Zucker, 1921; Shohl and Sato, 1923; Wiley *et al.*, 1933; Williamson and Freeman, 1957; Martin and Jones, 1961). The interpretation of these observations is complicated by the fact that metabolic alkalosis was produced by chronic administration of $NaHCO_3$, which may alter the state of extracellular fluid volume and, hence, may affect urinary calcium excretion. Marone *et al.* (1978) and Sutton *et al.* (1979) found that metabolic alkalosis in intact or TPTX dogs enhanced the tubular reabsorption of calcium relative to sodium. Studies in normal subjects and in patients with hypercalciuria have shown that oral bicarbonate loading is associated with a fall in urinary calcium excretion (Martin and Jones, 1961; Parfitt *et al.*, 1964; Edwards and Hodgkinson, 1965).

In a recent study in the rat, Marone and Sutton (1980) showed that acidosis potentiates and alkalosis impairs the calciuretic effects of furosemide. These observations suggest that the sites of action of metabolic acidosis or alkalosis and furosemide upon calcium reabsorption are different.

Chronic respiratory acidosis may increase (Gray *et al.*, 1973) and respiratory alkalosis may decrease (Siggard-Anderson, 1962) urinary calcium excretion.

7. *Dietary Intake*

Urinary calcium excretion increases after the ingestion of glucose (Lemann *et al.*, 1969, 1970b), most probably due to a decrease in the tubular reabsorption of this ion (Lemann *et al.*, 1970a). This effect is exaggerated in calcium oxalate stone-formers (Lemann *et al.*, 1969) and is not related to a fall in urinary pH; Lennon and Piering (1970) found that the effects of glucose and ammonium chloride ingestion on urinary calcium are additive. DeFronzo *et al.* (1976) have shown that insulin augments urinary calcium excretion; it is possible that glucose ingestion produces calciuria through its effect on insulin release.

The ingestion of rapidly metabolizable substances (Lindeman *et al.*, 1964, 1967), of alcohol (Kalbfleisch *et al.*, 1963) and of high protein diet (Margen and Calloway, 1967) also augment urinary excretion of calcium. The ingestion of fat has no effect (Lindeman *et al.*, 1967).

Urinary calcium is also affected by sodium intake (Kleeman *et al.*, 1964; Epstein, 1968). Modlin (1966) found a direct correlation between the 24-hr urinary excretion of calcium and sodium in a large number of normal subjects; under these experimental conditions, the urinary sodium undoubtedly reflects sodium intake. In that case the interrelationships between the renal handling of sodium and calcium described in acute studies would also exist on a day-to-day basis.

The renal excretion of calcium may vary with calcium intake but the relation is not close (Knapp, 1947). About 2–7% of the increment in calcium intake may appear in the urine (Peacock *et al.*, 1967). The augmentation in urinary calcium may be related to the rise in serum calcium (MacFaden *et al.*, 1965), which may suppress the activity of the parathyroid glands (Sherwood *et al.*, 1966) and increase filtered loads of calcium (Nordin *et al.*, 1967). A slow reduction in urinary calcium may continue to appear in the urine for days to weeks despite the ingestion of low calcium diet (Malm, 1963). It should be mentioned that patients with osteoporosis display little or no variations in urinary calcium following changes in the dietary intake of this ion (Whedon, 1959; Bahndarker and Nordin, 1962). This could be due to a decrease in intestinal calcium absorption in patients with osteoporosis.

Urinary calcium falls during the ingestion of a low magnesium diet and increases with high magnesium intake (Cunningham and Cunningham, 1938; Heaton and Parsons, 1961; Alcock and MacIntyre, 1964; Clark, 1968; Heaton, 1969).

During fasting, urinary calcium excretion increases (Drenick, 1972) and the administration of small amounts of sodium to fasting subjects augments urinary calcium output (Brickman *et al.*, 1970). The effect of fasting on urinary calcium excretion is rapidly reversed by refeeding with even a small amount of glucose (Drenick, 1972). The calciuria of fasting may be due to ketoacidosis of starvation, and Reidenberg *et al.* (1966) reported that administration of sodium bicarbonate blunted the calciuria.

8. Activity and Posture

Exercise decreases (Kattus *et al.*, 1949; Heaton and Hodgkinson, 1963) and prolonged immobilization (Deitrick *et al.*, 1948) increases urinary calcium excretion. The hypercalciuria of immobilization may be due to a relative increase in bone resorption. Patients with paraplegia, body casts, or other paralytic illnesses may have marked hypercalciuria and are predisposed to stone formation (Dunning and Plum, 1957). Oral phosphate (Goldsmith *et al.*, 1967) or thiazide (Griffith, 1971) administration may be helpful for the management of this type of hypercalciuria. Marked hypercalciuria has also been noted during weightlessness associated with space flights (Lutwak *et al.*, 1969).

9. Diurnal Variations

Urinary calcium displays a peak in its excretory rate during forenoon or midday, either coinciding or preceding the peak in sodium excretion (Heaton and Hodgkinson, 1963; Wesson, 1964; Toor *et al.*, 1965; Brisco and Ragan, 1966). The midday peak in calcium excretion is influenced by diet and may be reduced fasting (Heaton and Hodgkinson, 1963) or when food is given at 4-hr intervals around the clock (Loutit, 1965).

C. Effects of Hormones

1. Parathyroid Hormone

Data from clearance (Kleeman *et al.*, 1961; Massry *et al.*, 1968b), stop flow (Widrow and Levinsky, 1962), and micropuncture (Agus *et al.*, 1973) studies indicate that PTH enhances tubular transport of calcium and decreases C_{Ca}. The clearance of calcium rises during the first few hours after parathyroidectomy in rats (Talmage and Krantz, 1954) and dogs (Kleeman *et al.*, 1961) despite the fall in serum calcium; C_{Ca} is relatively high in humans with hypoparathyroidism (Kleeman *et al.*, 1961; Bethune *et al.*, 1968). The administration of parathyroid extract to humans or animals decreases urinary calcium excretion (Kleeman *et al.*, 1961; Bernstein *et al.*, 1963; Bethune *et al.*, 1968; Massry *et al.*, 1968b; Eisenberg, 1970), although others have observed either an increase or no change in C_{Ca} (Talmage and Kraintz, 1954; Pullman *et al.*, 1960; Gill *et al.*, 1967). The variability of these results may be related to an increase in plasma calcium, a rise in glomerular filtration rate, or augmented sodium excretion, all of which follow the administration of parathyroid extract. In patients with hypercalcemia, C_{Ca} for any given level of filtered load of calcium is lower in patients with hyperparathyroidism than in those with other hypercalcemic disorders (Kleeman *et al.*, 1961; Transbol *et al.*, 1970).

The exact site(s) in the nephron where PTH exerts its hypocalciuric effect is not fully delineated. However, most investigators agree that this action of the hormone is located at distal segments of the nephron. The stop flow studies of Widrow and Levinsky (1962) and the clearance experiments of Massry *et al.* (1968b) suggested that PTH augments calcium reabsorption of distal parts of the renal tubule. Agus *et al.* (1973), utilizing micropuncture techniques, found that PTH decreases the reabsorption of both calcium and sodium in the proximal tubule, but the final urinary excretion of calcium is reduced with little change in urinary sodium. Their data are consistent with PTH enhancing tubular calcium transport in the distal nephron. Costanzo and Windhager (1978a) utilizing microperfusion technique, have obtained findings consistent with the site of action of PTH being in the distal convoluted tubule. Micropuncture data in the dog by Sutton *et al.* (1976) suggest an effect for PTH both before and after the distal micropuncture site. Recent studies indicate that PTH stimulates calcium transport in the cortical part of the thick ascending limb of the loop of Henle (Suki and Rouse, 1979; Bourdedu and Burg, 1979a; Shareghi and Agus, 1979). Other data suggest in the rat (Agus *et al.*, 1977) and in the hamster (Harris *et al.*, 1976) that this effect is mostly located in the collecting duct.

The action of PTH on proximal calcium reabsorption is probably mediated through the stimulation of adenylate cyclase and the production of cyclic AMP, since the administration of dibutyryl cyclic AMP causes similar effects (Agus *et al.*, 1973). The influence of PTH on calcium reabsorption in the distal nephron is not linked with sodium transport. Indeed, the relationship between C_{Ca} and C_{Na} is altered during deficiency or excess of PTH. Although the mechanisms of action of PTH in the distal nephron are not yet delineated, data by Burnatowska *et al.* in the hamster (1977) suggest that the effect of PTH in the distal nephron may also be mediated by cyclic AMP.

2. *Calcitonin*

The effects of pharmacologic doses of calcitonin on calcium excretion appear to be species related. The hormone decreases calcium excretion in rats (Pechet *et al.*, 1967; Rasmussen *et al.*, 1967). Calcitonin has no effect on electrolyte excretion in the dog (Clark and Kenny, 1969), but Pak *et al.* (1970) reported that calcitonin administration to TPTX dogs increased urinary calcium excretion. In normal subjects and in patients with hypoparathyroidism, calcitonin produces calciuria (Singer *et al.*, 1969; Cochran *et al.*, 1970; Paillard *et al.*, 1972). It is of interest that hypercalciuria has not been reported in patients with medullary carcinoma of the thyroid, in spite of markedly elevated blood levels of calcitonin (Melvin and Tashjian, 1968).

Paillard *et al.* (1972) have provided data suggesting that calcitonin inhibits sodium reabsorption in the proximal tubule; calcium transport may also be inhibited at this site. The membrane of the renal tubular cells in cortex and outer medulla contains receptors for calcitonin (Marx *et al.*, 1972). The binding between the hormone and its receptors activates renal adenylate cyclase, this is followed by a series of steps that culminate in the action of calcitonin on electrolyte transport (Kurokawa *et al.*, 1974).

3. *Adrenal Steroids*

The effects of elevated blood levels of adrenal steroids on urinary calcium excretion depend on the duration of the state with excess hormone.

a. Glucocorticoids. The acute administration of glucocorticoids to animals (Massry *et al.*, 1967a) or to man (Lemann *et al.*, 1970a) has no effect on calcium excretion, but chronic administration usually causes calcium excretion to rise (Pechet *et al.*, 1959; Laake, 1960; Collins *et al.*, 1962). Thus, patients with Cushing syndrome have high urinary calcium excretion that falls after adrenalectomy (Molinatti *et al.*, 1960). The hypercalciuria in states with chronic excess of glucocorticoids is probably not due to an action of the hormones on the kidney but rather due to increased mobilization of calcium from bone.

b. Mineralocorticoids. Urinary calcium excretion is not affected by acute administration of mineralocorticoids to dogs (Massry *et al.*, 1967a) or man (Lemann *et al.*, 1970a). Thus, the mechanisms for sodium transport, which are stimulated by mineralocorticoids in the distal nephron, are dissociated from those

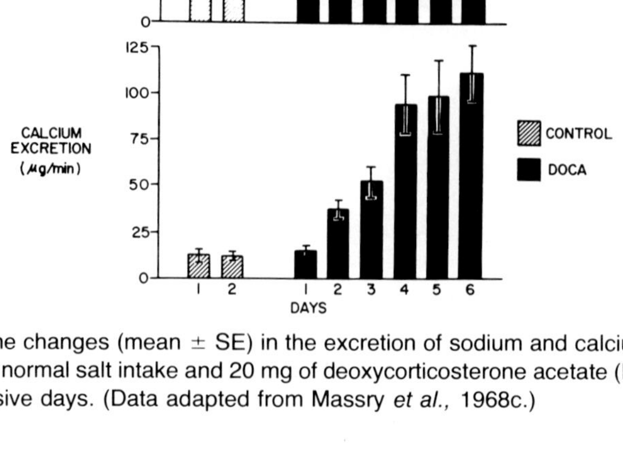

Fig. 14. The changes (mean ± SE) in the excretion of sodium and calcium observed in dogs receiving normal salt intake and 20 mg of deoxycorticosterone acetate (DOCA) per day over 6 successive days. (Data adapted from Massry *et al.*, 1968c.)

for calcium transport. The acute administration of mineralocorticoids alters the usual relationship between C_{Ca} and C_{Na}.

The chronic administration of mineralocorticoids to dogs (Massry *et al.*, 1968c) and rats (Suki *et al.*, 1968) has been shown to produce a marked increase in urinary calcium excretion. Although in these studies the mineralocorticoids had no effect during the first 2 days, calcium excretion gradually increased thereafter (Fig. 14). The change in urinary calcium coincided with the escape from the hormonal effect on sodium excretion. It has been suggested that the sodium retention that occurs with mineralocorticoid administration leads to chronic ECVE, which then causes a decrease in the tubular reabsorption of calcium, resulting in calciuria. High urinary calcium excretion has also been noted in patients with primary aldosteronism.

4. *Thyroid Hormone*

Hyperthyroidism is associated with hypercalciuria, and urinary calcium excretion is reduced in patients with hypothyroidism (Aub *et al.*, 1929; Krane *et al.*, 1956; Kleeman *et al.*, 1958; Cook *et al.*, 1959). The mechanisms underlying the changes in urinary calcium excretion during altered states of thyroid gland function are not known. The phenomenon may be related to the effects of thyroid hormone on bone metabolism. In hyperthyroidism, the negative calcium balance and presumed loss of calcium from skeleton probably account for the hypercalciuria. Many patients with thyrotoxicosis may have hypercalcemia, which would inhibit the activity of the parathyroid glands and lead to a further decrease in tubular reabsorption of calcium. At present, it is not known whether the thyroid hormone has a direct effect on the tubular transport of calcium.

5. *Growth Hormone*

The effect of this hormone on the renal excretion of calcium appears to be opposite that of parathyroid hormone. The administration of growth hormone augments the urinary excretion of calcium (Ikkos *et al.*, 1959). This effect of growth hormone may have clinical significance in that patients with acromegaly often shown hypercalciuria and may develop renal stones, presumably related in part to this renal effect (Bauer and Aub, 1941; DeGennes *et al.*, 1961). Since the serum calcium level is not affected by growth hormone, the renal effect of the hormone is presumably related to altered tubular reabsorption of calcium.

6. *Vitamin D*

Large doses of vitamin D may directly inhibit calcium transport by the nephron (Litvak *et al.*, 1958), but Bernstein *et al.* (1963) failed to confirm this. Furthermore, Ney *et al.* (1968) found that calcium excretion fell during the first 2–25 hr after vitamin D administration to rachitic dogs, while serum calcium did not change. Six days later, urinary calcium increased as serum calcium levels were rising. These observations suggest that vitamin D may enhance the tubular reabsorption of calcium, but such an effect could not be observed as the concentration of serum calcium rises. Indeed, Costanzo *et al.* (1974) found that vitamin D_3 produced a decrease in urinary excretion in D-deficient rats.

Puschett *et al.* (1972) and Nseir *et al.* (1978) reported that the acute administration of large doses of $25(OH)D_3$ produced a fall in the fraction of filtered calcium excreted in TPTX dogs. This effect occurred in the presence of antidiuretic hormone with or without the presence of PTH. Sutton *et al.* (1975a) reported that $25(OH)D_3$ enhances calcium reabsorption in the distal tubule. Puschett *et al.* (1972) also found that acute administration of $1,25(OH)_2D_3$ reduces the fractional excretion of calcium in the dogs. In contrast, long-term administration of small amounts of $1,25(OH)_2D_3$ to parathyroidectomized rats increased urinary calcium excretion (Rizzoli *et al.*, 1977).

IV. ROLE OF THE KIDNEY IN THE MAINTENANCE OF SERUM CALCIUM

It is generally accepted that three processes are involved in the control of the concentration of serum calcium. These include the interchange between the skeleton and blood, intestinal calcium absorption, and renal tubular reabsorption of calcium. However, controversy exists regarding the relative contribution of each of these mechanisms to the overall process of maintaining the concentration of serum calcium within the normal limits.

Nordin and Peacock (1969) and Nordin *et al.* (1972) maintain that the kidney is the main regulator of the concentration of serum calcium. They attributed the hypercalcemia of primary hyperparathyroidism to the increased tubular reabsorption of calcium produced by the excess blood levels of PTH. They also propose that the fall in the concentration of serum calcium after the surgical removal of parathyroid adenoma is due to increased urinary excretion of calcium secondary to a decrease in its tubular reabsorption which occurs as a consequence of the fall in the blood levels of PTH. Moreover, they claim that the hypocalcemia observed in early renal failure is due to a decrease in the tubular reabsorption of calcium. These authors base their interpretations and conclusions on the correlation between changes in calcium excretion (per 100 ml GFR) and serum calcium levels.

Several clinical and experimental observations vitiate these arguments of Nordin and his colleagues. If the loss of calcium in the urine plays a paramount role in the maintenance of serum calcium, its absolute excretion rather than the excretion per 100 ml GFR would be the determinant factor. Patients with early renal failure often show both reduced absolute calcium excretion and low excretion per 100 ml GFR (Lichtwitz and Parlier, 1965; Popovtzer *et al.*, 1970). As renal failure progresses, calcium excretion per 100 ml GFR increases, but total urinary calcium excretion remains very low (Popovtzer *et al.*, 1969). It seems very unlikely, therefore, that losses of calcium by the kidney could be responsible for the hypocalcemia in these patients. Second, severe hypocalcemia occurs within 1–3 days in patients with oliguric acute renal failure (Massry *et al.*, 1974). These patients develop hypocalcemia in the absence of urinary calcium losses. This indicates that other mechanisms are responsible for the hypocalcemia. Indeed, in a series of studies carried out in our laboratory, we demonstrated the critical role of the skeletal resistance to the calcemic action of PTH in the genesis of the hypocalcemia in patients with early and advanced chronic renal failure (Massry *et al.*, 1973; Llach *et al.*, 1975) and in those with acute renal failure (Massry *et al.*, 1974). Third, reduced tubular reabsorption of calcium may be the cause of enhanced calcium excretion in some patients with idiopathic hypercalciuria (Coe *et al.*, 1973), yet serum calcium levels of these patients are normal and may even be slightly elevated. Fourth, parathyroidectomy (Kleeman *et al.*, 1961) or suppression of the parathyroid glands by hypermagnesemia (Massry *et al.*, 1970a) is followed by a far greater decrease in serum calcium than can be accounted for by the urinary losses during the time of the observation. Finally, Garty *et al.* (1973) evaluated the role of the kidney in the recovery from acute hypercalcemia, as well as its role in the fall of serum calcium during the first 10 hr after total parathyroidectomy. The concentration of calcium in the blood of dogs was elevated by the infusion of 25 mg Ca^{2+}/kg body weight administered over 20 min. Blood levels of calcium rose to 18–20 mg/100 ml and returned to control values by the end of 7 hr. This occurred even though urinary calcium excretion accounted for only 10–17% of the infused calcium load. The same response was observed in dogs with bilateral ureteral ligation. Also, the magnitude of fall in the blood calcium level during the first 10 hr after total parathyroidectomy was the same in dogs with intact renal function as in those with bilateral ureteral ligation.

Although these observations contradict the hypothesis of Nordin and his associates, this is not to say that the kidneys are not involved in the regulation of the serum calcium level. In this reviewer's opinion, the interaction between bone and its extracellular bathing fluid is the process most responsible for the maintenance of the serum calcium within normal values; both gut and kidney contribute to this overall regulatory process.

V. URINARY CALCIUM IN PATIENTS WITH RENAL FAILURE

Hypocalciuria is almost always present in patients with renal failure and has been noted even in the early stages of renal insufficiency (Lichtwitz and Parlier, 1965; Better *et al.*, 1967; Friis *et al.*, 1968; Popovtzer *et al.*, 1970). Occasionally, however, patients with renal failure due to chronic pyelonephritis or polycytic kidney disease may lose sizeable amounts of calcium in their urine (Coburn *et al.*, 1969).

In patients with early renal failure, the fraction of filtered calcium excreted is also low but increases as renal failure progresses (Popovtzer *et al.*, 1969, 1970). From these observations it would seem that factors controlling the renal handling of calcium may differ at various stages of renal failure. Data from our laboratory indicate that the changes in the fractional calcium excretion are not related to the level of serum calcium. In early renal failure, both hypocalciuria and the decreased fractional excretion of calcium may result from the high circulating levels of parathyroid hormone, which acts to increase tubular reabsorption and to reduce urinary excretion of calcium. With more advanced renal failure, the increase in fractional excretion of calcium correlates very closely with that of sodium (Popovtzer *et al.*, 1979). This relationship is almost identical to that observed in normal dogs undergoing extracellular volume expansion with saline infusion (Massry *et al.*, 1967b; Brickman *et al.*, 1971). The existence of a hormonal factor that depresses the tubular reabsorption of sodium and calcium has been suggested, and the factor found in the plasma of uremic patients (Bourgoignie *et al.*, 1972) may be responsible for the decreased fractional reabsorption of sodium and calcium. In these circumstances, the effect of parathyroid hormone in reducing fractional excretion of calcium is probably overcome.

The interdependence between the clearances of sodium and calcium persists in patients undergoing maintenance hemodialysis who have only vestigial renal function and form small amounts of urine (Coburn *et al.*, 1969). Also, we found an increased fractional excretion of both calcium and sodium and interdependence between the renal handling of these two ions during the diuretic phase of acute renal failure; the slope for the correlation between their fractional excretions was 0.95 and did not differ from that seen during extracellular fluid volume expansion or noted in patients with advanced chronic renal failure.

Patients with the nephrotic syndrome have hypocalciuria even if their renal function is normal (Scriver, 1928; Emerson and Beckman, 1945; Jones *et al.*, 1967; Goldstein *et al.*, 1977). These patients have strong tendencies to retain calcium (hypocalcemia and secondary hyperparathyroidism) and sodium. These factors may contribute to their hypocalciuria. The effect of furosemide on the renal handling of calcium in these patients has been discussed earlier in this chapter.

VI. HYPERCALCIURIA

It is not easy to define the normal range for urinary calcium excretion since it is influenced by the many variables listed in Table II. Available data indicate that in 90% of healthy individuals, the daily urinary excretion of calcium is less than

TABLE II

Factors Affecting Daily Urinary Calcium Excretion

1. Dietary intake of calcium (Knapp, 1947; Nordin and Smith, 1965; Davis *et al.*, 1970)
2. Diurinal variations (Heaton and Hodgkinson, 1963; Briscoe and Ragan, 1966; Carruthers *et al.*, 1974)
3. Feeding patterns with an increase in the efficiency of intestinal calcium absorption with divided regimen (Phang *et al.*, 1968)
4. Seasonal variations (Robertson *et al.*, 1974) not entirely accounted for by changes in calcium intake or in blood levels of $25(OH)D_3$ (McLaughlin *et al.*, 1974)
5. Sex, with its effect presumably due to variations in lean body mass since relating calcium excretion to that of creatinine reduces the sex differences (Nordin *et al.*, 1967)
6. Age, with its effect secondary to reduction in intestinal absorption of calcium and/or the fall in GFR that accompanies aging
7. Dietary intake of sodium (Modlin, 1966), magnesium (Clark, 1968), phosphorus (Farquharson *et al.*, 1931), and possibly oxalate (Robertson and Morgan, 1972)
8. Impairment in renal function (Lichtwitz and Parlier, 1965; Popovtzer *et al.*, 1970)

250 mg in females and less than 300 mg in males with a calcium intake of 800 ± 200 mg/day (Hodgkinson and Pyrah, 1958). These values have, therefore, been suggested as the upper limits of daily urinary excretion. Only 5% of normal men or women have 24-hr urinary calcium outputs greater than that, whereas 30% of calcium stone formers will exceed these upper limits (Hodgkinson and Pyrah, 1958). Coe (1977) has introduced the term of "marginal hypercalciuria" to be applied to patients (11% of calcium stone formers) whose urinary calcium excretion is greater than 150 mg per gram of urinary creatinine and who benefit from therapy designed to reduce urinary calcium excretion.

A multitude of clinical disorders are associated with hypercalciuria (Table III). The major clinical significance of hypercalciuria is its relation to the genesis of renal stones. It has been estimated that 20–33% of the patients with renal calcium stones have hypercalciuria (Melick and Henneman, 1958; Albuquerque *et al.*, 1962). However, most patients with renal stones and hypercalciuria have no obvious cause for an increase in urinary calcium excretion and have therefore been described as having idiopathic hypercalciuria. Henneman *et al.* (1958) reported that idiopathic hypercalciuria occurs predominantly in males; their serum calcium level is normal and thus serum phosphorus tends to be low; they usually form calcium phosphate or oxalate stones.

Although the pathogenesis of idiopathic hypercalciuria is not fully understood, at least four pathogenetic factors may be operative, either singly or in various combinations. These include (a) increased bone reresorption (*resorptive hypercalciuria*), (b) increased intestinal absorption of calcium (*absorptive hypercalciuria*), (c) renal leak of calcium (*renal hypercalciuria*), and (d) renal leak of

TABLE III

Clinical Disorders Associated with Hypercalciuria

1. Increased gastrointestinal absorption
High calcium intake
Hypervitaminosis D
Sarcoidosis
Idiopathic hypercalciuria
2. Increased bone resorption relative to accretion
Primary hyperparathyroidism
Malignancy associated with hypercalcemia
Carcinoma with bone metastases
Hypervitaminosis D
Sarcoidosis
Hyperthyroidism
Cushing syndrome (exogenous or endogenous)
Renal tubular acidosis
Paget's disease
Phosphate depletion
Immobilization
Juvenile osteoporosis
Multiple myeloma
3. Decreased tubular reabsorption of calcium
Renal tubular acidosis
Fanconi syndrome
Phosphate depletion
Hypoparathyroidism with normal serum calcium
Medullary sponge kidney
Primary aldosteronism
High salt intake
High magnesium intake
Chronic furosemide administration
Idiopathic hypercalciuria
? Acromegaly

phosphate (*hypophosphatemic hypercalciuria*). The various tests and parameters that are helpful in the differential diagnosis of these forms of hypercalciuria are given in Table IV.

A. Resorptive Hypercalciuria

Liberman *et al.* (1968) performed calcium balances and radiokinetic studies using ^{47}Ca in patients with idiopathic hypercalciuria. They found increased rates of calcium turnover and suggested that a disturbance in bone metabolism may contribute to the hypercalciuria. Pak *et al.* (1975) described patients with hyperparathyroidism, increased bone resorption and hypercalciuria. These indi-

TABLE IV

Differential Diagnosis of Hypercalciuria[a]

	Resorptive hypercalciuria	Absorptive hypercalciuria	Renal hypercalciuria		Hypophosphatemic (hypercalciuria)
			2° Hyperparathyroidism	3° Hyperparathyroidism	
Serum calcium	nl or ↑	nl	nl	nl	nl
After calcium load	nl or ↑	nl	nl	nl or ↑	nl
Serum PTH	↑	nl or ↓	↑	↑	nl or ↓
After calcium load	↑	nl or ↓	nl	↑	nl or ↓
Serum phosphorus	nl or ↓	nl	nl or ↓	nl or ↓	↓
Serum $1,25(OH)_2D_3$	nl or ↑	nl or ↑	nl or ↑	nl or ↑	↑
Urine calcium					
Normal diet	>250 mg	>250 mg	>250 mg	>250 mg	>250 mg
Urine calcium					
Low calcium diet	>200 mg	<200 mg	>200 mg	>200 mg	>200 mg
Urine calcium					
Fasting	>0.11 mg/gm cr	<0.11 mg/gm cr	>0.11 mg/gm cr	>0.11 mg/gm cr	>0.11 mg/gm cr
After Calcium Load	>0.2 mg/gm cr	>0.2 mg/gm cr	>0.2 mg/gm cr	>0.2 mg/gm cr	>0.2 mg/gm cr
Urine cAMP					
Fasting	>4 μmole/gm cr	<4.2 μmole/gm cr	>4 μmole/gm cr	>4 μmole/gm cr	<4 μmole/gm cr
After calcium load	>4 μmole/gm cr	<4.2 μmole/gm cr	<4 μmole/gm cr	>4 μmole/gm cr	<4 μmole/gm cr
Renal phosphate					
Absorption-fasting	↓	nl	nl or ↓	nl or ↓	↓
Absorption-calcium load	↓	nl	nl	nl or ↓	↓
Urine hydroxyproline					
fasting	↑	nl	↑	↑	↑
After calcium load	↑	nl	nl	↑	nl
After phosphate load	↑	nl	↑	↑	↑

[a] nl, Normal value; cr, creatinine. By permission from Suki (1980).

viduals have normal serum calcium, elevated levels of PTH, increased urinary calcium and cyclic AMP excretion during fasting. Calcium loading failed to reduce blood PTH levels or urinary cyclic AMP excretion. Since these patients have normocalcemic hyperparathyroidism, it is surprising that they have hypercalciuria in the face of normal serum calcium and elevated PTH levels. It is possible that these patients have primarily a renal calcium leak and the increased urinary losses of calcium produced secondary hyperparathyroidism, which then progressed to adenoma of the parathyroid glands.

B. Absorptive Hypercalciuria

The patients with this type of hypercalciuria absorb more calcium than they need to keep a zero body calcium balance; the excess calcium is excreted by the kidney as a consequence of increased filtered loads of calcium and a decrease in blood levels of PTH (Henneman *et al.*, 1958; Harrison, 1959; Parfitt *et al.*, 1964; Caniggia *et al.*, 1965; Pak *et al.*, 1972, 1974b). The mechanisms that have led to intestinal calcium hyperabsorption are unknown.

About 30–80% of patients with idiopathic hypercalciuria have increased jejunal calcium absorption (Brannan *et al.*, 1979). Their serum calcium, is normal, their serum PTH low to normal, and their urinary calcium excretion is also normal. Cyclic AMP and hydroxyproline during fasting are normal or low. About one-third of the patients have elevated blood levels of $1,25(OH)_2D_3$ (Kaplan *et al.*, 1977). After the ingestion of food or following a calcium load, their serum calcium will increase more than in normal subjects. Blood PTH will therefore fall. These events in turn will be followed by an increase in urinary calcium excretion.

C. Renal Hypercalciuria

The patients with this type (Chapter 4, Vol. III) of hypercalciuria have a primary defect in renal tubular reabsorption of calcium resulting in increased losses of calcium in the urine, fall in serum calcium, and secondary hyperparathyroidism. The rise in blood PTH levels will depress the tubular reabsorption of phosphate and lower serum phosphorus levels. The fall in the latter could be associated with increased mobilization of calcium from bone and/or increased production of $1,25(OH)_2D_3$ which, in turn, may enhance intestinal calcium absorption. These events would increase the calcium load reaching the kidney and augment the degree of the hypercalciuria. About 20–65% of patients with idiopathic hypercalciuria may have a renal calcium leak (Pak *et al.*, 1974b, 1975).

Several lines of evidence support a renal leak of calcium as a cause for the hypercalciuria. Edwards and Hodgkinson (1965) found an increase in the renal clearance of calcium, while its filtered load was appreciably below normal. Eknoyan *et al.* (1972) found that patients with idiopathic hypercalciuria have a renal tubular leak of sodium; since the tubular reabsorption of sodium and calcium is interrelated, they suggested that a renal calcium leak is responsible for the hypercalciuria. Coe *et al.* (1973) provide further support for the renal calcium leak concept. These authors found elevated blood levels of PTH in patients with idiopathic hypercalciuria receiving unrestricted diet. The suppression of the hypercalciuria with thiazide therapy was associated with a fall in the blood levels of PTH to normal. Finally, the induction of hypercalciuria with furosemide administration caused a rise in blood levels of PTH. Although Pak *et al.* (1974b) could not confirm these observations in their patients, they found few patients that are similar to those described by Coe *et al.* (1973).

Evidence against a primary renal leak of calcium has been provided by Peacock and Nordin (1968), who found no decrease in tubular reabsorption of calcium in hypercalciuric subjects when tubular reabsorption of calcium was studied at different levels of filtered calcium. In addition, the slope of urinary calcium in relation to dietary intake was found to be steeper in patients with hypercalciuria, but the theoretical excretion at zero intake was normal. This would indicate adequate renal conservation of calcium in the absence of a dietary calcium load. Finally, the observation by Finn *et al.* (1970) that urinary excretion of calcium was normal in a transplant recipient who received a kidney from a donor with idiopathic hypercalciuria is not consistent with the renal calcium leak hypothesis.

In patients with hypercalciuria due to primary renal calcium leak, the blood levels of calcium are normal to low, those of phosphorus are low, and those of PTH are elevated. During fasting, the urinary excretion of calcium, cyclic AMP, and hydroxyproline are increased. Calcium loading is followed by an increase in calcium excretion, a decrease in urinary cyclic AMP and hydroxyproline and a fall in blood PTH. Bordier *et al.* (1977) reported that half of their patients with renal hypercalciuria developed tertiary hyperparathyroidism; calcium loading in this subgroup of patients failed to lower blood PTH or decrease hydroxyproline excretion.

D. Hypophosphatemic Hypercalciuria

A primary defect in renal tubular reabsorption of phosphate may be present in a subgroup of patients with idiopathic hypercalciuria; this defect could be responsible for the augmented urinary losses of calcium (Bordier *et al.*, 1977; Gray *et al.*, 1977; Shen *et al.*, 1977). The increased urinary losses of phosphate produces hypophosphatemia, which could be associated with augmented production of $1,25(OH)_2D_3$, enhanced intestinal absorption of calcium, and increased mobilization of calcium from bone; consequently, hypercalciuria will ensue. Also, hypophosphatemia and phosphate depeletion, per se, decrease tubular reabsorption of calcium.

In these patients, the levels of serum phosphorus and PTH are low. During fasting, urinary excretion of calcium and hydroxyproline are elevated and urinary cyclic AMP is low.

E. Treatment of Hypercalciuria

Two therapeutic modalities that reduce the urinary excretion of calcium have been used in the management of patients with hypercalciuria and renal calculi. These include benzothiazide diuretics (Yendt *et al.*, 1966, 1970) and oral phosphate (Bernstein and Newton, 1966; Thomas and Miller, 1967). Yendt *et al.* (1966, 1970) favor the use of hydrochlorothiazide, 50 mg twice daily, which causes a substantial decrease in urinary calcium excretion; this treatment is quite effective in reducing the incidence of renal stones. The mechanisms by which chronic thiazide therapy produces hypocalciuria have already been discussed. Chronic thiazide therapy could produce impotence in the male patient. Oral treatment with salts of inorganic phosphate also has been effective in treating the hypercalciuria and lowering the incidence of stones in these patients (Fleisch *et al.*, 1964). It is necessary to give 1–3 gm of elemental phosphorus per day in the form of sodium or potassium salts. Such therapy may cause troublesome diarrhea which limits its use.

Cellulose phosphate, which binds calcium in the intestine, has been used in the management of absorptive hypercalciuria (Pak *et al.*, 1974a). The dose is 10–15 gm per day given orally in divided doses of 5 gm each. The patients should also receive supplementation of 100–200 mg of magnesium per day since cellulose phosphate binds magnesium as well and causes a decrease in urinary magnesium excretion. This in turn could be hazardous since urinary magnesium is a potent inhibitor of crystalization in urine.

ACKNOWLEDGMENT

The author wishes to express his thanks to Ms. Gracy Fick and Ms. Melinda Ayers for their assistance in the preparation of this manuscript.

REFERENCES

Agus, Z.S. (1978). Renal transport of calcium. Uptade. *In* "Homeostasis of Phosphate and Other Minerals" (S.G. Massry, E. Ritz, and A. Rapado, eds.), pp. 37–49. Plenum, New York.

Agus, Z.S., Gardner, L.B., Beck, L.H., and Goldberg, M. (1973). Effects of parathyroid hormone on renal tubular reabsorption of calcium, sodium and phosphate. *Am. J. Physiol.* **224,** 1143–1148.

Agus, Z.S., Chiu, P.J.S., and Goldberg, M. (1975). Regulation of urinary calcium excretion in the rat. *Am. J. Physiol.* **232,** F545–549.

Ahumada, J.J., and Massry, S.G. (1971). Renal vasodilatation. Effect on renal handling of phosphate. *Clin. Sci.* **41,** 109–121.

Albright, F., Bauer, W., Claflin, D., and Cockrill, J.R. (1932). Studies in parathyroid physiology. III. The effect of phosphate ingestion in clinical hyperparathyroidism. *J. Clin. Invest.* **11,** 411–435.

Albuquerque, P.F., Forster, R., and Zanandrea, B. (1962). Etiological factors in urolithiasis. A clinical analysis of 275 cases. *Trans. Am. Assoc. Genito-Urinary Surgeons* **54,** 45–49.

Alcock, N., and MacIntyre, I. (1964). Some effects of magnesium depletion on calcium metabolism in the rat. *Clin. Sci.* **26,** 219–225.

Almeida, A.L.J., Kudo, L.H., and Rocha, A.S. (1978). Calcium transport in isolated perfused pars recta of proximal tubule. *Abstr. Int. Congr. Nephrol., 7th, 1978* E-16.

Antoniou, L.D., Eisner, G.M., Slatkoff, L.M., and Lilienfield, L.S. (1969). Relationship between sodium and calcium transport in the kidney. *J. Lab. Clin. Med.* **74,** 410–420.

Atchley, D.W., Loeb, R.F., Richards, D.W., Jr., Benedict, E.M., and Driscoll, M.E. (1933). On diabetic acidosis: A detailed study of electrolyte balances following the withdrawal and reestablishment of insulin therapy. *J. Clin. Invest.* **12,** 297–326.

Aub, J.C., Bauer, W., Heath, C., and Ropes, M. (1929). Studies of calcium and phosphorus metabolism. III. The effects of thyroid hormone and thyroid disease. *J. Clin. Invest.* **7,** 97–137.

Bauer, W., and Aub, J.C. (1941). Studies of calcium and phosphorus metabolism XVI. The influence of pituitary gland. *J. Clin. Invest.* **20,** 295–301.

Beck, L.H., and Goldberg, M. (1973). Effects of acetazolamide and parathyroidectomy on renal transport of sodium, calcium and phosphate. *Am. J. Physiol.* **224,** 1136–1142.

Ben-Isaac, C., Massry, S.G., Rosenfeld, S., Kleeman, C.R., and Bick, M. (1975). Evidence for humoral factor responsible for the hypercalciuria of phosphate depletion. *Clin. Res.* **23,** 134.

Bernstein, D., Kleeman, C.R., and Maxwell, M.H. (1963). The effect of calcium infusions, parathyroid hormone, and vitamin D on renal clearnace of calcium. *Exp. Biol. Med.* **112,** 353–355.

Bernstein, D.S., and Newton, R. (1966). The effect of oral sodium phosphate on the formation of renal calculi and on idiopathic hypercalciuria. *Lancet* **2,** 1105–1107.

Bethune, J.E., Turpin, R.A., and Inoue, H. (1968). Effect of parathyroid extract on divalent ion excretion in man. *J. Clin. Endocrinol. Metab.* **28,** 673–678.

Better, O.S., Kleeman, C.R., Gonick, H.C., Varrady, P.D., and Maxwell, M.H. (1967). Renal handling of calcium, magnesium, and inorganic phosphate in chronic renal failure. *Isr. J. Med. Sci.* **3,** 60–79.

Bhandarkar, S.S., and Nordin, B.E.C. (1962). Effect of low calcium diet on urinary calcium in osteoporosis. *Br. Med. J.* **1,** 145–147.

Blythe, W.B., Gitelman, H.J., and Welt, L.G. (1968). Effect of expansion of thc extracellular space on the rate of urinary excretion of calcium. *Am. J. Physiol.* **214,** 52–57.

Bordier, P., Ryckewart, A., Gueris, J., and Rasmussen, H. (1977). On the pathogenesis of so-called idiopathic hypercalciuria. *Am. J. Med.* **63,** 398–409.

Bourdeau, J.E., and Burg, M.B. (1979a). Effect of parathyroid hormone on calcium transport in the cortical thick ascending limb of Henle's loop. *Clin. Res.* **27,** 410A.

Bourdeau, J.E., and Burg, M.B. (1979b). Voltage dependence of calcium transport in the thick ascending limb of Henle's loop. *Am. J. Physiol.* **236,** F357.

Bourgoignie, J.J., Hwang, K.H., Espinel, C., Klahr, S., and Bricker, N.S. (1972). A natriuretic factor in the serum of patients with chronic uremia. *J. Clin. Invest.* **51,** 1514–1527.

Brannan, P.G., Morawski, S., Pak, C.Y.C., and Fordtran, J.S. (1979). Selective jejunal hyperabsorption of calcium in absorptive hypercalciuria. *N. Engl. J. Med.* **66,** 425–428.

Brickman, A.S., Drenick, E.J., Fisler, J., and Coburn, J.W. (1970). The effect of sodium supplementation on divalent cation during prolonged fasting. *Clin. Res.* **18,** 183.

Brickman, A.S., Massry, S.G., and Coburn, J.W. (1971). Calcium deprivation and renal handling of calcium during repeated saline infusion. *Am. J. Physiol.* **220,** 44–48.

Brickman, A.S., Massry, S.G., and Coburn, J.W. (1972). Changes in serum and urinary calcium during treatment with hydrochlorothiazide, studies on mechanisms. *J. Clin. Invest.* **51,** 945–954.

Brickman, A.S., Coburn, J.W., Massry, S.G., and Norman, A.W. (1974). 1,25 dihydroxyvitamin D_3 in normal man and patients with renal failure. *Ann. Intern. Med.* **80,** 161–168.

Brisco, A.M., and Ragan, C. (1966). Diurnal variations in calcium and magnesium excretion in man. *Metab., Clin. Exp.* **15,** 1002–1010.

Buckle, R.H., Care, A.D., Cooper, C.W., and Gitelman, H.J. (1968). The influence of plasma magnesium concentration on parathyroid hormone secretion. *J. Endocrinol.* **42,** 529–534.

Burg, M., and Green, N. (1973). Function of thick ascending limb of Henle's loop. *Am. J. Physiol.* **224,** 659–668.

Burnatowska, M.A., Harris, C.A., Sutton, R.A.L., and Dirks, J.H. (1977). Effects of PTH and cAMP on renal handling of calcium, magnesium, and phosphate in the hamster. *Am. J. Physiol.* **233,** F514–518.

Caniggia, A., Gennari, C., and Cesari, L. (1965). Intestinal absorption of ^{45}Ca in stone-forming patients. *Br. Med. J.* **1,** 427–430.

Carruthers, B.M., Copp, D.H., and McIntosh, H.W. (1974). Diurnal variations in the urinary excretion of calcium and phosphate and its relation to blood levels. *J. Lab. Clin. Med.* **63,** 959–968.

Chase, L.R., and Aurbach, G.D. (1967). Parathyroid function and renal excretion of 3′,5′ adenylic acid. *Proc. Natl. Acad. Sci. U.S.A.* **58,** 518–525.

Chase, L.R., Fedak, S.A., and Aurbach, G.D. (1969). Activation of skeletal adenyl cyclase by parathyroid hormone, in vitro. *Endocrinology* **84,** 761–768.

Clark, I. (1968). Effects of magnesium ions on calcium and phosphorus metabolism. *Am. J. Physiol.* **214,** 348–356.

Clark, J.D., and Kenny, A.D. (1969). Hog thyrocalcitonin in the dog. Urinary calcium, phosphorus, magnesium and sodium responses. *Endocrinology* **104,** 1089–1100.

Coburn, J.W., and Massry, S.G. (1970). Changes in serum and urinary calcium during phosphate depletion: Studies on mechanisms. *J. Clin. Invest.* **49,** 1619–1629.

Coburn, J.W., Popovtzer, M.M., Massry, S.G., and Kleeman, C.R. (1969) The physicochemical state and renal handling of divalent ions in chronic renal failure. *Arch. Intern. Med.* **124,** 302–311.

Coburn, J.W., Massry, S.G., and Kleeman, C.R. (1970). The effect of calcium infusion on renal handling of magnesium with normal and reduced glomerular filtration rate. *Nephron* **7,** 131–143.

Coburn, J.W., Hartenbower, D.L., and Massry, S.G. (1971). Modification of calciuretic effect of extracellular volume expansion by phosphate infusion. *Am. J. Physiol.* **220,** 377–383.

Cochran, M., Peacock, M., Sacks, G., and Nordin, B.E.C. (1970). Renal effects of calcitonin. *Br. Med. J.* **1,** 135–137.

Coe, F.L. (1977). Treated and intreated recurrent calcium nephrolithiasis in patients with idiopathic hypercalciuria, hyperuricosuria or no metabolic disorder. *Ann. Intern. Med.* **87,** 404–410.

Coe, F.L., Canterbury, J.M., Firpo. J.J., and Reiss, E. (1973). Evidence for secondary hyperparathyroidism in idiopathic hypercalciuria. *J. Clin. Invest.* **52,** 134–142.

Collins, E.J., Garrett, E.R., and Johnston, R.L. (1962). Effect of adrenal steroids on radiocalcium metabolism in dogs. *Metab., Clin. Exp.* **11,** 716–726.

Cook, P.B., Nassim, J.R., and Collins, J. (1959). The effect of thyrotoxicosis upon the metabolism of calcium, phosphate and nitrogen. *Q. J. Med.* **28,** 505–529.

Costanzo, L.S., and Weiner, I.M. (1974). On the hypocalciuric action of chlorothizaide. *J. Clin. Invest.* **54,** 628–637.

Costanzo, L.S., and Windhager, E.E. (1978a). Effect of parathyroid hormone (PTH) and cyclic AMP on calcium (Ca)-sodium (Na) transport in the distal tubule. *Proc. Am. Soc. Nephrol.* **11,** 4A.

Costanzo, L.S., and Windhager, E.E. (1978b). Calcium and sodium transport by the distal convoluted tubule of the rat. *Am. J. Physiol.* **235,** F492.

Costanzo, L.S., Sheehe, P.R., and Weiner, I.M. (1974). Renal actions of vitamin D in D-deficient rats. *Am. J. Physiol.* **226,** 1490–1495.

Cuisinier-Gleizes, P., Thomasset, M., Sainteny-Debove, F., and Mathieu, H. (1976). Parathyroid hormone and bone resorption in the growing rat. *Calcif. Tissue Res.* **20,** 235–249.

Cunningham, I.J., and Cunningham, M.M. (1938). Dietary magnesium and urinary calculi. *N. Z. J. Sci. Technol.* **19,** 529–535.

Davis, R.H., Morgan, D.B., and Rivilin, R.S. (1970). The excretion of calcium in the urine and its relation to calcium intake, sex and age. *Clin. Sci.* **39,** 1–12.

Day, H.G., and McCollum, E.V. (1939). Mineral metabolism, growth and symptomatology of rats on a diet extremely deficient in phosphorus. *J. Biol. Chem.* **130,** 269–283.

DeFronzo, R.A., Goldberg, M., and Agus, A.Z. (1976). The effect of glucose and insulin on renal electrolyte transport. *J. Clin. Invest.* **58,** 83–90.

DeGennes, L., Bricaire, H., Tourneur, R., Moreau, L., and Boutelier, D. (1931). Lithiase shinale cher un acromiégale. Rôle de l'hormone somatotrope dans le mécanisme de l'hypercalciurie. *J. Urol. Nephrol.* **67,** 75–77.

Deitrick, J.E., Whedon, G.D., and Shorr, R. (1948). Effects of immobilization upon various metabolic and physiologic functions of normal man. *Am. J. Med.* **4,** 3–136.

Demartini, F.E., Briscoe, A.M., and Ragan, C. (1967). Effect of ethacrynic acid on calcium and magnesium excretion. *Proc. Soc. Exp. Biol. Med.* **124,** 320–324.

DeRouffignac, C., Morel, F., Moss, N., and Roinel, N. (1973). Micropuncture study of water and electrolyte movements along the loop of Henle is psammomys with special reference to magnesium, calcium and phosphorus. *Pfluegers Arch.* **334,** 309–326.

DiBona, G. (1971). Effect of hypercalcemia on renal tubular sodium handling in the rat. *Am. J. Physiol.* **220,** 49–53.

Dirks, J.H., Cirksena, W.J., and Berliner, R.W. (1965). The effect of saline infusion on sodium reabsorption by the proximal tubule of the dog. *J. Clin. Invest.* **44,** 1160–1170.

Dominguez, J.H., Gray, R.W., and Lemann, J., Jr. (1976). Dietary phosphate deprivation in women and men. Effects on mineral and acid balances, parathyroid hormone and the metabolism of 250H Vitamin D. *Endocrinol. Metab.* **43,** 1056–1068.

Drenick, E.J. (1972). The effects of acute and prolonged fasting and refeeding on water, electrolyte, and acid-base metabolism. *In* "Clinical Disorders of Fluid and Electrolyte Metabolism" (M.H. Maxwell and C.R. Kleeman, eds.), pp. 1117–1137. McGraw-Hill, New York.

Duarte, C.G. (1968). Effects of ethacrynic acid and furosemide on urinary calcium, phosphorus and magnesium. *Metab., Clin. Exp.* **17,** 867–876.

Duarte, C.G., and Bland, J.H. (1965). Calcium, phosphorus and uric acid clearances after intravenous administration of chlorothiazide. *Metab., Clin. Exp.* **14,** 211–219.

Duarte, C.G., and Watson, J.F. (1967). Calcium reabsorption in proximal tubule of the dog nephron. *Am. J. Physiol.* **212,** 1355–1360.

Dubb, J.W., Goldberg, M., and Agus, Z.S. (1977). Tubular effects of acute metabolic acidosis in the rat. *J. Lab. Clin. Med.* **90,** 318.

Dunning, M.F., and Plum, F. (1957). Hypercalciuria following poliomyelitis. *Arch. Intern. Med.* **99,** 716–731.

Edwards, B.R., Baer, P.G., Sutton, R.A.L., and Dirks, J.H. (1973). Micropuncture study of diuretic effects on sodium and calcium reabsorption in the dog nephron. *J. Clin. Invest.* **52,** 2418–2427.

Edwards, B.R., Sutton, R.A.L., and Dirks, J.H. (1974). Effect of calcium infusion on renal tubular reabsorption in the dog. *Am. J. Physiol.* **227,** 13–18.

Edwards, N.A., and Hodgkinson, A. (1965). Studies of renal function in patients with idiopathic hypercalciuria. *Clin. Sci.* **29,** 327–338.

Eisenberg, E. (1970). Effects of serum calcium level and parathyroid extracts on phosphate and calcium excretion in hypoparathyroid patients. *J. Clin. Invest.* **44,** 942–946.

Eknoyan, G., Suki, W.N., and Martinez-Maldonado, M. (1970). Effect of diuretics on urinary excretion of phosphate, calcium and magnesium in thyroparathyroidectomized dogs. *Clin. Med.* **76,** 257–266.

Eknoyan, G., Dichosis, C., Martinez-Maldonado, M., and Suki, W.N. (1972). On the mechanism of renal wasting of calcium in idiopathic hypercalciuria. *Clin. Res.* **20,** 592.

Emerson, K., and Beckman, W.W. (1945). Calcium metabolism in children with nephrosis. I. A description of an abnormality in calcium metabolism in children with nephrosis. *J. Clin. Invest.* **24,** 504–572.

Epstein, F.H. (1968). Calcium and the kidney. *Am. J. Med.* **45,** 700–714.

Farquharson, R.F., Salter, W.T., Tibbets, D.M., and Aub, J.C. (1931). Studies on calcium and phosphorus metabolism. XIII. The effect of the ingestion of phosphorus on the excretion of calcium. *J. Clin. Invest.* **10,** 221–249.

Finn, W.F., Cerilli, G.J., and Ferris, T.F. (1970). Transplantation of a kidney from a patient with idiopathic hypercalciuria. *N. Engl. J. Med.* **283,** 1450–1454.

Fischer, F., and Hastrup, B. (1954). Cortisone and calcium balance (effect of calcium, vitamin D and methylandrostenediol). *Acta Endocrinol. (Copenhagen)* **16,** 141–148.

Frick, A., Rumrick, G., Ulrich, K.J., and Lassiter, W.E. (1965). Microperfusion study of calcium transport in the proximal tubule of the rat kidney. *Pfluegers Arch. Gesamte Physiol. Menschen Tiere* **286,** 109–117.

Friis, T., Hahnemann, S., and Weeke, E. (1968). Serum calcium and serum phosphorus in uremia during administration of sodium phytate and aluminum hydroxide. *Acta Med. Scand.* **183,** 497–505.

Fromter, E., and Gersner, K. (1974). Free flow potential profile along rat kidney proximal tubule. *Pfluegers Arch.* **351,** 69–83.

Garty, J., Nito, H., and Massry, S.G. (1973). The role of the kidney in the control of serum calcium. *Clin. Res.* **21,** 688.

Gill, J.R., Jr., Bell, N.H., and Bartter, F.C. (1967). Effect of parathyroid extract on magnesium excretion in man. *J. Appl. Physiol.* **22,** 136–138.

Givens, M.H., and Mendel, L.B. (1917). Studies in calcium and magnesium metabolism. I. The effects of base and acid. *J. Biol. Chem.* **31,** 421–433.

Gold, L.W., Massry, S.G., Rothman, C.M., and Coburn, J.W. (1973). Effect of phosphate depletion on renal handling of calcium and sodium. *Clin. Res.* **21,** 282.

Goldberg, M., Agus, Z.S., and Goldfarb, A. (1976). Renal handling of phosphate, calcium and magnesium. *In* "The Kidney" (B.M. Brenner and F.C. Rector, Jr., eds.), Vol. 1, pp. 334–390. Saunders, Philadelphia, Pennsylvania.

Goldfarb, S., Westby, G.R., Goldberg, M., and Agus, Z.S. (1977). Renal tubular effects of chronic phosphate depletion. *J. Clin. Invest.* **59,** 770–779.

Goldsmith, R.S., Woodhouse, C.F., Ingbar, S.J., and Segal, D. (1967). The effect of phosphate supplements in patients with fracture. *Lancet* **1,** 687–690.

Goldstein, D.A., Yoshitaka, O., Kiyoshi, K., and Massry, S.G. (1977). Blood levels of 25-hydroxyvitamin D in patients with nephrotic syndrome. *Ann. Intern. Med.* **87,** 664–667.

Gonda, A., Wong, N., Seely, J.F., and Dirks, J.H. (1969). The role of hemodynamic factors on urinary calcium and magnesium excretion. *Can. J. Physiol. Pharmacol.* **47,** 619–626.

Grabie, M., Lau, K., Agus, Z.S., Goldberg, M., and Goldfarb, S. (1978). Role of parathyroid hormone in the hypercalciuria of chronic phosphate depletion. *Miner. Electrolyte Metab.* **1,** 279–287.

Gray, R.W., Wilz, D.R., Caldas, A.E., and Lemann, J., Jr. (1977). The importance of phosphate in regulating plasma 1,25$(OH)_2$-vitamin D levels in humans: Studies in healthy subjects, in calcium stone formers and in patients with primary hyperparathyroidism. *J. Clin. Endocrinol. Metab.* **45,** 299–306.

Gray, S.P., Morris, J.E.W., and Brooks, C.F. (1973). Renal handling of calcium, magnesium, inorganic phosphate and hydrogen ions during prolonged exposure to elevated carbon diozide concentration. *Clin. Sci. Mol. Med.* **45,** 751–764.

Greenwald, I. (1945). The effect of phosphate on the solubility of calcium carbonate and of bicarbonate on the solubility of calcium and magnesium phosphate. *J. Biol. Chem.* **161,** 697–704.

Greenwald, I., Redish, J., and Kibrick, A.C. (1940). Dissociation of calcium and magnesium phosphates. *J. Biol. Chem.* **135,** 65–76.

Griffith, D.P. (1971). Immobilization hypercalciuria: Treatment and the possible pathophysiologic mechanisms. *Aerosp. Med.* **42,** 1322–1324.

Gutmann, Y., and Gottschalk, C.Y. (1966). Micropuncture study of the effect of calcium on sodium transport in the rat kidney. *Isr. J. Med. Sci.* **2,** 243–245.

Harris, C.A., Baer, P.G., Cherito, E., and Dirks, J.H. (1974). Composition of mammalian glomerular filtrate. *Am. J. Physiol.* **227,** 972–976.

Harris, C.A., Burnatowska, M., Sutton, R.A.L., and Dirks, J.H. (1976). Evidence for parathyroid hormone (PTH) enhancement of calcium and magnesium reabsorption in the terminal nephron segment of the hamster. *Clin. Res.* **24,** 410 A.

Harrison, A.R. (1959). Some results of metabolic investigations in cases of renal stone. *Br. J. Urol.* **31,** 398–403.

Heaton, F.W. (1969). The kidney and magnesium homeostasis. *Ann. N. Y. Acad. Sci.* **16,** 775–785.

Heaton, F.W., and Hodgkinson, A. (1963). External factors affecting diurnal variations in electrolyte excretion with particular reference to calcium and magnesium. *Clin. Chim. Acta* **8,** 246–254.

Heaton, F.W., and Parsons, F.M. (1961). The metabolic effect of high magnesium intake. *Clin. Sci.* **21,** 273–284.

Hebert, L.A., Lemann, J., Petersen, J.R., and Lennon, E.J. (1966). Studies of the mechanism by which phosphate infusion lowers serum calcium concentration. *J. Clin. Invest.* **45,** 1886–1894.

Henneman, P.H., Benedict, D.H., Forbes, A.P., and Dudley, H.R. (1958). Idiopathic hypercalcemia. *N. Engl. J. Med.* **259,** 802–807.

Higgins, B.A., Massim, J.R., Collins, J., and Hilb, A. (1964). The effect of bendrofluazide on urine calcium excretion. *Clin. Sci.* **27,** 457–462.

Hodgkinson, A., and Pyrah, L.N. (1958). The urinary excretion of calcium and inorganic phosphate in 344 patients with calcium stone of renal orogin. *Br. J. Surg.* **46,** 10–18.

Howard, P.J., Wilde, W.S., and Malvin, R.L. (1959). Localization of renal calcium transport. Effect of calcium load and of gluconate anion on water and potassium. *Am. J. Physiol.* **197,** 337–341.

Howards, S.S., Davis, B.B., Knox, F.G., Wright, F.S., and Berliner, R.W. (1968). Depression of fractional sodium reabsorption by the proximal tubule of the dog without sodium diuresis. *J. Clin. Invest.* **47,** 1561–1572.

Hulley, S.B., Goldsmith, R.S., and Ingbar, S.H. (1969). Effect of renal arterial and systemic infusion of phosphate on urinary calcium excretion. *Am. J. Physiol.* **217,** 1570–1571.

Ikkos, D., Lufft, R., and Geinzell, C.A. (1959). The effect of human growth hormone in man. *Acta Endocrinol. (Copenhagen)* **32,** 341–361.

Imai, M. (1978). Calcium transport across the rabbit thick ascending limb of Henle's loop perfused in vitro. *Pfluegers Arch.* **374,** 255–263.

Jahan, I., and Pitts, R.F. (1948). Effect of parathyroid on renal tubular reabsorption of phosphate and calcium. *Am. J. Physiol.* **155,** 42–49.

Jamison, R.L., Frey, N.R., and Lacy, F.B. (1974). Calcium reabsorption in the thin loop of Henle. *Am. J. Physiol.* **227,** 745–751.

Jones, J.H., Peters, D.K., Morgan, D.B., Coles, G.A., and Mallick, N.P. (1967). Observations on calcium metabolism in the nephrotic syndrome. *Q. J. Med.* **36,** 301–302.

Jorgensen, F.S. (1971). The effect of bendroflumethiazide (Centyl) on the renal excretion of calcium and aosium in normal, parathyroidectomized, thyroidectomized and thyroparathyroidectomized rats. *Acta Pharmacol. Toxicol.* **30,** 296–307.

Kalbfleisch, J.M., Lindeman, R.D., Ginn, H.E., and Smith, W.O. (1963). Effects of ethanol administration on urinary excretion of magnesium and other electrolytes in alcoholic and normal subjects. *J. Clin. Invest.* **42,** 1471–1475.

Kaplan, R.A., Haussler, M.R., Deftos, L.J., Bone, J., and Pak, C.Y.C. (1977). The role of 1-alpha, 25-dihydroxy vitamin D in the mediation of intestinal hyperabsorption of calcium in primary hyperparathyroidism and absorptive hypercalcemia. *J. Clin. Invest.* **59,** 756–760.

Kattus, A.A., Sinclair-Smith, B., Genest, J., and Newman, E.V. (1949). The effect of exercise on the renal mechanism of electrolyte excretion in normal subjects. *Bull. Johns Hopkins Hosp.* **84,** 344–368.

Kleeman, C.R., Tuttle, S., and Basset, S.H. (1958). Metabolic observations in a case of thyrotoxicosis with hypercalciuria. *J. Clin. Endocrinol. Metab.* **18,** 477–491.

Kleeman, C.R., Bernstein, D., Rockney, R., Dowling, J.T., and Maxwell, M.H. (1961). Studies on the renal clearance of diffusible calcium and the role of the parathyroid glands on its regulation. *Yale J. Biol. Med.* **34,** 1–30.

Kleeman, C.R., Bohannan, J., Bernstein, D., Ling, S., and Maxwell, M.H. (1964). Effect of variations in sodium intake on calcium excretion in normal humans. *Proc. Soc. Exp. Biol. Med.* **115,** 29–32.

Knapp, E.L. (1947). Factors influencing the urinary excretion of calcium in normal subjects. *J. Clin. Invest.* **26,** 182–202.

Krane, S.M., Brownell, G.L., Stanbury, J.B., and Corrigan, H. (1956). The effect of thyroid disease on calcium metabolism in man. *J. Clin. Invest.* **35,** 874–877.

Kreusser, W.J., Kurokawa, K., Aznar, E., Massry, S.G. (1978). Phosphate depletion: Effect on renal inorganic phosphorus and adenine nucleotide, urinary phosphate and calcium, and calcium balance. *Miner. Electrolyte Metab.* **1,** 30–42.

Kuntziger, H., Amiel, C., Roinel, N., and Morel, F. (1974). Effects of parathyroidectomy and cyclic AMP on renal transport of phosphate, calcium, and magnesium. *Am. J. Physiol.***227,** 905–911.

Kupfer, S., and Kosovsky, J.D. (1965). Effects of cardiac glycosides on renal tubular transport of calcium, magnesium, inorganic phosphate and glucose in the dog. *J. Clin. Invest.* **44,** 1132–1143.

Kurokawa, K., Nagata, N., Sasaki, M., and Nakaue, K. (1974). Effect of calcitonin on the concentration of adenosine 3′,5′-cyclic monophosphate in rat kidney in vivo and in vitro. *Endocrinology* **94,** 1514–1518.

Laake, H. (1960). The action of corticosteroid on the renal reabsorption of calcium. *Acta Endocrinol. (Copenhagen)* **34,** 60–64.

Lamberg, B.A., and Kuhlback, B. (1959). Effect of chlorothiazide and hydrochlorothiazide on the excretion of calcium in urine. *Scand. J. Clin. Lab. Invest.* **11,** 351–357.

Lassiter, W.F., Gottschalk, C.W., and Mylle, M. (1963). Micropuncture study of renal tubular reabsorption of calcium in normal rodents. *Am. J. Physiol.* **204,** 771–775.

Lavan, J.N. (1969). The effect of oral ammonium chloride on the urinary excretion of calcium, magnesium and sodium in man. *Ir. J. Med. Sci.* 223–227.

Lechene, C., Abraham, E., and Warner, R. (1975). Effect of sulfate loading on ionic distribution along the rat nephron. *Clin. Res.* **23,** 432A.

LeGrimellec, C. (1975). Micropuncture study along the proximal convoluted tubule: Electrolyte absorption in first convolutions. *Pfluegers Arch.* **354,** 133–150.

LeGrimellec, C., Roinel, N., and Morel, F. (1973). Simultaneous Mg, Ca, P, K, Na and Cl analysis in rat tubular fluid. I. During perfusion of either inulin of ferrocyanide. *Pfluegers Arch.* **340,** 181–196.

LeGrimellec, C., Roinel, N., and Morel, F. (1974). Simultaneous Mg, Ca, P, K and Cl analysis in rat tubular fluid. IV. During acute Ca plasma loading. *Pfluegers Arch.* **346,** 189–204.

LeGrimellec, C., Poujeol, P., and DeRouffignac, C. (1975). H^3 inulin and electrolyte concentrations in Bowman's capsule in rat kidney. Comparison with artificial ultrafiltration. *Pfluegers Arch.* **354,** 117–131.

Lemann, J., Jr., Litzow, J.R., and Lennon, E.J. (1967). Studies of the mechanism by which chronic metabolic acidosis augments urinary calcium excretion in man. *J. Clin. Invest.* **45,** 1318–1328.

Lemann, J., Jr., Piering, W.F., and Lennon, E.J. (1969). Possible role of carbohydrate induced calciuria in calcium oxalate stone formation. *N. Engl. J. Med.* **280,** 232–237.

Lemann, J., Jr., Piering, W.F., and Lennon, E.J. (1970a). Studies of the acute effects of aldosterone and cortisol on the interrelationship between renal sodium, calcium and magnesium excretion in normal man. *Nephron* **7,** 117–130.

Lemann, J., Jr., Lennon, E.J., Piering, W.F., Prier, E.L., Jr., and Ricanati, E.S. (1970b). Evidence that glucose ingestion inhibits net tubular reabsorption of calcium and magnesium in man. *J. Lab. Clin. Med.* **75,** 578–585.

Lennon, E.J., and Piering, W.F. (1970). A comparison of the effects of glucose ingestion and NH_4Cl acidosis on urinary calcium and magnesium excretion in man. *J. Clin. Invest.* **49,** 1458–1465.

Liberman, U.A., Sperling, O., Atsmon, A., Frank, M., Modan, M., and deVries, A. (1968). Metabolic and calcium kinetic studies in idiopathic hypercalciuria. *J. Clin. Invest.* **47,** 2580–2590.

Lichtwitz, A., and Parlier, R. (1965). Calcium et maladies metaboliques de l'os. III. *In* "Rein et Metabolism du Calcium a l'Etat Pathologique." Expansion Scientifique Francaise, Paris.

Lindeman, R.D., Ginn, H.E., Kalbfleisch, J.M., and Smith, W.O. (1964). Effect of galactose on urinary electrolyte excretion in man. *Proc. Soc. Exp. Biol. Med.* **115,** 264–267.

Lindeman, R.D., Adler, S., Yungst, M.J., and Beard, E.S. (1967). Influence of various nutrients on urinary divalent cation excretion. *J. Lab. Clin. Med.* **70,** 236–245.

Litvak, J., Moldawer, M.P., Forbes, A.P., and Henneman, P.H. (1958). Hypocalcemic hypercalciuria during vitamin D and dihydrotachysterol therapy. *J. Clin. Endocrinol. Metab.* **18,** 246–252.

Llach, F., Massry, S.G., Singer, F.R., Kurokawa, K., Kaye, J.H., and Coburn, J.W. (1975). Skeletal resistance to endogenous parathyroid hormone in patients with early renal failure: A possible cause for secondary hyperparathyroidism. *J. Clin. Endocrinol. Metab.* **41,** 339–345.

Lotz, V.M., Zisman, E., and Bartter, F.C. (1968). Evidence for a phosphorusdepletion syndrome in man. *N. Engl. J. Med.* **278,** 409–415.

Loutit, J.F. (1965). Diurnal variation in urinary excretion of calcium and strontrium. *Proc. R. Soc. London, Ser. B* **162,** 458–472.

Lutwak, L., Whedon, G.D., Lachance, P.A., Reid, J.M., and Lipscomb, H.S. (1969). Mineral electrolyte and nitrogen balance studies of the Gemini-VII fourteen-day orbital space flight. *J. Clin. Endocrinol. Metab.* **29,** 1140–1156.

MacFaden, I.J., Nordin, B.E.C., Smith, D.A., Wayne, D.J., and Rae, S.L. (1965). Effect of variation in dietary calcium on plasma calcium and urinary excretion of calcium. *Br. Med. J.* **1,** 161–164.

McIntosh, H.W., and Seraglia, M. (1963). Effect of acetazolamide and triple sulfonamide on citrate and calcium excretion. *Can. Med. Assoc. J.* **89,** 1332–1333.

McLaughlin, F., Fairney, A., Lester, E., Raggatt, R.R., Brown, D.J., and Witts, M.R. (1974). Seasonal variations in serum 25-hydroxycholecalciferol in healthy people. *Lancet* **1,** 536–538.

Malm, O.J. (1963). Adaptation to alterations in calcium intake. *In* "Transfer of Calcium and Strontium across Biologic Membranes" (R.H. Wasserman, ed.). Academic Press, New York.

Margen, S., and Calloway, D.H. (1967). Effect of dietary protein on urinary calcium. *Fed. Proc., Fed. Am. Soc. Exp. Biol.* **26,** 629.

Marone, C.C., and Sutton, R.A.L. (1980). Effects of furosemide on calcium and sodium excretion during acute metabolic acidosis and alkalosis in the rat. *Miner. Electrolyte Metab.* **4,** 62–67.

Marone, C.C., Wong, N.L.M., Sutton, R.A.L., and Dirks, J.H. (1978). Renal calcium handling in chronic metabolic acidosis and alkalosis in the conscious dog. *Clin. Res.* **26,** 470A.

Martin, H.E., and Jones, R. (1961). The effect of NH_4Cl and $NaHCO_3$ on the urinary excretion of Mg, Ca and phosphate. *Am. Heart J.* **62,** 206–210.

Marx, S.J., Woodard, C.J., and Aurback, G.D. (1972). Calcitonin receptors of kidney and bone. *Science* **178,** 999–1000.

Massry, S.G., Coburn, J.W., Chapman, L.W., and Kleeman, C.R. (1967a). The acute effect of adrenal steroids on the interrelationship between the renal excretion of sodium, calcium and magnesium. *J. Lab. Clin. Med.* **70,** 563–570.

Massry, S.G., Coburn, J.W., Chapman, L.W., and Kleeman, C.R. (1967b). Effect of NaCl infusion on urinary Ca^{++} and Mg^{++} during reduction in their filtered load. *Am. J. Physiol.* **213,** 1218–1224.

Massry, S.G., Popovtzer, M.M., Chapman, L.W., and Kleeman, C.R. (1968a). Effect of potassium infusion and intravenous diamox on the interdependence between the renal handling of sodium, calcium and magnesium. *Clin. Res.* **16,** 391.

Massry, S.G., Coburn, J.W., Chapman, L.W., and Kleeman, C.R. (1968b). Role of serum Ca, parathyroid hormone, and NaCl infusion on renal Ca and Na clearances. *Am. J. Physiol.* **214,** 1403–1409.

Massry, S.G., Mueller, E., Silverman, A.G., and Kleeman, C.R. (1968c). Inorganic phosphate treatment of hypercalcemia. *Arch. Intern. Med.* **121,** 307–312.

Massry, S.G., Coburn, J.W., and Kleeman, C.R. (1970a). Evidence for suppression of parathyroid gland by hypermagnesemia. *J. Clin. Invest.* **49,** 1619–1629.

Massry, S.G., Ahumada, J.J., Coburn, J.W., and Kleeman, C.R. (1970b). Effect of $MgCl_2$ infusion on urinary Ca and Na during reduction in their filtered loads. *Am. J. Physiol.* **219,** 881–885.

Massry, S.G., and Ahumada, J.J. (1972). Renal vasodilatation. Studies on the site of action in the nephron. *Clin. Sci.* **42,** 535–543.

Massry, S.G., and Coburn, J.W. (1973). The hormonal and non-hormonal control of renal excretion of calcium and magnesium. *Nephron* **10,** 66–112.

Massry, S.G., and Kleeman, C.R. (1972). Calcium and magnesium excretion during acute rise in glomerular filtration rate. *J. Lab. Clin. Med.* **80,** 654–664.

Massry, S.G., Coburn, J.W., Lee, D.B.N., Jowsey, J., and Kleeman, C.R. (1973). Skeletal resistance to parathyroid hormone in renal failure: Study on 105 human subjects. *Ann. Intern. Med.* **78,** 357–364.

Massry, S.G., Arieff, A.I., Coburn, J.W., Palmieri, G.B., and Kleeman, C.R. (1974). Divalent ion metabolism in patients with acute renal failure: Studies on the mechanism of hypocalcemia. *Kidney Int.* **5,** 437–445.

Melick, R.A., and Henneman, P.H. (1958). Clinical and laboratory studies of 207 consecutive patients in a kidney stone clinic. *N. Engl. J. Med.* **259,** 307–314.

Melvin, K.E.W., and Tashjian, A.H., Jr. (1968). The syndrome of excessive thyrocalcitonin produced by medullary carcinoma of the thyroid. *Proc. Natl. Acad. Sci. U.S.A.* **59,** 1216–1222.

Meyer, W.A., Brautbar, N., Montcalm, A., and Massry, S.G. (1979). Effects of thiazides on urinary and serum calcium during phosphate depletion. *Proc. Am. Soc. Nephrol.* **12,** 37A.

Modlin, M. (1966). The interrelation of urinary calcium and sodium in normal adults. *Invest. Urol.* **4,** 180–189.

Molinatti, G.M., Camanni, F., and Olivett, M. (1960). A study on the metabolism of calcium in the hyperadrenocortical syndrome. *Acta Endocrinol. (Copenhagen)* **34,** 323–334.

Moore, P.F. (1968). The effects of diazoxide and henzothiazide diuretics upon phosphodiesterase. *Ann. N.Y. Acad. Sci.* **150,** 256–260.

Murayama, Y., Morel, F., and LeGrimellec, C. (1972). Phosphate, calcium and magnesium transfer in proximal tubules and loops of Henle, as measured by single nephron microperfusion experiments in the rat. *Pfluegers Arch.* **333,** 1–16.

Ney, R.L., Kelly, G., and Bartter, F.C. (1968). Actions of vitamin D independent of the parathyroid glands. *Endocrinology* **82,** 760–766.

Nordin, B.E.C., and Peacock, M. (1969). Role of the kidney in regulation of plasma calcium. *Lancet* **2,** 1280–1283.

Nordin, B.E.C., and Smith, D.A. (1965). "Diagnostic Procedures in Disorders of Calcium Metabolism," pp. 27–34. Churchill, London.

Nordin, B.E.C., Hodgkinson, A., and Peacock, M. (1967). The measurement and the meaning of urinary calcium. *Clin. Orthop. Relat. Res.* **52,** 293–322.

Nordin, B.E.C., Peacock, M., and Wilkinson, R. (1972). The relative importance of gut, bone, and kidney in the regulation of serum calcium. *In* "Calcium, Parathyroid Hormone and the Calcitonins" (R.V. Talmage and D.L. Munson, eds.), p. 263. Excerpta Medica, Amsterdam.

Nseir, N.I., Szramowski, J., and Puschett, J.B. (1978). Mechanism of renal tubular effects of 25 hydroxy and 1,25-dihydroxyvitamin D in the absence of parathyroid hormone. *Miner. Electrolyte Metab.* **1,** 48–56.

Paillard, F., Ardaillou, R., Malendin, H., Fillastre, J.P., and Prier, S. (1972). Renal effects of salmon calcitonin in man. *J. Lab. Clin. Med.* **80,** 200–216.

Pak, C.Y.C., Ruskin, B., and Casper, A. (1970). Renal effects of porcine thyrocalcitonin in the dog. *Endocrinology* **87,** 262–270.

Pak, C.Y.C., East, D.A., Sanzenbacher, L.J., Delea, C.S., and Bartter, F.C. (1972). Gastrointestinal calcium absorption in nephrolithiasis. *J. Clin. Endocrinol. Metab.* **35,** 261–270.

Pak, C.Y.C., Delea, C.S., and Bartter, F.C. (1974a). Successful treatment of recurrent nephrolithiasis (calcium stones) with cellulose phosphate. *N. Engl. J. Med.* **290,** 175–180.

Pak, C.Y.C., Okata, M., Lawrence, F.C., and Snyder, W. (1974b). The hypercalciurias: Causes, parathyroid function and diagnostic criteria. *J. Clin. Invest.* **54,** 387–400.

Pak, C.Y.C., Kaplan, R., Bone, H:., Townsend, J., and Waters, O. (1975). A simple test for the diagnosis of absorptive, resorptive and renal hypercalciuria. *N. Engl. J. Med.* **292,** 497–500.

Parfitt, A.M. (1969). The acute effects of mersalyl, chlorothiazide and mannitol on the renal excretion of calcium and other ions in man. *Clin. Sci.* **36,** 267–282.

Parfitt, A.M. (1972). The interactions of thiazide diuretics with parathyroid hormone and vitamin D. Studies in patients with hypoparathyroidism. *J. Clin. Invest.* **51,** 1879–1888.

Parfitt, A.M., Higgins, B.A., Nassum, J.R., Collins, J.A., and Hilb, A. (1964). Metabolic studies in patients with hypercalciuria. *Clin. Sci.* **27,** 463–473.

Peacock, M., and Nordin, B.E.C. (1968). Tubular reabsorption of calcium in normal and hypercalciuric subjects. *J. Clin. Pathol.* **21,** 353–358.

Peacock, M., Hodgkinson, A., and Nordin, B.E.C. (1967). Importance of dietary calcium in the definition of hypercalciuria. *Br. Med. J.* **3,** 469–471.

Pechet, M.M., Bowers, B., and Bartter, F. (1959). Metabolic studies with a new series of 1,4-diene steroids. II. Effects on normal subjects prednisone, prednisolone and 9-α-fluoroprednisolone. *J. Clin. Invest.* **38,** 691–701.

Pechet, M.M., Bobadilla, E., Caroll, E.L., and Hesse, R.H. (1967). Regulation of bone resorption and bone formation. Influences of thyrocalcitonin, parathyroid hormone, neutral phosphate and vitamin D_3. *Am. J. Med.* **43,** 696–710.

Phang, I.M., Kales, A.N., and Hahn, T.J. (1968). Effect of divided calcium intake on urinary calcium excretion. *Lancet* **2,** 84–85.

Popovtzer, M.M., Massry, S.G., Coburn, J.W., and Kleeman, C.R. (1969). The interrelationship between sodium, calcium and magnesium excretion in advanced renal failure. *J. Lab. Clin. Med.* **73,** 763–771.

Popovtzer, M.M., Schainuck, L.I., Massry, S.G., and Kleeman, C.R. (1970). Divalent ion excretion in chronic kidney disease. Relation to degree of renal insufficiency. *Clin. Sci.* **38,** 297–307.

Porter, R.H., Cox, B.G., Heaney, D., Hostetter, T.H., Stinebaugh, P.J., and Suki, W.N. (1978). Treatment of hypoparathyroid patients with chlorothalidone. *N. Engl. J. Med.* **298,** 577–581.

Pullman, T.N., Lavender, A.R., Aho, I., and Rasmussen, H. (1960). Direct renal action of a purified parathyroid extract. *Endocrinology* **67,** 570–582.

Puschett, J.B., Moranz, J., and Kurnick, W.S. (1972). Evidence for a direct action of cholecalciferol and 25-hydroxycholecalciferol on the renal transport of phosphate, sodium and calcium. *J. Clin. Invest.* **51,** 373–385.

Quamme, G.A., and Dirks, J.H. (1978). Effects of magnesium (Mg) on calcium (Ca) and Mg transport in the rat. A microperfusion study. *Proc. Int. Congr. Nephrol., 7th, 1978,* p. E12.

Quamme, G.A., Wong, N.L.M., Sutton, R.A.L., and Dirks, J.H. (1975). Interrelationship of chlorothiazide and parathyroid hormone. A micropuncture study. *Am. J. Physiol.* **229,** 200–205.

Quamme, G.A., O'Callaghan, T., Wong, N.L.M., Sutton, R.A.L., and Dirks, J.H. (1976). Hypercalciuria in the phosphate depleted dog. A micropuncture study. *Proc. Am. Soc. Nephrol.* **9,** 6.

Rasmussen, H., Anast, C., and Arnaud, C. (1967). Thyrocalcitonin, EGTA, and urinary electrolyte excretion. *J. Clin. Invest.* **46,** 746–752.

Reidenberg, M.D., Haag, B.L., Channick, B.J., Shuman, C.R., and Wilson, T.G.G. (1966). The response of bone to metabolic acidosis in man. *Metab., Clin. Exp.* **15,** 236–241.

Reidenberg, M.M., Levy, R.W., and Cucinotta, A.J. (1968). Hypercalciuria during acidosis in hypoparathyroidism. *Proc. Soc. Exp. Biol. Med.* **127,** 1–3.

Rizzoli, R., Fleisch, H., and Bonjour, J.P. (1977). Effect of thyroparathyroidectomy on calcium metabolism in the rat. Role of 1,25-dihydroxyvitamin D_3. *Am. J. Physiol.* **223,** E160–E164.

Robertson, W.G., and Morgan D.B. (1972). The distribution of urinary calcium excretion in normal persons and stone formers. *Clin. Chim. Acta* **37,** 503–508.

Robertson, W.G., Gallagher, J.C., Marshal, D.H., Peacock, M., and Nordin, B.E.C. (1974). Seasonal variation in urinary excretion of calcium. *Br. Med. J.* **4,** 436–437.

Rocha, A.S., and Kokko, J.P. (1973). Sodium, chloride and water transport in medullary thick ascending limb of Henle. Evidence for active chloride transport. *J. Clin. Invest.* **52,** 612–623.

Rocha, A.S., Magaldi, J.B., and Kokko, J.P. (1977). Calcium and phosphate transport in isolated segment of rabbit Henle's loop. *J. Clin. Invest.* **59,** 975–984.

Rouse, D., and Suki, W.N. (1978). Calcium transport in the superficial straight proximal tubule (SPR). *Clin. Res.* **27,** 430A.

Samiy, A.H.E., Brown, J.L., Globus, D.L., Kessler, R.H., and Thompson, D.D. (1960). Interrelation between renal transport system of magnesium and calcium. *Am. J. Physiol.* **198,** 559–602.

Scriver, W. de M. (1928). Observations on the excretion of calcium ion in two cases of nephrosis treated with parathyroid extract. *J. Clin. Invest.* **6,** 115–125.

Seely, J.H., and Dirks, J.H. (1969). Micropuncture and diuretics. *Annu. Rev. Pharmacol.* **9,** 73–84.

Seldin, D.W., Eknoyan, G., Suki, W.N., and Rector, F.C., Jr. (1966). Localization of diuretic action from the pattern of water and electrolyte excretion. *Ann. N.Y. Acad. Sci.* **139,** 328–343.

Senft, G., Munske, K., Schultz, G., and Hoffman, M. (1968). Der Einfluss von Hydrochlorothiazide und anderen sulfonamidierten Diuretica auf die 3′-5′ AMP-phosphodiesterase-Activität in der Rattenniere. *Arch. Pharmal. Exp. Pathol.* **259,** 344–359.

Shareghi, G.R., and Agus, Z.S. (1979). PTH sensitive magnesium transport in the rabbit cortical thick ascending limb of Henle (CTAL). *Proc. Am. Soc. Nephrol.* **12,** 67A.

Shareghi, G.R., and Stoner, L.C. (1978). Calcium transport across segment of the rabbit distal nephron in vitro. *Am. J. Physiol.* **235,** F367.

Shen, F.H., Baylink, D.J., Nielson, R.L., Sherrard, J.J., Ivey, J.L., and Haussler, M.R. (1977). Increased serum 1,25-dihydroxyvitamin D in idiopathic hypercalciuria. *J. Lab. Clin. Med.* **90,** 955–962.

Sherwood, L.M., Potts, J.T., Jr., Care, A.D., Mayer, G.P., and Aurbach, G.D. (1966). Evaluation by radioimmunoassay of factors controlling the secretion of parathyroid hormone. *Nature (London)* **209,** 52–57.

Shohl, A.T., and Sato, A. (1923). Acid-base metabolism. II. Mineral metabolism. *J. Biol. Chem.* **58,** 257–266.

Sigaard-Anderson, O. (1962). Acute experimental acid-base disturbances in dogs. *Scand. J. Clin. Lab. Invest.* **66,** Suppl., 1–20.

Singer, F.R., Woodhouse, N.J.Y., Parkinson, D.K., and Joplin, G.F. (1969). Some acute effects of administered procine calcitonin in man. *Clin. Sci.* **37,** 181–190.

Sotornik, I., Schuck, O., and Stribrna, J. (1969). Influence of diuretics on renal calcium excretion. *Experientia* **25,** 591–592.

Stein, J.H., Rector, F.C., Jr., and Seldin, D.W. (1968). The effect of acute metabolic acidosis on proximal tubular sodium reabsorption in the rat. *Clin. Res.* **16,** 65.

Stein, J.H., Osgood, R.W., Boonjarern, S., and Ferris, T.F. (1973).

Stoerk, H.C., and Carnes, W.H. (1945). The relation of the dietary Ca: P ratio to serum calcium and to parathyroid volume. *J. Nutr.* **29,** 43–50.

Suki, W.N. (1979a). Effects of diuretics on calcium metabolism. *Miner. Electrolyte Metab.* **2,** 125–129.

Suki, W.N. (1979b). Calcium transport in the pars recta and the loop of Henle. *In* "Health and Disease" (S.G. Massry, E. Ritz, and H. Jahn, eds.), Plenum, New York (in press).

Suki, W.N. (1980). Hypercalciuria: Diagnosis and management. *Contrib. Nephrol.* (in press).

Suki, W.N., and Rouse, D. (1979). Heterogenicity of calcium transport in medullary and cortical segments of the thick ascending limb of Henle. *Proc. Am. Soc. Nephrol.* **12,** 70A.

Suki, W.N., Schwettmann, R.S., Rector, F.C., Jr., and Seldin, D.W. (1968). Effect of chronic mineralocorticoid administration on calcium excretion in the rat. *Am. J. Physiol.* **215,** 71–74.

Suki, W.N., Eknoyan, G., Rector, F.C., Jr., and Seldin, D.W. (1969). The renal diluting and concentrating mechanisms in hypercalcemia. *Nephron* **6,** 50–61.

Sutton, R.A.L., and Dirks, J.H. (1977). Renal handling of calcium: Overview. *In* "Phosphate Metabolism" (S.G. Massry and E. Ritz, eds.), pp. 15–27. Plenum, New York.

Sutton, R.A.L., and Dirks, J.H. (1978). Renal handling of calcium. *Fed. Proc., Fed. Am. Soc. Exp. Biol.* **37,** 2112–2119.

Sutton, R.A.L., Edwards, B.R., Wong, N.L.M., Baer, P.G., and Dirks, J.H. (1972). Thiazide diuretics: Differential effect on distal tubule calcium and sodium transport. *J. Clin. Invest.* **51,** 94a.

Sutton, R.A.L., Wong, N.L.M., and Dirks, J.H. (1975a). 25 hydroxy vitamin D ($25OHD_3$): Enhancement of distal tubular calcium reabsorption in the dog. *Proc. Am. Soc. Nephrol.* **8,** 8.

Sutton, R.A.L., Wong, N.L.M., and Dirks, J.H. (1975b). The hypercalciuria of metabolic acidosis. A specific impairment of distal calcium reabsorption. *Clin. Res.* **23,** 434A.

Sutton, R.A.L., Wong, N.L.M., and Dirks, J.H. (1976). Effects of parathyroid hormone on sodium and calcium transport in the dog nephron. *Clin. Sci. Mol. Med.* **51,** 345.

Sutton, R.A.L., Wong, N.L.M., and Dirks, J.H. (1979). Effects of metabolic acidosis and alkalosis on sodium and calcium transport in the dog kidney. *Kidney Int.* **15,** 520–533.

Talmage, R.V., and Kraintz, F.W. (1954). Progressive changes in renal phosphate and calcium excretion in rats following parathyroidectomy or parathyroid administration. *Proc. Soc. Exp. Biol. Med.* **87,** 263–267.

Thomas, W.C., and Miller, G.H. Jr. (1967). Inorganic phosphates in the treatment of renal calculi. Mod. Treat. 4, 494–504.

Thompson, R.B., Kaufman, C.E., and DeScala, V.A. (1971). Effect of renal vasodilatation on divalent ion excretion and Trn PAH in anesthetized dogs. *Am. J.Physiol.* **221,** 1097–1104.

Toor, M., Massry, S.G., Katz, A.I., and Agmon, J. (1965). Diurnal variations in the composition of blood urine of man living in hot climates. *Nephron* **2,** 334–354.

Transbol, R., Hornum, I., Hahnemann, S., Hauser, E., Ohlenschlaeger, H. Diemer, H., and Lockwood, K. (1970). Tubular reabsorption of calcium in the differential diagnosis of hypercalcemia. *Acta Med. Scand.* **188,** 505–522.

Ullrich, K.J., Rumrick, G., and Kloss, S. (1976). Acute Ca^{2+} reabsorption in the proximal tubule of the rat kidney. *Pfluegers Arch.* **364,** 223–228.

Walser, M. (1961a). Calcium clearance as a function of sodium clearance in the dog. *Am. J. Physiol.* **200,** 1099–1104.

Walser, M. (1961b). Ion association. VII. Dependence of calciuresis on natriuresis during sulfate infusion. *Am. J. Physiol.* **201,** 773–796.

Walser, M. (1971). Calcium-sodium interdependence in renal transport. *In* "Renal Pharmacology" (J.W. Fisher and E.J. Cafruny, eds.), pp. 21–43. Appleton, New York.

Walser, M., and Trounce, J.R. (1961b). Effects of diuresis and diuretics upon the renal tubular transport of aklaline earth cations. *Biochem. Pharmacol.* **8,** 157.

Wesson, L.G., Jr. (1962). Magnesium, calcium and phosphate excretion during osmotic diuresis in the dog. *J. Lab. Clin. Med.* **60,** 422–433.

Wesson, L.G., Jr. (1964). Electrolyte excretion in relation to diurnal cycles of renal function. Plasma electrolyte concentration and aldosterone secretion before and salt and water balance changes in normotensive subjects. *Medicine (Baltimore)* **43,** 547–592.

Whedon, G.D. (1959). Effects of high calcium intake on bones, blood and soft tissues; relation of calcium intake to balance in osteoporosis. *Fed. Proc., Fed. Am. Soc. Exp. Biol.* **18,** 1112–1118.

Widrow, S.H., and Levinsky, N.G. (1962). The effect of parathyroid extract on renal tubular calcium reabsorption in the dog. *J. Clin. Invest.* **41,** 2151–2159.

Wiley, F.H., Wiley, L.L., and Walter, D.S. (1933). The effects of ingestion of sodium, potassium, and ammonium chloride and sodium bicarbonate on the metabolism of inorganic salt and water. *J. Biol. Chem.* **101,** 83–92.

Williamson, B.J., and Freeman, S. (1957). Effect of acute changes in acid-base balance on renal calcium excretion in dogs. *Am. J. Physiol.* **191,** 384–387.

Wong, N.L.M., Quamme, G.A., Sutton, R.A.L., and Dirks, J.H. (1978). The effects of mannitol on divalent ion transport in the kidney. *Proc. Int. Congr. Nephrol., 7th, 1978* p. E12.

Yendt, E.R., Gagne, R.J.A., and Cohanim, M. (1966). The effects of thiazides in idiopathic hypercalciuria. *Am. J. Med. Sci.* **251,** 449–460.

Yendt, E.R., Guay, G.F., and Garcia, D.A. (1970). The use of thiazides in the prevention of renal calculi. *Can. Med. Assoc. J.* **102,** 614–620.

Young, V.F., Lofgreen, G.P., and Luick, J.R. (1966). The effect of phosphorus depletion and of calcium and phosphorus intake on the endogenous excretion of these elements by sheep. *Br. J. Nutr.* **20,** 795–805.

Zucker, T.F. (1921). The relation of acid base equilibrium in the body to relation of phosphorus and calcium. *Proc. Soc. Exp. Biol. Med.* **18,** 272–275.

5

Collagen Biosynthesis and Degradation

MARVIN L. TANZER

I. INTRODUCTION*

Interest in connective tissue research has expanded exponentially in the past 25 years as illustrated by the publication of numerous symposia, monographs, review journals, and special articles. This chapter will attempt to provide the broad framework and important benchmarks of a burgeoning field without imposing the details of the specialist upon the reader.

*This review was completed in August, 1978.

Disorders of Mineral Metabolism, Vol. II

ISBN 0-12-135302-8

Collagen provides an extracellular framework for multicellular animals in which a scaffolding of fibers has the basic form of an organ and provides tissue tensile strength. Collagen apparently evolved when multicellular animals developed; the protein has not been identified in unicellular animals. The collagenous architecture occurs in many forms such as reticulin, tendon, dermis, capsules, ligaments, basement membranes, cartilage, cornea, vitreous humor, bone, tooth, and intervertebral discs. Nature has tailored the connective tissues in higher animals to fulfill specific functions by integrating in collagen other components such as mineral, elastin, mucopolysaccharides, water, and glycoproteins. Thus, a tendon, which is mostly collagenous in composition, has high tensile strength approaching that of fine steel wire, whereas hyaline cartilage, which contains an equal mixture of collagen and mucopolysaccharides, is quite resistant to compressive forces. The versatility of collagen is exemplified by the fact that it is common to all of the connective tissues and is the most abundant protein in vertebrates, comprising 25–30% of the body protein. Most of the collagen is accounted for by bones, skin, and tendons. However, all tissues are supported by a collagenous framework that connects adjacent structures such as skeletal muscle to bone, bone to bone, and parenchymal organ to fascia.

The prominent role of collagen in tissue strength and form has aroused substantial interest in its structure and metabolism as well as its participation in embryological development, an area that has received increasing attention. Detailed knowledge of collagen structure and metabolism has led to new insights into the molecular mechanisms and pathophysiology of diseases that affect connective tissues. These include hereditary disorders and, more recently, acquired diseases that have a prominent fibrotic component.

Comprehensive reviews include a monograph that describes the major connective tissue components in contemporary terms (Mathews, 1975) and another that describes collagen biochemistry in great detail (Ramachandran and Reddi, 1976). Recent reviews have focused upon connective tissue components (Hall, 1963–1976), collagen biosynthesis (Grant and Jackson, 1976), genetically distinct collagens (Miller, 1976), immunology of collagen (Beard *et al.*, 1977), and biochemical defects in connective tissue diseases (Uitto and Lichtenstein, 1976).

II. EVOLUTIONARY AND TISSUE DISTRIBUTION OF COLLAGENS

Collagen may be defined as a protein with a unique conformation which is detected by its wide-angle X-ray diffraction pattern. The specific diffraction pattern is generated by the helical folding of the individual collagen polypeptides into a coil, with three such coils being wrapped in a supercoil (Fig. 1). The resultant cylindrical molecule is packed into a polymeric network that forms

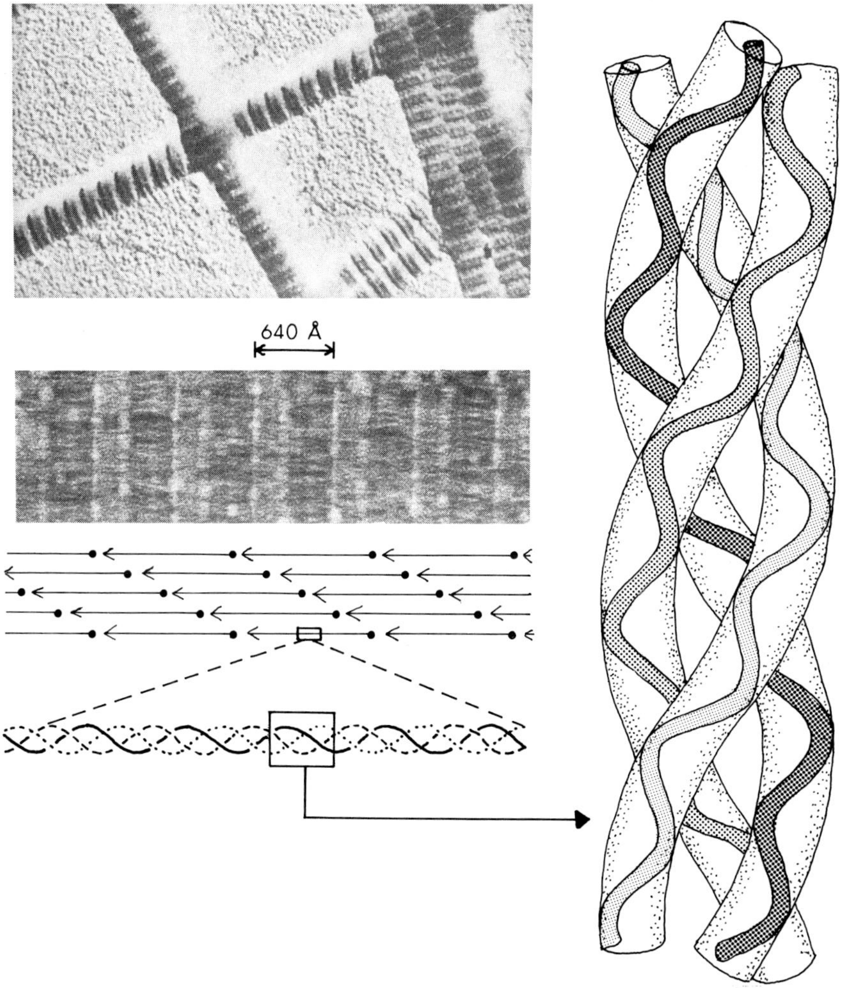

Fig. 1. Levels of organization of collagen. The shadow-cast electron micrograph at upper left illustrates the repetitive 64-nm periodicity. This periodicity and the finer banding are shown in the stained electron micrograph at middle left. Below this micrograph is an interpretation of molecular packing, showing collagen molecules as arrows in the "quarter stagger" packing mode. The triple-helical coiling is shown below and, in more detail on the right. (Adapted from Dickerson and Geis, 1969.)

ropes, cables, filaments, sheets, membranes, and capsules. Although the constituent molecules are structurally similar in all tissues, collagen has genetically distinct polypeptide chains (see below). Glycine comprises one-third of the total amino acid residues in all collagen chains and it occurs at every third locus. Thus, the basic repeat is Gly-x-y, and x and y are often proline and hydroxyproline. These cyclic amino acids allow the individual polypeptide chains to coil into the collagen helix, while hydroxyproline imparts stability to the triple-chain molecular structure (see below). One consequence of the three-chain, coiled-coil structure is that the polypeptides closely approach each other, allowing no internal room for the amino acid side chains, which are located on the exterior of the molecule. This arrangement places all of the side chains in direct contact with the solvent and tissue environment, whereas most proteins have some residues located in "interior" regions due to folding of polypeptide chains. Thus, collagen molecules can be pictured as resembling test tube brushes, with a central core and external bristles. This arrangement allows for maximal interaction between collagen molecules in the fibril as well as between fibrils and other connective tissue constituents.

A major unsolved problem of collagen structure is the manner in which the molecules are arranged in the three-dimensional fibrillar network (Fig. 1). Electron microscopic and low angle X-ray diffraction studies suggest that collagen molecules have a regular lateral alignment, with molecules displaced from one another by about one-fourth of their length (Fig. 1). There is no end-to-end abutment but there seem to be gaps of about 40 nm between the ends. Some other structural feature must be included in the model of collagen fibrillar organization to allow proper packing in three dimensions; such a modification was proposed by Smith (1968) to be a microfibrillar unit of five collagen molecules. This basic unit is thought to be the building block for higher levels of organization. At the present time there are several different models for microfibrillar organization and packing, none of which entirely fits all of the available data (Miller, 1976; Veis and Yuan, 1975). Further refinements of X-ray diffraction and data processing are now being used as well as newer methods of obtaining spatial arrangements, e.g., neutron diffraction.

The structural repeat of the collagen polypeptides Gly-x-y is a linear transcript of the encoded genetic sequences. Subsequent to translational expression of these sequences in nascent chains, several covalent modifications occur intracellularly. Certain proline residues are hydroxylated at position 4 to yield 4-hydroxyproline, and less often, at position 3 to produce the equivalent 3-hydroxyproline. A limited number of lysine residues are hydroxylated on carbon 5, to produce hydroxylysine. These latter hydroxyl groups are the site of further modification, with stepwise addition of galactose to form *O*-galactosylhydroxylysine, followed by glucose to yield the disaccharide. Sequence studies of collagen polypeptides have elucidated the location of these modified amino acids as well as confirming that glycine occurs at every third locus (Fietzek and Kuhn, 1976; Piez, 1976). The data also show that 4-hydroxyproline invariably occurs at the y position while 3-hydroxyproline seems to be restricted to the x position.

The functional role of 4-hydroxyproline has long been a source of puzzlement to collagen chemists. Early work of Gustavson (1955) suggested that this unusual amino acid played a role in stabilizing collagen molecular structure. This concept has now gained wide acceptance because new data indicate that unhydroxylated collagen has a significantly lower denaturation temperature than normal collagen (Berg and Prockop, 1973a; Jiminez *et al.*, 1973). Furthermore, there is a linear relationship between hydroxyproline content and the denaturation temperature. The precise manner by which a hydroxyl group on the proline ring can affect collagen stability is not clear, but several models of hydrogen bonding have been suggested (Ramachandran and Ramakrishnan, 1976). Since 3-hydroxyproline is a minor constituent in most vertebrate collagens, its role is probably minimal in stabilizing molecular structure, but this remains to be determined. The total hydroxyproline content of a specific collagen is fairly constant, although the degree of hydroxylation at a given proline locus may be quite variable (Bornstein, 1967).

The hydroxylysine content of collagens is quite variable and appears to be influenced by different biological factors (Barnes *et al.*, 1974). The modification of hydroxylysine to its aldehyde equivalent (see below) and of lysine to lysine aldehyde is important for the development of covalent cross-links in the collagen polymer. Indirect evidence suggests that the cross-links formed from hydroxylysine may be more stable than those derived from lysine (Eyre and Glimcher, 1973). Whether the glycosylation of hydroxylysine is an important factor in such stability is not known. Since the degree of lysine hydroxylation is quite variable, glycosylation is also variable. In addition, the extent of mono- and disaccharide formation varies independently of hydroxylysine content (Pinnell *et al.*, 1971). The functional role of these sugars in the collagen molecule is not known, although their location has been established in some collagen polypeptides that have been sequenced (Aguilar *et al.*, 1973). Since the sugars are relatively bulky, they may be important in affecting the mode of collagen polymerization (Morgan *et al.*, 1970).

The foregoing discussion has focused only on that portion of the collagen molecule which has the definitive collagen sequence, Gly-x-y, necessary to develop the collagen conformation. However, collagen molecules, as isolated from the polymeric tissue structures, have variable lengths of polypeptides extending beyond the typical collagen sequence. These extensions, originally called telopeptides (Schmitt, 1964), occur at both NH_2- and COOH-termini (Fietzek and Kuhn, 1976; Piez, 1976) and their length varies with the source of collagen as well as with the degree of adventitious proteolysis that occurs during collagen isolation (Rauterberg, 1973). Approximately 10–25 amino acids are present in noncollagen sequences, which cannot assume the collagen helical coil. These extensions are antigenically more potent than the collagen sequence (Timpl, 1976; Beard *et al.*, 1977) and are the major site of the aldehydes derived from lysine or hydroxylysine residues although the extension peptides are not collagenous. They are generated from the longer extensions of procollagen that are edited by processing enzymes (Grant and Jackson, 1976). It has been shown that procollagen may not be efficiently edited in some tissues, producing a population of molecules which contain extension peptides of varying lengths (Veis *et al.*, 1972).

A. Variations in the Molecular Nature of Collagenous Proteins

As discussed above, collagen conformation is unique, arising from its primary structural repeat of Gly-x-y. Since collagen is universally distributed throughout multicellular animals, various lengths of the basic molecular structure may exist. There appear to exist no theoretical constraints on minimal or maximal length for the molecules to assume the collagen conformation. Indeed, studies of synthetic collagen-like polypeptides have shown that these polypeptides adopt the triple-helical structure, although the chains are much shorter than collagen α-chains (Bhatnager and Rapaka, 1976). Most collagens from vertebrate and invertebrate animals are similar in molecular size. Notable exceptions occur among the cuticle collagens of invertebrates (Tanzer, 1978), which appear to have both the shortest and longest molecular forms (5.2×10^3 and 1.5×10^6 daltons, respectively). In contrast, most collagens are 3×10^5 daltons, although there is some variation depending upon the particular genetic type (see below). Recently, nonfibrous proteins have been shown to contain regions of collagenous primary structure and, in one case, indirect evidence suggests that the triple-helical conformation has been adopted. This protein, the C1q component of circulating complement, has been completely characterized in terms of molecular structure (Porter, 1977). The model (Fig. 2) shows substantial regions of collagen structure, alternating with noncollagen regions. The function of such collagenous

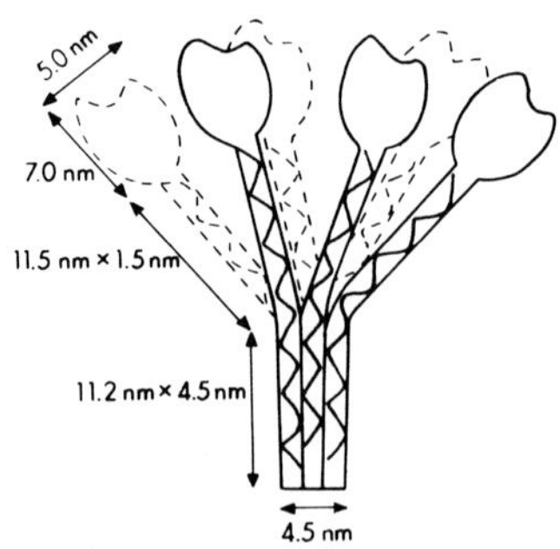

Fig. 2. The postulated model of molecular architecture of human complement subcomponent, Clq. Note that each of the six components contains three polypeptides, with eighteen polypeptides per molecule. The stalks of each component are mostly collagenous and believed to be organized in the collagen triple-helix. This triple-helix begins after a short noncollagen region at the base of the stalk and joins a long, globular region at the tip of the stalk. (Adapted from Reid and Porter, 1976.)

regions in a large, circulating protein may be a specific binding region for other complement components.

Another example, less well documented, of collagenous structure in a noncollagen protein, is of certain acetylcholinesterases (Silman, 1976). These enzymes, found in the membranes of the electric organ of electric fish, are large molecules that appear to have intramembranous and extramembranous domains (Lwebuga-Mukase *et al.*, 1976). The intramembranous portion contains a substantial amount of collagen-like protein, as defined by amino acid composition and susceptibility to highly purified bacterial collagenase. This enzyme probe is highly specific and has detected collagenous proteins in the salivary gland (Oppenheim *et al.*, 1971). The recognition that collagen structure can be an integral part of nonfibrous proteins opens a novel aspect of the role of collagen and may uncover other biological functions for such a unique protein conformation.

B. Genetic Isotypes of Collagen

Four different types of collagen that differ in their subunit composition have been identified in higher animals. Type I collagen, the best characterized, has the subunit composition $[\alpha 1(\text{I})]_2\ \alpha 2$. The molecular nomenclature indicates there are two identical $\alpha 1(\text{I})$ subunits and one dissimilar $\alpha 2$ subunit. This latter chain is unique to type I collagen and also distinguishes it from the other genetic types which contain only identical subunits. Type I collagen is widely distributed in skin, bone, tendon, and ligaments from which it can be partially extracted by nondenaturing solvents. Most structural information about collagen was obtained from type I because until recently it was the only known collagen. The discovery of type II collagen (Miller and Matukas, 1969) immediately raised the question concerning the number of potential collagen isotypes.

Type II collagen has the molecular structure $[\alpha 1(\text{II})]_3$; it has been isolated primarily from cartilagenous tissues (Miller, 1976). Since the subunit $\alpha 1(\text{II})$ more closely resembles $\alpha 1(\text{I})$ than $\alpha 2$ it was given a designation that indicates this similarity. Type II collagen has been extracted from cartilage by inhibiting covalent crosslinking or by using proteases such as pepsin that partially cleave the cross-linked noncollagen regions (Miller, 1971a). The isolated collagen can be purified by differential salt precipitation and ion-exchange chromatography (Miller, 1971b). Type II differs from type I collagen in its large content of hydroxylysine and glycosylated hydroxylysine (Miller, 1972). The most compelling evidence to indicate that the $\alpha 1(\text{II})$ subunit is genetically distinct comes from cleavage of the polypeptide at its methionine residues with the reagent CNBr. A linear peptide map of the cleaved pieces, relating them to the original chain, shows the map to contain unique cleavage sites, compared to the $\alpha 1(\text{I})$ and $\alpha 2$ subunits (Miller, 1976). Although some methionines are at identical loci in both $\alpha 1(\text{I})$ and $\alpha 1(\text{II})$ chains, other loci are quite different. Moreover, the amino acid sequences of fragments from identical regions of both $\alpha 1$ chains show there are differences at many positions.

Although type II collagen predominates in cartilagenous tissues, the biological role of this specificity is as yet unclear. The fibers of type II collagen are often narrow (10–20 nm) and often do not show a clear pattern of cross-striations (Bonucci, 1971). Similarly, narrow fibers seem to predominate when type II collagen is reconstituted *in vitro* and hence are likely to be intrinsic to this collagen (Stark *et al.*, 1972). Since type II collagen has a high content of glycosylated hydroxylysines, this carbohydrate may affect the extent of polymerization, but data in support of this notion are not convincing (Spiro, 1969).

Type III collagen is found in skin, aorta, and uterine leiomyoma and has been detected in other tissues in small amounts (Epstein, 1974; Chung and Miller, 1974). Similar to type II collagen, type III contains three identical subunits and is called $[\alpha 1(III)]_3$. Type III collagen usually contains more hydroxyproline and glycine than types I and II. In addition it differs qualitatively from the other two types in that it contains cysteine, an amino acid not previously believed to be present in collagen (Miller, 1976). Type III collagen can be obtained from tissues with the aid of nondenaturing extractants. Limited cleavage with pepsin yields much greater amounts of type III than by means of extraction (Epstein, 1974; Chung and Miller, 1974). Fractionation of type III and type I collagens is readily accomplished by differential salt precipitation or by ion-exchange chromatography (Byers *et al.*, 1974; Timpl *et al.*, 1975). A unique feature of type III collagen is the presence of intramolecular disulfide bridges, joining the three chains (Lenaers and Lapiere, 1975). These cross-links can be severed by disulfide reduction; the cysteine residues (two per chain) are located in the COOH-terminal portion of the subunit, within the terminal 100 residues (Chung *et al.*, 1974). Sequence studies indicate that the cysteines are within the primary structure of collagen (Miller, 1976).

Type III collagen is usually found in tissues that also contain type I collagen, but type III fibers are generally reticular (Gay *et al.*, 1975a). Reticulin often has separate histological locations, distinct from type I in the same tissues (Gay *et al.*, 1975b). The genesis of narrow diameter fibers from type III collagen cannot be due to carbohydrate excess, as postulated for type II. The specific biologic functions of type III collagen are obscure; its reticular network may allow for resilience and elasticity but no physical measurements have been reported to support this speculation.

Type IV collagen has been isolated from certain basement membranes (Kefalides, 1971) but has not been as completely characterized as the other collagen types. Partly this is because it is difficult to obtain enough purified basement membranes from lens capsules or renal glomeruli to yield the requisite amount of pure type IV collagen via limited proteolysis with pepsin. The molecular shorthand for type IV collagen is $[\alpha 1(IV)]_3$. Of the four collagens, type IV contains the highest amounts of 4- and 3-hydroxyproline and of hydroxylysine. The latter is extensively glycosylated, i.e., three or four times more than in type II collagen (Kefalides, 1973). Basement membrane collagen also appears larger than the other types of collagen, with a subunit molecular weight approaching 1.6×10^5 (Minor *et al.*, 1976). At present, there is uncertainty whether basement membranes contain only a single collagen type or whether other α chains also exist (Burgeson *et al.*, 1976). Recent studies suggest that collagenous chains smaller than α subunits may also be present in type IV collagen (Ohno *et al.*, 1975; Chung *et al.*, 1976). Type IV collagen does not seem to form typical striated fibrils *in situ,* as shown by electron microscopy of intact or isolated basement membranes (Pierce, 1970). However, it is possible to demonstrate morphologic structures using partially purified type IV collagen (Olsen *et al.*, 1973b), and some reports indicate that typical striated fibrils can be generated under certain conditions (Carlson *et al.*, 1978).

Other forms of collagen seem to be synthesized under special conditions. Thus, a molecule of $[\alpha 1(I)]_3$ collagen is found in cultures of chondrocytes previously exposed to bromodeoxyuridine, in aging chondrocytes and in collagen-synthesizing sarcomas (Moro and Smith, 1977). Collagen molecules containing new types of subunits have been detected in human placenta and in teratoma cell cultures (Burgeson *et al.*, 1976; Little *et al.*, 1977). It is not known how many different types of collagen subunits exist.

III. GENE EXPRESSION OF PROCOLLAGEN AND ITS POSTTRANSLATIONAL ENZYMES

The four established collagen types have been shown to be synthesized in precursor form, as procollagen molecules (Fig. 3). The best characterized procollagen is type I, which contains a procollagen NH_2-terminal extension approaching 2×10^4 molecular weight and a COOH-terminal extension approaching 3.5×10^4 molecular weight. However, these values are constantly being revised as the apparent size of procollagen increases each year; the protein is quite susceptible to proteolysis, leaving variable lengths of the extension peptides (Martin *et al.*, 1975).

Since at least five different collagen polypeptides exist, the questions of chromosomal localization, gene regulation, and molecular assembly arise. Which chromosomes contain the genetic information for each collagen polypeptide? Information bearing on this point is now available. Cell hybridization studies have shown that human chromosome No. 17 contains the coding information for the $\alpha 1(I)$ and $\alpha 2$ chains of type I collagen (Sundar Raj *et al.*, 1977); type III collagen is encoded on other chromosomes.

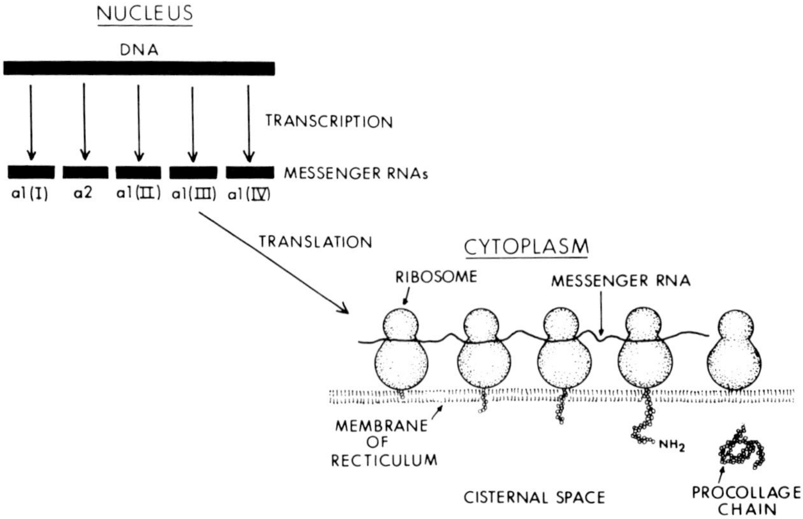

Fig. 3. Hypothetical pathway for procollagen polypeptide biosynthesis in which monocistronic codons are illustrated. The procollagen nascent chains traverse the endoplasmic reticulum where hydroxylation and glycosylation modifications occur.

Many cells in culture express more than one collagen type (Church *et al.*, 1973). Fibroblasts have been shown to produce types I and III collagen, in constant proportion, maintaining the proportion after subculturing (Hance and Crystal, 1977). Use of specific antibodies shows that individual fibroblasts produce these two collagen types (Gay *et al.*, 1976). Similar studies show that individual chondrocytes produce types I and II collagen, with the proportion changing as the culture conditions change (von der Mark and von der Mark, 1977). The mechanisms by which cells regulate collagen expression are obscure, although variables such as cyclic nucleotides and viral transformation do alter the expression (Peterkofsky and Prather, 1974; Hata and Peterkofsky, 1977). If different chromosomes encode for the individual subunits, a complex system of gene expression must exist. Theoretically, a total of 35 different collagen molecules could be assembled from the five known subunits, and it is not known how molecules are correctly assembled.

Similar considerations apply to the enzymes which modify collagen structure. The hydroxylation of procollagen by prolyl and lysyl hydroxylases involves three different enzymes (Prockop *et al.*, 1976) (the 3 and 4 isomers of hydroxyproline arise via different enzymes). Glycosylation of hydroxylysine occurs via galactosyl- and glucosyltransferases (Kivirikko and Risteli, 1976). Recent evidence indicates that the procollagen extensions contain typical glycoprotein oligosaccharides, glucosamine, galactosamine, and mannose (Clark and Kefalides,

1976). These presumably arise via step-wise addition of activated intermediates, similar to other glycoproteins (Hughes, 1976). Thus, a series of glycosylating enzymes is required, each of which might be specific for procollagens. Other modifications, which are either extracellular or mediated at the cell surface, include removal of the procollagen extensions and oxidative deamination of lysine and hydroxylysine to yield the cross-link precursor aldehydes. Obviously many enzymes are involved in the posttranslational modifications of procollagen (Fig. 4).

Since some of the enzymes are quite specific for collagen, the question arises whether they are coordinately expressed when a specific collagen gene is activated. Conceivably, one might have procollagen operons which are encoded for procollagen and its specific modification enzymes. There is no evidence supporting such a concept, but one might argue that the marked variation in degree of posttranslational changes is consistent with procollagen-specific isoenzymes. Thus, the variations in hydroxylation, glycosylation, and procollagen processing which occur for each type of collagen could have a tightly controlled regulatory basis.

The need to coordinate a large number of intracellular modifications of procollagen may account for the relatively slow assembly time that has been reported for collagen subunits in surviving organ cultures (Vuust and Piez, 1972); it is not

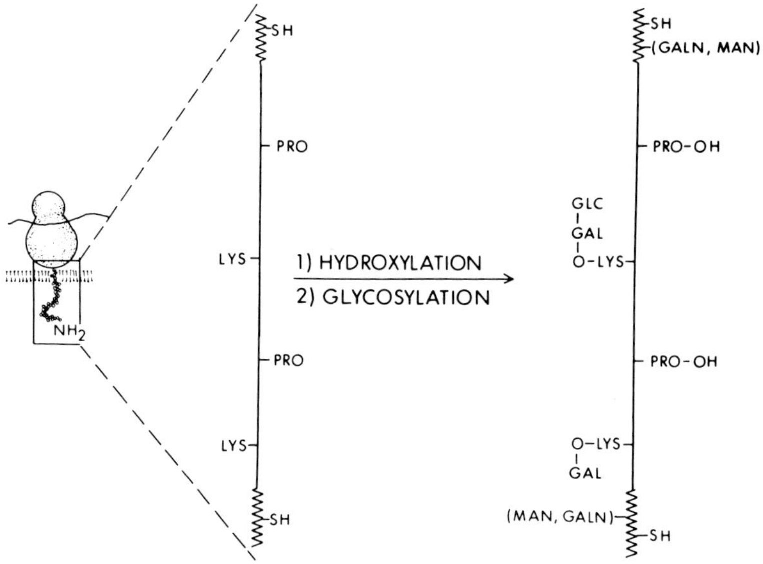

Fig. 4. Modifications of procollagen to form hydroxylated and glycosylated amino acid derivatives. These modifications occur on the nascent chains as they pass through the endoplasmic reticulum shown below the ribosome.

known whether these assembly times also obtain *in vivo*. Prolyl and lysyl hydroxylation, as well as hydroxylysine glycosylation, take place on the growing nascent chain (Brownell and Veis, 1975). This could also contribute to the slow chain growth rate, since hydroxyproline often constitutes 10% of the total residues and hydroxylysine reaches 4% of the total residues in some collagens.

Inasmuch as procollagen appears to move through the cell by the pathway followed by other export proteins, amino sugars and neutral sugars are probably added to the extension peptides en route (Hughes, 1976). These additions therefore would not affect the time of nascent chain growth, but could increase the total transit time through the cell. Interestingly, the transit time is much longer in cultured cartilage cells as compared to cultured fibroblasts (Dehm and Prockop, 1973). Cells of the lens require even longer time periods before secreted procollagen appears in the culture medium (Grant *et al.*, 1972). The reason for this is not clear. One explanation may be that the procollagen must be coiled into triple-helical form before it can be secreted from the cell (Prockop *et al.*, 1976; Grant and Jackson, 1976).

IV. TRANSLATIONAL EXPRESSION OF PROCOLLAGEN

Since the apparent size of procollagen continues to grow with each passing year, one cannot be certain of the size of the primary translation product. Furthermore, very large collagens with subunits approaching 5×10^5 molecular weight are found in some species of animals; such species also contain collagens of "normal" size, with subunits of 1×10^5 molecular weight (Tanzer, 1978). There thus appears to exist no upper limit that restricts the size of collagenous polypeptides. This being the case, an argument can be made for a relationship between (1) collagens of different sizes and (2) between current procollagen structures and those large chains which are collagenous from end to end (Kimura and Tanzer, 1977).

Present evidence indicates there is a separate procollagen mRNA for the proα1 and proα2 chains (Fig. 3) (Rowe *et al.*, 1978). Polyribosome sizes containing presumptive procollagen mRNA support these results (Kerwar *et al.*, 1972).

Radiolabeling studies of procollagen show that the extension peptides contain cysteine, that the COOH-terminal peptides are joined by disulfide linkages and that tryptophan is present only in the COOH-terminal extensions (Tanzer *et al.*, 1974). Amino acid compositions have been reported for NH_2- and COOH-terminal extensions, but there is considerable variability in the data, perhaps reflecting impurities or species differences (Martin *et al.*, 1975). Procollagen containing only NH_2-terminal extensions has been purified from the skins of mutant, dermatosparaxic animals that lack one of the processing enzymes (Hanset and Lapiere, 1974). The sequence of the extension has been determined for the $\alpha1(I)$ chain. Interestingly, this sequence of amino acids contains a short collagen section of 36 amino acids along its length (Becker *et al.*, 1976). This section is not directly contiguous with the main collagen section. Recently the pro-$\alpha2$ extension has also been shown to have a very considerable collagenous section (Becker *et al.*, 1977). Thus, the current model of procollagen structure shows repetitive, alternating regions of collagen and noncollagen sequence. This situation is similar to C1q structure (see Fig. 2), albeit that this molecule only has one collagenous sequence and two noncollagenous sequences.

Speculation concerning the biological roles of the noncollagen regions of procollagen has been widespread. Thus, it has been stated that the noncollagen regions facilitate molecular assembly of nascent chains and helical coiling, assist in intracellular translocation and secretion, prevent intracellular polymerization into fibers, or induce correct alignment of molecules into extracellular fibrils. There is no current experimental evidence to support any of these hypotheses.

The conversion of nascent procollagen to procollagen containing the proper helical conformation has been studied by pulse-chase experiments (Uitto and Prockop, 1974). The experiments were aimed at elucidating the temporal relationships of helical coiling, disulfide bond formation, and hydroxyproline formation. Parallel changes were detected in all three functions, with the hydroxyproline appearing prior to helix formation and disulfide bonding. It was postulated that disulfide bonding in some way facilitated helical coiling once sufficient numbers of hydroxyproline residues were present to impart stability to the coiled collagen (Fig. 5). Although the evidence supporting the stabilizing role of hydroxyproline is convincing (Rosenbloom *et al.*, 1973; Berg and Prockop, 1973a), the studies provide no direct support for the role of disulfide bridges in facilitating procollagen helical conformation.

The hydroxylation of collagen proline and lysine was studied for many years, long before procollagen was recognized in 1971 (see Martin *et al.*, 1975). Understanding the enzymology of these hydroxylations has proceeded slowly, primarily because highly purified enzymes were not available until relatively recently (Berg and Prockop, 1973b). The mechanistic details of the reactions are still in dispute, but the cofactors and cosubstrates have been identified (see Cardinale and Udenfriend, 1974). Molecular oxygen is incorporated into the hydroxyl group, while α-ketoglutarate is converted to succinate and carbon dioxide during each turnover of the enzyme (Rhoads and Udenfriend, 1968). Ferrous ions are a cofactor, as is ascorbic acid, but this latter cofactor can be replaced by other reducing agents and is therefore nonspecific. The hydroxylating enzyme has been purified to homogeneity, is an oligomer of 230,000 molecular weight and consists of two identical protomers (Berg and Prockop, 1973b). Each protomer seems to have nonidentical subunits. On electron microscopy the enzyme appears as an interlocked pair of V-shaped units (Olsen *et al.*, 1973a).

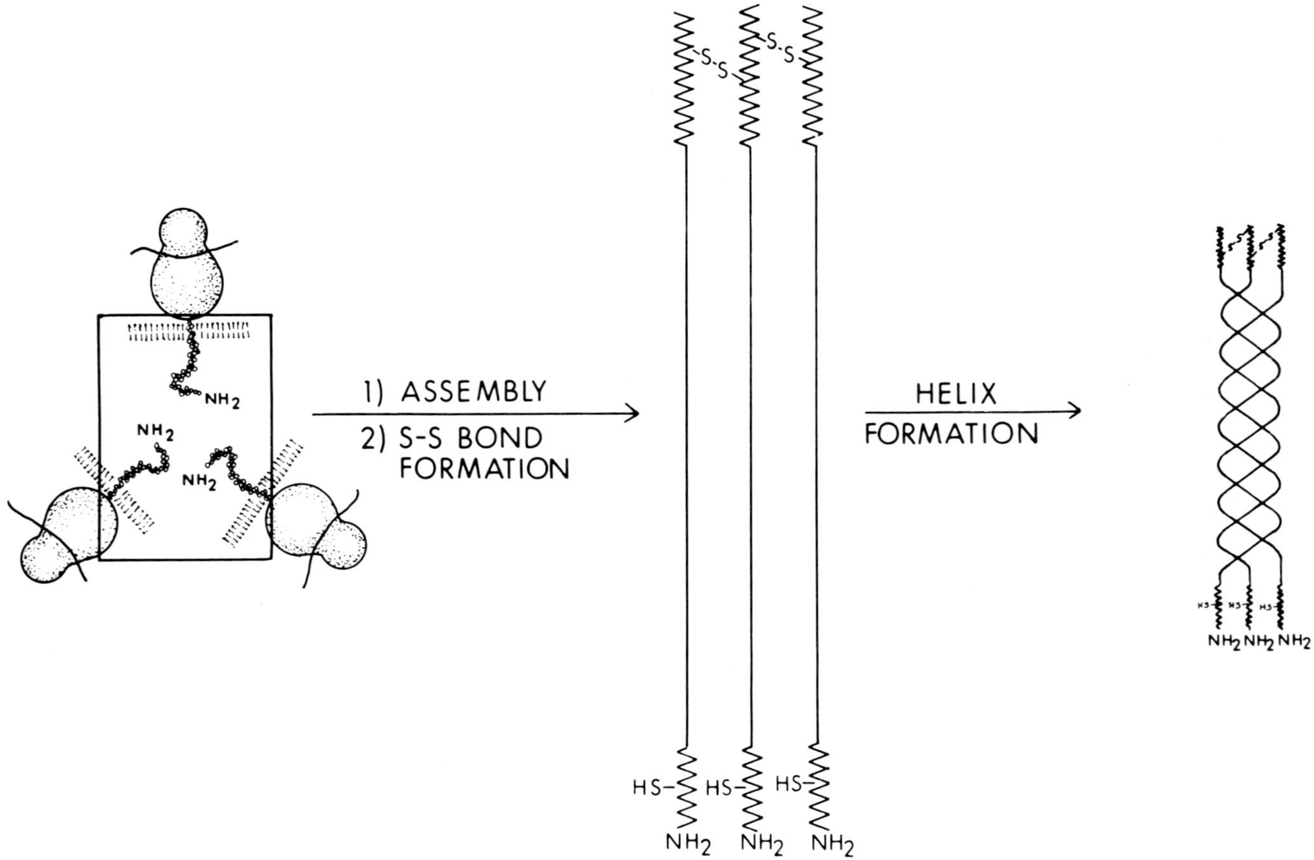

Fig. 5. Hypothetical pathway for procollagen molecule formation. Three nascent chains are shown converging beneath the endoplasmic reticulum to form a procollagen molecule which becomes disulfide-linked and partially helical.

In cell cultures, the enzyme, as detected by immunological methods (Gribble *et al.*, 1969) occurs in an inactive form. The amount of cross-reacting protein remains constant from early culture periods through late stages when enzyme activity appears (McGee *et al.*, 1971). Both lactate and ascorbate will activate the enzyme (Levene *et al.*, 1974; Comstock and Udenfriend, 1970) and ascorbate favors aggregation of the enzyme protomers into active oligomers (Stassen *et al.*, 1973).

The role of hydroxyproline in collagen structure and secretion has also been studied by using proline analogs that do not become hydroxylated. These studies generally indicate that collagens which contain the analogs are secreted at a slower rate than normal (Uitto and Prockop, 1974), appear unstable, and may not adopt the correct conformation. Some of the analogs have no effect on either prolyl hydroxylase activity or on the secretory pathway; rather, it appears that slower secretion is related to either procollagen conformation or to structural instability of the procollagen (Harsh *et al.*, 1972; Uitto *et al.*, 1972).

In summary, most of the evidence from studies using hydroxylation inhibitors or proline analogs indicates that proline hydroxylation in procollagen is necessary for suitable rates of procollagen secretion. Furthermore, hydroxyproline is needed to form a stable, triple-helical procollagen that somehow is "recognized" by the cell and then secreted.

Prolyl hydroxylase is believed to be located in the rough endoplasmic reticulum, as shown by the biochemical analysis of subcellular fractions (Cutroneo *et al.*, 1974). In addition, electron microscope studies with ferritin-labeled antibodies directed against the enzyme showed that the ferritin became deposited within the cisternae of the endoplasmic reticulum (Olsen *et al.*, 1973c). Therefore, the nascent procollagen is thought to be hydroxylated as it enters the cisternal space (Diegelmann *et al.*, 1973) (see Fig. 4).

Lysine hydroxylation is known to be mediated by a specific enzyme, distinct from prolyl hydroxylase (Miller, 1971; Kivirikko and Prockop, 1972). The cofactor and cosubstrate requirements of lysyl hydroxylase are identical to prolyl hydroxylase; this implies that the reaction mechanism may be similar for both enzymes. Lysine hydroxylation differs from proline hydroxylation in that it takes place both in the collagen and the noncollagen sequences (Fietzek and Kuhn, 1976; Piez, 1976); many lysine residues are incompletely hydroxylated (but hydroxylation can be increased by adding the enzyme to a thermally denatured substrate, Kivirikko *et al.*, 1973); there is a decrease of lysine hydroxylation, especially in the noncollagen regions, with age (Barnes *et al.*, 1974). On the other hand, the lysyl hydroxylase like the prolyl hydroxylase is found in the rough endoplasmic reticulum-derived fractions, when subcellular extracts are assayed (Guzman *et al.*, 1976).

Glycosylation of the hydroxyl group of hydroxylysine is highly variable, both with respect to the extent of this modification and the addition of just galactose or both galactose and glucose. Recent efforts have been directed at purifying these glycosyltransferases to homogeneity, following their initial detection and partial characterization (Spiro and Spiro, 1971; Myllylä *et al.*, 1976; Risteli *et al.*, 1976). The partially purified enzymes are specific for hydroxylysine, require a Mn^{2+} cofactor and use the nucleotide-sugar as substrate. Addition of the glucose residue requires prior addition of the galactose to hydroxylysine. Dithiothreitol activates and *p*-mercuribenzoate inhibits the enzymes (Myllylä *et al.*, 1976; Risteli *et al.*, 1976). Since glycosylation has been shown to occur on nascent peptides (Brownell and Veis, 1975), the enzymes are probably located in the endoplasmic reticulum. Thus, at least four modifying enzymes are present in the endoplasmic reticulum in close proximity to procollagen nascent chains (see Fig. 4).

The particular hydroxylysines that become glycosylated are not known in great detail, but sequence work has localized four such sites (Morgan *et al.*, 1970; Aguilar *et al.*, 1973). There is an arginine residue in close proximity to the hydroxylysine in three of these sequences, but no site-specific role of this residue has been shown. The role of collagen conformation in substrate availability is controversial; the more recent data suggest that glucose addition is prevented by the helical collagen structure (Myllylä *et al.*, 1975).

The presence in procollagen of disulfide bonds, though supported only by indirect evidence because sequence studies that show the number and location of the disulfide bridges have not yet been done, is widely accepted. Thus, chromatography or electrophoresis in the presence of disulfide-bond-cleaving reagents converts trimeric to monomeric components (Goldberg *et al.*, 1972), radioactive cysteine is incorporated into procollagen (Fessler *et al.*, 1975) and amino acid analysis of procollagen subunits demonstrates cysteine (Bornstein *et al.*, 1972). Procollagens type I and II clearly fall into the disulfide-bonded precursor status (Miller, 1976). However, since the types III and IV collagens already contain cysteine and disulfides, it is not certain that the procollagen forms have additional cysteines and disulfide links. These proteins may be held *in situ* by intermolecular disulfide bonds and the common use of proteases to liberate the molecules may leave substantial segments of the secreted protein remaining in the extracellular space. As noted above in type III collagen, two cysteine residues have been located near the COOH-terminal region of the α-subunit. In type IV collagen, some evidence suggests the disulfide bridges are near the NH_2-terminus (Kefalides, 1975). In type I procollagen, both NH_2 and COOH extensions contain cysteine, but only the COOH ones are in interchain bridges (Fessler *et al.*, 1975). In type I procollagen isolated from dermatosparaxic animals, the cysteines form intrachain disulfide bonds (Timpl *et al.*, 1973). Detailed analysis of the COOH-terminal extension peptides of type I procollagen has shown them to be linked by disulfide bridges and to be larger than the NH_2-terminal peptides (Fessler *et al.*, 1975). Recent studies suggest the same may be true of type II procollagen (Merry *et al.*, 1976).

Collagen helix formation may not be a prerequisite for disulfide bonding (Schofield *et al.*, 1974). Subcellular fractionation studies suggest that the disulfide bridges appear during translocation of procollagen from ribosome to smooth endoplasmic reticulum, probably in the cisternae of the endoplasmic reticulum (Harwood *et al.*, 1973). Recently, two different approaches have shown that procollagen nascent chains can assume a collagen helical conformation while attached to polyribosomes (Brownell and Veis, 1976, 1977). If this phenomenon occurs during procollagen biosynthesis then disulfide bridges would form after the correct conformation is reached; this would obviate any role of S–S bonds in helix formation. Other studies have shown that normal molecular assembly and secretion of procollagen may require an intact COOH-terminal extension (Rosenbloom *et al.*, 1976). Thus, the interrelationships of helical folding, disulfide bridging, translocation and secretion of procollagen are not resolved and more detailed, incisive studies are needed (Fig. 5).

V. INTRACELLULAR PATHWAY OF PROCOLLAGEN TRANSLOCATION

Proteins destined for export are synthesized by prokaryotic and eukaryotic cells. The latter have a more complex intracellular organization, as they contain nuclei and a highly developed, organized cytoplasm. Consequently, any proteins synthesized in the cytoplasm must traverse a series of membrane-defined regions. The clearest model of translocation and secretion has been elucidated in the case of pancreatic enzymes, although there are differences concerning the details (Palade, 1975; Rothman, 1975). Basically, exported protein moves along defined intracellular structures (Fig. 6) and is then released from the cell surface.

Historically, several routes for procollagen translocation and secretion have been proposed, based largely upon autoradiography of a variety of labeled, collagen-synthesizing tissues and cells (see Veis and Brownell, 1975) from different animal species. It is not surprising, therefore, that the results did not agree. Moreover, many of the cells synthesize and secrete macromolecules other than procollagen and also produce more than one genetic type of procollagen, not necessarily by the same pathway. Recent studies have focused on more specialized cells such as corneal epithelium, odontoblasts, and osteoblasts (Hay and Dodson, 1973; Weinstock and Leblond, 1974). These cells have well-defined cytoplasmic organelles and the odontoblasts, in particular, are attractive because like pancreatic acinar cells they are polarized. Use of autoradiography in these specialized cells has reinforced the microscopic observations and indicates that procollagen translocation and secretion follow the route taken by other exported proteins. Studies with ferritin-labeled antibodies which provide a specific label for the cells (Olsen and Prockop, 1974; Nist *et al.*, 1975) have reinforced these observations.

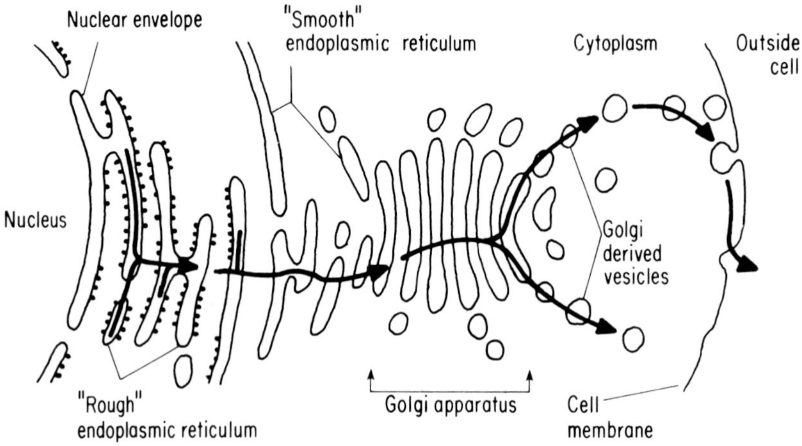

Fig. 6. Hypothetical pathway of procollagen biosynthesis and secretion. The intact procollagen passes through a series of membranous conduits after emerging across the endoplasmic reticulum. Note that it is not necessary for any additional membranes to be crossed in order to be secreted by this pathway. (Adapted from Watson, 1976; copyright 1976, 1970, 1965 by W. A. Benjamin, Inc., Menlo Park, California.)

Subcellular fractionation techniques, modeled on the pancreatic system using inhibitor probes, have been applied to collagen-synthesizing cells (Harwood *et al.,* 1976). At the level of nascent chains, use of puromycin suggests a vectorial discharge into the microsomal lumen (Harwood *et al.,* 1974). Earlier work had shown that most of the collagen polysomes were membrane-associated and sedimented from cellular lysates at low centrifugal forces (Diegelmann *et al.,* 1973). Translocation through subcellular compartments was followed with the aid of pulse-chase experiments done in both tendon and cartilage cells (Harwood *et al.,* 1976). Both types of cells were found to have a similar pathway, i.e., rough to smooth microsomal fractions to the exterior; but the transit times were slower in cartilage cells by about 10 min. The reasons for this difference are not known.

Agents that are known to disrupt microtubules, such as colchicine and vinblastine, interfere with procollagen secretion (see Veis and Brownell, 1975). Agents that interfere with energy metabolism, such as deoxyglucose and uncouplers of oxidative phosphorylation, also affect procollagen secretion (see Grant and Jackson, 1976). Recent use of tunicamycin, an agent thought specifically to prevent amino sugar addition to glycoproteins, has yielded conflicting results on procollagen secretion (Duksin and Bornstein, 1977; Housley *et al.,* 1980). In summary, these various studies are consistent with the proposed pathway of procollagen secretion (Fig. 6) and suggest that microtubules may be important in the process.

VI. EXTRACELLULAR POSTTRANSLATIONAL MODIFICATIONS

Once procollagen reaches the cell surface it undergoes additional modifications, being converted to collagen in some cases (at least for type I) and also serving as substrate for the aldehyde-producing enzyme, lysyl oxidase (Siegel, 1974). In the case of type I procollagen it appears that most of the molecules are processed to remove the extension peptides (Fig. 7). However, since procollagen subunits are found in some abundance in bovine and rat skin (Veis *et al.,* 1972, 1973), the conversion process is not highly efficient. Furthermore, it appears that type IV procollagen is not processed (Minor *et al.,* 1976), nor is it known if type III is processed (Goldberg, 1977) since this collagen is usually obtained subsequent to pepsin digestion of suitable tissues (Epstein, 1974; Chung and Miller, 1974). Type II procollagen does appear to undergo conversion to collagen (Uitto, 1977), although it should be noted that type II collagen has most often been characterized after its release from cartilage by the action of proteases (see Miller, 1976). The end regions of collagen, previously termed telopeptides, have important effects on *in vitro* fibrogenesis (Davison, 1973), but it is not clear how long these regions usually are *in situ* or how important they are in the fibrogenesis of each collagen type.

The cleavage of the extension peptides in type I procollagen has been followed in some model systems (Fessler *et al.,* 1975; Davidson *et al.,* 1975). It appears that the NH_2-terminal extension is removed first, followed by the COOH-

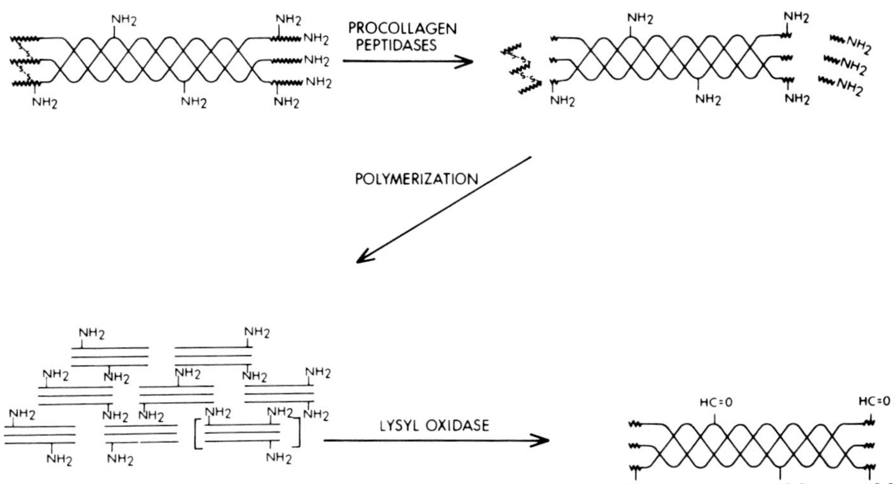

Fig. 7. Extracellular modifications of procollagen to yield cross-linked fibers. A sequential pathway of proteolytic processing, self-assembly into collagen polymers, and enzymatic conversion of limited numbers of ϵ-NH_2 groups into aldehydes is shown.

terminal extension (Fig. 7). Thus, at least two enzymes must be involved. The released COOH-terminal segment has been detected in culture media as a disulfide linked trimer (Sherr *et al.*, 1973). An enzyme, procollagen peptidase, was isolated and characterized (Kohn *et al.*, 1974); it requires calcium as a cofactor and makes a single endopeptidic cleavage between the NH_2-terminal procollagen extension and the type I collagen. The enzyme activity cannot be detected in mutant animals who have dermatosparaxis (Lapiere *et al.*, 1971). A similar protease was detected in other tissues (Bornstein *et al.*, 1972) but has not been characterized. The enzyme appears to be extracellular since it is found in the media of cultured cells (Layman and Ross, 1973). Relatively little is known about processing enzymes for the COOH-terminal region at the present time. The fate of the cleaved extension peptides is not known, although several roles have been proposed, including some type of feedback regulation of collagen biosynthesis.

The enzyme lysyl oxidase has been purified to apparent homogeneity and its mechanism of action has been studied (Fig. 7; Siegel, 1974). It should be noted that standard purification schemes use high concentrations of urea throughout the workup. This may yield a modified enzyme because of cyanate reaction with enzyme NH_2 groups (Stark *et al.*, 1960). Indeed, various "forms" of the enzyme have been reported (Stassen, 1976), as well as several curious kinetic properties, including equal efficiency on quite different substrates such as collagen and elastin (Siegel and Fu, 1976). The enzyme requires Cu^{2+} ion as a cofactor, is irreversibly inhibited by aminonitriles, and appears to be more efficient on reconstituted collagen fibrils than in collagen solutions. The aldehyde oxygen seems to be derived from O_2 rather than H_2O (Siegel *et al.*, 1970) but more definitive evidence is needed on this point. It appears that procollagen can serve as a substrate for lysyl oxidase since dermatosparaxic procollagen does contain aldehydes (Fujii *et al.*, 1976).

VII. FIBRIL FORMATION AND MATURATION

There is a paucity of information about the details of *in vivo* fibrogenesis, primarily because there are so many variables. An *in vitro* model of fibrogenesis, using purified collagen, has been exploited for many years (see Gross, 1974) and the various factors of solvent environment, temperature, and pH have been examined. This model system also has the interesting feature that the reconstituted collagen fibrils undergo progressive insolubility in the test tube, analogous to *in vivo* phenomena (Gross, 1964). One component in the development of such insolubility is the formation of covalent cross-links between adjacent molecules (Tanzer, 1973). These bridges arise from spontaneous condensation of the collagen aldehydes with other collagen amino acids (Fig. 8). Inhibition or blockage of the aldehydes prevents cross-link formation as does lack of correct fibril forma-

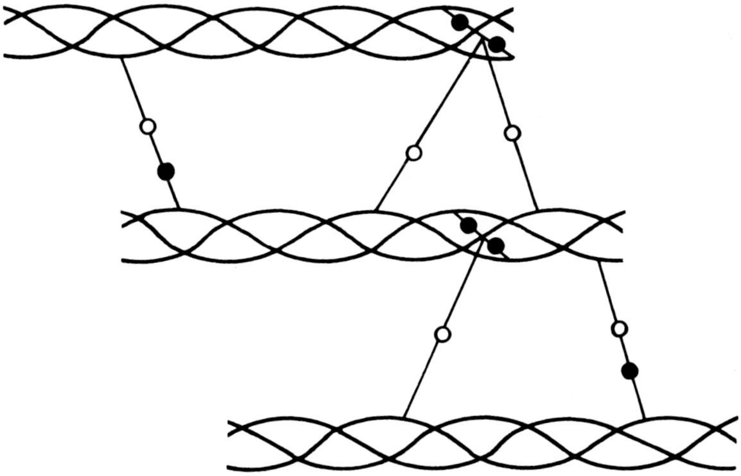

Fig. 8. Details of collagen cross-linking. Three collagen molecules in a quarter-stagger packing arrangement are shown bridged by cross-links of various complexity. The dark circles are aldehydes and the light circles are other amino acid functional groups that have formed cross-links with the aldehydes.

tion. The chemical structures of the cross-links appear to become modified with time (Fujii and Tanzer, 1974) and two such "mature" cross-links have been isolated and characterized (Housley *et al.*, 1975; Fujimoto *et al.*, 1977; Fujimoto and Moriguchi, 1978). No enzymatic mediation seems to be involved in cross-link formation. Recent data on the distribution of cross-links in the fibers support the quarter-stagger model of packing and cross-links have been found that join various regions of adjacent collagen molecules (Stimler and Tanzer, 1976).

The great diversity of architecture of collagenous fibers, from amorphous basement membrane to highly organized, orthogonal arrays such as the cornea, emphasizes the complexity of the protein organization. Most collagen, once deposited in the extracellular space, has a long lifetime, often lasting the life of the animal (Thompson and Ballou, 1956). Active turnover does occur in some tissues, particularly bone, which is being constantly remodeled, at least in young animals (Glimcher, 1976). The age-dependent changes in collagen cross-linking and insolubility may be involved in affecting the rate of turnover but there are no data bearing directly on this point.

VIII. COLLAGEN DEGRADATION

The proteolysis of collagen fibers is effectively carried out by clostridial collagenases which degrade collagen into very small peptides (see Seifter and Harper, 1971). However, the collagenolytic enzymes that normally occur in

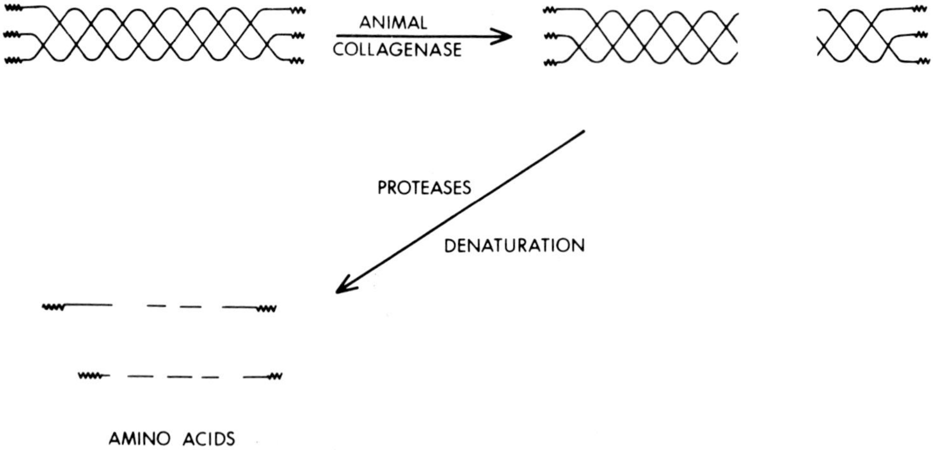

Fig. 9. Hypothetical pathway of collagen degradation. An initial endopeptidic cleavage by animal collagenase is followed by denaturation and proteolysis by other enzymes.

higher animals do not seem to resemble the bacterial counterparts. The collagenases of eukaryotes all seem to have similar specificity, namely they cleave the collagen molecule at about one-fourth the distance internal to the COOH-terminus (Gross, 1974). All three collagen polypeptides are clipped at similar loci, whether initially in fibrils or in solution (McCroskery *et al.,* 1975). Such collagenases have been found to be widely distributed in the tissues of higher animals, have different molecular properties, and arise from various cell types (Harris and Krane, 1974). The collagen substrate influences the rate of digestion in that the different genetic types of collagen have varying susceptibilities to a given collagenase (see Weiss, 1976) and the introduction of chemical cross-links into the collagen polymer alters the rate of digestion at different temperatures (Harris and Farrell, 1972). The reaction products are soluble under conditions that occur *in vivo* and have a lower denaturation temperature than the original substrate (Sakai and Gross, 1967). However, since most substrate molecules are cross-linked in the fibers, it is believed that other proteases, which attack the noncollagen cross-linked telopeptides as well as the denatured products of collagenase digestion, are also important (Fig. 9; Weiss, 1976). Present evidence indicates that the collagenases are present in tissues in a zymogen form which is activated by limited proteolysis (Harper *et al.,* 1971). Collagenase activity is often inhibited by EDTA, sulfhydryl reagents, and serum proteins (Gross, 1976), which may therefore play a regulatory role, but this is conjectural. In summary, the isolation of specific eukaryotic collagenases has markedly advanced our understanding of collagen degradation and will enable future work to focus closely upon regulatory aspects of this phenomenon.

IX. BIOCHEMICAL AND MOLECULAR ASPECTS OF COLLAGEN ALTERATIONS IN DISEASE PROCESSES

The tissue expression of collagen is clearly very complicated, involving multiple genes, post-translational modifications, secretory pathways, polymerization into specific fibrils, followed by time-dependent changes in the fibrils, and finally a degradative pathway. Genetic lesions may affect either single or multiple steps in the pathway, depending upon the arrangment of information in the genome (see above). Several hereditary disorders of connective tissue have been reported to have a molecular basis.

The Ehlers–Danlos syndrome has been divided into seven clinical categories and some of these have been found to contain alterations in collagen expression. Determination of the amino acid composition of aortic tissue of patients with group IV Ehlers–Danlos indicated that these patients have a low collagen content while peptide mapping suggested that type III collagen was deficient (Pope *et al.*, 1975). Skin fibroblasts from such patients, when placed in culture, expressed little type III collagen (Gay *et al.*, 1976).

In osteogenesis imperfecta, fibroblasts from one fetus, when placed in culture, indicated a predominance of type III collagen synthesis, compared to type I (Penttinen *et al.*, 1975). Similar studies, on other patient's tissues, were also reported for a patient with features of both osteogenesis imperfecta and Marfan's syndrome (Müller *et al.*, 1975).

At the posttranslational level, other abnormalities have been detected. In Ehlers–Danlos group VI there is a marked decrease of hydroxylysine in skin collagen and low levels in the collagens of other tissues (Pinnell *et al.*, 1972). Hydroxyproline levels were normal in all tissues and cell culture studies have shown that lysyl hydroxylase activity was 10–14% of normal (Krane *et al.*, 1972). The cross-linking profile of the tissues was abnormal, with deficiency in hydroxylysine-derived cross-links and the appearance of compounds which presumably are lysine-derived cross-links (Eyre and Glimcher, 1972).

In contrast, excess hydroxylysine has been found in a patient with osteogenesis imperfecta (Trelstad *et al.*, 1977). The skin and cartilage collagens contained high levels of hydroxylysine, but no other molecular abnormalities were detected; no alterations in genetic types of collagen were noted in contrast to the studies noted above. Other studies of this disorder suggests a change in content of collagen types (Sykes *et al.*, 1977) and a change in cross-linking toward a more immature state (Fujii and Tanzer, 1977).

Ehlers–Danlos patients of the group V category have been examined and their fibroblasts in culture have diminished levels of lysyl oxidase activity (DiFerrante *et al.*, 1975). Increased solubility of collagen from these cultures was noted.

Studies of collagen from patients with Ehlers–Danlos syndrome, group VII, have shown that there is a prominent amount of procollagen present (Lichtenstein *et al.*, 1973). This is thought to be procollagen with just the NH_2-terminal extensions; the patient's fibroblasts in culture showed a diminished level of procollagen peptidase. The total amount of collagenous proteins produced in culture was greater than normal; this suggests some regulatory disturbance. This disorder may be related to dermatosparaxis, a congenital defect in the conversion of procollagen to collagen which occurs in cattle (Hanset and Ansay, 1967) and sheep (Helle and Ness, 1972). The skin of these animals mostly contains procollagen that has been processed to the point of retaining the NH_2-terminal extension (Lenaers *et al.*, 1971). As noted above, there is no detectable procollagen peptidase in the skin (Lapiere *et al.*, 1971). The collagen fibrils appear normal on lateral section but in cross-section are ribbons rather than cylinders (O'Hara *et al.*, 1970). Reconstituted fibrils have a similar appearance and produce an abnormal cross-linking profile (Bailey and Lapiere, 1973).

Another animal model is that of aneurysm-prone mice, which have defective cross-linking of collagen and elastin (Rowe *et al.*, 1974). Lower levels of lysyl oxidase occur in the connective tissues (Rowe *et al.*, 1977), which would provide a rational basis for impaired crosslinking.

An induced disease of cross-linking, phenotypically similar, is experimental lathyrism (Tanzer, 1965). This disorder is produced by administering aminonitriles which irreversibly inhibit lysyl oxidase (Narayanan *et al.*, 1972). Another phenotypically similar, induced disease is copper deficiency, which, similar to lathyrism, has profound effects on the strength of connective tissues (Carnes, 1968). Copper deficiency impairs the activity of lysyl oxidase which requires Cu^{2+} as a cofactor (Siegel *et al.*, 1970). Menkes kinky hair syndrome, which has widespread clinical features including those affecting connective tissues (Danks *et al.*, 1972), is thought to be due to a genetic defect in copper absorption (Danks *et al.*, 1973). Presumably, lysyl oxidase activity is abnormal in this syndrome. Finally, homocystinuria, a hereditary disorder of the metabolism of sulfur-containing amino acids, is thought to affect connective tissues by binding of homocysteine to the aldehydes which form cross-links (Kang and Trelstad, 1973). However, it appears more likely that an intermediate type of cross-link accumulates that does not progress to maturity (Siegel, 1977).

A number of acquired diseases have been thought to involve collagen metabolism by producing an imbalance in synthetic and degradative rates. Collagen accumulates in scleroderma, cirrhosis, pulmonary fibrosis, hypertrophic scars, and keloids. Indeed, scar production in any tissue is a late response to injury and the fibrotic tissue then interferes with normal parenchymal function. Studies of cultured cells from patients with scleroderma show increased rates of collagen synthesis (LeRoy, 1974), but the mechanisms have not been deciphered. Many investigators are now focusing their attention on collagen metabolism in acquired disorders looking for biochemical changes and underlying mechanisms. Hopefully, rational therapeutic interference might then be designed. This burgeoning area of research is beyond the scope of this review but recent information has been correlated (Kivirikko and Risteli, 1976). The interplay between the advances in collagen biology, chemistry and pathology which has occurred in the past several years may now produce progress in the understanding of acquired diseases.

REFERENCES

Aguilar, J. H., Jacobs, H. G., Butler, W. T., and Cunningham, L. W. (1973). The distribution of carbohydrate groups in rat skin collagen. *J. Biol. Chem.* **248,** 5106–5113.

Bailey, A. J., and Lapiere, C. M. (1973). Effect of an additional peptide extension of the N-terminus of collagen from dermatosparactic calves on the cross-linking of the collagen fibers. *Eur. J. Biochem.* **34,** 91–96.

Barnes, M. J., Constable, B. J., Morton, L. F., and Royce, P. M. (1974). Age related variations in hydroxylation of lysine and proline in collagen. *Biochem. J.* **139,** 461–468.

Beard, H. K., Faulk, W. P., Conochie, L. B., and Glynn, L. E. (1977). Some immunological aspects of collagen. *Prog. Allergy* **22,** 45–106.

Becker, U., Timpl, R., Helle, O., and Prockop, D. J. (1976). NH_2-terminal extensions on skin collagen from sheep with a genetic defect in conversion of procollagen into collagen. *Biochemistry* **15,** 2853–2862.

Becker, U., Helle, O., and Timpl, R. (1977). Characterization of the amino-terminal segment in procollagen pα2 chain from dermatosparactic sheep. *FEBS Lett.* **73,** 197–200.

Berg, R. A., and Prockop, D. J. (1973a). The thermal transition of a non-hydroxylated form of collagen. Evidence for a role for hydroxyproline in stabilizing the triple helix of collagen. *Biochem. Biophys. Res. Commun.* **52,** 115–120.

Berg, R. A., and Prockop, D. J. (1973b). Affinity column purification of protocollagen proline hydroxylase from chick embryos and further characterization of the enzyme. *J. Biol. Chem.* **248,** 1175–1182.

Bhatnagar, R. S., and Rapaka, R. S. (1976). Synthetic polypeptide models of collagen: Synthesis and applications. *In* "Biochemistry of Collagen" (G. N. Ramachandran and A. H. Reddi, eds.), pp. 479–523. Plenum, New York.

Bonucci, E. (1971). The locus of initial calcification in cartilage and bone. *Clin. Orthop. Relat. Res.* **78,** 108–139.

Bornstein, P. (1967). Comparative sequence studies of rat skin and tendon collagen. I. Evidence for incomplete hydroxylation of individual prolyl residues in the normal proteins. *Biochemistry* **6,** 3082–3093.

Bornstein, P., Ehrlich, H. P., and Wyke, A. W. (1972). Procollagen: Conversion of the precursor to collagen by a neutral protease. *Science* **175,** 544–546.

Brownell, A. G., and Veis, A. (1975). Intracellular location of the glycosylation of hydroxylysine of collagen. *Biochem. Biophys. Res. Commun.* **63,** 371–377.

Brownell, A.G., and Veis, A. (1976). Intracellular location of triple helix formation of collagen. Enzyme probe studies. *J. Biol. Chem.* **251,** 7137–7143.

Brownell, A. G., and Veis, A. (1977). Triple-helix formation on ribosome-bound nascent chains of procollagen: Deuterium-hydrogen exchange studies. *Proc. Natl. Acad. Sci. U.S.A.* **74,** 902–905.

Burgeson, R. E., El Adli, F. A., Kaitila, I. I., and Hollister, D. W. (1976). Fetal membrane collagens: Identification of two new collagen alpha chains. *Proc. Natl. Acad. Sci. U.S.A.* **73,** 2579–2583.

Byers, P. H., McKenney, K. H., Lichtenstein, J. R., and Martin, G. R. (1974). Preparation of type III procollagen and collagen from rat skin. *Biochemistry* **13,** 5243–5248.

Cardinale, G., and Udenfriend, S. (1974). Prolyl hydroxylase. *Adv. Enzymol.* **41,** 245–300.

Carlson, E. C., Brendel, K., and Meezan, E. (1978). Striated collagen fibrils derived from ultrastructurally pure isolated basal lamina. *In* "Biology and Chemistry of Basement Membranes" (N. A. Kefalides, ed.), pp. 31–41. Academic Press, New York.

Carnes, W. H. (1968). Copper and connective tissue metabolism. *Int. Rev. Connect. Tissue Res.* **4,** 197–232.

Chung, E., and Miller E. J. (1974). Collagen polymorphism: Characterization of molecules with the chain composition $[\alpha 1(III)]_3$ in human tissues. *Science* **183,** 1200–1201.

Chung, E., Keele, E. M., and Miller, E. J. (1974). Isolation and characterization of the cyanogen bromide peptides from the α1(III) chain of human collagen. *Biochemistry* **13,** 3459–3464.

Chung, E., Rhodes, R. K., and Miller, E. J. (1976). Isolation of three collagenous components of probable basement membrane origin from several tissues. *Biochem. Biophys. Res. Commun.* **71,** 1167–1174.

Church, R. L., Tanzer, M. L., and Lapiere, C. M. (1973). Identification of two distinct species of procollagen synthesized by a clonal line of calf dermatosparactic cells. *Nature (London), New Biol.* **244,** 188–190.

Clark, C. C., and Kefalides, N. A. (1976). Studies on the carbohydrate moieties of procollagen. The incorporation of isotopically-labeled mannose and glucosamine into the pro-peptides of procollagen secreted by matrix-free chick embryo cells. *Proc. Natl. Acad. Sci. U.S.A.* **73,** 34–38.

Comstock, J. P., and Udenfriend, S. (1970). Effect of lactate on collagen proline hydroxylase activity in cultured L-929 fibroblasts. *Proc. Natl. Acad. Sci. U.S.A.* **66,** 552–557.

Cutroneo, K. R., Guzman, N. A., and Sharawy, M. M. (1974). Evidence for a subcellular vesicular site of collagen prolyl hydroxylation. *J. Biol. Chem.* **249,** 5989–5994.

Danks, D. M., Campbell, P. E., Stevens, B. J., Mayne, V., and Cartwright, E. (1972). Menke's kinky-hair syndrome: An inherited defect in copper absorption with widespread effects. *Pediatrics* **50,** 188–201.

Danks, D. M., Cartwright, E., Stevens, B. J., and Townley, R. R. W. (1973). Menke's kinky-hair disease: Further definition of the defect in copper transport. *Science* **179,** 1140–1142.

Davidson, J. M., McEneany, L. S. G., and Bornstein, P. (1975). Intermediates in the limited proteolytic conversion of procollagen to collagen. *Biochemistry* **14,** 5188–5194.

Davison, P. F. (1973). Homeostasis in extra cellular tissues: Insights from studies on collagen. *CRC Crit. Rev. Biochem.* **1,** 201–245.

Dehm, P., and Prockop, D. J. (1973). Biosynthesis of cartilage procollagen. *Eur. J. Biochem.* **35,** 159–166.

Dickerson, R. E., and Geis, I. (1969). "The Structure and Action of Proteins." Harper & Row, New York.

Diegelmann, R. F., Bernstein, L., and Peterkofsky, B. (1973). Cell-free collagen synthesis on membrane-bound polysomes of chick embryo connective tissues and the localization of prolyl hydroxylase on the polysome-membrane complex. *J. Biol. Chem.* **248,** 6514–6521.

DiFerrante, N., Leachman, R. D., Angelini, P., Donnelly, P. V., Francis, G., and Almazan, A. (1975). Lysyl oxidase deficiency in Ehlers-Danlos syndrome type V. *Connect. Tissue Res.* **3,** 49–53.

Duksin, D., and Bornstein, P. (1977). Impaired conversion of procollagen to collagen by fibroblasts and bone treated with tunicamycin, an inhibitor of protein glycosylation. *J. Biol. Chem.* **252,** 955–962.

Epstein, E. H., Jr. (1974). $[\alpha 1(III)]_3$ human skin collagen. Release by pepsin digestion and preponderance in fetal life. *J. Biol. Chem.* **249,** 3225–3231.

Eyre, D. R., and Glimcher, M. J. (1972). Reducible cross-links in hydroxylysine-deficient collagens of a heritable disorder of connective tissue. *Proc. Natl. Acad. Sci. U.S.A.* **69,** 2594–2598.

Eyre, D. R., and Glimcher, M. J. (1973). Analysis of a crosslinked peptide from calf bone collagen: Evidence that hydroxylysyl glycoside participates in the crosslink. *Biochem. Biophys. Res. Commun.* **52,** 663–671.

Fessler, L. I., Morris, N. P., and Fessler, J. H. (1975). Procollagen: Biological scission of amino and carboxyl extension peptides. *Proc. Natl. Acad. Sci. U.S.A.* **72,** 4905–4909.

Fietzek, P. P., and Kuhn, K. (1976). The primary structure of collagen. *Int. Rev. Connect. Tissue Res.* **7,** 1–60.

Fujii, K., and Tanzer, M. L. (1974). Age related changes in the reducible cross-links of human tendon collagen. *FEBS Lett.* **43,** 300–302.

Fujii, K., and Tanzer, M. L. (1977). Osteogenesis imperfecta: Biochemical studies of bone collagen. *Clin. Orthop. Relat. Res.* **124,** 271–277.

Fujii, K., Tanzer, M. L., and Cooke, P. H. (1976). Collagen fibrogenesis and the formation of complex crosslinks. *J. Mol. Biol.* **106,** 223–227.

Fujimoto, D., and Moriguchi, T. (1978). Pyridinoline, a non-reducible crosslink of collagen. Quantitative determination, distribution and isolation of a crosslinked peptide. *J. Biochem. (Tokyo)* **83,** 863–867.

Fujimoto, D., Akiba, K., and Nakamura, N. (1977). Isolation and characterization of a fluorescent material in bovine achilles tendon collagen. *Biochem. Biophys. Res. Commun.* **76,** 1124–1129.

Gay, S., Fietzek, P. P., Remberger, K., Eder, M., and Kuhn, K. (1975a). Liver cirrhosis: Immunofluorescence and biochemical studies demonstrate two types of collagen. *Klin. Wochenschr.* **53,** 205–208.

Gay, S., Balleison, L., Remberger, K., Fietzek, P. P., Adelmann, B. C., and Kuhn, K. (1975b). Immunohistochemical evidence for the presence of collagen type III in human arterial walls, arterial thrombi and in leukocytes incubated with collagen *in vitro*. *Klin. Wochenschr.* **53,** 899–902.

Gay, S., Martin, G. R., Muller, P. K., Timpl, R., and Kuhn, K. (1976). Simultaneous synthesis of types I and III collagen by fibroblasts in culture. *Proc. Natl. Acad. Sci. U.S.A.* **73,** 4037–4040.

Glimcher, M. J. (1976). Composition, structure, and organization of bone and other mineralized tissues and the mechanism of calcification. *In* "Handbook of Physiology," Parathyroid Gland (R. O. Greep and E. B. Astwood, eds.), Sect. 7, Vol. VII, pp. 25–116. Am. Physiol. Soc., Baltimore, Maryland.

Goldberg, B. (1977). Kinetics of processing of type I and type III procollagens in fibroblast cultures. *Proc. Natl. Acad. Sci. U.S.A.* **74,** 3322–3325.

Goldberg, B., Epstein, E. H., Jr., and Sherr, C. J. (1972). Precursors of collagen secreted by cultured human fibroblasts. *Proc. Natl. Acad. Sci. U.S.A.* **69,** 3655–3659.

Grant, M. E., and Jackson, D. S. (1976). The biosynthesis of procollagen. *Essays Biochem.* **12,** 77–113.

Grant, M. E., Kefalides, N. A., and Prockop, D. J. (1972). The biosynthesis of basement membrane collagen in embryonic chick lens. I. Delay between the synthesis of polypeptide chains and the secretion of collagen by matrix-free cells. *J. Biol. Chem.* **247,** 3539–3544.

Gribble, T. J., Comstock, J. P., and Udenfriend, S. (1969). Collagen chain formation and peptidyl proline hydroxylation in monolayer tissue cultures of L-929 fibroblasts. *Arch. Biochem. Biophys.* **129,** 308–316.

Gross, J. (1964). Thermal denaturation of collagen in the dispersed and solid state. *Science* **143,** 960–961.

Gross, J. (1974). Collagen biology: Structure, degradation and disease. *Harvey Lect.* **68,** 351–432.

Gross, J. (1976). Aspects of the animal collagenases. *In* "Biochemistry of Collagen" (G. N. Ramachandran and A. H. Reddi, eds.), pp. 275–375. Plenum, New York.

Gustavson, K. H. (1955). The function of hydroxyproline in collagens. *Nature (London)* **175,** 70–74.

Guzman, N. A., Rojas, F. J., and Cutroneo, K. R. (1976). Collagen lysyl hydroxylation occurs within the cisternae of the rough endoplasmic reticulum. *Arch. Biochem. Biophys.* **172,** 449–454.

Hall, D. A. (1963–1976). "International Review of Connective Tissue Research," Vol. 1–7. Academic Press, New York.

Hance, A. J., and Crystal, R. G. (1977). Rigid control of synthesis of collagen types I and III by cells in culture. *Nature (London)* **268,** 152–154.

Hanset, R., and Ansay, M. (1967). Dermatosparaxie (peau déchirée) chez le veau: Un défaut général du tissu conjonctif, de nature héréditaire. *Ann. Med. Vet.* **7,** 451–470.

Hanset, R., and Lapiere, C. M. (1974). Inheritance of dermatosparaxis in the calf. A genetic defect of connective tissues. *J. Hered.* **65,** 356–358.

Harper, E., Bloch, K., and Gross, J. (1971). The zymogen of tadpole collagenase. *Biochemistry* **10,** 3035–3041.

Harris, E. D., and Farrell, M. E. (1972). Resistance to collagenase: A characteristic of collagen fibrils crosslinked by formaldehyde. *Biochim. Biophys. Acta* **278,** 133–141.

Harris, E. D., and Krane, S. M. (1974). Collagenases. *N. Engl. J. Med.* **291,** 557–563; 605–609; 652–661.

Harsh, M., Murphy, L., and Rosenbloom, J. (1972). Metabolism by isolated fibroblasts of abnormal collagens containing analogues of proline or lysine. *FEBS Lett.* **26,** 48–52.

Harwood, R., Grant, M. E., and Jackson, D. S. (1973). The subcellular location of inter-chain disulfide bond formation during procollagen biosynthesis by embryonic chick tendon cells. *Biochem. Biophys. Res. Commun.* **55,** 1188–1196.

Harwood, R., Grant, M. E., and Jackson, D. S. (1974). Secretion of procollagen: Evidence for the transfer of nascent polypeptides across microsomal membranes of tendon cells. *Biochem. Biophys. Res. Commun.* **59,** 947–954.

Harwood, R., Grant, M. E., and Jackson, D. S. (1976). The route of secretion of procollagen. The influence of α,α' bipyridyl, colchicine and antimycin A on the secretory process in embryonic chick tendon and cartilage cells. *Biochem. J.* **156,** 81–90.

Hata, R., and Peterkofsky, B. (1977). Specific changes in the collagen phenotype of BALB 3T3 cells as a result of transformation by sarcoma viruses or a chemical carcinogen. *Proc. Natl. Acad. Sci. U.S.A.* **74,** 2933–2937.

Hay, E. D., and Dodson, J. W. (1973). Secretion of collagen by corneal epithelium. I. Morphology of the collagenous products produced by isolated epithelia grown on frozen-killed lens. *J. Cell Biol.* **57,** 190–213.

Helle, O., and Ness, N. N. (1972). A hereditary skin defect in sheep. *Acta Vet. Scand.* **13,** 443–445.

Housley, T. J., Tanzer, M. L., Henson, E., and Gallop, P. M. (1975). Collagen crosslinking: Isolation of hydroxyaldol-histidine, a naturally-occurring cross-link. *Biochem. Biophys. Res. Commun.* **67,** 824–830.

Housley, T. J., Rowland, F. N., Ledger, P. W., Kaplan, J., and Tanzer, M. L. (1980). Effects of tunicamycin on the biosynthesis of procollagen by human fibroblasts. *J. Biol. Chem.* **255,** 121–128.

Hughes, R. C., ed. (1976). Biosynthesis of glycoproteins. *In* "Membrane Glycoproteins," pp. 182–228. Butterworth, London.

Jiminez, S., Harsch, M., and Rosenbloom, J. (1973). Hydroxyproline stabilizes the triple helix of chick tendon collagen. *Biochem. Biophys. Res. Commun.* **52,** 106–114.

Kang, A. H., and Trelstad, R. L. (1973). A collagen defect in homocystinuria. *J. Clin. Invest.* **52,** 2571–2578.

Kefalides, N. A. (1971). Isolation of a collagen from basement membranes containing three identical α chains. *Biochem. Biophys. Res. Commun.* **45,** 226–234.

Kefalides, N. A. (1973). Structure and biosynthesis of basement membranes. *Int. Rev. Connect. Tissue Res.* **6,** 63–104.

Kefalides, N. A. (1975). Basement membranes: Structural and biosynthetic considerations. *J. Invest. Dermatol.* **65,** 85–92.

Kerwar, S. S., Kohn, L. D., Lapiere, C. M., and Weissbach, H. (1972). *In vitro* synthesis of procollagen on polysomes. *Proc. Natl. Acad. Sci. U.S.A.* **69,** 2727–2731.

Kimura, S., and Tanzer, M. L. (1977). Nereis cuticle collagen: Isolation and characterization of two distinct subunits. *Biochemistry* **16,** 2554–2560.

Kivirikko, K. I., and Prockop, D. J. (1972). Partial purification and characterization of protocollagen lysine hydroxylase from chick embryos. *Biochim. Biophys. Acta* **258,** 366–379.

Kivirikko, K. I., and Risteli, L. (1976). Biosynthesis of collagen and its alterations in pathological states. *Med. Biol.* **54,** 159–186.

Kivirikko, K. I., Ryhanen, L., Anttinen, H., Bornstein, P., and Prockop, D. J. (1973). Further hydroxylation of lysyl residues in collagen by protocollagen lysyl hydroxylase *in vitro*. *Biochemistry* **12,** 4966–4971.

Kohn, L. D., Isersky, C., Zupnik, J., Lenaers, A., Lee, G., and Lapiere, C. M. (1974). Calf tendon procollagen peptidase: Its purification and endopeptidase mode of action. *Proc. Natl. Acad. Sci. U.S.A.* **71,** 40–44.

Krane, S. M., Pinnell, S. R., and Erbe, R. W. (1972). Lysyl-protocollagen hydroxylase deficiency in fibroblasts from siblings with hydroxylysine deficient collagen. *Proc. Natl. Acad. Sci. U.S.A.* **69,** 2899–2903.

Lapiere, C. M., Lenaers, A., and Kohn, L. D. (1971). Procollagen peptidase: An enzyme excising the coordination peptides of procollagen. *Proc. Natl. Acad. Sci. U.S.A.* **68,** 3054–3058.

Layman, D. L., and Ross, R. (1973). The production and secretion of procollagen peptidase by human fibroblasts in culture. *Arch. Biochem. Biophys.* **157,** 451–456.

Lenaers, A., and Lapière, C. M. (1975). Type III procollagen in skin. *Biochim. Biophys. Acta* **400,** 121–131.

Lenaers, A., Ansay, M., Nusgens, G. V., and Lapière, C. M. (1971). Collagen made of extended α-chains, procollagen in genetically defective dermatosparactic calves. *Eur. J. Biochem.* **23,** 533–543.

LeRoy, E. C. (1974). Increased collagen synthesis by scleroderma skin fibroblasts *in vitro*. A possible defect in the regulation or activation of the scleroderma fibroblast. *J. Clin. Invest.* **54,** 880–889.

Levene, C. I., Aled, J. J., Prynne, C. J., and Bates, C. J. (1974). The activation of protocollagen proline hydroxylase by ascorbic acid in cultured 3T6 fibroblasts. *Biochim. Biophys. Acta* **338,** 29–36.

Lichtenstein, J. R., Martin, G. R., Kohn, L. D., Byers, P. H., and McKusick, J. A. (1973). Defect in conversion of procollagen to collagen in a form of Ehlers-Danlos syndrome. *Science* **182,** 298–300.

Little, C. D., Church, R. L., Miller, R. A., and Ruddle, F. H. (1977). Procollagen and collagen produced by a teratocarcinoma-derived cell line, TSD4: Evidence for a new molecular form of collagen. *Cell* **10,** 287–295.

Lwebuga-Mukase, J. S., Lappi, S., and Taylor, P. (1976). Molecular forms of acetylcholinesterase from *Torpedo Californica:* Their relationship to synaptic membranes. *Biochemistry* **15,** 1425–1434.

McCroskery, P. A., Richards, J. F., and Harris, E. D. (1975). Purification and characterization of a collagenase extracted from rabbit tumors. *Biochem. J.* **152,** 131–142.

McGee, J. O'D., Langness, U., and Udenfriend, S. (1971). Immunological evidence for an inactive precursor of collagen proline hydroxylase in cultured fibroblasts. *Proc. Natl. Acad. Sci. U.S.A.* **68,** 1585–1589.

Martin, G. R., Byers, P. H., and Piez, K. A. (1975). Procollagen. *Adv. Enzymol.* **42,** 167–191.

Mathews, M. B. (1975). Macromolecular structure and evolution. *In* "Connective Tissue," pp. 1-306. Springer-Verlag, Berlin and New York.

Merry, A. H., Harwood, R., Woolley, D. E., Grant, M. E., and Jackson, D. S. (1976). Identification and partial characterization of the non-collagenous amino- and carboxy-terminal extension peptides of cartilage procollagen. *Biochem. Biophys. Res. Commun.* **71,** 83–90.

Miller, A. (1976). Molecular packing in collagen fibrils. *In* "Biochemistry of Collagen" (G. N. Ramachandran and A. H. Reddi, eds.), pp. 85–136. Plenum, New York.

Miller, E. J. (1971a). Collagen cross-linking: Identification of two cyanogen bromide peptides containing sites of intermolecular cross-link formation in cartilage collagen. *Biochem. Biophys. Res. Commun.* **45,** 444–451.

Miller, E. J. (1971b). Isolation and characterization of a collagen from chick cartilage containing three identical α chains. *Biochemistry* **10,** 1652–1659.

Miller, E. J. (1972). Structural studies on cartilage collagen employing limited cleavage and solubilization with pepsin. *Biochemistry* **11,** 4903–4909.

Miller, E. J. (1976). Biochemical characteristics and biological significance of the genetically-distinct collagens. *Mol. Cell. Biochem.* **13,** 165–192.

Miller, E. J., and Matukas, V. J. (1969). Chick cartilage collagen: A new type of $\alpha 1$ chain not present in bone or skin of the species. *Proc. Natl. Acad. Sci. U.S.A.* **64,** 1264–1268.

Miller, R. L. (1971). Chromatographic separation of the enzymes required for hydroxylation of lysine and proline residues in protocollagen. *Arch. Biochem. Biophys.* **147,** 339–342.

Minor, R. R., Clark, C. C., Strause, E. L., Koszalka, T. R., Brent, R. L., and Kefalides, N. A. (1976). Basement membrane procollagen is not converted to collagen in organ cultures of parietal yolk sac endoderm. *J. Biol. Chem.* **251,** 1789–1794.

Morgan, P. H., Jacobs, H. G., Segrest, J. P., and Cunningham, L. W. (1970). A comparative study of glycopeptides derived from selected vertebrate collagens. A possible role of the carbohydrate in fibril formation. *J. Biol. Chem.* **245,** 5042–5048.

Moro, L., and Smith, B. D. (1977). Identification of collagen $\alpha 1$(I) trimer and normal type I collagen in a polyoma virus-induced mouse tumor. *Arch. Biochem. Biophys.* **182,** 33–41.

Müller, P. K., Lemmen, C., Gay, S., and Meigel, W. N. (1975). Disturbance in the regulation of the type of collagen synthesized in a form of osteogenesis imperfecta. *Eur. J. Biochem.* **59,** 97–104.

Myllylä, R., Risteli, L., and Kivirikko, K. I. (1975). Glucosylation of galactosylhydroxylysyl residues in collagen *in vitro* by collagen glucosyltransferase. Inhibition by triple-helical conformation of the substrate. *Eur. J. Biochem.* **58,** 517–521.

Myllylä, R., Risteli, L., and Kivirikko, K. I. (1976). Collagen glucosyltransferase. Partial purification and characterization of the enzyme from whole chick embryos and chick embryo cartilage. *Eur. J. Biochem.* **61,** 59–67.

Narayanan, A. S., Siegel, R. C., and Martin, G. R. (1972). On the inhibition of lysyl oxidase by β-aminopropionitrille. *Biochem. Biophys. Res. Commun.* **46,** 745–751.

Nist, C., von der Mark, K., Hay, E. D., Olsen, B. R., Bornstein, P., Ross, R., and Dehm, P. (1975). Location of procollagen in chick corneal and tendon fibroblasts with ferritin-conjugated antibodies. *J. Cell Biol.* **65,** 75–87.

O'Hara, P. J., Read, W. K., Romane, W. M., and Bridges, C. H. (1970). A collagenous tissue dysplasia of calves. *Lab. Invest.* **23,** 307–314.

Ohno, M., Riquetti, P., and Hudson, B. G. (1975). Bovine renal glomerular basement membrane. Isolation and characterization of a glycoprotein component. *J. Biol. Chem.* **250,** 7780-7787.

Olsen, B. R., and Prockop, D. J. (1974). Ferritin-conjugated antibodies used for labeling of organelles involved in the cellular synthesis and transport of collagen. *Proc. Natl. Acad. Sci. U.S.A.* **71,** 2033-2037.

Olsen, B. R., Berg, R. A., Kivirikko, K. I., and Prockop, D. J. (1973a). Structure of protocollagen proline hydroxylase from chick embryos. *Eur. J. Biochem.* **35,** 135-147.

Olsen, B. R., Alper, R., and Kefalides, N. A. (1973b). Structural characterization of a soluble fraction from lens-capsule basement membrane. *Eur. J. Biochem.* **38,** 220-228.

Olsen, B. R., Berg, R. A., Kishida, Y., and Prockop, D. J. (1973c). Collagen synthesis: Localization of prolyl hydroxylase in tendon cells detected with ferritin-labeled antibodies. *Science* **182,** 825-827.

Oppenheim, F. G., Hay, D. I., and Franzblau, C. (1971). Proline-rich proteins from human parotid saliva. I. Isolation and partial characterization. *Biochemistry* **10,** 4233-4238.

Palade, G. (1975). Intracellular aspects of the process of protein synthesis. *Science* **189,** 347-357.

Penttinen, R. P., Lichtenstein, J. R., Martin, G. R., and McKusick, V. A. (1975). Abnormal collagen metabolism in cultured cells in osteogenesis imperfecta. *Proc. Natl. Acad. Sci. U.S.A.* **72,** 586-589.

Peterkofsky, B., and Prather, W. B. (1974). Increased collagen synthesis in Kirsten sarcoma virus-transformed BALB 3T3 cells grown in the presence of dibutyryl cyclic AMP. *Cell* **3,** 291-299.

Pierce, G. B. (1970). Epithelial basement membrane: Origin, development and role in disease. *In* "Chemistry and Molecular Biology of the Intercellular Matrix" (E. A. Balazs, ed.), Vol. 1, pp. 471-506. Academic Press, New York.

Piez, K. A. (1976). Primary structure. *In* "Biochemistry of Collagen" (G. N. Ramachandran and A. H. Reddi, eds.), pp. 1-44. Plenum, New York.

Pinnell, S. R., Fox, R., and Krane, S. M. (1971). Human collagens: Differences in glycosylated hydroxylysines in skin and bone. *Biochim. Biophys. Acta* **229,** 119-122.

Pinnell, S. R., Krane, S. M., Kenzora, J. E., and Glimcher, M. J. (1972). A heritable disorder of connective tissue. Hydroxylysine-deficient collagen disease. *N. Engl. J. Med.* **286,** 1013-1020.

Pope, F. M., Martin, G. R., Lichtenstein, J. R., Penttinen, R., Gerson, B., Rowe, D. W., and McKusick, V. A. (1975). Patients with Ehlers-Danlos syndrome type IV lack type III collagen. *Proc. Natl. Acad. Sci. U.S.A.* **72,** 1314-1316.

Porter, R. R. (1977). Structure and activation of the early components of complement. *Fed. Proc., Fed. Am. Soc. Exp. Biol.* **36,** 2191-2196.

Prockop, D. J., Berg, R. A., Kivirikko, K. I., and Uitto, J. (1976). Intracellular steps in biosynthesis of collagen. *In* "Biochemistry of Collagen" (G. N. Ramachandran and A. H. Reddi, eds.), pp. 163-274. Plenum, New York.

Ramachandran, G. N., and Ramakrishnan, C. (1976). Molecular structure. *In* "Biochemistry of Collagen" (G. N. Ramachandran and A. H. Reddi, eds.), pp. 45-84. Plenum, New York.

Ramachandran, G. N., and Reddi, A. H., eds. (1976). "Biochemistry of Collagen." Plenum, New York.

Rauterberg, J. (1973). The C-terminal non-helical portion of the collagen molecule. *Clin. Orthop. Relat. Res.* **97,** 196-212.

Reid, K. B. M., and Porter, R. R. (1976). Subunit composition and structure of subcomponent C1q of the first component of human complement. *Biochem. J.* **155,** 19-23.

Rhoads, R. E., and Udenfriend, S. (1968). Decarboxylation of α-ketoglutarate coupled to collagen proline hydroxylase. *Proc. Natl. Acad. Sci. U.S.A.* **60,** 1473-1478.

Risteli, L., Myllylä, R., and Kivirikko, K. I. (1976). Partial purification and characterization of collagen galactosyltransferase from chick embryos. *Biochem. J.* **155,** 145-153.

Rosenbloom, J., Harsch, M., and Jiminez, S. (1973). Hydroxyproline content determines the denaturation temperature of chick tendon collagen. *Arch. Biochem. Biophys.* **158,** 478–484.

Rosenbloom, J., Endo, R., and Harsch, M. (1976). Termination of procollagen chain synthesis by puromycin. Evidence that assembly and secretion require a COOH-terminal extension. *J. Biol. Chem.* **251,** 2070–2076.

Rothman, S. S. (1975). Protein transport by the pancreas. *Science* **190,** 747–753.

Rowe, D. W., McGoodwin, E. B., Martin, G. R., Sussman, M. D., Grahn, D., Faris, B., and Franzblau, C. (1974). A sex-linked defect in the cross-linking of collagen and elastin associated with the mottled locus in mice. *J. Exp. Med.* **139,** 180–192.

Rowe, D. A., McGoodwin, E. B., Martin, G. R., and Grahn, D. (1977). Decreased lysyl oxidase activity in the aneurysm-prone, mottled mouse. *J. Biol. Chem.* **252,** 939–942.

Rowe, D. W., Moen, R. C., Davidson, J. M., Byers, P. H., Bornstein, P. and Palmiter, R. D. (1978). Correlation of procollagen mRNA levels in normal and transformed chick embryo fibroblasts with different rates of procollagen synthesis. *Biochemistry* **17,** 1581–1590.

Sakai, T., and Gross, J. (1967). Some properties of the products of reaction of tadpole collagenase with collagen. *Biochemistry* **6,** 518–528.

Schmitt, F. O. (1964). Telopeptide control of tropocollagen interaction dynamics. *Fed. Proc., Fed. Am. Soc. Exp. Biol.* **23,** 618–622.

Schofield, J. D., Uitto, J., and Prockop, D. J. (1974). Formation of interchain disulfide bonds and helical structure during biosynthesis of procollagen by embryonic tendon cells. *Biochemistry* **13,** 1801–1806.

Seifter, S., and Harper, E. (1971). The collagenases. *In* "The Enzymes" (P. D. Boyer, ed.), 3rd ed., Vol. 3, pp. 649–697. Academic Press, New York.

Sherr, C. J., Taubman, M. B., and Goldberg, B. (1973). Isolation of a disulfide-stabilized, three chain polypeptide fragment unique to the precursor of human collagen. *J. Biol. Chem.* **248,** 7033–7038.

Siegel, R. (1974). Biosynthesis of collagen crosslinks: Increased activity of purified lysyl oxidase with reconstituted collagen fibrils. *Proc. Natl. Acad. Sci. U.S.A.* **71,** 4826–4830.

Siegel, R. C. (1977). Collagen cross-linking. Effect of D-penicillamine on cross-linking *in vitro*. *J. Biol. Chem.* **252,** 254–259.

Siegel, R. C., and Fu, J. C. C. (1976). Collagen cross-linking. Purification and substrate specificity of lysyl oxidase. *J. Biol. Chem.* **251,** 5779–5785.

Siegel, R. C., Pinnell, S. R., and Martin, G. R. (1970). Cross-linking of collagen and elastin. Properties of lysyl oxidase. *Biochemistry* **9,** 4486–4492.

Silman, I. (1976). Molecular structure of acetylcholinesterase. *Trends Biochem. Sci.* **1,** 225–227.

Smith, J. W. (1968). Molecular pattern in native collagen. *Nature (London)* **219,** 157–158.

Spiro, R. G. (1969). Characterization and quantitative determination of the hydroxylysine-linked carbohydrate units of several collagens. *J. Biol. Chem.* **244,** 602–612.

Spiro, R. G., and Spiro, M. J. (1971). Studies on the biosynthesis of the hydroxylysine-linked disaccharide unit of basement membranes and collagens. III. Tissue and subcellular distribution of glycosyltransferases and the effect of various conditions on the enzyme levels. *J. Biol. Chem.* **246,** 4919–4925.

Stark, G. R., Stein, W. H., and Moore, S. (1960). Reactions of the cyanate present in aqueous urea with amino acids and proteins. *J. Biol. Chem.* **235,** 3177–3181.

Stark, M., Miller, E. J., and Hühn, K. (1972). Comparative electron-microscopic studies on the collagens extracted from cartilage, bone and skin. *Eur. J. Biochem.* **27,** 192–196.

Stassen, F. L. H. (1976). Properties of highly purified lysyl oxidase from embryonic chick cartilage. *Biochim. Biophys. Acta* **438,** 49–60.

Stassen, F. L. H., Cardinale, G. J., and Udenfriend, S. (1973). Activation of prolyl hydroxylase in L-929 fibroblasts by ascorbic acid. *Proc. Natl. Acad. Sci. U.S.A.* **70,** 1090–1093.

Stimler, N. P., and Tanzer, M. L. (1976). Location of the intermolecular cross-linking sites in collagen. *In* "Protein Crosslinking, Nutritional and Medical Consequences" (M. Friedman, ed.), pp. 675–697. Plenum, New York.

Sundar Raj, C. V., Church, R. L., Klobutcher, L. A., and Ruddle, F. H. (1977). Genetics of the connective tissue proteins. Assignment of the gene for human type I procollagen to chromosome 17 by analysis of cell hybrids and microcell hybrids. *Proc. Natl. Acad. Sci. U.S.A.* **74,** 4444–4448.

Sykes, B., Francis, M. J. O., and Smith, R. (1977). Altered relation of two collagen types in osteogenesis imperfecta. *N. Engl. J. Med.* **296,** 1200–1203.

Tanzer, M. L. (1965). Experimental lathyrism. *Int. Rev. Connect. Tissue Res.* **3,** 91–112.

Tanzer, M. L. (1973). Cross-linking of collagen. *Science* **180,** 561–566.

Tanzer, M. L. (1978). The biological diversity of collagenous proteins. *Trends Biochem. Sci.* **3,** 15–17.

Tanzer, M. L., Church, R. L., Yaeger, J. A., Wampler, D. E., and Park, E. D. (1974). Procollagen: Intermediate forms containing several types of peptide chains and non-collagen peptide extensions at NH_2 and COOH ends. *Proc. Natl. Acad. Sci. U.S.A.* **71,** 3009–3013.

Thompson, R. C., and Ballou, J. E. (1956). Studies of metabolic turnover with tritium as a tracer. V. The predominantly non-dynamic state of body constituents in the rat. *J. Biol. Chem.* **223,** 795–809.

Timpl. R. (1976). Immunological studies on collagen. *In* "Biochemistry of Collagen" (G. N. Ramachandran and A. H. Reddi, eds.), pp. 319–376. Plenum, New York.

Timpl, R., Wick, G. Furthmayr, H., Lapiere, C. M., and Kuhn, K. (1973). Immunochemical properties of procollagen from dermatosparactic calves. *Eur. J. Biochem.* **32,** 584–591.

Timpl, R., Glanville, R. W., Nowack, H., Wiedemann, H., Fietzek, P. P., and Kuhn, K. (1975). Isolation, chemical and electron microscopical characterization of neutral salt soluble type III collagen and procollagen from fetal bovine skin. *Hoppe-Seyler's Z. Physiol. Chem.* **356,** 1783–1792.

Trelstad, R. L., Rubin, D., and Gross, J. (1977). Osteogenesis imperfecta congenita. Evidence for a generalized molecular disorder of collagen. *Lab. Invest.* **36,** 501–508.

Uitto, J. (1977). Biosynthesis of type II collagen. Removal of amino- and carboxy-terminal extensions from procollagen synthesized by chick embryo cartilage cells. *Biochemistry* **16,** 3421–3429.

Uitto, J., and Lichtenstein, J. R. (1976). Defects in the biochemistry of collagen in diseases of connective tissue. *J. Invest. Dermatol.* **66,** 55–79.

Uitto, J., and Prockop, D. J. (1974). Biosynthesis of cartilage procollagen. Influence of chain association and hydroxylation of prolyl residues on the folding of the polypeptides into the triple-helical conformation. *Biochemistry* **13,** 4586–4591.

Uitto, J., Dehm, P., and Prockop, D. J. (1972). Incorporation of cis-hydroxyproline into collagen by tendon cells. Failure of the intracellular collagen to assume a triple-helical conformation. *Biochim. Biophys. Acta* **278,** 601–605.

Veis, A., and Brownell, A. G. (1975). Collagen biosynthesis. *CRC Crit. Rev. Biochem.* **3,** 417–453.

Veis, A., and Yuan, L. (1975). Structure of the collagen microfibril. A four-stranded overlap model. *Biopolymers* **14,** 895–900.

Veis, A., Anesey, J., Garvin, J. E., and Dimuzio, M. T. (1972). High molecular weight collagen. A long-lined intermediate in the biogenesis of collagen fibrils. *Biochem. Biophys. Res. Commun.* **48,** 1404–1411.

Veis, A., Anesey, J., Yuan, L., and Levy, S. J. (1973). Evidence for an NH_2-terminal extension in high molecular weight collagens from mature bovine skin. *Proc. Natl. Acad. Sci. U.S.A.* **70,** 1464–1467.

von der Mark, K., and von der Mark, H. (1977). Immunological and biochemical studies of collagen type transition during *in vitro* chondrogenesis of chick limb mesodermal cells. *J. Cell Biol.* **73,** 736–747.

Vuust, J., and Piez, K. A. (1972). A kinetic study of collagen biosynthesis. *J. Biol. Chem.* **247,** 856–862.

Watson, J. D. (1976). "Molecular Biology of the Gene," 3rd ed. Benjamin, Menlo Park, California.

Weinstock, M., and Leblond, C. P. (1974). Synthesis, migration and release of precursor collagen by odontoblasts as visualized by radioautography after [^{3}H] proline administration. *J. Cell Biol.* **60,** 92–127.

Weiss, J. B. (1976). Enzymic degradation of collagen. *Int. Rev. Connect. Tissue Res.* **7,** 102–157.

6

Parathyroid Hormone

JAN A. FISCHER

Disorders of Mineral Metabolism, Vol. II

ISBN 0-12-135302-8

I. INTRODUCTION

It is the purpose of this chapter to attempt to relate the regulation of the secretion and the metabolism of parathyroid hormone (PTH) to an analysis of serum PTH levels in disorders of mineral metabolism. Circulating PTH levels can only be interpreted in relation to the serum calcium concentration, which is the most important regulator of the PTH secretion. The consequent biological and pathophysiological alterations at the level of the skeleton and the kidney have been extensively covered recently (Rasmussen and Bordier, 1974; Borle, 1974; Aurbach and Heath, 1974; Parsons, 1976). They are briefly summarized and mainly alluded to when required for the understanding of the pathogenesis and the diagnosis of disorders of the parathyroid glands.

II. CHEMISTRY OF PARATHYROID HORMONE

Human, bovine, and porcine PTH consist of single polypeptide chains of 84 amino acid residues (Fig. 1). Bovine PTH (bPTH) was isolated by Rasmussen and Craig (1959) and by Aurbach in 1959 and the primary structure determined by Brewer and Ronan (1970) as well as by Niall *et al.* in 1970. Two isohormones differing in some structural detail from bPTH have also been isolated (Keutmann *et al.*, 1971). Porcine PTH (pPTH) was purified (Littledike and Hawker, 1967) and isolated (Woodhead *et al.*, 1971), and the amino acid sequence determined (Sauer *et al.*, 1974). It differs in seven amino acid residues from bPTH-(1–84) (Fig. 1).

The biological activity of bPTH (as measured by a rise in serum calcium in thyroparathyroidectomized rats) was similar to that of pPTH, whereas the adenylate cyclase activity of the rat cortical enzyme was somewhat lower with pPTH as compared to bPTH (Littledike and Hawker, 1967; Woodhead *et al.*, 1971). Mild oxidation with hydrogen peroxide destroyed the biological, but not the immunological activity of bovine and porcine PTH (Rasmussen and Craig, 1961; Tashjian *et al.*, 1964b; Woodhead *et al.*, 1971; O'Riordan *et al.*, 1974). The biological activity of extracted bPTH is more extensively treated in Sections V and VI.

Human parathyroid hormone (hPTH) was isolated in pure form by Brewer *et al.* (1972), who also determined the amino acid sequence of the amino-terminal residues 1–34. Subsequently, hPTH was also isolated by Keutmann *et al.* (1974) and an alternative structure differing in three amino acid residues for the NH_2-terminal sequence was proposed by Niall *et al.* (1974). The reason for the discrepancies is not clear. The complete amino acid sequence of hPTH-(1–84) was subsequently reported by Keutmann *et al.* (1978) (Fig. 1). The structures of bovine and human PTH-(1–84) (with the single exception of the amino acid at residue 76) reported by Niall *et al.* (1974) and Keutmann *et al.* (1978), re-

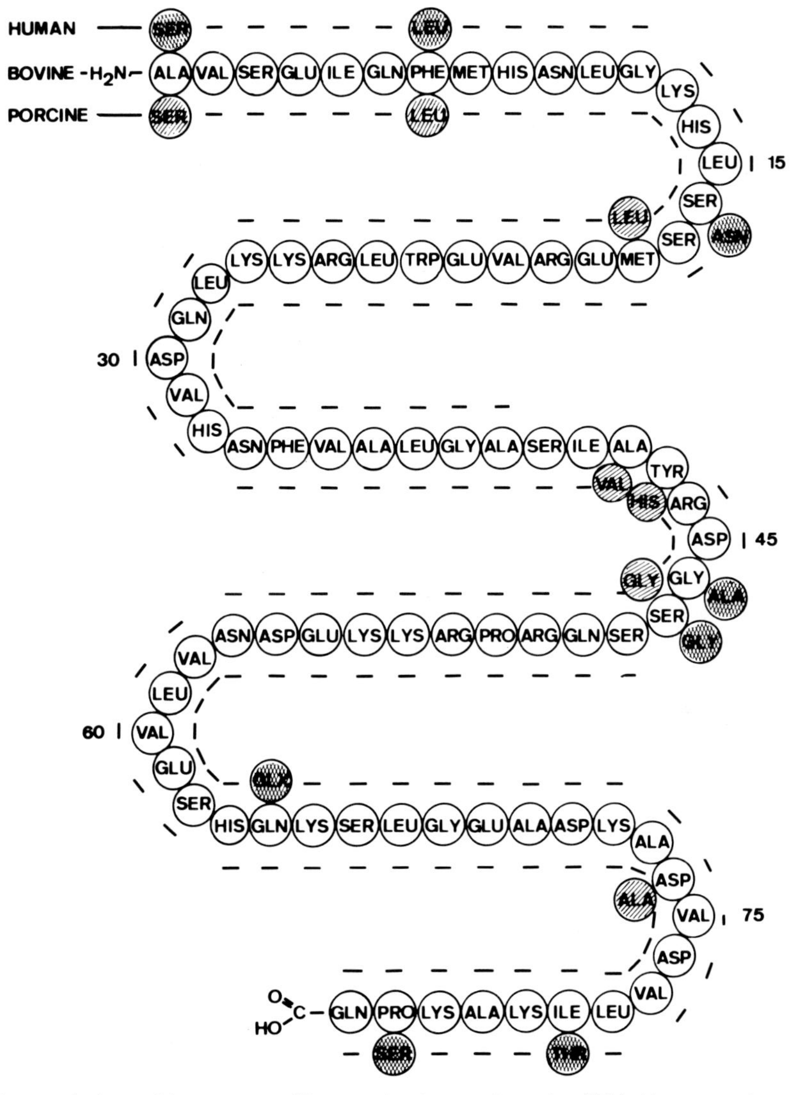

Fig. 1. Amino acid sequence of human, bovine, and porcine PTH. Human and porcine PTH differ from bovine PTH in the amino acids represented in crosshatched and hatched circles, respectively. (Adapted from Habener *et al.,* 1977b and Keutmann *et al.,* 1978.)

spectively, have been confirmed by analysis of the sequence of desoxyribonucleic acids coding for the precursors of the two hormones (Kronenberg *et al.,* 1979; Hendy *et al.,* 1981).

The biological activity of hPTH-(1–84) has so far been only assayed in the renal cortical adenylate cyclase assay. In rat cortical membranes bPTH-(1–84) showed higher biological activity as compared to hPTH-(1–84) (Tregear *et al.*, 1974; Di Bella *et al.*, 1976), whereas with human cortical membranes these hormones showed similar activities (Di Bella *et al.*, 1976).

In addition to the intact PTH-(1–84) biosynthetic precursors and NH_2- and COOH-terminal fragments of PTH-(1–84) have been identified in bovine parathyroid glands and human parathyroid tumors. Large molecular weight forms include preproparathyroid hormone (PreProPTH) and proparathyroid hormone (ProPTH) with 31 and 6 additional amino acids, respectively, at the NH_2-terminal end of PTH-(1–84). The six additional amino acids of ProPTH are identical in the bovine and the human molecules (Fig. 2) (Hamilton *et al.*, 1974; Jacobs *et al.*, 1974; Habener *et al.*, 1978). Suggestive evidence of the presence of larger molecular weight immunoreactive PTH species than hPTH-(1–84) has been obtained in the incubation medium of human parathyroid explant cultures and in the peripheral circulation on gel filtration analysis (Habener *et al.*, 1971; Canterbury and Reiss, 1972; Martin *et al.*, 1973; Fischer *et al.*, 1974). An immunoreactive PTH species larger than hPTH-(1–84) appears to be a predominant component in the serum of some patients with ectopic hyperparathyroidism (Benson *et al.*, 1974a). Definitive experiments to prove the existence of large molecular weight forms outside of the parathyroid glands have not been carried out.

A smaller molecular weight PTH fragment, which retained the calcium mobilizing and the phosphaturic activity of the intact hormone, was isolated by Rasmussen *et al.* (1964c). Biologically active fragments have been identified as bPTH-(1–29) and -(1–65), whereas fragment 1–20 obtained by tryptic cleavage was biologically inactive (Keutmann *et al.*, 1972; Murray *et al.*, 1975). NH_2- and COOH-terminal fragments were also extracted from human parathyroid tumors whose sequence remains to be determined (Silverman and Yalow, 1973; Di Bella *et al.*, 1978). Intact PTH-(1–84) and a COOH-terminal fragment with a molecular weight of about 7000 appear to be the major circulating PTH species and NH_2-terminal fragment(s) represent minor components. The fragments are secreted by the parathyroid glands (Flueck *et al.*, 1977), but also are generated in peripheral organs such as the liver and the kidney (Canterbury *et al.*, 1975; Martin *et al.*, 1976; Hruska *et al.*, 1977) (see Sections III and IV).

A biologically active NH_2-terminal tetratriacontapeptide of bPTH was synthesized by Potts *et al.* (1971). This synthetic peptide has a comparable potency to bPTH-(1–84) on a molar basis both *in vitro* (activation of renal adenylate cyclase in the rat) and *in vivo* (increase in serum calcium in chicken) (Tregear *et al.*, 1973). The fragment 1–26 was biologically inactive, whereas with the fragments 1–27 rat adenylate cyclase activity could be stimulated at 2% of the potency of native bPTH-(1–84). The NH_2-terminal residues alanine and valine are essential for biological activity since the synthetic peptide containing residues 3–34 is

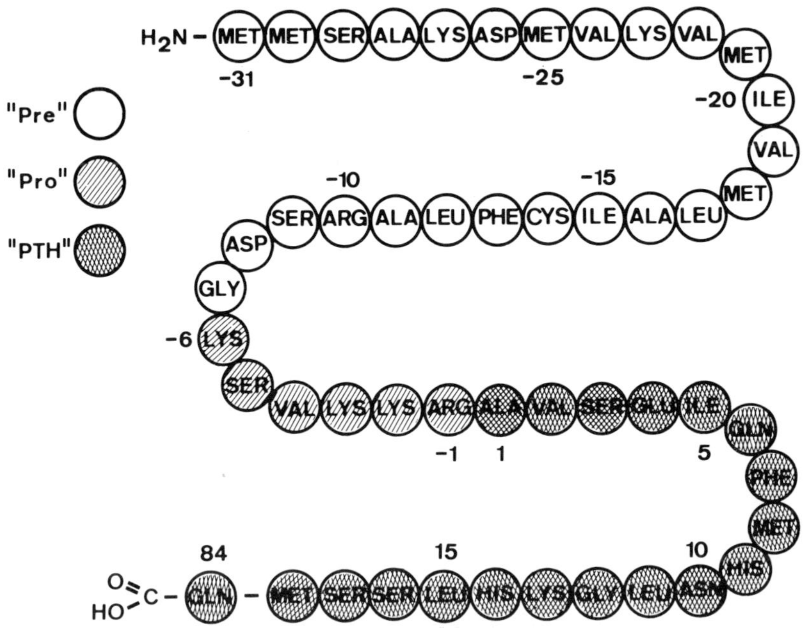

Fig. 2. Amino acid sequence of bovine PreProPTH. The numbers refer to the polypeptide numbering system, beginning with −31 at the NH_2-terminus of PreProPTH. The sequence of ProPTH begins at the amino acid residue −6 and of bPTH-(1-84) at 1. (Adapted from Habener *et al.,* 1978.)

inactive. This suggests that the minimal chain length important for biological activity lies between residues 1–27 and 1–34. Interestingly, bPTH-(3–34) presumably binds to membranes, but it has inhibitory properties in the presence of biologically active synthetic peptides (Goltzman *et al.,* 1975). Oxidation of native bPTH-(1–84) or of synthetic bPTH-(1–34) resulted in virtually complete loss of biological activity, whereas an analog having the two methionines replaced by norleucines retained the biological activity (Rosenblatt *et al.,* 1976).

Human PTH-(1–34) based on the sequence obtained by Niall *et al.* (1974) was synthesized (Tregear *et al.* (1974), and it was found to be equally biologically active as bPTH-(1–34) in the chick hypercalcemia and renal adenylate cyclase assay, but less active in the rat renal adenylate cyclase assay (Tregear *et al.,* 1974; Martin *et al.,* 1974). Substitution of the NH_2-terminal serine with alanine yielded an analog with comparable *in vitro* activity to bPTH-(1–34) in the rat (Tregear and Potts, 1975). All these studies support the notion that the biological properties of the various synthetic and extracted PTH peptides are not only defined by their chemical structures but also tend to vary with the biological system or animal species used.

III. BIOSYNTHESIS AND SECRETION OF PARATHYROID HORMONE

A. Biosynthesis

Biosynthetic precursors having molecular weights larger than PTH-(1–84) have been isolated and partially characterized with amino acid incorporation experiments. PreProPTH was originally identified in a cell-free extract of wheat germ as the translation product of an mRNA isolated from calf and hyperplastic human parathyroid tissues (Kemper *et al.*, 1974a; Habener *et al.*, 1975b). Furthermore, deoxyribonucleic acid complementary in sequence to the mRNA for PreProPTH was synthesized using reverse transcriptase (Kronenberg *et al.*, 1977). Kemper *et al.* (1976) and Kemper (1976) have presented evidence that the normal initiator codon *in vivo* is present; this suggests that PreProPTH has been identified in parathyroid cells as the earliest biosynthetic product. PreProPTH contains 31 additional amino acid residues at the NH_2-terminal end of PTH-(1–84) (Fig. 2) (Habener *et al.*, 1978). PreProPTH appears to be converted to ProPTH within seconds after completion of its synthesis on the rough endoplasmic reticulum (Habener *et al.*, 1977a).

Proparathyroid hormone has also been identified as a biosynthetic precursor in parathyroid slices (Kemper *et al.*, 1972; Cohn *et al.*, 1972). ProPTH consists of 90 amino acid residues with six residues being attached to the NH_2-terminal end of PTH-(1–84) (Fig. 2). ProPTH was identified radioimmunologically in bovine and human parathyroid tissue extracts but not in the venous effluent of the parathyroid glands (Habener *et al.*, 1974a, 1976). ProPTH comprises 5% of immunoreactive PTH in bovine glands and 50% in human tumors (Habener *et al.*, 1976). ProPTH is converted to PTH-(1–84) by proteolytic cleavage within about 20 min after its first appearance in the tissue (Chu *et al.*, 1973; Habener *et al.*, 1974b). The converting enzyme is probably a trypsin-like substance, since the pancreatic trypsin *in vitro* selectively cleaved the ProPTH–PTH-(1–84) bond (Goltzman *et al.*, 1976a). The converting activity appears to be associated with the particulate fraction of parathyroid homogenates (MacGregor *et al.*, 1976). [^{3}H]leucine-labeled ProPTH and PTH were sequentially visualized by radioautographic grain counts over the rough endoplasmic reticulum, the Golgi complex, and in an area rich in secretory granules close to the plasma membrane. The conversion of ProPTH to PTH-(1–84) takes place at the Golgi region (Habener *et al.*, 1979). Lysosomes associated with the destruction of secretory granules and proteolytic degradation of PTH-(1–84) by parathyroid extracts represent additional loci for PTH secretion and metabolism (Shannon and Roth, 1974; Fischer *et al.*, 1972; Chu *et al.*, 1973; Habener *et al.*, 1975a). Intact hPTH-(1–84), but also its COOH- and NH_2-terminal fragments have been detected in the venous effluent of the parathyroid glands. Since all amounts were higher in the venous effluent as compared to the peripheral circulation, it appears that the parathyroid glands secrete NH_2- and COOH-terminal PTH fragments in addition to intact PTH-(1–84) (Flueck *et al.*, 1977). Morrissey *et al.* (1980) have demonstrated the presence of PTH-(34–84) and -(37–84) in the incubation medium of dispersed porcine parathyroid cells. Nevertheless, PTH-(1–84) appears to be the most important biologically active PTH form secreted *in vivo* by the parathyroid glands (Habener *et al.*, 1971; Flueck *et al.*, 1977).

B. Control Points of the Secretion

Potential and documented control points of PTH synthesis and secretion are summarized in Fig. 3. However, in most cases it is not yet known whether the effects are direct or indirect. The most important regulator is the extracellular ionized calcium concentration (control point 6). In magnesium deficiency the secretion is suppressed (control point 7). The contribution of other regulators such as the adrenergic nervous system, catecholamines, and the D vitamins is not yet well defined.

Certain conditions, such as calcium- and/or a vitamin D deficiency, or chronic renal failure tend to lower the serum calcium concentration. As a consequence the parathyroid glands are stimulated to produce a greater hormonal output and show hyperplastic enlargement, with the chief cells on morphological grounds showing evidence of increased hormone synthesis and secretion (for a detailed review of the ultrastructural changes, see Roth and Raisz, 1966; Roth and Capen, 1974). Already within 48 hr after bilateral nephrectomy, hypertrophy and hyperplasia occur (Talmage *et al.*, 1960). Furthermore, a significant difference between deoxyribonucleic acid synthesis rates in high and low calcium media was observed in organ culture within 3 hr (Lee and Roth, 1975) (control point 1). As a consequence, the uptake and incorporation of amino acids in the parathyroid glands was increased (Raisz, 1967) (control point 2). Chu *et al.* (1973) demonstrated in rat gland extracts that at least the initial biosynthesis of ProPTH appeared not to be influenced by varying dietary calcium intakes, whereas the synthesis of PTH-(1–84) was inversely related to the dietary calcium contents. The authors demonstrated that under conditions of low compared to high dietary calcium intake, there was a greater efficiency of the conversion of ProPTH to PTH-(1–84) due to less degradation of ProPTH and PTH-(1–84). Newly synthesized PTH-(1–84) appears to be preferentially secreted during incubation of bovine parathyroid slices in 1.25 m*M* as compared to 2.5 m*M* calcium *in vitro* (MacGregor *et al.*, 1975). These findings have been extended, and it was shown that low calcium stimulates the secretion both of stored and newly synthesized PTH, whereas cyclic adenosine monophosphate (cyclicAMP) and isoprotorenol enhance the release of preexisting hormone only (Morrissey and Cohn, 1979). However, the biosynthesis of ProPTH seemed not to be affected by changes of

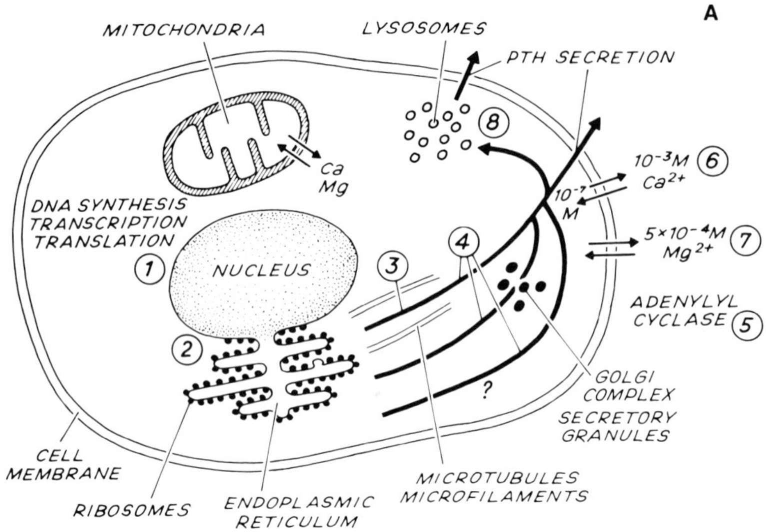

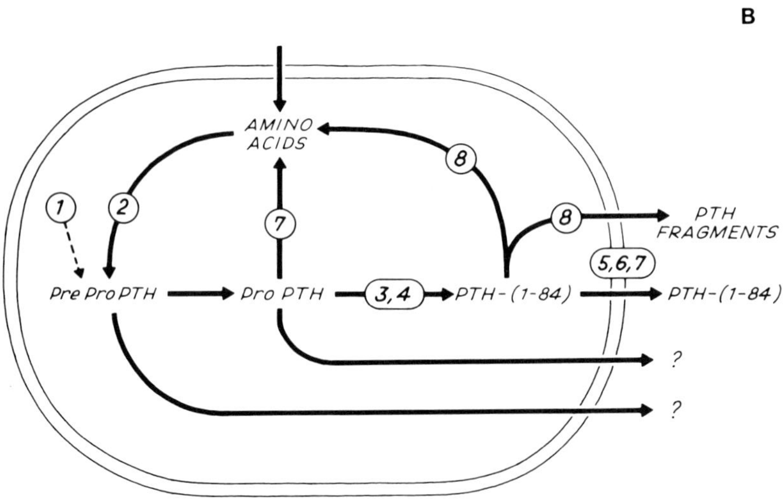

Fig. 3. Biosynthesis and control points (numbers) of PTH formation and pathways within parathyroid cells. A, morphology; B, biosynthetic scheme (for details see text).

the calcium concentration in the incubation medium of dispersed porcine parathyroid cells (Morrissey and Cohn, 1978). In contrast to these findings, we have demonstrated using dispersed bovine parathyroid cells, a more marked incorporation of radioactive amino acids into ProPTH and PTH-(1–84) at low than at high calcium concentrations (Moran *et al.*, 1981) (control point 2).

Habener *et al.* (1974b) were unable to detect a difference in the conversion of ProPTH to PTH-(1–84) *in vitro* with varying calcium concentrations (0.5–5.0 m*M*) in the incubation medium of bovine parathyroid slices. The calcium ionophores A23187 and X537A specifically blocked the conversion of ProPTH to PTH at the level of the Golgi complex and as a consequence suppressed PTH secretion (Habener *et al.*, 1977b) (control point 4). Moreover, the calcium ionophore A23187 inhibited the release of both cyclic AMP and PTH from dispersed parathyroid cells (Brown *et al.*, 1980). On the other hand, verapamil, which inhibits calcium transport across plasma membranes, stimulated the secretion of PTH *in vitro* (Ramp *et al.*, 1979).

Fischer *et al.* (1972) have, furthermore, demonstrated that [^{131}I]bPTH-(1–84) was more rapidly destroyed by parathyroid extracts in the presence of 1 m*M* $CaCl_2$ in the incubation medium as compared to 5 m*M* EDTA (control point 8). Habener *et al.* (1974b) have indicated that in 2–3 m*M* calcium concentrations, up to 40% of [^{3}H]PTH was neither secreted by nor stored in the glands, but was instead degraded within the tissue. Morphological evidence obtained *in vitro* and *in vivo* suggests that PTH is degraded in lysosomal bodies under conditions of decreased parathyroid secretory function with hypercalcemia or high calcium in the incubation medium (Capen, 1971; Oldham *et al.*, 1971).

Furthermore, the secretion of COOH-terminal fragments by the parathyroid glands may be related to the serum concentration of calcium. Indeed Hanley *et al.* (1978) and Mayer et al. (1979) have presented evidence that the amounts of COOH-terminal fragments in the perfusate of bovine parathyroid slices and in the venous effluent of parathyroid glands are proportionally higher at high than at low calcium concentrations, suggesting that the cleavage of human PTH-(1–84) within parathyroid cells is calcium-related. Moreover, we have demonstrated proportionally higher amounts of COOH-terminal PTH fragments in the peripheral blood of hypercalcemic patients with primary hyperparathyroidism as compared to hypocalcemic patients with secondary hyperparathyroidism and normal renal function (Dambacher *et al.*, 1979). On the other hand, the conversion of intact [^{131}I]bPTH-(1–84) to smaller molecular weight, biologically active fragments by parathyroid extracts appears to be preferentially stimulated in the presence in the incubation medium of 1 m*M* EDTA as compared to 1 m*M* $CaCl_2$, whereas fragments were not degraded in the presence of EDTA (Fischer *et al.*, 1972).

Analysis by gel filtration and electrophoresis revealed that in addition to PTH-(1–84), a large fraction of the amino acids were incorporated into a 150,000 molecular weight glycoprotein that did not react with antibodies raised to PTH. This protein, whose function is at present unknown, was released into the incubation medium of parathyroid explants kept *in vitro* and comprised up to 50% of the total secreted proteins (Au *et al.*, 1970; Sherwood *et al.*, 1970b; Kemper *et al.*, 1974b; Morrissey *et al.*, 1978; Morrissey and Cohn, 1978; Moran *et al.*, 1981); the biosynthesis and secretion *in vitro* is inversely related to the calcium concentration. Recently, the parathyroid secretory protein has been isolated and partially characterized (Takatsuki *et al.*, 1981).

Parathyroid responses are not only inversely related to the extracellular calcium, but possibly also to magnesium concentrations (Care *et al.*, 1966). However, changes in the magnesium concentration between 0.2 and 1.7 m*M* were without effect on bPTH-(1–84) synthesis *in vitro* (Hamilton *et al.*, 1971). Furthermore, PTH levels in plasma are normal or decreased in hypocalcemic patients with magnesium deficiency and it appears that some extracellular magnesium concentration (>0.4 m*M*) is required for PTH release from the glands (Fig 4) (Anast *et al.*, 1972) (control point 7).

Coincident with an increased secretion of PTH *in vitro* caused by falls in the extracellular calcium and/or magnesium concentrations, there was an increased release of cyclic AMP (Abe and Sherwood, 1972; Sherwood and Abe, 1972a)

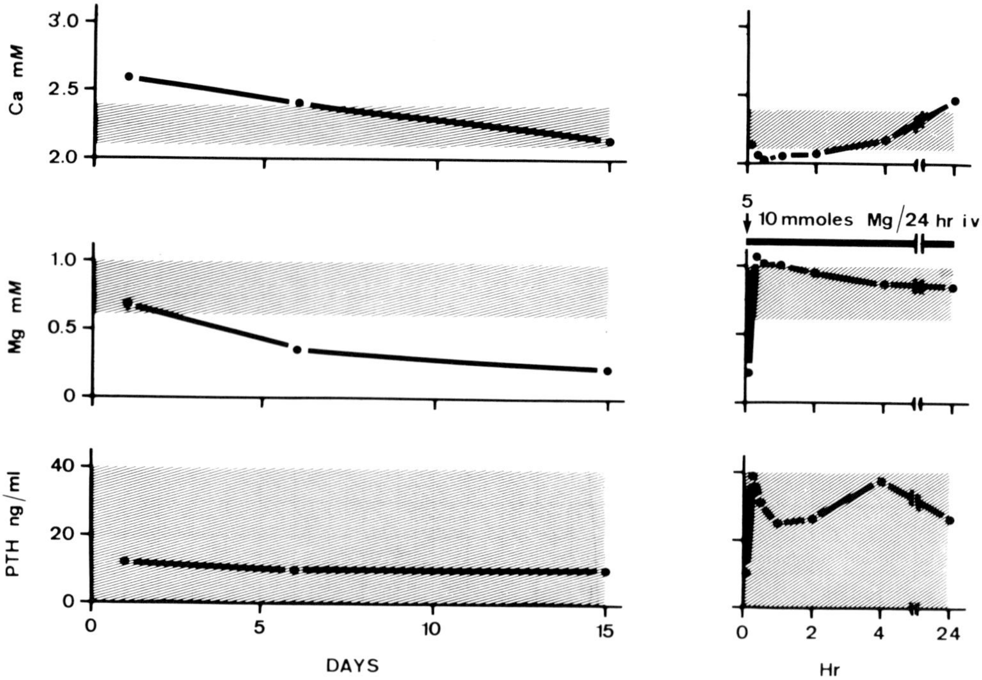

Fig. 4. Serum calcium, magnesium, and PTH levels before and after the intravenous administration of magnesium chloride in a hypomagnesemic 3.2-year-old girl with hypomagnesemia and reduced intestinal magnesium absorption. Carboxyl terminal immunoreactive PTH as determined with [^{131}I]bPTH-(1-84), antibodies to PTH (guinea pig 1 *M*, diluted 1:100,000), and a human tissue culture standard (C-72). The shaded areas indicate the normal adult range. Serum PTH is low in hypomagnesemia in relation to the low normal serum level of calcium, and serum PTH levels are raised in response to iv magnesium. (From E. Signer and J. A. Fischer, unpublished.)

(control point 5). Half-maximal inhibition of adenylyl cyclase activity was achieved in the presence of 3×10^{-3} and $10^{-2} M$ magnesium with 10^{-6} and $10^{-3} M$ calcium, respectively (Dufresne and Gitelman, 1972; Matsuzaki and Dumont, 1972). Moreover, calmodulin regulated phosphodiesterase activity has been demonstrated in parathyroid tissue (Willgoss *et al.*, 1980, Brown, 1980).

Besides low extracellular calcium and magnesium levels dibutyryl cyclic AMP, aminophylline, β-adrenergic catecholamines and calcitonin stimulate PTH secretion (Sherwood and Abe, 1972b; Williams *et al.*, 1973; Bowser *et al.*, 1975; Brown *et al.*, 1977a; Fischer *et al.*, 1971, 1973c). Epinephrine, calcitonin and glucagon also stimulated adenylate cyclase activity of parathyroid homogenates (Dufresne and Gitelman, 1972; Matsuzaki and Dumont, 1972; Brown *et al.*, 1977b). The presence of adrenergic nerve terminals close to parathyroid cells (Altenähr, 1971; Yeghiayan *et al.*, 1972; Norberg *et al.*, 1975) suggests a possible role for catecholamines released by the autonomic nervous system in the physiological regulation of PTH secretion. Brown *et al.* (1977b) have localized β-adrenergic receptors on isolated parathyroid cells with [^{125}I]hydroxybenzylpindolol as ligand, and, furthermore, demonstrated coupling between the binding of iodohydroxybenzylpindolol, and the stimulation of cyclic AMP levels and of the adenylate cyclase activity, as well as of PTH release. PTH responses to epinephrine were transient, whereas the stimulation of cyclic AMP apparently continued unabated (Brown *et al.*, 1977a; Hanley *et al.*, 1980). Cyclic AMP responses to low calcium were only 3% of the stimulation obtained with isoproterenol, suggesting that factors other than cyclic AMP may be important for the calcium-mediated PTH release (Brown *et al.*, 1977a). For a detailed analysis of relationships between the catecholamines and calcium regulated PTH secretion see Section III,C.

Calcitonin also stimulates adenylate cyclase activity in homogenates of parathyroid glands. This suggests that the PTH response to calcitonin is mediated by cyclic AMP (Dufresne and Gitelman, 1972). Since calcitonin may depress the cytoplasmic calcium concentration within parathyroid cells (MacManus and Whitfield, 1970; Borle, 1975), it may act by stimulating adenylate cyclase activity. This in turn would increase cyclic AMP levels within parathyroid cells.

1,25-$(OH)_2D_3$ was accumulated in chick parathyroid glands (Henry and Norman, 1975) and cytoplasmic and nuclear binding components for 25-$(OH)D_3$ and 1,25-$(OH)_2D_3$ have been identified in this tissue (Haddad *et al.*, 1976; Hughes and Haussler, 1978). These findings, together with the isolation of a calcium-binding protein from parathyroid glands (Oldham *et al.*, 1974), suggest that 1,25-$(OH)_2D_3$ may be involved in the transport of calcium into parathyroid cells. For the role of vitamin D and of its metabolites on PTH responses see Section III,C.

Compounds that interfere with microtubular function such as colchicine and vinblastine lowered the conversion of ProPTH to PTH-(1–84), whereas cytochalasine B which inhibits microfilaments was ineffective (Kemper *et al.*, 1975) (control point 3). Colchicine and vinblastine, however, did not inhibit the release of PTH *in vivo* (Chanard *et al.*, 1977). Common ultrastructural findings in response to stimulation of PTH secretion by low calcium, vitamin A, and cytochalasin B suggest that these agents may act through a similar mechanism (Chertow *et al.*, 1975b; 1977).

Major control points of the calcium-regulated PTH secretion may include hormone synthesis and degradation within parathyroid cells (Fig. 3). An additional control point appears to be the adenylate cyclase of the parathyroid cells. Some minimum extracellular magnesium concentration is required for the release of the hormone. The detailed contribution of catecholamines and of the D-vitamins to the regulation of secretion is at present unknown. The pathogenesis of "autonomous" primary hyperparathyroidism and the regulation of the parathyroid tissue mass in the absence of known stimulators remains to be demonstrated.

C. Regulation of Parathyroid Hormone Responses

Raisz (1963b) was the first to study the feedback regulation of the parathyroids by extracellular calcium concentrations. He did this by maintaining parathyroid explants for 48 hr in tissue culture. PTH levels were assessed in a bioassay, where the release of ^{45}Ca from embryonic bone was determined. The inverse relationship between extracellular calcium concentrations and biologically active PTH was demonstrated. However, the parathyroid glands were cultured for 24–48 hr, which precluded the study of the regulation of rapid responses seen *in vivo*. On gel filtration analysis fractions co-eluting with bPTH-(1–84) were responsible for the increased ^{45}Ca release in the presence of 0.75 m*M* calcium (Au *et al.*, 1970). Similar fractions produced marked hypercalcemia *in vivo* in chickens (Feinblatt *et al.*, 1975). In other *in vitro* and in most of the *in vivo* studies PTH levels were determined radioimmunologically. These measurements usually include a mixture of intact PTH-(1–84) and of its fragments. Since PTH fragments have been demonstrated in the venous effluent of the parathyroid glands *in vivo*, it is possible that fragments seen in the medium of parathyroid explants are secreted by the glands and are not necessarily artefacts of the culture conditions (Flueck *et al.*, 1977; Sherwood *et al.*, 1970b; Arnaud *et al.*, 1971b; Hanley *et al.*, 1978). On the other hand, PTH in the peripheral circulation represents the difference between that secreted by the glands and that metabolized in peripheral organs. Under these circumstances it is preferable to use the term PTH response for peripherally measured PTH levels rather than to imply that a given plasma level reflects secretion only. Studies such as those by Mayer *et al.* (1976, 1979; Mayer and Hurst, 1978a), who measured PTH levels in the venous effluent of bovine parathyroid glands in response to various regulators, may come closest to measuring regulation of hormone secretion. However, in the Mayer studies individual samples included PTH that had been produced in 5–15 min periods. Such intervals are probably too long for the study of the acute response that occurred within seconds and minutes (Fischer *et al.*, 1973a,c; Blum *et al.*, 1974b). The perifusion of parathyroid pieces or dispersed cells *in vitro,* where secretory responses occuring within min can be estimated, appears to be the most suitable system mimicing PTH secretion *in vivo* (Hanley *et al.*, 1980; Dempster *et al.*, 1981). Ultimately, it will be necessary to integrate the information obtained on PTH responses *in vivo* and *in vitro* with studies on the metabolism of PTH within parathyroid cells and in peripheral organs (see Sections III,A and IV).

1. Calcium

Secretory responses of the parathyroid glands are inversely related to the extracellular ionized calcium concentration (Sherwood *et al.*, 1966; Care *et al.*, 1966; Fischer *et al.*, 1973a). During an acute fall of the plasma calcium concentration caused by ethyleneglycol-bis(β-aminoethyl ether)-N,N'-tetraacetate (EGTA) infusions in cows *in vivo,* PTH was released from the parathyroid glands within less than 20 sec (Blum *et al.*, 1974b). The release of PTH was already stimulated by small (0.1 mg/dl) falls in the plasma calcium concentration. The magnitude of PTH responses was determined by decrements of the plasma calcium concentration of up to 1.2 mg/dl. When the decrement was greater, PTH responses did not rise further (Fig. 5). A similar type of relationship was demonstrated in cows with postparturient hypocalcemia (Blum *et al.*, 1974a), in rats kept on calcium- and vitamin D-deficient diets (Bronner *et al.*, 1976) and in newborn infants (Wieland *et al.*, 1978). More direct evidence that extracellular calcium concentrations over a narrow range are inversely related to PTH secretion came from measurements obtained by Mayer and Hurst (1978a) in the venous parathyroid effluent. Parathyroid hormone responses were not fully suppressed in the presence of high extracellular calcium concentrations (Mayer *et al.*, 1976). The secreted nonsuppressible PTH could represent in part biologically inactive breakdown products. During calcium infusions in patients with primary hyperparathyroidism the COOH-terminal fragments thought to be biologically inactive, remained in the circulation for hours (von Lilienfeld-Toal *et al.*, 1976). In fact, there is evidence that presumably biologically inactive COOH-terminal PTH fragments are preferentially secreted at a high calcium concentration (Hanley *et al.*, 1978; Mayer *et al.*, 1979).

The PTH responses during sustained hypocalcemia are biphasic. Initially, there occurs a rapid and burst-like release of PTH, followed by a second phase during which hormone release is sustained. The second phase has not been seen in the catecholamine induced PTH responses (Blum *et al.*, 1978).

Parathyroid hormone levels are related to the phosphate intake. Oral administration of phosphate has resulted in increased PTH levels, while plasma ionized and total calcium concentrations tended to decrease (Reiss *et al.*, 1970; Jowsey *et al.*, 1974). Small increases in serum phosphate have been found to increase PTH levels in patients with phosphate diabetes (Fanconi *et al.*, 1974). During

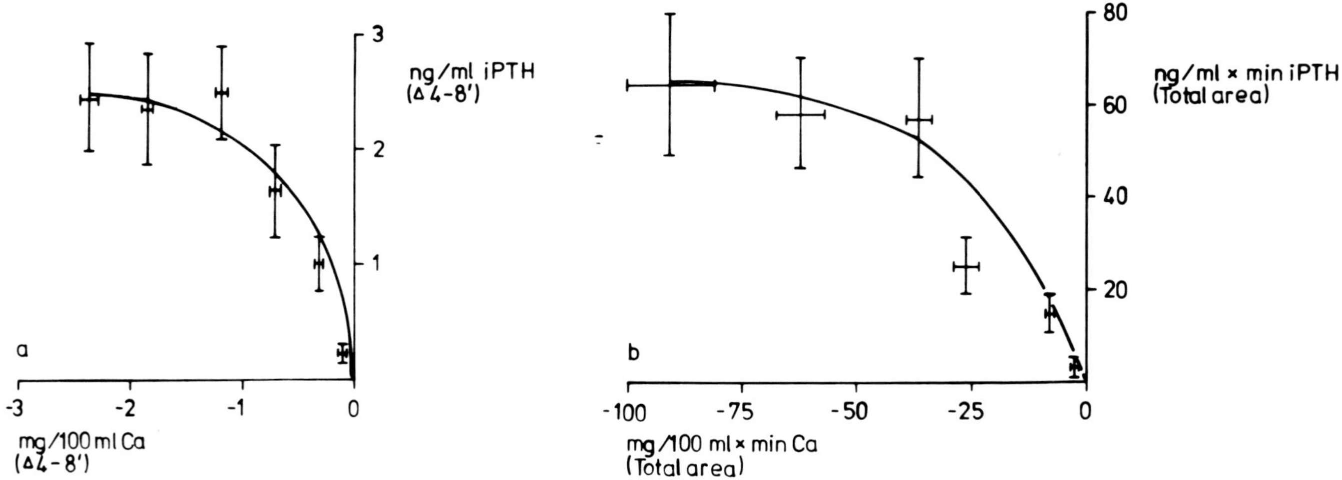

Fig. 5. Relationship between the degree of hypocalcemia during infusions with EGTA and peak PTH responses (left), and total decremental change of calcium and total incremental PTH output (right). Amino terminal immunoreactive PTH as determined with [^{131}I]bPTH-(1-84), antibodies to bPTH (chicken 12 *M*, diluted 1:2000) and bPTH-(1-84) as standard. (From Blum *et al.*, 1974b.)

dietary phosphate deprivation, both PTH and calcium levels tended to fall (Dominguez *et al.*, 1976). Phosphate deprivation is an important factor in the prevention of secondary hyperparathyroidism of chronic renal failure (Slatopolsky *et al.*, 1971). During phosphate infusions serum phosphate increases, serum ionized (and total) calcium decrease, and PTH levels are stimulated (Sherwood *et al.*, 1968; Fischer *et al.*, 1973a). Calcium infusions suppress the phosphate-induced release of PTH. PTH responses to phosphate are reciprocally related to changes in the serum ionized calcium concentration, and it appears unlikely that phosphate stimulates PTH secretion directly.

2. *Magnesium*

The effects of changes in the extracellular magnesium concentration are qualitatively comparable to those produced by calcium when studied in parathyroid explants, low-magnesium-stimulating and high-magnesium-suppressing PTH responses (Sherwood *et al.*, 1966, 1970a; Oldham *et al.*, 1971). PTH measurements in parathyroid explant cultures and in the venous drainage of parathyroid glands have, furthermore, shown that, on a molar basis, magnesium is 2–3 times less effective than calcium in suppressing PTH responses (Habener and Potts, 1976; Mayer and Hurst, 1978b). Following magnesium infusions *in vivo* PTH levels were suppressed in spite of concomitant hypocalcemia (J. W. Blum and J. A. Fischer, unpublished observations). Severe magnesium deficiency (serum magnesium < 1.0 mg/dl) is characterized by hypocalcemia accompanied by low PTH levels. If magnesium is infused under these conditions, PTH levels are paradoxically raised (Fig. 4) (Anast *et al.*, 1972; David *et al.*, 1975; Chase and Slatopolsky, 1974; Signer *et al.*, 1975; Anast *et al.*, 1976). Comparable results have been obtained *in vitro* (Takatsuki *et al.*, 1980). The results suggest that some levels of extracellular magnesium are required for an adequate secretory response of the parathyroid glands. Magnesium is not only required at the level of the parathyroid glands but also for the end-organs of PTH, where calcemic and phosphaturic responses have been found impaired (Estep *et al.*, 1969; Levi *et al.*, 1974; Rude *et al.*, 1976; Freitag *et al.*, 1979).

3. *Catecholamines and Calcitonin*

With the exception of a low serum calcium concentration, epinephrine appears to be the most powerful stimulator of PTH secretion *in vivo*. The PTH responses of cows to epinephrine were as sensitive as their plasma glucose and free fatty acid responses (Fischer *et al.*, 1973c). Stimulation of the PTH release by isoproterenol and suppression by propranolol point to the existence of β-adrenergic receptors of parathyroid cells (Brown *et al.*, 1977b). PTH responses to epinephrine were suppressed in hypercalcemic animals (Fischer *et al.*, 1973c; Kukreja *et al.*, 1976b). On the other hand, epinephrine enhanced the PTH release induced by a hypocalcemia and thus appeared to modulate the effect of hypocalcemia. In contrast to the biphasic PTH response to sustained hypocalcemia, prolonged epinephrine infusions initially produced only a release of PTH (Blum *et al.*, 1978). Similarly, the addition of catecholamines to the incubation medium of parathyroid explants or cells stimulated PTH release (Sherwood and Abe, 1972b; Williams *et al.*, 1973; Brown *et al.*, 1977a). PTH responses to isoproterenol *in vitro* were also transient (Brown *et al.*, 1977b; Hanley *et al.*, 1980). Thereafter, the receptors to catecholamines became refractory to additional stimuli and desentization took place. PTH responses to hypocalcemia and to catecholamines thus appear mediated by different, but closely related mechanisms of the parathyroid cells.

Dopamine, as well as β-adrenergic catecholamines, have been shown to stimulate cyclic AMP production in parathyroid cells and to induce PTH release *in vitro* and *in vivo* (Brown *et al.*, 1977c; Blum *et al.*, 1979b).

All these results have been obtained in respect to the exogenous administration of possibly pharmacological amounts of catecholamines. The physiological importance of catecholamines as regulators of PTH secretion remains to be assessed. Preliminary evidence that endogenous catecholamines stimulate the release of PTH comes from experiments of Blum *et al.* (1979a), who demonstrated an increase of epinephrine and norepinephrine as well as of PTH levels, when cows were subjected to treadmill exercise. Hypoglycemia that presumably stimulated epinephrine release in man caused increased PTH levels, even though calcium and magnesium concentrations remained unchanged (Shah *et al.*, 1975).

Calcitonin has been found to stimulate the release of PTH in parathyroid explant cultures (Fischer *et al.*, 1971). In patients with medullary carcinoma of the thyroid diffuse hyperplasia of the parathyroid glands has been observed as part of the multiple endocrine neoplasia, type 2 (Steiner *et al.*, 1968). PTH levels were paradoxically raised in some of these patients during calcium infusions, together with the expected increase in calcitonin (Deftos and Parthemore, 1974). This observation suggests that calcitonin may also have a direct effect on PTH response. The detailed physiological role of catecholamines and of calcitonin in the regulation of secretion of PTH remains to be determined.

4. *The D Vitamins*

In vitamin D-deficiency rickets PTH blood levels are elevated both in hypocalcemic and in normocalcemic patients (Arnaud *et al.*, 1972; Joffe *et al.*, 1972; Fischer *et al.*, 1973b). Moreover, PTH levels can be reduced to normal by treatment with vitamin D_3, raising serum calcium levels, but also without altering the serum ionized or total calcium concentrations (Fischer *et al.*, 1973b). Consequently, vitamin D may act to inhibit PTH secretion.

Exogenous 1,25-$(OH)_2D_3$ decreases serum PTH in normal men and in patients with renal insufficiency and elevated serum calcium (Llach *et al.*, 1977; Brickman *et al.*, 1974; Binswanger *et al.*, 1979). Concerning direct effects of

$1,25\text{-}(OH)_2D_3$, conflicting results have, however, been obtained. Thus, in pharmacological amounts it appears to directly suppress (Chertow *et al.*, 1975a) or to stimulate (Canterbury *et al.*, 1978) PTH levels, whereas the inhibition of parathyroid gland weight and of PTH secretion by $24,25\text{-}(OH)_2D_3$ may be physiologically important (Bates *et al.*, 1975; Henry *et al.*, 1977; Canterbury *et al.*, 1978). In intact rats kept on low calcium diet PTH levels and duodenal calcium transport were raised, the synthesis of $1,25\text{-}(OH)_2D_3$ having presumably increased (Grubenmann *et al.*, 1978). Consequently, at least in the rat, the effect of endogenous $1,25\text{-}(OH)_2D_3$ in suppressing PTH release may be unimportant.

5. *Parathyroid Tissue Mass*

Suggestive evidence for the concept that an increase in parathyroid tissue leads to raised PTH levels came from the hypercalcemia seen in rats with multiple isologous parathyroid transplants (Gittes and Raddé, 1966). Consequently, one cause for increased PTH levels may be an increase in gland mass. The hypercalcemia caused by increased PTH levels is apparently unable to inhibit PTH secretion adequately. The picture thus resembles so called "autonomous" secretion of PTH seen in primary hyperparathyroidism. Even so, calcium infusions will decrease PTH levels in patients with primary hyperparathyroidism, and EDTA or phosphate infusions will raise PTH in such patients as well as *in vitro* (Reiss and Canterbury, 1969; Murray *et al.*, 1972; Binswanger and Fischer, 1974; Lockefeer *et al.*, 1974; Birnbaumer *et al.*, 1977; Habener, 1978; Brown *et al.*, 1978). In conclusion, PTH levels are inadequately suppressed in hypercalcemic patients with primary hyperparathyroidism; the etiology of the increased tissue mass causing raised PTH secretion remains unknown.

6. *Additional Potential Regulators*

Au (1976) has demonstrated a direct effect of cortisol on PTH release in rat parathyroid cultures. Cortisol in pharmacological amounts injected into intact rats caused parathyroid hyperplasia and an increase in serum PTH levels with no corresponding change in calcium (Williams *et al.*, 1974). Comparable studies have been performed in man (Fucik *et al.*, 1975). The decreased bone mass seen in rats treated with cortisol, however, appears to be unrelated to the presence of the parathyroid glands (Kukreja *et al.*, 1976a). Furthermore, adrenalectomy prevented the fall of the plasma calcium in thyroparathyroidectomized rats (Williams *et al.*, 1974). A rare cause of hypercalcemia in man is acute Addison's disease, a condition that corresponds to the functional removal of the adrenal cortex. The hypocalcemic effect of cortisol may be an additional cause of secondary hyperparathyroidism which could then be prevented by acute adrenalectomy. Since pharmacological amounts of cortisol are required to demonstrate an effect on PTH secretion, the physiological importance of this regulatory principle remains to be demonstrated.

Growth hormone may be a stimulator of PTH secretion. Rats receiving injections of bovine growth hormone showed a progressive increase in both serum PTH and calcium after the second week; at 6 weeks the weight of the parathyroid gland had increased slightly (Lancer *et al.*, 1976).

Somatostatin was shown to suppress serum PTH levels *in vivo* in rats and monkeys, whereas in man somatostatin, in amounts that suppress plasma glucagon levels, was ineffective (Hargis *et al.*, 1978; Deftos *et al.*, 1976).

IV. METABOLISM OF PARATHYROID HORMONE

Intact PTH-(1–84) is metabolized in peripheral organs but also by parathyroid tissue. The relative contribution of PTH fragments directly secreted by the parathyroid glands to the peripheral circulation is as yet unknown (see Section III,A).

A. *In Vitro*

Parathyroid hormone is rapidly metabolized in broken cell preparations of the liver and the kidney (Fang and Tashjian, 1972; Martin *et al.*, 1969a; Fischer *et al.*, 1972; Fujita *et al.*, 1973a; Londos and Bronner, 1973; Catherwood and Singer, 1974). Indeed, the proteolytic degradation of bPTH-(1–84) into NH_2- and COOH-terminal fragments takes place in Kupffer cells and not in hepatocytes (Segre *et al.*, 1981b). Incubation of $[^{125}I]$bPTH-(1–84) with purified canine renal plasma membranes or isolated kidney tubules resulted in the generation of the 7000-molecular weight COOH-terminal fragment, the predominant PTH species found in the peripheral circulation of patients with primary hyperparathyroidism (Catherwood and Singer, 1974). The conversion of radioiodinated bPTH-(1–84) to its fragments by a crude liver extract was accelerated and the degradation of the fragments retarded by EDTA (Fischer *et al.*, 1972). These findings have been extended by Canterbury *et al.*, (1975), who demonstrated in the course of a liver perfusion that bPTH-(1–84) was metabolized into a biologically active 3500 molecular weight NH_2-terminal and biologically inactive 7000 and 3000 molecular weight COOH-terminal fragments. This conversion is activated by low calcium concentrations. Similar fragments were also generated within 5 min after the addition of bPTH-(1–84) to the perfused isolated canine kidney (Hruska *et al.*, 1977). The degradation of bPTH-(1–84) and of its fragments was inversely related to the calcium concentration in the perfusate. The physiological relevance of these findings remains to be demonstrated. Oldham *et al.* (1978), on the other hand, have demonstrated in kidney perfusion experiments that more intact PTH is extracted by the kidney at high than at low calcium concentrations. The results might explain the proportionally higher amounts of

COOH-terminal PTH fragments in hypercalcemic patients with primary hyperparathyroidism as compared to hypocalcemic patients with secondary hyperparathyroidism and normal renal function (Dambacher *et al.*, 1979). Biologically active NH_2-terminal fragments are bound to receptors located on the contraluminal side of tubular epithelial cells, and biologically inactive COOH-terminal fragments are presumably removed by glomerular filtration and tubular reabsorption (Shlatz *et al.*, 1975; Martin *et al.*, 1977). Specific and physiologically important sites of degradation of PTH, if present, remain to be localized.

The biological significance of the fragments produced by the kidney remains to be delineated. In view of the comparable stimulation of adenylate cyclase activity of renal cortical membranes by intact PTH-(1–84) and by its NH_2-terminal fragments (see Section II), the question arises as to whether PTH-(1–84) has to be metabolized in order to become biologically active, or whether the intact hormone interacts with these sites prior to its metabolic breakdown. Goltzman *et al.* (1976b; Goltzman, 1978) have presented preliminary evidence that bPTH-(1–84) stimulated adenylate cyclase activity in renal cortical and skeletal membranes directly without having to be cleaved into PTH fragments. Martin *et al.* (1978), on the other hand, have shown that synthetic bPTH-(1–34) is much more active in stimulating cyclic AMP production by isolated perfused bone than intact bPTH-(1–84). The authors implied that peripheral cleavage of the intact hormone into NH_2-terminal fragments may be a prerequisite for biological activity at the level of the skeleton.

Finally, the metabolic degradation of bPTH-(1–84) in bovine plasma or human serum is negligible for up to 24 hr (Hunziker *et al.*, 1977). PTH fragments are generated in peripheral organs *in vivo* but not in the plasma.

B. *In Vivo*

The rate of elimination of PTH from the circulation is assessed either following the exogenous administration of bPTH-(1–84) or the removal of human parathyroid tumors, or as a result of calcium infusions.

When administered iv, bPTH-(1–84) is metabolized within minutes into NH_2- and COOH-terminal fragments. The initial cleavage takes place at sites between amino acid residues 30 and 40 resulting in the generation of a 7000 molecular weight COOH- and a 3500-molecular-weight NH_2-terminal fragment. COOH-terminal fragments have been clearly visualized (Segre *et al.*, 1974; Hunziker *et al.*, 1977), whereas Hunziker *et al.* (1977) also noted a NH_2-terminal fragment. By subjecting pooled fractions containing the 7000 molecular weight fragment to sequence analysis and identifying the number of cycles required before release of radioactivity located at the tyrosine residue at position 43, Segre *et al.* (1974, 1976, 1977) localized the cleavage of the intact hormone at sites between residues 34 and 38. The synthetic bPTH-(28–48) was found to be an inhibitor of the *in vivo* cleavage of bPTH-(1–84) when administered simultaneously with the intact hormone (Rosenblatt *et al.*, 1977). Disappearance rates of intact bPTH-(1–84) and of the NH_2-terminal fragments were similar, whereas COOH-terminal fragments remained in the circulation longer. However, there is no evidence to support the notion that COOH-terminal fragments persist in the circulation very long (Hruska *et al.*, 1975; Segre *et al.*, 1974; Hunziker *et al.*, 1977). The NH_2-terminal fragment may correspond to the biologically active NH_2-terminal 3500 molecular weight, and the COOH-terminal fragments to the biologically inactive 3500 and 7000 molecular weight COOH-terminal PTH forms that Canterbury *et al.* (1975) generated when they perfused rat livers with bPTH-(1–84). Intact hPTH-(1–84) was essentially undetectable 30 min after patients with primary hyperparathyroidism had been parathyroidectomized. At the same time hPTH fragments were clearly visualized (Canterbury and Reiss, 1972).

The PTH excreted in the urine, if any, has not been adequately examined so far with biochemical and immunochemical methods. A hypercalcemic PTH-like material has been found, but not characterized in urine (Bethune and Turpin, 1968). Patients with surgically verified primary hyperparathyroidism appear to excrete more of this principle than normal subjects. The material was undetectable in patients with hypoparathyroidism. PTH excretion by the bile also has not been investigated. Our discussion of the metabolism of PTH by the liver and by the kidney *in vivo* is therefore limited to the observations made in the venous effluents of the two organs. Indeed, arteriovenous PTH concentration differences of exogenous and endogenous hormone have been demonstrated in liver and kidney (Singer *et al.*, 1975; Catherwood *et al.*, 1976; Corvilain *et al.*, 1977; Hruska *et al.*, 1981). According to Martin *et al.* (1976, 1978) only intact PTH-(1–84) is metabolized by the liver, and no hepatic uptake of fragments can be demonstrated, whereas the skeleton removes PTH fragments. The kidney, on the other hand, removes both intact hormone and PTH fragments from the circulation.

Another approach to the study of PTH metabolism is to localize exogenously adminstered hormone by histological techniques. Ten minutes after the iv injection of [^{125}I]- or [^{3}H]bPTH-(1–84) there was high deposition in the kidney with most of the activity localized in the proximal convoluted tubules of rats and dogs (de Kretser *et al.*, 1970; Nordquist and Palmieri, 1974; W. F. Neuman *et al.*, 1975a). By immunofluorescence PTH was found to be present only in the cytoplasm of renal tubules, whereas electron autoradiographic studies showed most of the labeled hormone to be located in the mitochondria of proximal tubular cells. Additional sites as revealed by autoradiographic techniques, are the periosteal and endosteal cells adjacent to the bone matrix (W. F. Neuman *et al.*, 1975a). However, whether the intracellular localization of PTH is related to functional sites of the hormone or to its degradation is not yet known.

All these studies serve as background for the quantitative analysis of the plasma kinetics of exogenously administered PTH-(1–84), or the disappearance of endogenous PTH after parathyroidectomy or during calcium infusions. In studies performed up to 1969, half-lives of disappearance of nonlabeled or of radioiodinated bPTH-(1–84) injected iv into normal human subjects, rats, dogs and cows, and of endogenous PTH after removal of parathyroid tumors in patients with primary hyperparathyroidism varied between 10 and 30 min (Melick *et al.*, 1965; Sherwood *et al.*, 1968; Martin *et al.*, 1969b; Melick and Martin, 1969; Buckle, 1969). In subsequent studies, half-lives of the disappearance of iv administered bPTH-(1–84) of 2–9 min were observed in dogs, chickens, and calves, and of endogenous bPTH during calcium infusions of 2–4 min in cows (Blum *et al.*, 1974b, 1978; Hruska *et al.*, 1975; Singer *et al.*, 1975; W. F. Neuman *et al.*, 1975b; Hunziker *et al.*, 1977). In some of the studies through 1969, early timed blood samples were not obtained. These are essential to a precise determination of the half-lives of PTH. The disappearance rates of endogenous PTH as measured after parathyroidectomy, or of iv administered bPTH-(1–84) are longer than normal in nephrectomized patients, dogs, and rats (Berson and Yalow, 1968; Melick and Martin, 1969; Martin *et al.*, 1969b; Hruska *et al.*, 1975; Papapoulos *et al.*, 1977; Freitag *et al.*, 1978). After hepatectomy and nephrectomy the clearance of bPTH-(1–84) is more markedly reduced than after nephrectomy alone (Segre *et al.*, 1981a). Moreover, both the hepatic and renal uptake of intact PTH are reduced in dogs with chronic renal failure (Hruska *et al.*, 1981). These observations point to the liver and the kidney as important catabolic and/or excreting site of the hormone described above. In the majority of these studies measurements of radioactive or immunoreactive blood PTH included a mixture biologically active and inactive intact PTH-(1–84) and its fragments. They therefore yielded information on the overall metabolism of the hormone and its fragments, but did not differentiate between biologically active and inactive forms.

An important contribution has come from the study of Goldsmith *et al.* (1973), who demonstrated that the rate of disappearance of endogenous hPTH during calcium infusions was prolonged in patients with chronic renal insufficiency, when serum PTH was measured with a radioimmunoassay system that recognized COOH-terminal fragments in addition to intact PTH-(1–84). Comparable results were obtained by Silverman and Yalow (1973), who demonstrated that intact hPTH-(1–84) levels decreased reversibly during calcium infusions in a patient with chronic renal insufficiency, while the amounts of circulating COOH-terminal PTH fragments remained practically unchanged. Furthermore, during calcium infusions in patients with secondary hyperparathyroidism due to chronic renal failure, intact hPTH-(1–84) disappeared from the circulation, while biologically inactive COOH-terminal fragments remained clearly visible (Born *et al.*, 1980).

In conclusion, intact PTH-(1–84) is metabolized *in vivo* to NH_2- and COOH-terminal fragments within minutes. According to Martin *et al.* (1976) intact PTH is metabolized by the liver and kidney, whereas PTH fragments are mainly extracted by the kidney. In renal insufficiency PTH remains in the circulation longer than in normal subjects, thus pointing to the kidney as an important metabolic and/or excretory site of the hormone.

V. BIOLOGICAL EFFECTS OF PARATHYROID HORMONE

The mechanism of action and the biological effects of PTH have been the subject of several reviews (Aurbach and Heath, 1974; Borle, 1974; Parsons, 1976; Rasmussen and Bordier, 1974). A considerable number of results obtained on the biological effects of PTH are not necessarily relevant for an understanding of the physiology and the pathophysiology of the hormone until the biological properties of circulating endogenous PTH can be evaluated in more detail. Nevertheless, the different sites of action are summarized with particular emphasis on the mechanism of action of the hormone.

A. Actions on the Kidney

1. Mechanism of Action

At the cellular level PTH binding and stimulation of cyclic AMP formation have been documented. The specific binding of [^{125}I]bPTH-(1–84) and -(1–34) and of [^{3}H]bPTH-(1–84) to plasma membranes from bovine renal cortex and rat kidney has been demonstrated (Sutcliffe *et al.*, 1973; Di Bella *et al.*, 1974; Zull *et al.*, 1977). The concentrations of bPTH-(1–84) and -(1–34) for half-maximal inhibition of binding of labeled hormone as well as half-maximal activation of 3′,5′-adenylyl cyclase are several orders of magnitude higher than circulating PTH levels (Di Bella *et al.*, 1974; Nissenson and Arnaud, 1979, Nissenson *et al.*, 1981). Biologically inactive oxidized PTH failed to inhibit the binding of labeled bPTH-(1–84) or to activate the adenylate cyclase. The enzyme from plasma membrane fractions of rat renal cortex was activated by PTH, whereas the enzyme from the renal medulla was activated by vasopressin (Chase and Aurbach, 1968).

PTH-sensitive adenylate cyclase activity has been found in rat and rabbit glomeruli (Sraer *et al.*, 1974; Imbert *et al.*, 1974). As a possible consequence, the single nephron glomerular ultrafiltration rate is decreased in the presence of PTH as well as in hypercalcemic animals (Humes *et al.*, 1978; Ichikawa *et al.*, 1978). Segments of the kidney tubules mainly sensitive to PTH were insensitive to calcitonin (Chabardès *et al.*, 1975, 1976; Morel *et al.*, 1976). Furthermore, selective proteolysis by trypsin of membranes from the rat kidney cortex abolished the adenylate cyclase response to PTH, whereas stimulation by calcitonin and prostaglandin E_1 remained unaltered (Chase, 1975). The PTH-stimulated adenylate cyclase activity was found to be present in contraluminal but not in luminal rat kidney cortex membranes (Shlatz *et al.*, 1975). PTH added to the incubation medium of kidney slices *in vitro* and administered to thyroparathyroidectomized rats *in vivo* (DeRubertis and Craven, 1976; Sakai *et al.*, 1976) stimulated a cyclic AMP-dependent protein kinase activity in rat renal cortex. In contrast to the adenylate cyclase, which is predominantly localized at the contraluminal kidney membrane, the protein kinase(s) is localized at the brush border and may be important for the PTH mediated alterations of solute reabsorption in the proximal tubule (Kinne *et al.*, 1975). Kempson *et al.* (1981) have recently demonstrated that nicotinamide adenine dinucleotide can modulate the transport of inorganic phosphate across the renal luminal brush border membrane and across the proximal tubular wall. In fact, both PTH and dibutyryl cyclic AMP injected into the whole animal but not when applied *in vitro* inhibited the sodium-dependent phosphate uptake by isolated renal brush-border vesicles (Evers *et al.*, 1978). Furthermore, micropuncture data indicate that PTH applied to the contraluminal, but not to the luminal cell side of the proximal convoluted tubule had an inhibitory effect on fluid and glucose reabsorption; a similar inhibitory effect of cyclic AMP on the luminal cell side suggests that it was a mediator of the PTH effect (Baumann *et al.*, 1977).

The extracted bPTH-(1–84) and the synthetic NH_2-terminal bPTH-(1–34) fragment are equally potent in stimulating renal cortical adenylate cyclase activity (see Section II). On gel filtration of pooled sera from patients with primary hyperparathyroidism fractions co-eluting with intact hPTH-(1–84) and a presumably 4500–5000 molecular weight NH_2-terminal fragment stimulated the enzyme, whereas a 7000 molecular weight fragment, presumably a COOH-terminal, was inactive (Canterbury *et al.*, 1973). When PTH was administered to vitamin D-deficient rats, the urinary cyclic AMP and phosphate excretions were blunted; furthermore, a renal cortical adenylate cyclase from vitamin D- and/or calcium-deficient rats showed less activation by PTH than was observed with enzyme prepared from vitamin D-fed animals (Forte *et al.*, 1976; Carnes *et al.*, 1980). The blunted cyclic AMP response could be restored by treatment with calcium and vitamin D. The phosphaturic but not the cyclic AMP response to PTH was blunted in phosphate-deprived rats; this suggests that impaired phosphaturia would contribute to phosphate conservation (Steele, 1976).

In pseudohypoparathyroidism type I, an absent or reduced urinary cyclic AMP response to exogenous PTH was assumed to be the cause of the lack or deficient phosphaturic responses in these patients (Chase *et al.*, 1969b). However, during treatment with calcium or vitamin D the administration of PTH resulted in a normal fall of the tubular reabsorption of phosphate. This was not accompanied by a raised urinary cyclic AMP excretion (Kind *et al.*, 1973; Stögmann and Fischer, 1975). In this disease at least the role and the importance of cyclic AMP as mediator of the cellular responses to PTH remains to be delineated (see Section VII,F).

Besides cyclic AMP, calcium has been recognized as an important mediator of hormonal responses (Rasmussen, 1970). The concentration of the free calcium in the cytoplasm is probably only important for the regulation of the cellular activity. It is estimated to range between 10^{-6} and 10^{-8} M. Changes can usually only be assessed indirectly. This is shown by the measurement of calcium fluxes across the plasma membrane, and the membranes of mitochondria, microsomes and the reticular endothelial system. By making use of monkey kidney cells grown in tissue culture, Borle (1973) has demonstrated that PTH raised the influx end efflux of calcium across the cell membrane, as well as calcium efflux from mitochondria into the cytoplasm. An increased extrusion of calcium from isolated mitochondria *in vitro* had previously been demonstrated by DeLuca *et al.* (1962). Conversely, calcitonin primarily increased the retention of calcium by mitochondria (Borle, 1975). The free calcium concentration appears to be increased after PTH and decreased after the administration of calcitonin. According to these results the mitochondrial membrane appears to be a possible locus for the regulation of calcium transport and the transmission of the hormonal message of PTH and of calcitonin. This would imply, however, that polypeptide hormones can cross the cell membrane. Indeed, Nordquist and Palmieri (1974) have shown that labeled PTH, conserving at least partly its immunoreactive activity, can be localized in the cytoplasm of renal proximal tubular cells and that labeled PTH is found predominantly in mitochondria. The question as to whether PTH crosses the plasma membrane of kidney tubules remains to be resolved.

The relationships between the effect of PTH on the free calcium concentration in the cytoplasm and cyclic AMP are complex. In isolated renal tubules, PTH stimulated the formation of cyclic AMP and gluconeogenesis; in the absence of calcium in the incubation medium, only cyclic AMP was formed (Nagata and Rasmussen, 1970). After PTH injection, the increase in urinary cyclic AMP and phosphate excretion was less in calcium-infused than in control rats.

Calcium had no effect on phosphate excretion induced by dibutyryl cyclic AMP. Calcium inhibited the activation of renal cortical adenylate cyclase in response to PTH, but had no effect on the phosphodiesterase. It appears that the inhibition by calcium occurs at or before the step of PTH-dependent cyclic AMP generation in the kidney (Beck *et al.*, 1974). The addition of purified PTH to isolated kidney mitochondria produced an increased accumulation of magnesium, phosphate and potassium, a release of calcium and hydrogen ions, and a stimulation of respiration (Rasmussen *et al.*, 1964b). The changes are similar to those produced by the hormone on renal tubular function.

In view of the many different effects of PTH in kidney tubules a unifying concept as to whether PTH has one or several sites of action is still lacking. Possible candidates as common mediators for the biological responses to PTH include changes of the free calcium, cyclic AMP, phosphate, and magnesium concentrations and cyclic AMP-associated inhibition of carbonic anhydrase (Beck *et al.*, 1975; Knox *et al.*, 1976; Kinne and Schwartz, 1977).

2. *Biological Effects*

The truly biological effects of PTH have been reviewed extensively by Knox *et al.* (1973), Aurbach and Heath (1974), Borle (1974), and by Diaz-Buxo and Knox (1975), and they are only summarized in the present context. Early effects include an increase of the urinary cyclic AMP, followed by a raised phosphate excretion (Chase and Aurbach, 1967). The stimulation of the urinary excretion of phosphate is caused by a decreased tubular reabsorption in the proximal tubules, but probably also by a raised secretion of phosphate in the distal tubules, with the phosphate clearance occasionally exceeding the creatinine clearance (Webster *et al.*, 1967; Boudry al., 1975). The tubular reabsorption of calcium is increased under the influence of PTH (Nordin and Peacock, 1969).

Agus *et al.* (1973) have demonstrated that PTH inhibits the proximal tubular sodium reabsorption; but that the nonreabsorbed sodium was absorbed distally. The administration of PTH also caused a raised bicarbonate excretion, which, however, was not sufficient to cause metabolic acidosis. The effect was caused by an inhibition of proximal tubular reabsorption of bicarbonate (Karlinsky *et al.*, 1974; Bank and Aynedjian, 1976; Arruda *et al.*, 1977).

Finally, PTH caused a raised excretion of several amino acids and of glucose (Short *et al.*, 1974). Aminoaciduria is associated with some cases of hyperparathyroidism, but is not a constant feature. The tubular reabsorptive capacity (Tm/GFR) of glucose is raised in patients with hyperparathyroidism; however, there is a considerable overlap with control subjects (Halver, 1967). The effect is caused by an inhibition of the renal reabsorption of glucose and in closely related to the PTH induced inhibition of phosphate reabsorption (Harter *et al.*, 1974). Finally, Morris *et al.* (1971) have demonstrated a complex tubular dysfunction (reduced reabsorption of phosphate, amino acids, glucose, uric acid, and bicarbonate) in a patient with a hereditary fructose intolerance that may have been induced by PTH.

The administration of dibutyryl cyclic AMP into thyroparathyroidectomized rats mimics the effects of PTH leading to an inhibition of the tubular reabsorption of phosphate, bicarbonate, and sodium, and a stimulation of calcium and magnesium (Rasmussen *et al.*, 1968; Russell *et al.*, 1968; Agus *et al.*, 1971; Karlinsky *et al.*, 1974; Burnatowska *et al.*, 1977). The importance of cyclic AMP in the mediation of the cellular responses to PTH appears to be reasonably well established.

B. Actions on the Bone

1. *In Vitro*

The activation of skeletal adenylate cyclase by PTH and calcitonin is well established (Chase *et al.*, 1969a; Peck *et al.*, 1973; Heersche *et al.*, 1974). Moreover, a separation of PTH and calcitonin-sensitive from nonresponsive bone cells has been achieved (Wong and Cohn, 1974, 1975; Smith and Johnston, 1975; Nagata *et al.*, 1976; Luben *et al.*, 1976). Selective proteolysis by trypsin in membranes from rat fetal calvaria abolished the adenylate cyclase response to PTH, whereas the stimulation by calcitonin and prostaglandin E_2 remained unaltered (Chase and Obert, 1975). A separate effect of calcitonin must also be considered, since it blocked PTH- but also cyclic AMP-induced bone mobilization; this suggests that the inhibitory effect of calcitonin is on a step beyond adenylate cyclase activation by PTH (Rasmussen *et al.*, 1968). An increased uptake of [^{3}H]cytidine into ribonucleic acid has been observed in the presence of PTH, but also of a calcium-rich peritoneal fluid; presumably calcium can also act as a second messenger of this particular effect of PTH (Park and Talmage, 1968).

The administration of PTH causes an initial and transient uptake of radioactive calcium from the incubation medium by 5-day-old mouse calvaria. This rise in uptake occurs within minutes and is followed by the release of calcium over the next 3–4 hr (Robertson *et al.*, 1972). The simultaneous release of calcium and hydroxyproline from embryonic bone into the incubation medium and the formation of osteoclasts have been observed after 2–3 days (Gaillard, 1961; Raisz, 1965; Martin *et al.*, 1965). A parallel reduction of calvaria ash and hydroxyproline content suggests the simultaneous dissolution of bone mineral and collagen. PTH stimulated the release of calcium from devitalized bone by cultured osteoclast-type bone cells, but also by ascites carcinoma cells (Luben *et al.*, 1977; Tennenhouse *et al.*, 1966). Besides a stimulation of bone resorption, small amounts of hPTH-(1–34) appear to stimulate bone formation as evidenced on histological examination of mouse long bone rudiments (Gaillard *et al.*, 1977).

Additional direct or indirect effects of PTH include a decreased citrate decarboxylation, increased hyaluronate synthesis, activation of lysosomal enzymes, lactate production, decreased collagen synthesis, and stimulation of collagenase activity (Wolinsky and Cohn, 1969; Luben *et al.*, 1974; Vaes, 1967; Dietrich *et al.*, 1976; Sakamoto *et al.*, 1975). A PTH-induced synthesis of hyaluronate in fetal radii can be suppressed with calcitonin, whereas calcitonin has no effect on the decreased production of citrate. Presumably different cell types are involved in producing the two effects (Luben *et al.*, 1976).

2. *In Vivo*

The well known catabolic effects of PTH leading to chronic demineralization of bone and osteitis fibrosa have been amply documented. According to Rasmussen *et al.* (1964a), the release of calcium from the skeleton involves the stimulation of protein synthesis. PTH was ineffective in raising the serum calcium concentration above normal when rats were treated with actinomycin D. PTH was equally ineffective in raising serum calcium levels in a vitamin D-deficient hypoparathyroid patient and in vitamin D-deficient, parathyroidectomized rats (Gerblich *et al.*, 1977; Harrison *et al.*, 1958; Rasmussen *et al.*, 1963; Arnaud *et al.*, 1966). Vitamin D, but also parenteral calcium and dietary lactose, restored defective PTH responses (Rasmussen *et al.*, 1963; Au and Raisz, 1967; Gerblich *et al.*, 1977).

The administration of dibutyryl cyclic AMP to thyroparathyroidectomized rats mimics the effect of PTH, i.e., leading to rises in plasma calcium and to increased urinary calcium and hydroxyproline (Rasmussen *et al.*, 1968).

As a result of raised bone resorption, a negative calcium balance is found in patients with primary hyperparathyroidism and severe hypercalcemia (reviewed by Parsons, 1976). Histological examination of bone biopsies has revealed increased resorption in the majority of patients with primary hyperparathyroidism (Jowsey, 1966; Miravet *et al.*, 1969; Byers and Smith, 1971; Schenk *et al.*, 1973). The rate of bone resorption is, however, difficult to assess on histological grounds because functional properties of osteoclasts and of the bone resorbing surfaces are unknown. In addition to osteoclastic, osteocytic osteolysis appears to be another site of action of PTH. This results in localized demineralization and enhanced proteolytic activity; osteolysis can be suppressed with calcitonin (Bélanger and Rasmussen, 1968). As a result of increased bone resorption and collagenolysis the urinary excretion of hydroxyproline can be increased in patients with primary hyperparathyroidism.

Rasmussen and Bordier (1974) have suggested that the activities of osteoclasts and osteoblasts are directly related. They have proposed a sequential activation of preosteoclasts into osteoclasts, which would then be converted into preosteoblasts and osteoblasts. In short-term experiments, PTH induces an increased activation of new osteoprogenitor cells, an inhibition of the conversion of osteoclasts to osteoblasts, an increase in the activity of preexisting osteoclasts and a suppression of preexisting osteoblasts resulting in an increase in bone resorption and a decrease in bone formation. On the other hand, during long-term administration of moderate doses of PTH or in moderately severe primary hyperparathyroidism in man a secondary rise in the size of the osteoblast pool occurs, which usually appears sufficient to reestablish relative skeletal balance with a concomitant increase in bone remodelling.

Possible anabolic effects of PTH have been presented in detail in a recent review of Parsons (1976). The histological evidence comes from the quantitative morphometric analysis of bone biopsies obtained from patients with primary hyperparathyroidism (Jowsey, 1966; Byers and Smith, 1971; Schenk *et al.*, 1973). An increased extent of osteoid seams was a rather constant finding in hyperparathyroidism and presumed to result from vitamin D-deficiency (Woodhouse *et al.*, 1971; Bordier *et al.*, 1975). An increased number of osteoid seams can also be an expression of a raised matrix synthesis with an associated increase in the number of osteoblasts (Schenk *et al.*, 1973). The raised serum alkaline phosphatase and an increased accretion rate of nonradioactive strontium or labeled calcium represent suggestive evidence of a possible stimulation of bone formation (Dent and Harter, 1962; Fraser *et al.*, 1960; Lafferty and Pearson, 1963; Milhaud and Bourichon, 1964; Sammon *et al.*, 1970). Finally, focal areas of osteosclerosis is a well-known finding, particularly in patients with secondary hyperparathyroidism of chronic renal failure (Kaye *et al.*, 1960; Doyle, 1972; Campos *et al.*, 1976). It is less frequently found in patients with primary hyperparathyroidism (Genant *et al.*, 1975). In both intact and thyroparathyroidectomized rats, the administration of PTH resulted in an increased incorporation of [^{3}H]proline into bone hydroxyproline (Kalu *et al.*, 1970). Bone alkaline phosphatase and calcium-adenosine triphosphatase activities were also elevated and may be related to an increase in the metabolic activity of osteoblasts (Weisbrode *et al.*, 1974). The calcium balance is positive in some patients with moderate primary hyperparathyroidism and a small increase of serum calcium concentrations (reviewed by Parsons, 1976). These results served as rational for a long-term administration of hPTH-(1–34) in patients with postmenopausal osteoporosis (Reeve *et al.*, 1976a,b). Results so far have been disappointing.

C. Additional Sites of Action

The depressed intestinal calcium absorption in parathyroidectomized rats at high calcium intakes (Sammon *et al.*, 1970) may be indirect and caused by an inhibition of the formation of 1,25(OH)$_2$D$_3$ at the level of the kidney (Boyle *et al.*, 1971; Garabedian *et al.*, 1972; Rasmussen *et al.*, 1972). Reductions in serum phosphate concentrations that may be associated with hyperparathyroidism stimulate renal synthesis of 1,25(OH)$_2$D$_3$ in man (Gray *et al.*, 1977). The *in vitro* intestinal transport of calcium and phosphate as studied in everted intestinal loop preparations were reduced in parathyroidectomized rats and stimulated following injections into the whole animal of parathyroid extract (PTE) (Rasmussen and DeLuca, 1963; Lifshitz *et al.*, 1969). Similarly, in isolated intestinal mucosal cells PTH stimulated a sodium-dependent mechanism of calcium transport across the basal-lateral membranes (Birge *et al.*, 1974). bPTH appears to have no direct effect on the intestinal calcium absorption *in vitro* in embryonic chick duodenum (Corradino, 1976). Nevertheless, Vegt and de Ruijter (1977) have found a direct stimulating effect of PTH on the passive influx of calcium into rat epithelial intestinal cells. A direct effect of PTH on lysosomal enzyme release from isolated intestinal cells has recently been demonstrated (Nemere and Szego, 1981). Intestinal calcium transport may represent a physiologically important site of indirect [via 1,25(OH)D$_3$] or direct action of PTH.

Additional sites of action whose physiological importance has not yet been clearly documented include the parotid gland, the pituitary gland, the stomach, the liver, the lymphocytes, the red blood cells, adipose tissue, and the heart.

In the absence of changes in serum, PTH caused significant rises of salivary protein, calcium, and phosphorus concentrations in man (Schneider *et al.*, 1977). Without raising blood calcium levels, PTH stimulated gastrin secretion in the pig. This effect is suppressed with calcitonin (Bolman *et al.*, 1977). Moreover, PTH stimulated the release of prolactin in man (Isaac *et al.*, 1978).

An augmentation of arterial hepatic and renal flow occurred within 1 min after the injection of PTE or bPTH-(1–34) (Charbon and Hulstaert, 1974). Purified bPTH and synthetic bPTH-(1–34) caused a stimulation of liver adenylate cyclase (Chase *et al.*, 1969a; Moxley *et al.*, 1974; Canterbury *et al.*, 1974). The calcium influx was increased in the perfused rat liver 6 hr after the administration of PTE (Chausmer *et al.*, 1972). In the same preparation purified bPTH inhibited glycogen synthesis (Hems *et al.*, 1975). In hepatocytes the glucose output was stimulated (Moxley *et al.*, 1974). PTH stimulated phosphate uptake and glutamate oxidation in liver mitochondria (Rasmussen and DeLuca, 1963). Following partial hepatectomy in rats cell proliferation was inhibited in hypocalcaemic animals and stimulated by intraperitonal injections of PTH or calcium (Rixon and Whitfield, 1976).

Calcium and PTH promote cell division in the bone marrow and initiation of deoxyribonucleic acid synthesis and stimulation of the proliferation of rat thymocytes maintained *in vitro* (Perris and Whitfield, 1971; Whitfield *et al.*, 1971). The mitotic stimulation by PTH was inhibited by calcitonin (MacManus and Whitfield, 1970). In HeLa cells calcium uptake was increased with PTE in the incubation medium (Borle, 1968). On the other hand, intact bPTH-(1–84) inhibits erythropoiesis (Meytes *et al.*, 1981).

Werner and Löw (1973) have shown that lipolysis of rat adipose tissue can be stimulated by purified PTH and synthetic bPTH-(1–34); the effect appears to be mediated by cyclic AMP (Werner and Löw, 1973; Thajchayapong *et al.*, 1976). Similar results were obtained with human adipose tissue (Gozariu *et al.*, 1974; Sinha *et al.*, 1976; Kather and Simon, 1977).

Finally, PTH was shown to increase the rate of beating of cultured heart cells; the effect is probably due to calcium entry into cells (Bogin *et al.*, 1981).

VI. MEASUREMENTS OF PARATHYROID HORMONE LEVELS

A. Bioassay

1. In Vivo Assays

The hypercalcemic action of PTH had initially been quantitated by Collip and Clark (1925) in intact dogs. This assay has been widely used and remains the official USP (United States Public Health Service) method for the standardization

TABLE I

Bioassay of Parathyroid Hormone

Animal species	Parameter	Dose range: bPTH-(1–84) (μg)	Dose range: bPTH (USPU[a] MRCU)	Index of precision (λ)	Reference
In vivo					
Parathyroidectomized rat	Serum Ca	1–5	5–40	0.23 ± 0.05 (SD)	Munson (1961)
Chick	Serum Ca	—	1–10	0.08–0.21	Parsons *et al.* (1973)
Japanese quail	Serum Ca	—	0.5–6	0.10–0.34	Dacke and Kenny (1973)
In vitro					
Rat kidney cortex	Adenylate cyclase	0.07–0.56	0.14–1.13	0.03–0.27	Marcus and Aurbach (1969)
Dog kidney cortex	Adenylate cyclase	3×10^{-5}–10^{-4}	—	0.05–0.09	Nissenson *et al.* (1981)
Guinea pig kidney cortex	Glucose 6-phosphate dehydrogenase	5×10^{-9}–10^{-7}	—	ND[b]	Chambers *et al.* (1978)
Rat bone cells	Cyclic AMP content	0.001–1	0.002–2	ND	Peck *et al.* (1973)
Rat bone cells	Cyclic AMP content	10^{-8}–0.2	—	ND	Rodan and Rodan (1974)
Rat long bone	^{45}Ca release	—	0.01–1.0	ND	Raisz (1965)
Mouse calvaria	^{40}Ca release	—	0.01–1.0	0.08–0.35	Zanelli *et al.* (1969)
Mouse calvaria	^{40}Ca release	—	0.06–1.2	0.15–0.69	Webster *et al.* (1974)

[a] 2000–4000 USPU or MRCU correspond to 1 mg bPTH-(1–84) (Rasmussen and Craig, 1961; Tregear *et al.*, 1973).

[b] ND = not done

of commercial preparations in the United States. Subsequently, the most widespread method was based on the measurement of serum calcium levels 6 hr after parathyroidectomy and sc injection of PTH in rats (Munson, 1961). Its dose range amounts to about 1–5 μg bPTH-(1–84) or 5–40 USP units (Table I). Later hypercalcemic assays in intact chicks and Japanese quails have been introduced by Parsons *et al.* (1973) and Dacke and Kenny (1973), respectively. The dose range varied between 0.5 and 10 MRC (Medical Research Council) units, which correspond to the USP units described previously. Two thousand to 4000 USP or MRC units represent approximately 1 mg bPTH-(1–84) (Rasmussen and Craig, 1961; Tregear *et al.*, 1973). All these assay methods require large amounts of PTH as compared to circulating levels of bPTH-(1–84) which amount to about 10 pg/ml (Chambers *et al.*, 1978; Dambacher *et al.*, 1979; Goltzman *et al.*, 1980). The insensitivity of the assay methods can be partially explained by the administration of bPTH into species other than the bovine.

2. *In Vitro* Assays

In vitro assays can be much more sensitive than the conventional hypercalcemic *in vivo* assays. The results obtained do not necessarily reflect biological properties seen *in vivo* of the PTH administered. The most widely used assay is based on the stimulation of the rat kidney cortical adenylate cyclase activity (Marcus and Aurbach, 1969). Its dose range amounts to 0.14–1.13 USP units or 0.07–0.56 μg purified bPTH-(1–84). By making use of a comparable assay, Canterbury *et al.* (1973, 1975) have examined circulating immunoreactive PTH species in man and demonstrated that in addition to hPTH-(1–84) a NH_2-terminal fragment with a molecular weight of 4500–5000 was biologically active. Similar findings have been obtained in a cytochemical bioassay measuring the stimulation of glucose-6-phosphate dehydrogenase activity of the guinea-pig kidney cortex by bPTH in amounts of as low as 0.005–0.1 pg/ml, which has recently been introduced (Chambers *et al.*, 1978; Goltzman *et al.*, 1980). The sensitivity of the adenylate cyclase assay has been improved by the addition of guanosine triphosphate and its nonmetabolisable analog 5′-guanalylimidodiphosphate (Nissenson *et al.*, 1981).

Peck *et al.* (1973) have used rat bone cells whose sensitivity to PTH amounts to about 1 ng/ml. Rodan and Rodan (1974) detected an increased accumulation of cyclic AMP in freshly isolated bone cells already with 0.01 pg bPTH-(1–84). This effect was, however, also obtained with calcitonin and epinephrine. The release of ^{45}Ca from rat long bones was quantitated by Raisz (1963a) and of ^{40}Ca from mouse calvaria by Zanelli *et al.* (1969) and by Webster *et al.* (1974). The dose ranges amount to 0.01–1.2 USP or MRC units. Bone cells have so far never been used for the characterization of circulating PTH species.

The indices of precision (λ) are comparable in *in vivo* and *in vitro* assays and range between 0.03 and 0.69 (Table I).

B. Radioimmunoassay

Except for the recently introduced cytochemical bioassay (Chambers *et al.*, 1978; Goltzman *et al.*, 1980) circulating PTH levels have been estimated in normal subjects exclusively by radioimmunoassay. This requires sufficient sensitivity to measure PTH levels in the majority of normal subjects and to discriminate between the control and patients with hyperparathyroidism. Berson and Yalow (1966), when introducing the first clinically useful radioimmunoassay system for the measurement of PTH in human plasma, noted considerable overlap between PTH levels in control subjects and in patients with primary hyperparathyroidism. They were the first to point out that circulating PTH is immunoheterogeneous and PTH levels varied depending on the antisera used in the radioimmunoassay (Berson and Yalow, 1968). They also demonstrated that the use of different antisera yielded different half-lives of disappearance of endogenous immunoreactive PTH in patients after removal of parathyroid tumors. Depending on whether rapidly disappearing intact PTH or slowly removed fragments are recognized with the radioimmunoassay system used, apparent half-lives of disappearance of PTH vary from 1–3 min to several hours in man and in animals (Berson and Yalow, 1968; Buckle, 1969; Hunziker *et al.*, 1977).

With most radioimmunoassay systems currently in use there is some overlap in PTH levels in patients with primary hyperparathyroidism and in control subjects (Arnaud *et al.*, 1971c; Silverman and Yalow, 1973; Fischer *et al.*, 1974). Only Reiss and Canterbury (1968) demonstrated a clearcut discrimination of PTH levels in sera obtained from hypoparathyroid, normal and hyperparathyroid subjects. Silverman and Yalow (1973) and Arnaud *et al.* (1974) pointed out that discrimination between normal and hyperparathyroid subjects was relatively small with antibodies whose specificities were directed mainly to the NH_2-terminal region of hPTH-(1–84) and good with antibodies having specificities directed to the COOH-terminal region of the molecule. The different discrimination is probably related to measurement problems of immunoreactive PTH in normal subjects. We have obtained good discrimination of PTH levels between normal and hyperparathyroid subjects using a radioimmunoassay system, which predominantly recognizes the NH_2-terminal third of hPTH-(1–84), and intact PTH in patients with hyperparathyroidism on gel filtration analysis (Fischer *et al.*, 1981). With all the presently used radioimmunoassays the estimated levels of NH_2-terminal PTH in normal subjects are far higher than values obtained of intact PTH-(1–84) after gel filtration of serum, or in the cytochemical bioassay (Dambacher *et al.*, 1979; Goltzman *et al.*, 1980). Moreover, the proportional amounts of intact PTH-(1–84) are low, and the predominant circulating PTH components represent COOH-terminal fragments. Radioimmunoassays detecting only intact PTH-(1–84) require an unusual sensitivity for the measurement of circulating PTH in normal subjects. It seems therefore, that immunoreactive PTH levels of normal subjects are frequently artifactually raised, when measured in radioimmunoassays not detecting COOH-terminal PTH fragments.

The reason for the variation of immunoreactive PTH measurements is the ability of certain antisera to recognize a combination of intact hPTH-(1–84) and of its NH_2- and/or COOH-terminal fragments (Fig. 6). The levels of hPTH-(1–84) are higher in patients with primary or secondary hyperparathyroidism as compared to control subjects (Dambacher *et al.*, 1979). In relation to hPTH-(1–84) a 7000 molecular weight COOH-terminal fragment is the most important circulating immunoreactive species in hypercalcemic patients with primary hyperparathyroidism and in patients with chronic renal insufficiency. On the other hand, in hypocalcemic patients with secondary hyperparathyroidism and normal renal function, and in normal subjects, the 7000 molecular weight fragment is less abundant. During calcium infusion in patients with primary or

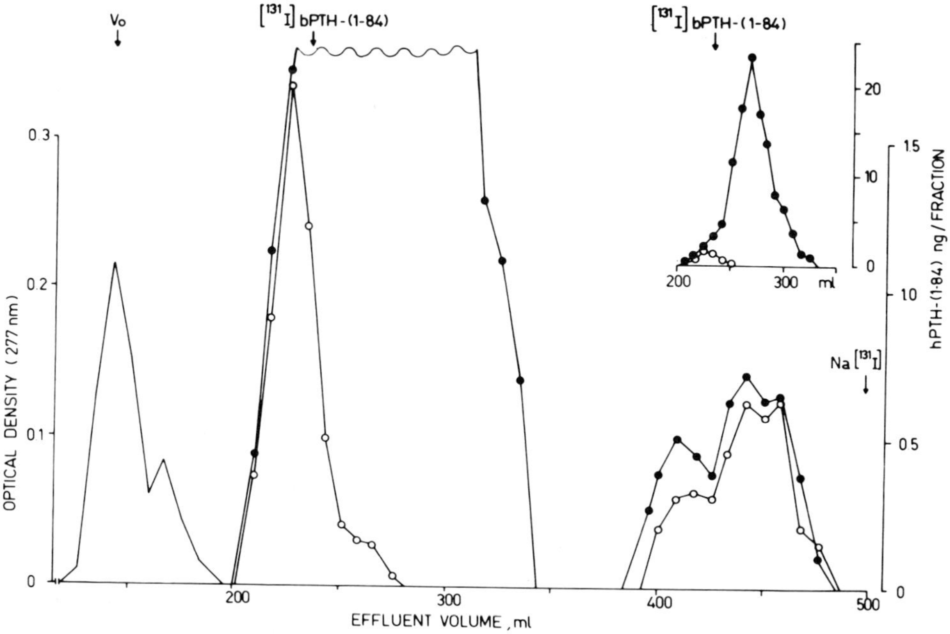

Fig. 6. Characterization of PTH from a patient with primary hyperparathyroidism by chromatography on Bio-Gel P-150. [^{131}I]bPTH-(1–84), and Na[^{131}I] were added as tracer to a 10-ml sample of serum; 2.5×100-cm column, 0.2 *M* ammonium acetate, pH 4.7, and human serum albumin 2.5 mg/ml as eluant. 15 ml/hr flow rate, 7.5-ml fractions. Serum PTH was measured with [^{131}I]bPTH-(1–84), anti-hPTH-(TCA) exhibiting specificity to COOH- (goat 3, day 306, diluted 1:1500) (●) and NH_2- (goat 16, day 810, diluted 1:15,000) (○) terminal parts of hPTH-(1–84), and hPTH-(1–84) G-100 as standard. Note that antibodies to NH_2-terminal parts of hPTH-(1–84) recognize the intact hPTH-(1–84) and small amounts of fragments, and antibodies to COOH-terminal parts predominantly fragments. (Adapted from Hunziker and Fischer, 1978.)

secondary hyperparathyroidism the rate of disappearance of intact hPTH-(1–84) was faster than that of its fragments (Canterbury and Reiss, 1972; Born *et al.*, 1980). Goldsmith *et al.* (1973) and Arnaud *et al.* (1974) demonstrated that a radioimmunoassay system with antigenic determinations directed to the NH_2-terminal parts of hPTH-(1–84) molecule was more suitable for the study of acute secretory activities in patients with renal insufficiency, since intact hPTH and its NH_2-terminal fragments disappeared faster from the circulation than the 7000 molecular weight COOH-terminal fragment. The detailed effect of changes in the extracellular calcium concentration on the secretion and metabolism of intact PTH and of its fragments remains to be evaluated (see Sections III and IV).

Although heterogeneity and the occurrence of several fragments in addition to intact PTH in the circulation can account for some of the problems related to radioimmunological measurements of serum PTH levels, methodological factors can produce artifacts and spurious results. For practical purposes several variables have to be considered for the development of a radioimmunoassay system in general and for human PTH in particular. They include the choice of the radioactive ligand, the specificity of the antibodies as regards the localization of the antigenic site on the PTH molecule, the immunodilution of the standard and of unknown samples, as well as nonspecific interferences by biological samples of the antigen-antibody reaction (Arnaud *et al.*, 1971a, 1974; Segre *et al.*, 1972; Silverman and Yalow, 1973; Fischer *et al.*, 1974, 1981).

In most of the diagnostically useful radioimmunassays, iodine labeled bPTH-(1–84) is used for the radioimmunological measurement of human PTH, since the intact hPTH-(1–84) is not available in sufficient quantities. The difference in the chemical structures of bPTH-(1–84) and hPTH-(1–84) presents a major obstacle in the analysis of the immunological properties of human PTH. Most of the radioimmunoassays used for the determination of circulating human PTH utilize antibodies raised to bPTH or pPTH, which cross-react with human PTH to a variable degree. Only rarely have strictly heterologous radioimmunoassay systems proved useful for measuring hPTH. Most antibodies to human tumor extracts raised in goats have recognized circulating PTH in hyperparathyroid patients, but not in all control subjects (Fischer *et al.*, 1974; Wieland *et al.*, 1979). Thus a major obstacle to a high affinity radioimmunoassay system measuring circulating hPTH in normal subjects is the unavailability of hPTH-(1–84).

VII. PARATHYROID HORMONE IN NORMAL SUBJECTS AND IN DISORDERS OF MINERAL METABOLISM

A. General Considerations

By themselves serum PTH measurements are of little use to the clinician and have to be related to other parameters, such as the serum calcium and phosphate, and the urinary excretion of cyclic AMP, calcium, and phosphate. The normal range of serum calcium levels is well defined (Keating *et al.*, 1969). However, overlaps of PTH levels in sera obtained from hypoparathyroid, normal, and hyperparathyroid subjects have been widely noted. In untreated hypoparathyroid patients (see Section VII,G), the serum calcium concentration is decreased, serum phosphate increased and serum PTH levels are undetectable or low. In patients whose hypocalcemia is unrelated to decreased parathyroid function, on the other hand, PTH levels are high normal or increased, levels characteristic of

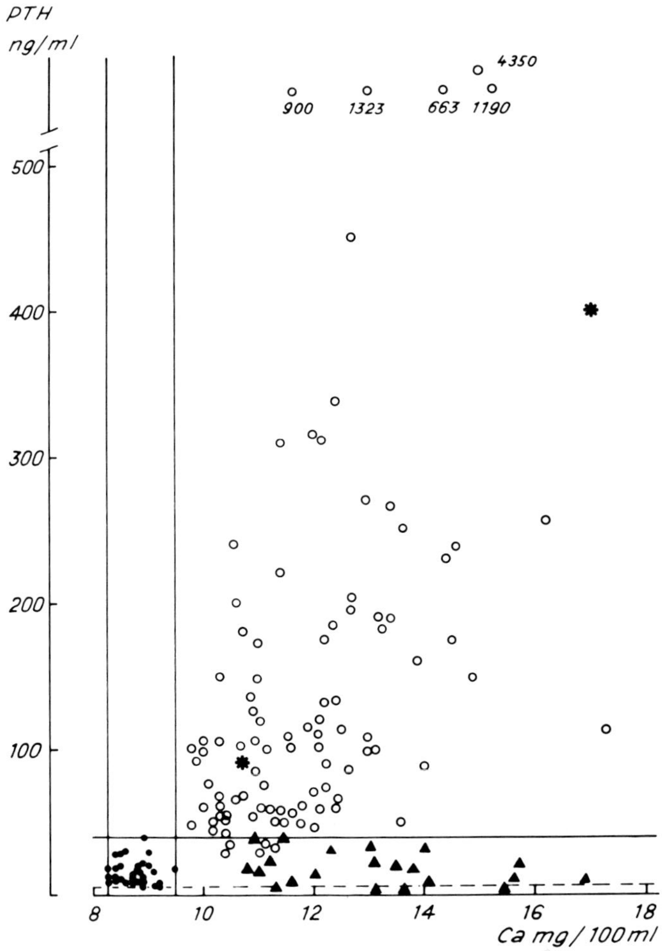

Fig. 7. Serum PTH as a function of calcium in control subjects (●), patients with primary hyperparathyroidism in the absense (○) and in the presence (∗) of a malignancy, and malignant tumors (▲). Carboxyl terminal PTH as determined with the radioimmunoassay system described in the legend to Fig. 4. The solid lines indicate the normal range and the broken line the sensitivity limits of the radioimmunoassay. (Adapted from Fischer *et al.,* 1976.)

secondary hyperparathyroidism (see Section VII,F). Thus, these two groups of hypocalcemic patients can be clearly differentiated with the aid of PTH measurements (Werder *et al.*, 1978). Toward the end of pregnancy (see Section VII,C) and in some patients with secondary hyperparathyroidism (see Section VII,F), PTH levels are increased, when the serum calcium is still in the normal range. In patients with primary hyperparathyroidism, serum calcium and PTH levels are raised by definition, whereas patients whose hypercalcemia is not caused by tumors of the parathyroid glands, PTH levels are slightly raised, normal or undetectable. Some of these patients suffer from ectopic hyperparathyroidism (Fig. 7) (see Section VII,E).

B. Normal Subjects

PTH levels are inversely related to serum calcium levels. A negative relationship between PTH and ionized or total serum calcium concentration indicates normally functioning PTH secretion (S. B. Arnaud *et al.*, 1973; C. D. Arnaud *et al.*, 1971c; Wieland *et al.*, 1978). In hypocalcemias induced by peroral administration of phosphate or volume expansion with iv saline, or after iv injections of calcitonin PTH levels were increased; conversely, iv calcium infusions decrease PTH levels and eliminate the phosphate induced rise of serum PTH (Reiss *et al.*, 1970; Arnaud *et al.*, 1971c; Shaw *et al.*, 1974). A diurnal rhythm of PTH serum levels with a nocturnal rise has been demonstrated both in control subjects and in patients with primary hyperparathyroidism; iv calcium infusions prevented the nocturnal rise (Arnaud *et al.*, 1971c; Jubitz *et al.*, 1972; Sinha *et al.*, 1975). Moreover, plasma PTH levels appear to be related to sleep stage cycles (Kripke *et al.*, 1978).

C. Pregnancy and Newborn Infants

Cushard *et al.* (1972a) have demonstrated a rise of PTH levels during the 36–40th week of pregnancy, even though the serum calcium remained in the normal range. Postpartum and during lactation, when the calcium losses were greatest, PTH returned to the normal range. Similar results have been obtained by Bouillon and de Moor (1973) and by Root *et al.* (1974).

PTH levels of newborn infants are generally determined in cord blood. At birth, calcium levels were found to be high and PTH levels low or undetectable (David and Anast, 1974; Wieland *et al.*, 1980). Within 48 hr the ionized and total plasma calcium levels decreased, even though PTH concentrations were still low; thereafter plasma PTH and calcium levels increased in parallel. Fairney (1975) also noted a rise of PTH levels between birth and the 6th day. In some infants older than 48 hr serum calcium remains decreased in the presence or slightly increased PTH levels as compared to the normal adult range (Wieland *et al.*, 1979). Exceptionally, the hypocalcemia lasts longer than the first week of life; in these cases permanent hypoparathyroidism becomes probable (Fanconi and Prader, 1967).

The transient functional hypoparathyroidism of the first days of life is probably caused by an increased calcium transport across the placenta, which is impermeable to maternal parathyroid hormone (Garel, 1972; M. W. Neuman *et al.*, 1975; Northrop *et al.*, 1977). Fetal parathyroid function appears, therefore, to be suppressed in the presence of a high extracellular calcium concentration. This is seen more dramatically in women known to be hyperparathyroid during pregnancy by neonatal hypocalcemia and tetany, death, or abortion in 80% of the pregnancies (Van Arsdel, 1955; Bocquetin *et al.*, 1973; Monteleone *et al.*, 1975; Delmeonico *et al.*, 1976). Relatively high serum ionized calcium levels were found by Tsang *et al.* (1973, 1975) in cord blood of premature infants and of children of diabetic mothers. The authors suggested that fetal hypercalcemia was the cause of the functional hypoparathyroidism seen subsequently in these infants.

The hypocalcemia may also be explained by a reduced responsiveness of the renal proximal tubules seen in normal newborn infants, where urinary cAMP and phosphate responses to PTH are decreased as compared to the third day of life and to adult subjects (Linarelli, 1972). Finally, plasma calcitonin levels are increased in neonatal infants and may contribute to the observed hypocalcemia (Cannarozzi *et al.*, 1976; Wieland *et al.*, 1980).

Exchange blood transfusions containing large amounts of phosphate and citrate have caused an increase of the complexed serum calcium and a fall of the ionized calcium. This was associated with a Q-oTc prolongation in the electrocardiogram, and as a consequence with a transient increase in PTH levels; the total serum calcium showed a slight increase which may reflect raised calcium mobilization (Wieland *et al.*, 1979). Wieland *et al.* (1979) also demonstrated that PTH responses during phosphate and citrate induced hypocalcemia were unrelated to the gestational age, whereas Tsang *et al.* (1973) described decreased stimulability of PTH secretion in premature infants.

D. Primary Hyperparathyroidism

Primary hyperparathyroidism is caused by a single or multiple adenoma, by a diffuse hyperplasia of all the parathyroid glands, or by a carcinoma. Multiple adenoma cannot always be differentiated from primary chief cell hyperplasia (Roth, 1971). The diffuse hyperplasia of the parathyroid glands can be encountered in familial hyperparathyroidism (Cutler *et al.*, 1964; Marx *et al.*, 1973, 1977; Goldsmith *et al.*, 1976). It may be part of a multiple endocrine neoplasia syndrome, where it is associated with tumors of the pancreatic islets, the adrenal cortex and the pituitary (Type 1), or with pheochromocytoma and medullary thyroid carcinoma and mucosal neuromas (Type 2) (Ballard *et al.*, 1964; Steiner *et al.*, 1968). In multiple endocrine neoplasia Type 2a hyperparathyroidism occurs frequently and mucosal neuromas only rarely, whereas in Type 2b (=

Type 3) mucosal neuromas are part of the syndrome and primary hyperparathyroidism occurs only exceptionally (Khairi *et al.*, 1975; Heath *et al.*, 1976). The syndrome is transmitted as an autosomal dominant trait with varying penetrance. The tendency is to claim a genetic defect in many of these tumors of neuroectodermal origin (Pearse and Takor, 1976). Alternatively, PTH secretion may be stimulated by catecholamines or by calcitonin (Parthemore and Deftos, 1979) (see Section III, C), or primary hyperparathyroidism induced by previous exposure to radiation of thyroid carcinoma (Tisell *et al.*, 1978). A special form of familial hyperparathyroidism, hypocalciuric hypercalcemia with a generally mild clinical course and absence of nephrolithiasis, usually does not require parathyroid surgery (Marx *et al.*, 1980).

From a functional point of view, PTH secretion is increased and as a consequence serum calcium levels are also raised. The abnormal tissue, however, responds to changes in calcium *in vitro* with a suppression of adenylate cyclase activity, which required higher amounts of calcium in membrane preparations from hyperfunctioning parathyroid glands as compared to normal parathyroid tissues (Bellorin-Font *et al.*, 1981). Moreover, PTH secretion was inversely related to the extracellular concentration (Birnbaumer *et al.*, 1977; Habener, 1978; Dietel *et al.*, 1978; Brown *et al.*, 1978). A hypocalcemia induced with EDTA or phosphate may stimulate PTH levels (Murray *et al.*, 1972; Binswanger and Fischer, 1974; Lockefeer *et al.*, 1974; Bouillon and de Moor, 1977). Varying results have been obtained with calcium infusions, where Murray *et al.* (1972) and Monchik *et al.* (1977) demonstrated a suppression of PTH levels in most of the patients studied with adenomatous primary hyperparathyroidism, whereas Reiss and Canterbury (1969) demonstrated a suppression of PTH levels in patients with primary hyperplasia only, but not in patients with parathyroid adenoma. These apparently conflicting results may be explained by altered secretory responses in the two forms of primary hyperparathyroidism. It must be emphasized, however, that adenomatous and hyperplastic hyperparathyroidism cannot always be differentiated on morphological grounds (Roth, 1971). In conclusion, it remains to be evaluated whether primary hyperparathyroidism represents only a functional defect of the PTH secretion or whether in some cases at least, it is also caused by a genetic defect.

Nephrolithiasis and nephrocalcinosis are the leading symptoms of primary hyperparathyroidism. Of 2980 patients with nephrolithiasis, about 7% suffer from hyperparathyroidism (Table II). On the other hand, a majority of patients with primary hyperparathyroidism (65%) suffer from nephrolithiasis and/or nephrocalcinosis; skeletal symptoms are encountered in 47% of 1267 cases (Table III). The serum concentration of $1,25(OH)_2D$ is frequently raised in patients with primary hyperparathyroidism; marked elevations are associated with a higher incidence of renal stones (Broadus *et al.*, 1980). With the advent of large scale screening methods for the measurement of serum calcium levels the average

TABLE II

Frequency of Primary Hyperparathyroidism in Patients with Nephrolithiasis

References	Nephrolithiasis (N)[a]	Primary hyperparathyroidism (N)[a]	Percentage
Beard and Goodyear (1950)	150	12	8.0
Milne (1954)	302	4	1.3
McIntosh *et al.* (1958)	50	5	10.0
Melick and Henneman (1958)	207	20	9.7
Fetter and McCuskey (1960)	172	6	3.5
McGeown (1960)	405	68	16.8
Hellström and Ivemark (1962)	481	29	6.0
Cottet *et al.* (1962)	288	9	3.1
Harrison (1964)	695	45	6.5
Coe and Kavalach (1974)	230	10	4.3
Total number	2980	208	7.0

[a] Number of patients.

TABLE III

Leading Symptoms in Patients with Primary Hyperparathyroidism

References	Patients (N)[a]	Nephrolithiasis and/or nephrocalcinosis		Skeletal symptoms	
		N[a]	Percentage	N[a]	Percentage
Norris (1947)	314	118	38	292	93
Albright and Reifenstein (1948)	64	52	81	35	55
Burk (1948)	10	6	60	9	90
Rienhoff (1950)	26	19	73	8	31
Lahey and Murphy (1953)	29	13	45	25	86
Richardson (1953)	11	9	82	9	82
Black (1953)	112	89	79	32	29
Bogdonoff *et al.* (1956)	27	21	78	11	41
McGeown and Morrison (1959)	53	48	91	4	8
Harrison (1960)	22	22	100	—	—
Hellström and Ivemark (1962)	138	119	86	60	43
Dent (1964)	125	84	67	38	30
Pyrah *et al.* (1966)	66	46	70	37	56
Johansson *et al.* (1972)	118	80	68	16	14
Kistler (1976)	152	98	64	23	15
Total number	1267	824	65	599	47

[a] N, number of patients.

annual incidence of primary hyperparathyroidism rose from 8 to 28 cases per 100,000 population in residents close to the Mayo Clinic, and the frequency of urolithiasis fell from 51 to 4% (Heath *et al.*, 1980).

The leading biochemical sign of primary hyperparathyroidism is an increase in serum calcium levels (Fig. 7, Arnaud *et al.*, 1971c). In some patients the leading symptom is extreme dehydration accompanied by severe hypercalcemia; in 118 of these cases reviewed by Kistler (1976) the mortality amounted to 47%.

Both the serum ionized and total calcium levels are increased in patients with primary hyperparathyroidism and the determination of the ionized calcium concentration offers no real advantage over the measurement of the serum total calcium level (Fischer *et al.*, 1974). Occasionally, in myeloma patients with hyperproteinemia, the total serum calcium concentration may be increased, even though the ionized calcium concentration is still within the normal range. In studies by Low *et al.* (1973) and by Muldowney *et al.* (1976) the apparent normal range of total serum calcium concentration exceeds our own "normal" range. Perhaps patients with borderline elevated total serum calcium levels are grouped in the normal range by these authors.

The diagnosis of primary hyperparathyroidism can be established in hypercalcemic patients with raised PTH levels. With clinically useful radioimmunoassays serum PTH levels are in the range of normal subjects in 5–20% of patients with primary hyperparathyroidism (Arnaud *et al.*, 1971c; Blair *et al.*, 1973; Conaway and Anast, 1974; Fischer *et al.*, 1974, 1981). In these patients serum PTH is usually higher than in patients with hypercalcemia due to tumors not originating from the parathyroid glands (Fig. 7) (Riggs *et al.*, 1971b; Benson *et al.*, 1974b; see Section VII,E). Interestingly, serum PTH levels were found increased in patients with hypercalcemia of immobilization and to be in the range of patients with primary hyperparathyroidism (Lerman *et al.*, 1977). With PTH levels in the

TABLE IV

Differential Diagnosis of Hypercalcemia

Primary (tertiary) hyperparathyroidism
Ectopic hyperparathyroidism
Lymphoma
Multiple myeloma
Other malignancies
Vitamin D intoxication
Sarcoidosis
Milk-alkali syndrome (Burnett syndrome)
Immobilization
Hyperthyroidism
Acute Addison's syndrome
Thiazide therapy
Vitamin A therapy
Laboratory error

normal range, causes of hypercalcemia other than abnormal parathyroid function have to be ruled out on clinical and biochemical grounds (Table IV). Normocalcemic primary hyperparathyroidism, which warrants surgical removal of parathyroid tumors, remains unproved (Arnaud *et al.*, 1971c; Fischer *et al.*, 1981). Normocalcemic hyperparathyroidism with hypercalciuria and nephrolithiasis is discussed in Section VII,F,5.

In addition to serum calcium and PTH measurements, the amount of cyclic AMP excreted in the urine has been established as a diagnostic tool, provided the urinary cyclic AMP excretion is related to the glomerular filtration rate (Fig. 8; Broadus *et al.*, 1977). The discrimination by urinary cyclic AMP measurements (expressed per 100 ml glomerular filtrate) between normal subjects and patients with primary hyperparathyroidism is about the same as by PTH radioimmunoassay. A similar discrimination between values for control subjects and patients with hyperparathyroidism is obtained when the nephrogenous cyclic AMP is calculated. Nephrogenous cyclic AMP represents the difference between the cyclic AMP filtered by the kidney and that excreted in the urine (Babka *et al.*, 1976; Drezner *et al.*, 1976a; Schmidt-Gayk *et al.*, 1977) and, according to Broadus *et al.* (1977), is expressed as nmol cyclic AMP per 100 ml glomerular filtrate. Nephrogenous cyclic AMP can be raised in normo- and in hypercal-

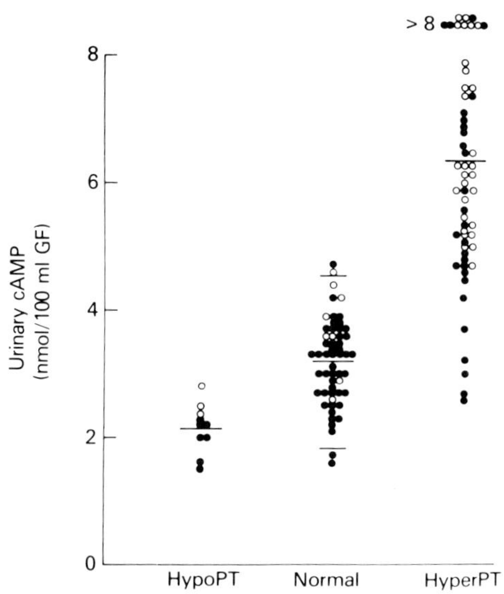

Fig. 8. Urinary cyclic AMP, expressed in nmol per 100 ml glomerular filtrate, in control subjects (Normal) and in patients with hypoparathyroidism (HypoPT) and primary hyperparathyroidism (HyperPT). The open circles represent subjects with renal impairment (mean GFR < 80 ml/min). The horizontal lines depict the mean values for the patients with hypoparathyroidism and primary hyperparathyroidism, and the control group is shown as mean ± 2 SD. (From Broadus *et al.*, 1977.)

cemic patients with tumors unrelated to the parathyroid glands (Stewart *et al.*, 1980; Rude *et al.*, 1981). This value is therefore less diagnostically useful than serum PTH measurements. In hyperthyroid patients the urinary cyclis AMP excretion is normal when related to 100 ml glomerular filtrate (Broadus, 1977).

Serum and urinary phosphate, whether expressed as the amount of phosphate reabsorbed in the tubule (the phosphate excretion index) or as the ratio of the maximum tubular reabsorptive capacity of phosphate to the glomerular filtration rate (Nordin and Bulusu, 1968; Bijvoet, 1969), are normal in most patients with surgically verified primary hyperparathyroidisim (Fig. 9; Binswanger and Fischer, 1978) Hence these indices cannot be used diagnostically (see also Pyrah *et al.*, 1966).

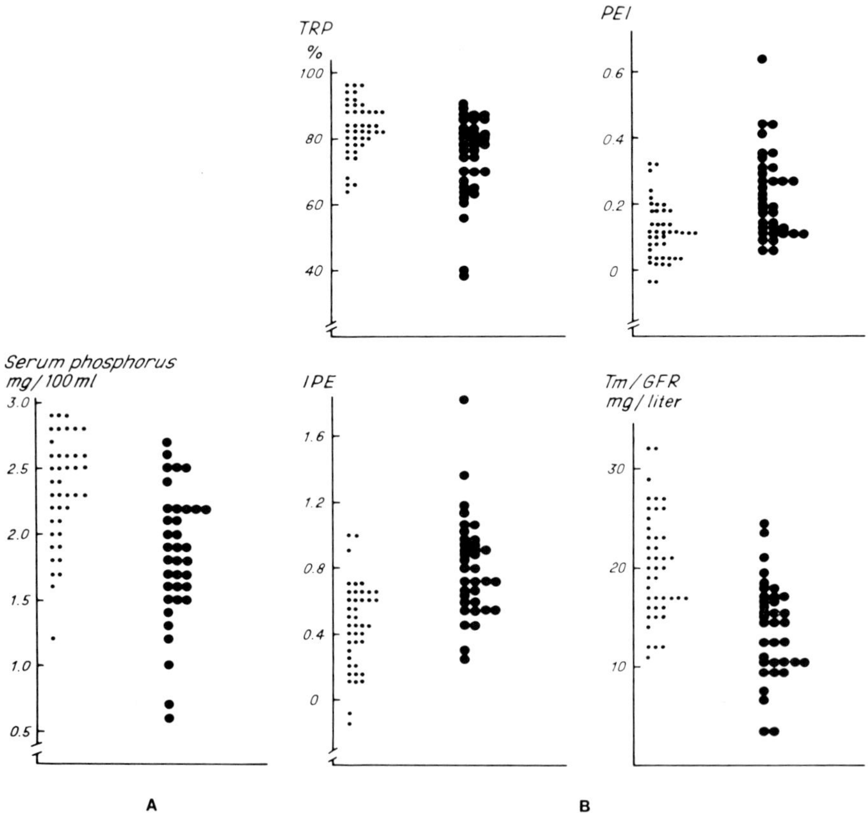

Fig. 9. A, serum phosphorus and B, urinary phosphate excretion [per cent tubular reabsorption of phosphate (TRP), phosphate excretion indices after Nordin and Bulusu (1968) (PEI, IPE), and the ratio of the maximal tubular reabsorptive capacity of phosphate and the glomerular filtration rate (Tm/GFR) (Bijvoet, 1969)]. Inorganic phosphorus was determined with a method using malachite green as indicator (Hohenwallner and Wimmer, 1973). Control subjects (○), and patients with primary hyperparathyroidism (●). (From Binswanger and Fischer, 1978.)

By measuring PTH levels in samples obtained by catheter from the parathyroid and thyroid venous effluents it is possible to locate a parathyroid tumor. This can be helpful to the surgeon, as it helps to differentiate a single adenoma from multiple abnormal glands. Correct localization however, is difficult in patients who have undergone unsuccessful surgery for hyperparathyroidism, inasmuch as their venous drainage has become abnormal (Bilezikian *et al.*, 1973; Eisenberg *et al.*, 1974). PTH measurements in the venous effluent for parathyroid localization may, furthermore, not be helpful, when a adenoma is localized at an aberrant place such as in the mediastinum, since the arterial supply may arise from the cervical area; in these cases the tumor can be localized arteriographically (Doppman *et al.*, 1977). Before localization studies are undertaken, it is necessary to establish primary hyperparathyroidism in peripheral blood, inasmuch as the effluent from normal glands also exhibits higher PTH levels than found peripherally (Shimkin and Powell, 1973).

Surgical removal of parathyroid tumors is the treatment of choice in primary hyperparathyroidism. Postoperatively, severe hypocalcemia and tetany may occur, especially in severe cases with marked bone involvement. A hypocalcemia may occasionally be the cause of temporarily raised serum PTH levels. Long-term longitudinal postoperative studies have rarely been undertaken. In a study on 52 patients who were successfully operated for primary hyperparathyroidism, the blood pressure rose and renal function continued to deteriorate, even though the serum calcium concentration had returned to the normal range (Britton *et al.*, 1971).

Total parathyroidectomy and autotransplantation or homotransplantation into the forearm muscle of an immunosuppressed patient have been used to treat diffuse parathyroid hyperplasia (Groth *et al.*, 1973; Wells *et al.*, 1975, 1976; Alveryd *et al.*, 1975). Some patients become hypocalcemic after this procedure and require vitamin D replacement therapy (Burnett *et al.*, 1977). It appears logical that an expert parathyroid surgeon considered this approach as "too much surgery" (Cope, 1976).

In so-called "biochemical" primary hyperparathyroidism with borderline increased serum calcium levels but normal kidney function and no clinical symptoms such as metabolically active nephrolithiasis, intractable ulcer, or pancreatitis, it remains debatable whether or not the parathyroid tumors should be removed surgically or whether treatment with phosphate or diuretics or no treatment at all can be considered (Purnell *et al.*, 1974). Preliminary results that centered on a 5-year course of "biochemical" hyperparathyroidism indicated that about 20% of 147 patients required surgical intervention, 20% dropped from the study, and 4% died before final evaluation. Thus, in a 5-year period it proved impossible to define criteria for surgical treatment.

The primary hyperparathyroidism of early infancy deserves special comment. Hyperparathyroidism in children below the age of 10 years is extremely rare; it is not even mentioned in 2980 cases evaluated and summarized by Pyrah *et al.* (1966), Johansson *et al.* (1972) and Kistler (1976). In primary hyperparathyroidism of early infancy, consanguinity is frequently described and the evidence favors autosomal recessive inheritance; the clinical course is extremely severe and the mortality in 11 cases summarized by Goldbloom *et al.* (1972) was 64%. Rhone (1975) reviewed seven cases of neonatal hyperparathyroidism; we have observed a similar patient with consanguinity of the parents and also alcaptonuria (Kind *et al.,* 1976). Diffuse hyperplasia of all four parathyroid glands was always demonstrated in these patients.

Parathyroid carcinoma occurs in 1–4% of the patients with primary hyperparathyroidism (Beahrs *et al.,* 1963; Schantz and Castleman, 1973; Kistler, 1976). Parathyroid carcinoma tends to invade the adjacent tissues and mitotic figures in varying numbers can almost always be identified; tumor cells may also invade vascular channels. In this condition PTH and serum calcium levels are very high. The diagnosis of a parathyroid carcinoma can only be established when metastases are present.

E. Ectopic Hyperparathyroidism

There is evidence that some cancers produce PTH or PTH-like substances causing hypercalcemia, which can be reversed on resection of the tumors (Tashjian *et al.,* 1964a; Goldberg *et al.,* 1964; Roof *et al.,* 1971; Riggs *et al.,* 1971b; Palmieri *et al.,* 1974). The predominant cancer associated with hypercalcemia is adenocarcinoma of the kidney: 9 of 17 cases, or 53%, according to Lipsett (1968), and 21 or 73 cases, or 29%, according to Omenn *et al.* (1969). Twenty of 73 cases of carcinoma were found to have originated in the lung (27%), 6 in the ovary (8%), and 5 in the pancreas (7%); the rest (29%) were distributed among various other organs (Omenn *et al.,* 1969). In all but two cases the lung cancer was of the squamous cell type. This is not true of adenocarcinoma or oat cell carcinoma; the latter two cell types are most frequently associated with osseous metastases, even though the patients were normocalcemic (Bender and Hansen, 1974). Hypercalcemia is also frequently associated with breast cancer (225 of 430 patients or 52%; Myers, 1973), which appears to be a relatively rare cause of ectopic PTH production (Omenn *et al.,* 1969; Mavligit *et al.,* 1971).

Parathyroid hormone production by the cancer tissue was recognized with the aid of an immunofluorescent technique (Palmieri *et al.,* 1974). A useful technique is the measurement of arteriovenous gradients of PTH in liver tissue with a primary hepatoma and in kidney with a hypernephroma (Knill-Jones *et al.,* 1970; Buckle *et al.,* 1970; Blair *et al.,* 1973). Cell culture of a renal carcinoma revealed PTH biosynthesis and release; in addition to intact PTH-(1–84), a basic PTH resembling ProPTH and labeled fragments were found in cells after incubation with radioactive amino acids (Greenberg *et al.,* 1973; Hamilton *et al.,* 1977). In the serum of some cancer patients a PTH-component larger than hPTH-(1–84) has been demonstrated, whereas PTH fragments occurred in smaller amounts than in patients with primary hyperparathyroidism (Benson *et al.*, 1974a).

According to Benson *et al.* (1974b) serum PTH levels were normal or close to normal in 95% of 108 hypercalcemic patients with malignant disease. They thus differentiated these from patients with primary hyperparathyroidism and generally raised PTH levels. The authors claim that normal levels of immunoreactive PTH, accompanied by malignancy, reflect an ectopic production of a PTH, which reacts poorly with the antibodies used. Most cases lack definitive proof that PTH originated from cancers unrelated to parathyroid glands rather than from parathyroid tissue. This appears particularly important, inasmuch as PTH secretion was not found to be fully suppressed in hypercalcemic calves (Mayer *et al.*, 1976). The issue is further complicated by the fact that patients with primary hyperparathyroidism have been reported to have a significantly higher incidence of carcinoma of the gastrointestinal tract, the breast, and thyroid (Kaplan *et al.*, 1971). In cases with raised serum PTH levels, the additional diagnosis of primary hyperparathyroidism could be established (Fig. 7).

F. Secondary Hyperparathyroidism

In patients with secondary hyperparathyroidism, serum PTH levels are raised in response to various factors known to stimulate PTH secretion (see Section III,C). Causes in man include nutritional calcium and vitamin D deficiency, disturbances of vitamin D metabolism, pseudohypoparathyroidism, and treatment with hypocalcemic agents such as calcitonin, which cause decreased bone resorption, and diuretic agents (e.g., furosemide) which produce a renal calcium loss. Among patients with secondary hyperparathyroidism decreased serum calcium concentrations, and in normocalcemic patients reduced calcium intake and raised calcium loss are the most important pathogenetic factors. The etiological role of factors other than calcium, such as the D-vitamins, catecholamines and abnormal PTH remains to be elucidated (Fischer and Blum, 1980; Nagant de Deuxchaisnes *et al.*, 1981). The only differential diagnoses represent primary and ectopic hyperparathyroidism, although there may be overlaps, largely because the etiology of raised PTH secretion remains to be determined in primary and in ectopic hyperparathyroidism (Table V).

1. Calcium and Vitamin D Deficiency and Altered Vitamin D Metabolism

This section will discuss patients with normal renal function and secondary hyperparathyroidism. Osteitis fibrosa and rickets are the leading symptoms of patients with nutritional calcium and vitamin D deficiency and intestinal malabsorption, as well as in disturbances of vitamin D metabolism, such as pseudovitamin D deficiency (Arnaud *et al.*, 1970, 1971c, 1972; Fanconi and Fischer,

TABLE V

Pathogenesis of Hyperparathyroidism

Form	Serum calcium	Pathogenesis: Undisputed	Pathogenesis: Questionable
Primary	↑	?	?
Secondary	↓	Hypocalcemia	Direct stimulation or lack of suppressing effects of D vitamins on PTH secretion; abnormal PTH (Secondary, Normocalcemic, Tertiary)
Normocalcemic	→	?	
Tertiary	↑	Preceding secondary hyperparathyroidism	

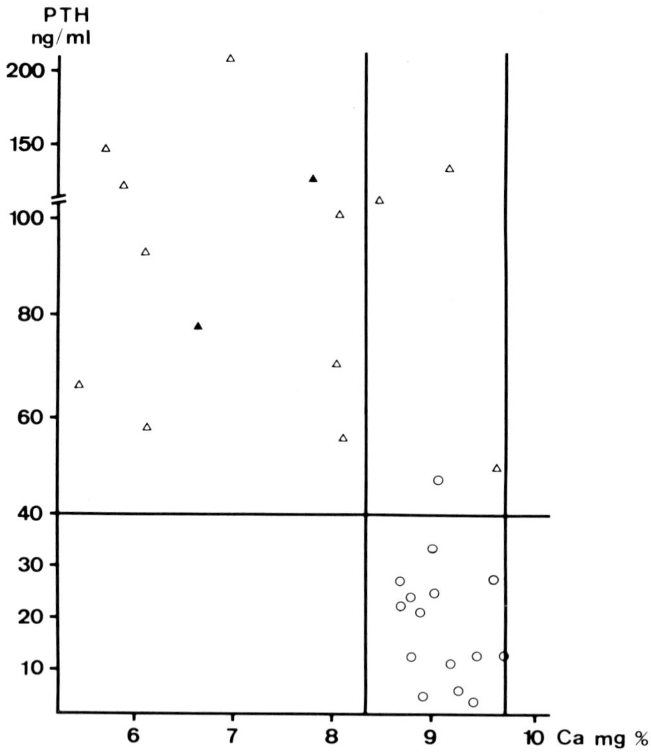

Fig. 10. Serum PTH as a function of calcium in patients with nutritional vitamin D deficiency rickets (△), pseudo-vitamin D deficiency rickets (▲), and hypophosphatemic vitamin D-resistant rickets (○). For details see Figs. 4 and 7. (From Fischer *et al.,* 1973b, and Fanconi *et al.,* 1974.)

1976; Kooh *et al.*, 1977). In all these conditions, serum calcium levels are frequently decreased, but sometimes normal, and serum PTH is increased (Fig. 10). Hypocalcemia is the best known stimulator of PTH secretion, but nutritional vitamin D deficiency or a defective conversion of $25(OH)D_3$ to $1,25(OH)_2D_3$ and $24,25(OH)_2D_3$ may represent additional causes of raised PTH secretion.

During treatment with vitamin D_3, serum calcium levels are normalized in hypocalcemic patients, and as a consequence PTH levels returned to the normal range. Serum PTH levels were, however, also increased in normocalcemic children whose serum PTH returned to the normal range even though serum ionized and total calcium levels remained practically unchanged; vitamin D_3 or its metabolites may therefore directly suppress PTH secretion (Fischer *et al.*, 1973b; see Section III,C).

Exceptionally, serum calcium levels are raised and tertiary hyperparathyroidism with partial ''autonomy'' of PTH secretion was assumed to be the cause of it (St. Goar, 1963; Clinicopathological Conference, 1972). Tertiary hyperparathyroidism, if it does exist, resembles primary hyperparathyroidism.

2. *Renal Hyperparathyroidism*

In patients with chronic renal insufficiency, secondary hyperparathyroidism causing osteitis fibrosa, osteomalacia, and soft tissue calcifications represents a major complication. The clinical, biochemical, and histological findings have been summarized in several studies (Stanbury and Lumb, 1966; Garner and Ball, 1966; Massry and Goldstein, 1978). PTH levels are inversely related to the renal clearance of inulin (Arnaud, 1973). Increased PTH levels may, however, also be caused by a decreased catabolism of the intact hormone and of its presumably biologically active and inactive fragments (see Section IV,B). The study of absolute PTH levels by radioimmunoassay may include biologically inactive, slowly metabolized hormone fragments. Immunoreactive PTH measurements are more meaningful, if obtained with assays recognizing predominantly intact PTH-(1–84), whose metabolism is faster than of COOH-terminal PTH fragments (Binswanger *et al.*, 1979; Born *et al.*, 1980). In patients with renal insufficiency, hypocalcemia is probably an early stimulus of PTH secretion, inasmuch as phosphate retention due to renal disease causes small and frequent falls of the total and ionized serum calcium concentrations (Slatopolsky *et al.*, 1971). This form of secondary hyperparathyroidism can be prevented in dogs by the prophylactic use of a low phosphate diet supplemented with 25-hydroxycholecalciferol (Rutherford *et al.*, 1977). In severe renal disease, PTH levels are often very high and the relationship between serum calcium and PTH may be obscured (Massry *et al.*, 1974; Bordier *et al.*, 1975; Binswanger *et al.*, 1979). PTH levels were found to be highest in patients on chronic hemodialysis with a high serum phosphate and a low dialysate calcium concentration (Fournier *et al.*, 1971). Another complication of secondary hyperparathyroid in uremic patients is an acidosis that may be caused by renal bicarbonate wastage. The degree of acidosis appears to be directly related to the level of circulating plasma PTH (Wallach *et al.*, 1972; Muldowney *et al.*, 1972). Additional factors may include a disturbance of vitamin D metabolism leading to a decreased synthesis of the dihydroxylated vitamin D metabolites.

A close relationship has been reported to exist between PTH levels on the one hand, and resorption surfaces and the number of osteoclasts per bone surface on the other. The latter two parameters were measured histomorphometrically on biopsies obtained from the iliac crest (Bordier *et al.*, 1975). The calcemic response to parathyroid extract was found to be significantly depressed in patients with chronic renal insufficiency and to be unrelated to the initial serum levels of calcium, phosphate and PTH; a depressed response was also seen in patients with subtotal parathyroidectomy (Massry *et al.*, 1973). Furthermore, the recovery from a hypocalcemic infusion induced with EDTA was slower in patients with chronic renal insufficiency and raised PTH levels, as compared to normal subjects (Llach *et al.*, 1975).

The treatment of chronic renal hyperparathyroidism involves three components: adequate calcium intake, dialysis against high concentrations of calcium (Fournier *et al.*, 1971) and magnesium (Pletka *et al.*, 1974), and administration of vitamin D or its metabolites, or dihydrotachysterol. Treatment with vitamin D_3, or 1,25-dihydroxycholecalciferol, has led to a lowering of serum PTH with serum calcium levels rising as a result of vitamin D repletion. Direct effects of vitamin D metabolites on PTH secretion remain to be demonstrated (Potter *et al.*, 1974; Bouillon *et al.*, 1975; Brickman *et al.*, 1974; Binswanger *et al.*, 1979). Treatment with dihydrotachysterol also improved hyperparathyroid bone disease in chronic renal insufficiency (Kaye *et al.*, 1970). Phosphate-binding agents are needed to reduce phosphate absorption so as to prevent soft tissue calcification. A subtotal parathyroidectomy is indicated in only exceptional circumstances when dealing with hypocalcemic patients with renal hyperparathyroidism. Hypercalcemia is a rarely observed complication of secondary hyperparathyroidism of chronic renal insufficiency; even in the presence of moderately increased serum PTH levels, vitamin D intoxication or causes other than hyperparathyroidism have to be ruled out before a surgical removal of hyperplastic parathyroid glands can be considered.

Following renal transplantation, serum PTH is lowered, but may not be normalized in some patients for several months or years (Schwartz *et al.*, 1970; David *et al.*, 1973; Kleerekoper *et al.*, 1975; Chatterjee *et al.*, 1976). Thus Pletka *et al.* (1976) found that PTH levels remained elevated in nearly two-thirds of 76 patients they had studied. Since renal function often does not return to normal in some of these patients, the increased PTH levels may be the result of a decrease in the renal degradation of PTH fragments. On the other hand, the hypercalcemia seen in about one-third of 160 patients (Schwartz *et al.*, 1970; David *et al.*, 1973; Kleerekoper *et al.*, 1975; Chatterjee *et al.*, 1976) probably is due to persistent hyperparathyroidism. Increased serum calcium levels may, however, also be caused by the use of phosphate-free antacids, which when taken in large amounts cause hypophosphatemia and hypercalcemia (Alfrey *et al.*, 1968). In spite of these reservations secondary hyperparathyroidism with marked bone involvement following renal transplantation has been demonstrated (Kleerekoper *et al.*, 1975). This condition is due to a persistence of enlarged parathyroids together with a return of normal 1,25$(OH)_2D_3$ synthesis following transplantation; it may additionally be due to the use of corticosteroids (Massry *et al.*, 1973; Fucik *et al.*, 1975). If the renal function deteriorates in the presence of increased serum calcium levels, a subtotal parathyroidectomy may be indicated.

In cases of acute renal failure with slight hypocalcemia during the polyuric phase, PTH was found to be increased in the presence of decreased serum levels of 25-hydroxycholecalciferol and 1,25$(OH)_2D_3$ (Pietrek *et al.*, 1978; Llach *et al.*, 1981). In some cases of severe hypercalcemia (of up to 17 mg/dl), there was no clear relationship to hyperparathyroidism, since PTH levels were close to the normal range and not related to the marked hypercalcemia (Tavill *et al.*, 1964; Leonard and Eichner, 1970; Wu *et al.*, 1972). A hypercalcemia was also noted in a patient with idiopathic hypoparathyroidism in acute renal failure (Chertow *et al.*, 1974).

3. *Hypophosphatemic Vitamin D-Resistant Rickets*

The question whether the high urinary phosphate excretion in this condition is caused by a secondary hyperparathyroidism or by a primary renal tubular leak of phosphate was answered by Arnaud *et al.* (1971a) when they demonstrated normal serum PTH levels in these patients (Fig. 10). Although several authors have reported increased PTH levels, these have turned out not to be high enough to support the alternative hypothesis that hypophosphatemia in this disease is due to secondary hyperparathyroidism (Lewy *et al.*, 1972; Fujita *et al.*, 1972; Reitz and Weinstein, 1973; Hahn *et al.*, 1975). Treatment with oral phosphate raises PTH levels in these patients and carries the risk of secondary hyperparathyroidism (Arnaud *et al.*, 1971a; Fanconi *et al.*, 1974). Some patients present with or develop a hypercalcemia that has required the surgical removal of parathyroid tumors (Talwalkar *et al.*, 1974; Kistler *et al.*, 1976; Kleerekoper *et al.*, 1977). The pathogenesis of hypophosphatemic rickets remains to be clearly evaluated. Glorieux and Scriver (1972) located the primary disturbance of phosphate transport in the kidney tubules and suggested the loss of a PTH-sensitive component of phosphate transport as the cause of it. Calcium infusions suppress the urinary phosphate excretion, whereas the iv administration of bPTH did not seem to lower the tubular reabsorption of phosphate. On the other hand, Hahn *et al.* (1975) have demonstrated a normal and Short *et al.* (1976) have demonstrated even exaggerated urinary responses of phosphate excretion to iv infusions of bovine PTH extracts. The exaggerated urinary response to parathyroid extract was, however, only seen when the renal tubular reabsorption of phosphate was suppressed with calcium infusions before the administration of the hormone.

In patients with a hereditary intolerance to fructose, ingestion of this sugar induced a proximal renal tubular dysfunction that included impairment of bicarbonate and calcium reabsorption in the tubule. In a patient with hypoparathyroidism, these changes were noted only when PTH was present (Morris, 1968; Morris *et al.*, 1971). Tubular reabsorption of phosphate may also be impaired and thus the picture may resemble a Fanconi syndrome in association with a renal acidification defect.

4. *Pseudohypoparathyroidism*

Pseudohypoparathyroidism was originally described by Albright *et al.* (1942) as a syndrome caused by an inability to respond to PTH. Characteristic clinical features include a short stature, brachymetacarpia and -tarsia, a round face, and obesity. Additional signs such as dental anomalies, mental retardation, and calcified basal ganglia are typical for hypoparathyroidism in general and not specific for pseudohypoparathyroidism (see Section VII,G). The laboratory findings are characteristic of hypoparathyroidism with decreased serum calcium and increased serum phosphate levels. In hypocalcemic patients with pseudohypoparathyroidism, serum PTH levels are normal or increased, whereas in true hypoparathyroidism PTH levels are undetectable or low in the presence of decreased serum calcium concentrations (Fig. 11, Table VI) (Chase *et al.*, 1969b; Frame *et al.*, 1972; Birkenhäger *et al.*, 1973; Lee *et al.*, 1968; Nusynowitz and Klein, 1973; Drezner *et al.*, 1973; Werder *et al.*, 1978).

Sometimes very high PTH values have been noted in normocalcemic cases of pseudohypoparathyroidism; in several of these patients, serum PTH was lowered to normal during calcium infusions that had raised the serum calcium to abnormally high levels (Werder *et al.*, 1978). The situation is thus similar to acquired vitamin D deficiency rickets. It is therefore possible that a disturbance of vitamin D metabolism has led to the raised PTH levels (see Section VII,F,1).

Inasmuch as PTH is raised in hypocalcemic patients and suppressed when they receive calcium infusions, an inadequate secretion of PTH does not appear to be the cause of clinical hypoparathyroidism encountered in these patients. The question then arises whether the end organ is unresponsive to PTH, the conventional hypothesis, or whether the parathyroid glands secrete an abnormal, biologically inactive peptide, or a factor interfering with the activity of biologically active PTH.

The finding that PTH acts via the adenylate cyclase system and that the urinary excretion of cyclic AMP cannot be stimulated with PTH in pseudohypoparathyroidism gave rise to the suggestion that the disorder may be the result of defective or absent PTH-sensitive receptors in bone and kidney (Chase *et al.*, 1969b). Indeed, in some patients the activity of a guanine nucleotide regulatory protein coupling the membrane receptor to the adenylate cyclase was found to be decreased in the kidney and in red blood cells (Drezner *et al.*, 1978; Levine *et al.*, 1980; Farfel *et al.*, 1980).

This hypothesis does not explain, why in some patients with pseudohypoparathyroidism the apparent resistance to the administration of exogenous parathyroid extract was abolished by treatment with vitamin D (Suh *et al.*, 1970; Kind *et al.*, 1973; Stögmann and Fischer, 1975). Moreover, in one patient, PTH-responsiveness was restored after surgical removal of four hyperplastic parathyroid glands (Nagant de Deuxchaisnes and Krane, 1978). In all these patients the urinary cyclic AMP excretion was not affected after an intravenous administration of a parathyroid extract, when the kidney tubules clearly responded with an increased urinary phosphate excretion and a concomitant decrease of the tubular reabsorption of phosphte; furthermore, serum calcium levels were raised in response to PTH (Bell *et al.*, 1972; Birkenhäger *et al.*, 1973; Kind *et al.*, 1973; Stögmann and Fischer, 1975; Nagant de Deuxchaisnes and Krane, 1978).

We have therefore measured circulating levels of PTH in patients with pseudohypoparathyroidism using a sensitive cytochemical bioassay of PTH (Nagant de Deuxchaisnes *et al.*, 1981). In all patients with pseudohypopara-

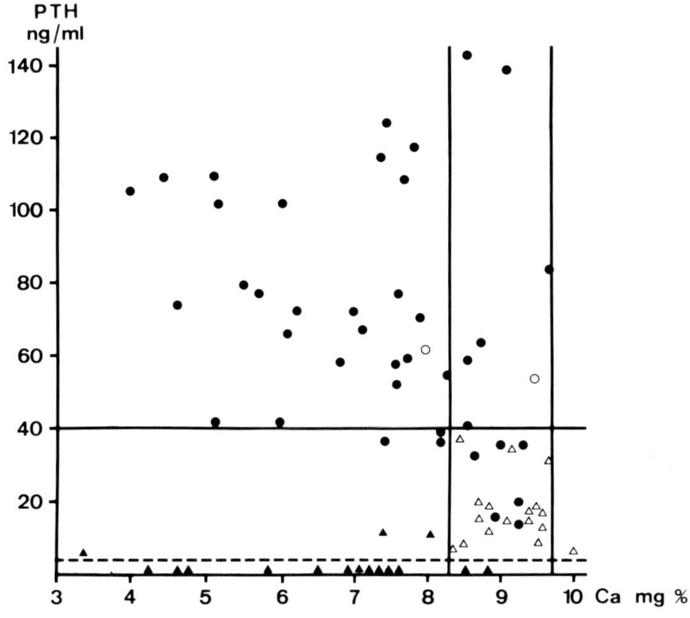

Fig. 11. Serum PTH as a function of calcium in patients with idiopathic hypoparathyroidism (▲), pseudohypoparathyroidism type I (●), and type II (○), and pseudopseudohypoparathyroidism (△). For details see Figs. 4 and 7. (Adapted from Werder *et al.*, 1978.)

TABLE VI

Pathogenesis of Hypoparathyroidism[a]

Form	Serum PTH	Pathogenesis: Undisputed	Pathogenesis: Questionable
Thyroid and parathyroid surgery, metastatic cancer invasion, infiltration (?)	$\downarrow\rightarrow$	Lack of PTH	
Functional (hypercalcemia of the mother in neonates, hypercalcemia unrelated to hyperparathyroidism)	$\downarrow\rightarrow$	Lack of PTH	
Idiopathic	$\downarrow\rightarrow$[a]	Lack of PTH	Autoimmune, branchial dysembryogenesis
Magnesium deficiency	$\downarrow\rightarrow$	Lack of PTH, end-organ unresponsiveness	
Pseudohypoparathyroidism	$\uparrow\rightarrow$[a]	End-organ unresponsiveness,	Abnormal PTH
Vitamin D deficiency, altered vitamin D metabolism	$\uparrow$		End-organ unresponsiveness
Antibodies to PTH[b]	Not measured	End-organ unresponsiveness	

[a] According to the definition in this chapter.
[b] Melick *et al.*, 1967.

thyroidism examined, the levels of immunoreactive PTH were in the hyperparathyroid range, whereas the bioactive levels were normal or close to the normal range. The finding that much of the immunoreactive circulating PTH may not be biologically active, may explain some of the clinical findings in this disease. Indeed, PTH receptors might be blocked or partially blocked, by the presence in the circulation of some patients with pseudohypoparathyroidism of a factor, such as an excess of apparently immunochemically intact, but biologically inactive PTH.

The resistance to PTH is presumably not caused by a defective conversion of intact PTH to PTH fragments, since purified bPTH-(1–84), and synthetic bPTH-(1–34) and hPTH-(1–34) all were equally ineffective in raising urinary cyclic AMP and phosphate excretions in pseudohypoparathyroidism (Neer *et al.*, 1977).

Thyroid-stimulating hormone responses to iv injections of thyrotropin-releasing hormone are exaggerated in patients with pseudohypoparathyroidism, but not in idiopathic hypoparathyroidism (Werder *et al.*, 1975). Patients with pseudohypoparathyroidism also have an impaired prolactin response to the administration of thyrotropin-releasing hormone (Carlson *et al.*, 1977). The question as to whether pseudohypoparathyroidism, hypothyroidism, and prolactin deficiency are caused by the same metabolic defect remains to be evaluated.

Drezner *et al.* (1973) have described yet another form of pseudohypoparathyroidism type II which, in contrast to type I, showed a normal urinary cyclic AMP response, but no rise in urinary phosphate or serum calcium. In pseudohypoparathyroidism type II the phosphaturic effect of a parathyroid extract can be restored during a calcium infusion (Rodriguez *et al.*, 1974).

In conclusion, pseudohypoparathyroidism is a form of secondary hyperparathyroidism with increased PTH levels. After the administration of exogenous PTH, some patients (type II) respond with increased urinary cyclic AMP excretion; in the large majority of patients, however, the cyclic AMP excretion remains unaltered (type I). The truly biological effects of exogenous PTH e.g. a stimulation of urinary phosphate excretion and a rise of serum calcium concentration, may be absent or present in patients with pseudohypoparathyroidism, and should not be used as diagnostic indices. The levels of $1,25(OH)_2D_3$ in the serum are sometimes decreased, but this is not pathogenetically important, as some patients with true hypoparathyroidism have also been reported to have low $1,25(OH)_2D$ levels (Haussler *et al.*, 1976; Drezner *et al.*, 1976b; Lund *et al.*, 1980). The classical dysmorphological signs originally described by Albright *et al.* (1942) may or may not be present in pseudohypoparathyroidism (Werder *et al.*, 1978). Finally, pseudohypoparathyroidism may be associated with hypothyroidism and prolactin deficiency. In view of the rather low biological activity of PTH in a cytochemical assay in the face of high immunoreactive PTH in patients with pseudohypoparathyroidism type I, it appears possible, that

PTH receptors might be blocked by the presence of a factor in the circulation (Nagant de Deuxchaisnes *et al.*, 1981). As yet it is not possible to propose a unifying hypothesis regarding the pathogenesis of this disease.

5. *Miscellaneous Forms of Secondary Hyperparathyroidism*

Hypocalcemia is the single most important cause of an increase in serum PTH levels. An example is the hypocalcemia induced by oral phosphate or calcitonin (Reiss *et al.*, 1970; Riggs *et al.*, 1971a). During acute extracellular fluid expansion serum calcium may be decreased and PTH increased (Shaw *et al.*, 1974). Intravenous calcium infusions, on the other hand, suppress PTH levels (Arnaud *et al.*, 1971c).

In patients with idiopathic hypercalciuria, PTH may be increased and the serum calcium (total and ionized) is normal (Coe *et al.*, 1973; Pak *et al.*, 1974). Furosemide treatment leads to a hypercalciuria and raised PTH levels even though the serum ionized calcium appears unchanged. Coe *et al.* (1973) have postulated that in the absence of hypocalcemia, hypercalciuria may be the cause of hyperparathyroidism. Bordier *et al.* (1977) presented some evidence for a primary renal calcium leak in these patients.

In patients with distal renal tubular acidosis, PTH levels were moderately increased; treatment with alkali caused decreased urinary calcium excretion and raised serum clacium levels; as a result, serum PTH was lowered (Gonick *et al.*, 1973; Coe and Firpo, 1975; Lee *et al.*, 1976). In acute metabolic acidosis induced with ammonium chloride there occurred a hypercalciuria, a fall in serum ionized calcium, and as a result a slight increase of PTH levels (Coe *et al.*, 1975).

Catecholamines are potent stimulators of PTH secretion (see Section III,C). In three patients with hypercalcemia and familial pheochromacytoma, adrenalectomy corrected the hypercalcemia and the increased PTH levels of one patient (Swinton *et al.*, 1972; Kukreja *et al.*, 1973; Gray and Gillon, 1976). However, hyperparathyroidism is rarely encountered in patients with pheochromocytoma (Miller *et al.*, 1975). Since epinephrine only stimulates transient PTH release, a chronic catecholamine excess may not necessarily cause hyperparathyroidism (Blum *et al.*, 1978). The administration of adrenergic agonists such as isoproterenol and epinephrine has led to an increase of PTH levels, whereas the β-adrenergic blocking agent propranolol suppressed PTH levels without apparently changing serum total calcium concentrations (Kukreja *et al.*, 1975). Furthermore, a hypoglycemic stress also stimulated PTH levels, suggesting that adrenergic stimuli may be physiologically important (Shah *et al.*, 1975). All these effects are unrelated to changes in serum calcium concentrations and appear to affect PTH secretion directly.

Parathyroid gland hyperplasia is occasionally encountered in patients with medullary carcinoma of the thyroid; in some patients calcium infusions have increased immunoreactive calcitonin levels, and as a possible consequence also PTH concentrations (Deftos and Parthemore, 1974). A possible direct effect of calcitonin and cortisol on PTH secretion have been observed in parathyroid explant cultures *in vitro* (Fischer *et al.*, 1971; Au, 1976). In patients treated with glucocorticoids serum PTH levels may also be increased with no changes occurring in the total serum calcium concentration (Fucik *et al.*, 1975).

Alternatively, hyperparathyroidism is part of a familial multiple endocrine neoplasia syndrome—type I, which includes tumors of the pancreatic islets, the adrenal cortex, and the pituitary, or type II, which includes pheochromocytoma and medullary thyroid carcinoma (Ballard *et al.*, 1964; Steiner *et al.*, 1968). The question as to whether the entire syndrome is transmitted as an autosomal dominant trait with varying penetrance, or whether hyperparathyroidism occurs secondary to catecholamine, calcitonin, or glucocorticoid excess or to changes in the serum calcium concentration remains to be elucidated.

In the large majority of patients with osteoporosis and crush fractures, PTH levels are essentially normal (Riggs *et al.*, 1973; Fujita *et al.*, 1973b). In some patients with quadriplegia due to spinal cord trauma, PTH levels were found increased (Arnstein *et al.*, 1973). Treatment of patients with postmenopausal osteoporosis with calcitonin led to a decrease in serum calcium and a consequent increase in PTH levels (Jowsey *et al.*, 1971). Calcium and vitamin D, on the other hand, caused increased serum calcium and decreased PTH concentrations (Riggs *et al.*, 1976). It appears unlikely, however, that in the majority of osteoporotic patients loss of bone mineral is due to increased PTH secretion (see also Chapter 2, Vol. III).

G. Hypoparathyroidism

In the context of this chapter true hypoparathyroidism means a total or partial deficiency of PTH secretion (Table VI, Fig. 11). In idiopathic hypoparathyroidism PTH levels are either undetectable or low as is serum calcium. Usually the serum phosphate concentration is increased and dental abnormalities, cataracts, mental retardation, and calcified basal ganglia may occur. The administration of exogenous PTH results in increased urinary output of cyclic AMP and phosphate, and in raised serum calcium levels (Ellsworth and Howard, 1934; Chase *et al.*, 1969b). Patients with hypoparathyroidism or pseudohypoparathyroidism (see Section VII,F) may be treated with vitamin D or its analogs or with low amounts of 1,25$(OH)_2D_3$ (Kooh *et al.*, 1975). In some patients with hypoparathyroidism, the circulating levels of 1,25$(OH)_2D_3$ are decreased (Haussler *et al.*, 1976; Land *et al.*, 1980).

In the following, several forms of true hypoparathyroidism are discussed in somewhat more detail.

1. *Parathyroidectomy and Invasion and Infiltration of Parathyroid Tissue*

The best-defined form of hypoparathyroidism with a lack of the hormone or insufficient secretion occurs after an inadvertent removal of parathyroid tissue during a thyroidectomy. In patients with a diffuse hyperplasia of all the parathyroid glands, a remaining half-gland is usually sufficient to maintain a normal serum calcium concentration. Profound hypocalcemia may occasionally result in patients with primary hyperparathyroidism from infarction of a parathyroid adenoma (Northcutt *et al.*, 1969). On occasion hypoparathyroidism occurs because of a metastatic invasion of more than 70% of the parathyroid glandular tissue (Horwitz *et al.*, 1972). Similarly, hemochromatosis may cause hypoparathyroidism through an infiltration of parathyroid tissue (MacDonald and Mallory, 1960; Sherman *et al.*, 1970).

2. *Functional Hypoparathyroidism*

The transient physiological functional hypoparathyroidism of the neonate and the more severe form with a hypercalcemia of the mother are discussed in Section VII,C.

Patients with extreme magnesium deficiency (serum magnesium < 1 mg/dl) are usually hypocalcemic and PTH levels are undetectable or low in the face of a decreased serum calcium concentrations (Anast *et al.*, 1972; Chase and Slatopolsky, 1974). The secretory responsiveness of the parathyroid glands can be restored with magnesium infusions, which paradoxically and transiently raise PTH levels (Fig. 4) (see Section III,C); thereafter, a normal inhibitory effect of the hypermagnesemia on PTH release occurs. Hypocalcemia occurs not only because of decreased parathyroid secretory function, but also because of a resistance of the end organs to the action of PTH (Anast *et al.*, 1972; Suh *et al.*, 1973; Estep *et al.*, 1969; Muldowney *et al.*, 1970; Woodward *et al.*, 1972; Paunier *et al.*, 1968; Connor *et al.*, 1972; Chase and Slatopolsky, 1974; Freitag *et al.*, 1979).

In some patients with hypocalcemia and acute pancreatitis PTH levels remain within a normal range even though the serum calcium was decreased; a relative parathyroid insufficiency may account for the hypocalcemia observed in this disease (Robertson *et al.*, 1976).

3. *Idiopathic Hypoparathyroidism*

In the present chapter idiopathic hypoparathyroidism is defined as a form of hypoparathyroidism with absent or decreased hormonal secretion. In our opinion it should not be distinguished from true hypoparathyroidism after parathyroidectomy. Untreated patients are hypocalcemic, and serum PTH levels are undetectable or low in the presence of a decreased serum calcium concentrations (Fig. 11). PTH levels in untreated hypocalcemic patients with pseudohypoparathyroidism and idiopathic hypoparathyroidism can be clearly differentiated (Werder *et al.*, 1978).

The patients respond to the exogenous administration of PTH with an increased urinary excretion of cyclic AMP and phosphate and raised serum calcium levels. These parameters do, however, not allow a clear differentiation between idiopathic and pseudohypoparathyroidism, since a normal cyclic AMP response to PTH is found by definition in pseudohypoparathyroidism type II. Furthermore, some truly biological responses can be encountered in a large number of patients with pseudohypoparathyroidism under certain conditions (see Section VII,F,4).

The pathogenesis of idiopathic hypoparathyroidism is unknown at present. In some cases, probably absent parathyroid glands are associated with an absent thymus, cardiovascular anomalies, and other defects of branchial origin (Di George, 1967; Nezelof *et al.*, 1975). Miller *et al.* (1972) introduced the term branchial dysembryogenesis for the syndrome. Other cases were associated with Addison's disease, pernicious anemia, Hashimoto's disease, primary ovarian failure, and monoliasis (Bronksy *et al.*, 1958; Kunin *et al.*, 1963; Kleerekoper *et al.*, 1974). Blizzard *et al.* (1966) noted antibodies to parathyroid tissue (not parathyroid hormone) in 38% of 72 patients with idiopathic hypoparathyroidism, in 26% of 92 patients with Addison's disease and in 12% with Hashimoto's thyroiditis as compared to 6% of 245 control patients, and suggested a possible autoimmune etiology of the disease. On rare occasions parathyroid tissue has been found to be infiltrated with lymphocytes (Craig *et al.*, 1955; Mitschke *et al.*, 1973).

4. *Sarcoidosis and Hyperthyroidism*

In the majority of patients with sarcoidosis, PTH levels were found to be low or undetectable regardless of whether the serum calcium was normal or increased (Cushard *et al.*, 1972b). This can be explained by an excessive formation of $1,25(OH)_2D$ and stimulation of intestinal calcium absorption causing suppression of PTH levels (Papapoulos *et al.*, 1979; Stern *et al.*, 1980) (see Section III,C).

Similar findings have been made in patients with hyperthyroidism, where the serum calcium was higher and PTH levels correspondingly lower than in hypothyroidism (Bouillon and de Moor, 1974; Burman *et al.*, 1976). Sarcoidosis and hyperthyroidism represent yet other forms of functional hypoparathyroidism, which is, however, never associated with a hypocalcemia. This does not rule out that primary hyperparathyroidism and sarcoidosis or hyperthyroidism sometimes coexist (Parfitt and Dent, 1970; Bergdahl, 1977).

ACKNOWLEDGMENTS

I would like to express my gratitude to Dr. F. Bronner, for valuable advice.

These studies have been supported by the Swiss National Science Foundation (Grants 3.941-0.78, 3.773-0.76).

REFERENCES

Abe, M., and Sherwood, L. M. (1972). Regulation of parathyroid hormone secretion by adenyl cyclase. *Biochem. Biophys. Res. Commun.* **48,** 396-401.

Agus, Z. S., Puschett, J. W., Senesky, D., and Goldberg, M. (1971). Mode of action of parathyroid hormone and cyclic adenosine 3′,5′-monophosphate on renal tubular phosphate reabsorption in the dog. *J. Clin. Invest.* **50,** 617-626.

Agus, Z. S., Gardner, L. W., Beck, L. H., and Goldberg, M. (1973). Effects of parathyroid hormone on renal tubular reabsorption of calcium, sodium, and phosphate. *Am. J. Physiol.* **224,** 1143-1148.

Albright, F., and Reifenstein, E. C., Jr. (1948). "The Parathyroid Glands and Metabolic Bone Disease." Williams & Wilkins, Baltimore, Maryland.

Albright, F., Burnett, C. H., Smith, P. H., and Parson, W. (1942). Pseudo-Hypoparathyroidism, an example of "Sebright-Bantam-Syndrome." Report of three cases. *Endocrinology (Baltimore)* **30,** 922-932.

Alfrey, A. C., Jenkins, D., Groth, C. G., Schorr, W. S., Gecelter, L., and Ogden, D. A. (1968). Resolution of hyperparathyroidism, renal osteodystrophy and metastatic calcification after renal homotransplantation. *N. Engl. J. Med.* **279,** 1349-1356.

Altenahr, E. (1971). Electron microscopical evidence for innervation of chief cells in human parathyroid gland. *Experientia* **27,** 1077.

Alveryd, A., El-Zawahry, M. D., Herlitz, P., and Nodenstam, H. (1975). Primary hyperplasia of the parathyroids. *Acta Chir. Scand.* **141,** 24-30.

Anast, C. S., Mohs, J. M., Kaplan, S. L., and Burns, T. W. (1972). Evidence for parathyroid failure in magnesium deficiency. *Science* **177,** 606-608.

Anast, C. S., Winnacker, J. L., Forte, L. R., and Burns, T. W. (1976). Impaired release of parathyroid hormone in magnesium deficiency. *J. Clin. Endocrinol. Metab.* **42,** 707-717.

Arnaud, C. D. (1973). Hyperparathyroidism and renal failure. *Kidney Int.* **4,** 89-95.

Arnaud, C. D., Rasmussen, H., and Anast, C. (1966). Further studies on the interrelationship between parathyroid hormone and vitamin D. *J. Clin. Invest.* **45,** 1955-1964.

Arnaud, C. D., Maijer, R., Reade, T., Scriver, C. R., and Whelan, D. T. (1970). Vitamin D dependency: An inherited postnatal syndrome with secondary hyperparathyroidism. *Pediatrics* **46,** 871-880.

Arnaud, C. D., Glorieux, F., and Scriver, C. R. (1971a). Serum parathyroid hormone in X-linked hypophosphatemia. *Science* **173,** 845-847.

Arnaud, C. D., Sizemore, G. W., Oldham, S. B., Fischer, J. A., Tsao, H. S., and Litteldike, E. T. (1971b). Human parathyroid hormone: Glandular and secreted molecular species. *Am. J. Med.* **50,** 630-638.

Arnaud, C. D., Tsao, H. S., and Littledike, T. (1971c). Radioimmunoassay of human parathyroid hormone in serum. *J. Clin. Invest.* **50,** 21-34.

Arnaud, C. D., Glorieux, F., and Scriver, C. R. (1972). Serum parathyroid hormone levels in acquired vitamin D deficiency of infancy. *Pediatrics* **49,** 837-840.

Arnaud, C. D., Goldsmith, R. S., Bordier, P. J., and Sizemore, G. W. (1974). Influence of immunoheterogeneity of circulating parathyroid hormone on results of radioimmunoassays of serum in man. *Am. J. Med.* **56,** 785–793.

Arnaud, S. B., Goldsmith, R. S., Strickler, G. B., McCall, J. T., and Arnaud, C. D. (1973). Serum parathyroid hormone and blood minerals: Interrelationship in normal children. *Pediatr. Res.* **7,** 485–493.

Arnstein, A. R., McCann, D. S., Blumenthal, F. S., and Prunty, J. (1973). Serum immunoreactive parathyroid hormone in patients with paralysis due to spinal cord trauma. *In* "Clinical Aspects of Metabolic Bone Disease" (W. Frame, A. M. Parfitt, and H. Duncan, eds.), pp. 253–256. Excerpta Medica, Amsterdam.

Arruda, J. A. L., Nascimento, L., Westenfelder, C., and Kurtzman, N. A. (1977). Effect of parathyroid hormone on urinary acidification. *Am. J. Physiol.* **232,** F429–F439.

Au, W. Y. W. (1976). Cortisol stimulation of parathyroid hormone secretion by rat parathyroid glands in organ culture. *Science* **193,** 1015–1017.

Au, W. Y. W., and Raisz, L. G. (1967). Restoration of parathyroid responsiveness in vitamin-D deficient rats by parenteral calcium or dietary lactose. *J. Clin. Invest.* **46,** 1572–1578.

Au, W. Y. W., Poland, A. P., Stern, P. H., and Raisz, L. G. (1970). Hormone synthesis and secretion by rat parathyroid glands in tissue culture. *J. Clin. Invest.* **49,** 1639–1646.

Aurbach, G. D. (1959). Isolation of parathyroid hormone after extraction with phenol. *J. Biol. Chem.* **234,** 3179–3181.

Aurbach, G. D., and Heath, D. A. (1974). Parathyroid hormone and calcitonin regulation of renal function. *Kidney Int.* **6,** 331–345.

Babka, J. C., Bower, R. H., and Sode, J. (1976). Nephrogenous cyclic AMP levels in primary hyperparathyroidism. *Arch. Intern. Med.* **136,** 1140–1144.

Ballard, H. S., Frame, B., and Hartsock, R. J. (1964). Familial multiple endocrinopeptic ulcer complex. *Medicine (Baltimore)* **43,** 481–516.

Bank, N., and Aynedjian, H. S. (1976). A micropuncture study of the effect of parathyroid hormone on renal bicarbonate reabsorption. *J. Clin. Invest.* **58,** 336–344.

Bates, R. F. L., Care, A. D., Peacock, M., Mawer, E. B., and Taylor, C. M. (1975). Inhibitory effect of 24,25-dihydroxycholecalciferol on parathyroid hormone secretion in the goat. *J. Endocrinol.* **49,** 6P (abstr.).

Baumann, K., Chan, Y.-L., Bode, F., and Papavassiliou, F. (1977). Effect of parathyroid hormone and cyclic adenosine 3′,5′-monophosphate on isotonic fluid reabsorption: Polarity of proximal tubular cells. *Kidney Int.* **11,** 77–85.

Beahrs, O. H., Peter Angelos, S., and Woolner, L. B. (1963). Carcinoma of the parathyroid gland. *Surg. Clin. North Am.* **43,** 1123–1127.

Beard, D. E., and Goodyear, W. E. (1950). Hyperparathyroidism and urolithiasis. *J. Urol.* **84,** 638–642.

Beck, N., Singh, H., Reed, S. W., and Davis, B. B. (1974). Direct inhibitory effect of hypercalcemia on renal actions of parathyroid hormone. *J. Clin. Invest.* **53,** 717–725.

Beck, N., Kim, K. S., Wolak, M., and Davis, B. B. (1975). Inhibition of carbonic anhydrase by parathyroid hormone and cyclic AMP in rat renal cortex *in vitro*. *J. Clin. Invest.* **55,** 149–156.

Bélanger, L. F., and Rasmussen, H. (1968). Inhibition of osteolytic osteolysis by thyrocalcitonin and some anti-growth factors. *In* "Parathyroid Hormone and Thyrocalcitonin (Calcitonin)" (R. V. Talmage and L. F. Bélanger, eds.), pp. 156–168. Excerpta Medica, Amsterdam.

Bell, N. H., Avery, S., Sinha, T., Clark, C. M., Jr., Allen, D. D., and Johnston C., Jr. (1972). Effects of dibutyryl cyclic adenosine 3′,5′-monophosphate and parathyroid extract on calcium and phosphorus metabolism in hypoparathyroidism and pseudohypoparathyroidism. *J. Clin. Invest.* **51,** 816–823.

Bellorin-Font, E., Martin, K. J., Freitag, J. J., Anderson, C., Sicard, G., Slatopolsky, E., and Klahr, S. (1981). Altered adenylate cyclase kinetics in hyperfunctioning human parathyroid glands. *J. Clin. Endocrinol. Metab.* **52,** 499–507.

Bender, R. A., and Hansen, H. (1974). Hypercalcemia in bronchogenic carcinoma. *Ann. Intern. Med.* **80,** 205–208.

Benson, R. C., Jr., Riggs, B. L., Pickard, B. M., and Arnaud, C. D. (1974a). Immunoreactive forms of circulating parathyroid hormone in primary and ectopic hyperparathyroidism. *J. Clin. Invest.* **54,** 175–181.

Benson, R. C., Jr., Riggs, B. L., Pickard, B. M., and Arnaud, C. D. (1974b). Radioimmunoassay of parathyroid hormone in hypercalcemic patients with malignant disease. *Am. J. Med.* **56,** 821–826.

Bergdahl, L. (1977). Hyperparathyroidism in thyrotoxicosis. *Am. J. Surg.* **133,** 206–210.

Berson, S. A., and Yalow, R. S. (1966). Parathyroid hormone in plasma in adenomatous hyperparathyroidism, uremia, and bronchogenic carcinoma. *Science* **154,** 907–909.

Berson, S. A., and Yalow, R. S. (1968). Immunochemical heterogeneity of parathyroid hormone in plasma. *J. Clin. Endocrinol. Metab.* **28,** 1037–1047.

Bethune, J. E., and Turpin, R. A. (1968). A study of urinary excretion of parathyroid hormone in man. *J. Clin. Invest.* **47,** 1583–1589.

Bijvoet, O. L. M. (1969). Relation of plasma phosphate concentration to renal tubular absorption of phosphate. *Clin. Sci.* **37,** 23–36.

Bilezikian, J. P., Dopman, J. L., Shimkin, P. M., Powell, D., Wells, S. A., Heath, D. A., Ketcham, A. S., Monchik, J., Mallette, L. E., Potts, J. T., Jr., and Aurbach, G. D. (1973). Preoperative localization of abnormal parathyroid tissue. *Am. J. Med.* **55,** 505–514.

Binswanger, U., and Fischer, J. A. (1974). Response of immunoreactive parathyroid hormone to intravenous phosphate infusion in primary hyperparathyroidism. *Klin. Wochenschr.* **52,** 30–32.

Binswanger, U., and Fischer, J. A. (1978). Laboratoriumsuntersuchungen bei Erkrankungen der Parathyreoidea. *In* "Klinik der inneren Sekretion" (A. Labhart, ed.), 3rd ed., pp. 889–900, 916–918. Springer-Verlag, Berlin and New York.

Binswanger, U., Fischer, J. A., Iselin, H., Oswald, N., Frei, D., and Willimann, P. (1978). 1,25-dihydroxycholecalciferol treatment of clinically asymptomatic renal osteodystrophy. *Miner. Electrolyte Metab.* **2,** 103–115.

Birge, S. J., Switzer, S. C., and Leonard, D. R. (1974). Influence of sodium and parathyroid hormone on calcium release from intestinal mucosal cells. *J. Clin. Invest.* **54,** 702–709.

Birkenhäger, J. C., Seldenrath, H. J., Hackeng, W. H. L., Schellekens, A. P. M., van der Veer, A. L. J., and Roelfsema, F. (1973). Calcium and phosphorus metabolism, parathyroid hormone, calcitonin and bone histology in pseudohypoparathyroidism. *Eur. J. Clin. Invest.* **3,** 27–34.

Birnbaumer, M. E., Schneider, A. B., Palmer, D., Hanley, D. A., and Sherwood, L. M. (1977). Secretion of parathyroid hormone by abnormal human parathyroid glands in vitro. *J. Clin. Endocrinol. Metab.* **45,** 105–113.

Black, B. M. (1953). "Hyperparathyroidism." Thomas, Springfield, Illinois.

Blair, A. J., Jr., Hawker, C. D., and Utiger, R. D. (1973). Ectopic hyperparathyroidism in a patient with metastatic hypernephroma. *Metab., Clin. Exp.* **22,** 147–154.

Blizzard, R. M., Chee, D., and Davis, W. (1966). The incidence of parathyroid and other antibodies in the sera of patients with idiopathic hypoparathyroidism *Clin. Exp. Immunol.* **1,** 119–128.

Blum, J. W., Mayer, G. P., and Potts, J. T., Jr. (1974a). Parathyroid hormone responses during spontaneous hypocalcemia and induced hypercalcemia in cows. *Endocrinology (Baltimore)* **95,** 84–92.

Blum, J. W., Fischer, J. A., Schwörer, D., Hunziker, W., and Binswanger, U. (1974b). Acute parathyroid hormone response: Sensitivity, relationship to hypocalcemia, and rapidity. *Endocrinology (Baltimore)* **95,** 753–759.

Blum, J. W., Fischer, J. A., Guillebeau, A., Hunziker, W. H., Binswanger, U., Picotti, G. B., and DaPrada, M. (1978). Parathyroid hormone responses to catecholamines and to changes of extracellular calcium in cows. *J. Clin. Invest.* **61,** 1113–1122.

Blum, J. W. Bianca, W., DaPrada, M., and Fischer, J. A. (1979a). Stimulation of plasma parathyroid hormone and catecholamine levels during stimulated high altitude and treadmill exercise in cattle. *Horm. Metab. Res.* **11,** 246–251.

Blum, J. W., Kunz, P., Fischer, J. A., Binswanger, U., Lichtensteiger, W., and DaPrada, M. (1979b). Parathyroid hormone response to dopamine in cattle. *Am. J. Physiol.* **239,** E255–E264.

Bocquetin, F., Safar, A., Aicardi, J., and Job, J.-C. (1973). Tétanie hypocalcémique néonatale chez deux enfants d'une mère hyperparathyroidienne. *Arch. Fr. Pédiatr.* **30,** 989–998.

Bogdonoff, M. D., Woods, A. H., White, J. E., and Engel, E. L. (1956). Hyperparathyroidism. *Am. J. Med.* **21,** 583–595.

Bogin, E., Massry, S. G., and Harary, I. (1981). Effect of parathyroid hormone on rat heart cells. *J. Clin. Invest.* **67,** 1215–1227.

Bolman, III, R. M., Cooper, C. W., Garner, S. C., Munson, P. L., and Wells, S. A., Jr. (1977). Stimulation of gastrin secretion in the pig by parathyroid hormone and its inhibition by thyrocalcitonin. *Endocrinology (Baltimore)* **100,** 1014–1021.

Bordier, P. J., Marie, T. J., and Arnaud, C. D. (1975). Evolution of renal osteodystrophy: Correlation of bone histomorphometry and serum mineral and immunoreactive parathyroid hormone values before and after treatment with calcium carbonate or 25-hydroxycholecalciferol. *Kidney Int.* **7,** 102–112.

Bordier, P. J., Ryckewart, A., Guéris, J., and Rasmussen, H. (1977). On the pathogenesis of so-called idiopathic hypercalciuria. *Am. J. Med.* **63,** 398–409.

Borle, A. B. (1968). Calcium metabolism in HeLa cells and the effects of parathyroid hormone. *J. Cell Biol.* **36,** 567–582.

Borle, A. B. (1973). Calcium metabolism at the cellular level. *Fed. Proc., Fed. Am. Soc. Exp. Biol.* **32,** 1944–1950.

Borle, A. B. (1974). Calcium and phosphate metabolism. *Annu. Rev. Physiol.* **36,** 361–390.

Borle, A. B. (1975). Regulation of cellular calcium metabolism and calcium transport by calcitonin. *J. Membr. Biol.* **21,** 125–146.

Born, W., Fischer, J. A., Paillard, F., Meyrier, A., and Ardaillou, R. (1980). Effects of calcium on distribution of parathyroid hormone forms in venous parathyroid effluent before and after renal transplantation. *Calcif. Tissue Int.* **31,** 72 (abstr.).

Boudry, J.-F., Troehler, U., Touabi, M., Fleisch, H., and Bonjour, J.-P. (1975). Secretion of inorganic phosphate in the rat nephron. *Clin. Sci.* **48,** 475–489.

Bouillon, R., and de Moor, P. (1973). Pathophysiological data obtained with a radioimmunoassay for human parathyroid hormone. *Ann. Endocrinol.* **34,** 657–667.

Bouillon, R., and de Moor, P. (1974). Parathyroid function in patients with hyperthyroidism and hypothyroidism. *J. Clin. Endocrinol. Metab.* **38,** 999–1004.

Bouillon, R., and de Moor, P. (1977). Parathyroid hormone secretion in primary hyperparathyroidism. *J. Clin. Endocrinol. Metab.* **45,** 261–269.

Bouillon, R., Verberckmoos, R., and de Moor, P. (1975). Influence of dialysate calcium concentration and vitamin D on serum parathyroid hormone during repetitive dialysis. *Kidney Int.* **7,** 422–432.

Bowser, E. N., Hargis, G. K., Henderson, W. J., and Williams, G. A. (1975). Parathyroid hormone secretion in the rat: Effect of aminophylline. *Proc. Soc. Exp. Biol. Med.* **148,** 344–346.

Boyle, I. T., Gray, R. W., and DeLuca, H. F. (1971). Regulation by calcium of *in vivo* synthesis of 1,25-dihydroxycholecalciferol and 21,25-dihydroxycholecalciferol. *Proc. Natl. Acad. Sci. U.S.A.* **68,** 2131–2134.

Brewer, H. B., Jr., and Ronan, R. (1970). Bovine parathyroid hormone: Aminoacid sequence. *Proc. Natl. Acad. Sci. U.S.A.* **67,** 1862–1869.

Brewer, H. B., Jr., Fairwell, T., Ronan, R., Sizemore, G. W., and Arnaud, C. D. (1972). Human parathyroid hormone: Amino-acid sequence of the amino-terminal residues 1–34. *Proc. Natl. Acad. Sci. U.S.A.* **69,** 3585–3588.

Brickman, A. S., Coburn, J. W., Norman, A. W., and Massry, S. G. (1974). Short-term effects of 1,25-dihydroxycholecalciferol on disordered calcium metabolism of renal failure. *Am. J. Med.* **57,** 28–33.

Britton, D. C., Johnston, I. D. A., Thompson, M. H., and Fleming, L. B. (1971). Renal function following parathyroid surgery in primary hyperparathyroidism. *Lancet* **2,** 74–75.

Broadus, A. E. (1977). Clinical cyclic nucleotide research. *Adv. Cyclic Nucleotide Res.* **8,** 509–548.

Broadus, A. E., Mahaffey, J. E., Bartter, F. C., and Neer, R. M. (1977). Nephrogenous cyclic adenosine monophosphate as a parathyroid function test. *J. Clin. Invest.* **60,** 771–783.

Broadus, A. E., Horst, R. L., Lang, R., Littledike, E. T., and Rasmussen, H. (1980). The importance of circulating 1,25-dihydroxyvitamin D in the pathogenesis of hypercalciuria and renal-stone formation in primary hyperparathyroidism. *N. Engl. J. Med.* **302,** 421–426.

Bronner, F., Golub, E. E., and Fischer, J. A. (1976). The effect of vitamin D on renal calcium clearance. *In* "Urolithiasis Research" (H. Fleisch, W. G. Robertson, L. H. Smith, and W. Vahlensieck, eds.), pp. 383–388. Plenum, New York.

Bronsky, D., Kushner, D. S., Dubin, A., and Snapper, J. (1958). Idiopathic hypoparathyroidism and pseudo-hypoparathyroidism. *Medicine (Baltimore)* **37,** 317–352.

Brown, E. M. (1980). Calcium-regulated phosphodiesterase in bovine parathyroid cells. *Endocrinology (Baltimore)* **107,** 1998–2003.

Brown, E. M., Hurwitz, S., and Aurbach, G. D. (1977a). Beta-adrenergic stimulation of cyclic AMP content and parathyroid hormone release from isolated bovine parathyroid cells. *Endocrinology (Baltimore)* **100,** 1696–1702.

Brown, E. M., Hurwitz, S., Woodward, C. J., and Aurbach, G. D. (1977b). Direct identification of beta-adrenergic receptors on isolated bovine parathyroid cells. *Endocrinology (Baltimore)* **100,** 1703–1709.

Brown, E. M., Carroll, R. J., and Aurbach, G. D. (1977c). Dopaminergic stimulation of cyclic AMP accumulation and parathyroid hormone release from dispersed bovine parathyroid cells. *Proc. Natl. Acad. Sci. U.S.A.* **74,** 4210–4213.

Brown, E. M., Brennan, M. F., Hurwitz, S., Windeck, R., Marx, S. J., Spiegel, A. M., Koehler, J. O., Gardner, D. G., and Aurbach, G. D. (1978). Dispersed cells prepared from human parathyroid glands: Distinct calcium sensitivity of adenomas vs. primary hyperplasia. *J. Clin. Endocrinol. Metab.* **46,** 267–276.

Brown, E. M., Gardner, D. G., and Aurbach, G. D. (1980). Effects of the calcium ionophore A23187 on dispersed bovine parathyroid cells. *Endocrinology (Baltimore)* **106,** 133–138.

Buckle, R. M. (1969). Radioimmunoassay of parathyroid hormone in primary hyperparathyroidism: Studies of the removal of parathyroid adenoma. *Br. Med. J.* **2,** 789–793.

Buckle, R. M., McMillan, M., and Mallinson, C. (1970). Ectopic secretion of parathyroid hormone by a renal adenocarcinoma in a patient with hypercalcemia. *Br. Med. J.* **4,** 724–726.

Burk, L. B. (1948). Hyperparathyroidism. *Am. J. Surg.* **76,** 404–411.

Burman, K. D., Monchik, J. M., Earll, J. M., and Wartofski, L. (1976). Ionized and total serum calcium and parathyroid hormone in hyperthyroidism. *Ann. Intern. Med.* **84,** 668–671.

Burnatowska, M. A., Harris, C. A., Sutton, R. A. L., and Dirks, J. H. (1977). Effect of PTH and cAMP on renal handling of calcium, magnesium, and phosphate in the hamster. *Am. J. Physiol.* **233,** F514–518.

Burnett, H. F., Thompson, B. W., and Barbour, G. L. (1977). Parathyroid autotransplantation. *Arch. Surg. (Chicago)* **112,** 373–379.

Byers, P. D., and Smith, R. (1971). Quantitative histology of bone in hyperparathyroidism. *Q. J. Med.* [*N.S.*] **40,** 471–486.

Campos, C., Arata, R. O., and Mautalen, C. A. (1976). Parathyroid hormone and vertebral osteosclerosis in uremic patients. *Metab. Clin. Exp.* **25,** 495–501.

Cannarozzi, D. B., Canale, D. D., and Donabedian, R. K. (1976). Hypercalcitonemia in infancy. *Clin. Chim. Acta* **66,** 387–392.

Canterbury, J. M., and Reiss, E. (1972). Multiple immunoreactive molecular forms of parathyroid hormone in human serum. *Proc. Soc. Exp. Biol. Med.* **140,** 1393–1398.

Canterbury, J. M., Levy, G. S., and Reiss, E. (1973). Activation of renal cortical adenylate cyclase by circulating immunoreactive parathyroid hormone fragments. *J. Clin. Invest.* **52,** 524–527.

Canterbury, J. M., Levy, G., Ruiz, E., and Reiss, E. (1974). Parathyroid hormone activation of adenylate cyclase in liver. *Proc. Soc. Exp. Biol. Med.* **147,** 366–370.

Canterbury, J. M., Bricker, L. A., Levy, G. S., Kozlovskis, P. L., Ruiz, E., Zull, J. E., and Reiss, E. (1975). Metabolism of bovine parathyroid hormone: Immunological and biological characteristics of fragments generated by liver perfusion. *J. Clin. Invest.* **55,** 1245–1253.

Canterbury, J. M., Lerman, S., Claflin, A. J., Henry, H., Norman, A., and Reiss, E. (1978). Inhibition of parathyroid hormone secretion by 25-hydroxycholecalciferol and 24,25-dihydroxycholecalciferol in the dog. *J. Clin. Invest.* **51,** 1375–1383.

Capen, C. C. (1971). Fine structural alterations of parathyroid glands in response to experimental and spontaneous changes of calcium in extracellular fluids. *Am. J. Med.* **50,** 598–611.

Care, A. D., Sherwood, L. M., Potts, J. T., Jr., and Aurbach, G. D. (1966). Evaluation by radioimmunoassay factors controlling the secretion of parathyroid hormone. Perfusion of the isolated parathyroid gland of the goat and sheep. *Nature (London)* **209,** 55–57.

Carlson, H. E., Brickman, A. S., and Bottazzo, E. F. (1977). Prolactin deficiency in pseudohypoparathyroidism. *N. Engl. J. Med.* **296,** 140–144.

Carnes, D. L., Nickols, A., Anast, C. S., and Forte, L. R. (1980). Regulation of renal adenylate cyclase by parathyroid hormone. *Am. J. Physiol.* **239,** E396–E400.

Catherwood, B. D., and Singer, F. R. (1974). Generation of a carboxyl-terminal fragment of bovine parathyroid hormone by canine renal plasma membranes. *Biochem. Biophys. Res. Commun.* **57,** 469–475.

Catherwood, B. D., Friedler, R. M., and Singer, F. R. (1976). Sites of clearance of endogenous parathyroid hormone in the vitamin D-deficient dog. *Endocrinology (Baltimore)* **98,** 228–232.

Chabardès, S. D., Imbert, M., Clique, A., Montégut, M., and Morel, F. (1975). PTH sensitive adenyl cyclase activity in different segments of the rabbit nephron. *Pfluegers Arch.* **354,** 229–239.

Chabardès, S. D., Imbert-Teboul, M., Montégut, M., Clique, A., and Morel, F. (1976). Distribution of calcitonin-sensitive adenylate cyclase activity along the rabbit kidney tubule. *Proc. Natl. Acad. Sci. U.S.A.* **73,** 3608–3612.

Chambers, D. J., Dunham, J., Zanelli, J. M., Parsons, J. A., Bitensky, L., and Chayen, J. (1978). A sensitive bioassay of parathyroid hormone in plasma. *Clin. Endocrinol. (Oxford)* **9,** 375–379.

Chanard, J., Black, R., Purkerson, M., Lewis, J., Klahr, S., and Slatopolsky, E. (1977). The effects of colchicine and vinblastine on parathyroid hormone secretion in the rat. *Endocrinology (Baltimore)* **101,** 1792–1800.

Charbon, G. A., and Hulstaert, P. F. (1974). Augmentation of arterial hepatic and renal flow by extracted and synthetic parathyroid hormone. *Endocrinology (Baltimore)* **95,** 621–626.

Chase, L. R. (1975). Selective proteolysis of the receptor for parathyroid hormone in renal cortex. *Endocrinology (Baltimore)* **96,** 70–76.

Chase, L. R., and Aurbach, G. D. (1967). Parathyroid function and the renal excretion of 3′,5′-adenylic acid. *Proc. Natl. Acad. Sci. U.S.A.* **58,** 518–525.

Chase, L. R., and Aurbach, G. D. (1968). Renal adenyl cyclase: Anatomic separate sites for parathyroid hormone and vasopressin. *Science* **159,** 545–548.

Chase, L. R., and Obert, K. A. (1975). Selective proteolysis of the receptor for parathyroid hormone in skeletal tissue. *Metab. Clin. Exp.* **24,** 1067–1071.

Chase, L. R., and Slatopolsky, E. (1974). Secretion and metabolic efficacy of parathyroid hormone in patients with severe hypomagnesimia. *J. Clin. Endocrinol. Metab.* **38,** 363–371.

Chase, L. R., Fedak, S. A., and Aurbach, G. D. (1969a). Activation of skeletal adenyl cyclase by parathyroid hormone *in vitro*. *Endocrinology (Baltimore)* **84,** 761–768.

Chase, L. R., Melson, G. L., and Aurbach, G. D. (1969b). Pseudohypoparathyroidism: Defective excretion of 3′,5′-AMP in response to parathyroid hormone. *J. Clin. Invest.* **48,** 1832–1844.

Chatterjee, S. N., Friedler, R. M., Berne, T. V., Oldham, S. B., Singer, F. R., and Massry, S. G. (1976). Persistent hypercalcemia after successful renal transplantation. *Nephron* **17,** 1–7.

Chausmer, A. B., Sherman, B. S., and Wallach, S. (1972). The effect of parathyroid hormone on hepatic cell transport of calcium. *Endocrinology (Baltimore)* **90,** 663–672.

Chertow, B. S., Plymate, S. R., and Becker, F. O. (1974). Vitamin D-resistant idiopathic hypoparathyroidism. *Arch. Intern. Med.* **133,** 838–840.

Chertow, B. S., Baylink, D. J., Wergedahl, J. E., Su, M. H. H., and Norman, A. W. (1975a). Decrease in serum immunoreactive parathyroid hormone in rats and in parathyroid hormone secretion *in vitro* by 1,25-dihydroxycholecalciferol. *J. Clin. Invest.* **56,** 668–678.

Chertow, B. S., Buschmann, R. J., and Henderson, W. J. (1975b). Subcellular mechanisms of parathyroid hormone secretion: Ultrastructural changes in response to calcium, vitamin A, vinblastine, and cytocholasin B. *Lab. Invest.* **32,** 190–200.

Chertow, B. S., Williams, G. A., Norris, R. M., Baker, G. R., and Hargis, G. K. (1977). Vitamin A stimulation of parathyroid hormone: Interactions with calcium, hydrocortisone, and vitamin E in bovine parathyroid tissues and effects of vitamin A in man. *Eur. J. Clin. Invest.* **7,** 307–314.

Chu, L. L. H., MacGregor, R. R., Anast, C. S., Hamilton, J. W., and Cohn, D. V. (1973). Studies on the biosynthesis of rat parathyroid hormone and proparathyroid hormone: Adaption of the parathyroid gland to dietary restriction of calcium. *Endocrinology (Baltimore)* **93,** 915–924.

Clinicopathological Conference (1972). Tertiary hyperparathyroidism - does it exist? *Am. J. Med.* **52,** 254–266.

Coe, F. L., and Firpo, J. J., Jr. (1975). Evidence for mild reversible hyperparathyroidism in distal renal tubular acidosis. *Arch. Intern. Med.* **135,** 1485–1489.

Coe, F. L., and Kavalach, A. G. (1974). Hypercalciuria and hyperuricosuria in patients with calcium nephrolithiasis. *N. Engl. J. Med.* **291,** 1344–1350.

Coe, F. L., Canterbury, J. M., Firpo, J. J., and Reiss, E. (1973). Evidence for secondary hyperparathyroidism in idiopathic hypercalciuria. *J. Clin. Invest.* **52,** 134–142.

Coe, F. L., Firpo, J. J., Jr., Hollandsworth, D. L., Segil, L., Canterbury, J. M., and Reiss, E. (1975). Effect of acute and chronic metabolic acidosis on serum immunoreactive parathyroid hormone in man. *Kidney Int.* **8,** 262–273.

Cohn, D. V., MacGregor, E. R., Chu, L. L. H., Kimmel, J. R., and Hamilton, J. W. (1972). Calcemic fraction-A: Biosynthetic peptide precursor of parathyroid hormone. *Proc. Natl. Acad. Sci. U.S.A.* **69,** 1521–1525.

Collip, J. B., and Clark, E. P. (1925). Further studies of the physiological actions of parathyroid hormone. *J. Biol. Chem.* **64,** 485–507.

Conaway, H. H., and Anast, C. S. (1974). Double-antibody radioimmunoassay for parathyroid hormone. *J. Lab. Clin. Med.* **83,** 129–138.

Connor, T. B., Toskes, P., Mahaffey, J., Martin, L. G., Williams, J. B., and Walser, M. (1972). Parathyroid function during chronic magnesium deficiency. *Johns Hopkins Med. J.* **131,** 100–117.

Cope, O. (1976). Hyperparathyroidism - too little, too much surgery? *N. Engl. J. Med.* **295,** 100–102.

Corradino, R. A. (1976). Parathyroid hormone and calcitonin: No direct effect on vitamin D_3-mediated, intestinal calcium absorptive mechanism. *Horm. Metab. Res.* **8,** 485–488.

Corvilain, J., Manderlier, T., Struyven, J., Fuss, M., Bergans, A., Nijs, N., and Brauman, H. (1977). Metabolism of human PTH by the kidney and the liver. *Horm. Metab. Res.* **9,** 239–242.

Cottet, J., Vittu, C. H., and Canarelli, G. (1962). Calciuries et lithiases urinaires. *In* "Rein et foie," Vol. 4, Part 2, pp. 29–54. Vittel, France.

Craig, J. M., Schiff, L. M., and Boone, J. E. (1955). Chronic moniliasis associated with Addison's disease. *Am. J. Dis. Child.* **89,** 669–683.

Cushard, W. G., Jr., Creditor, M. A., Canterbury, J. M., and Reiss, E. (1972a). Physiologic hyperparathyroidism in pregnancy. *J. Clin. Endocrinol. Metab.* **34,** 767–771.

Cushard, W. G., Jr., Simon, A. B., Canterbury, J. M., and Reiss, E. (1972b). Parathyroid function in sarcoidosis. *N. Engl. J. Med.* **286,** 395–398.

Cutler, R. E., Reiss, E., and Ackerman, L. V. (1964). Familial hyperparathyroidism. *N. Engl. J. Med.* **270,** 859–865.

Dacke, C. G., and Kenny, A. D. (1973). Avian bioassay methods for parathyroid hormone. *Endocrinology (Baltimore)* **92,** 463–470.

Dambacher, M. A., Fischer, J. A., Hunziker, W. H., Born, W., Moran, J., Roth, H.-R., Delvin, E. E., and Glorieux, F. H. (1979). Distribution of circulating immunoreactive components of parathyroid hormone in normal subjects and in patients with primary and secondary hyperparathyroidism: the role of kidney and of the serum calcium concentration. *Clin. Sci.* **57,** 435–443.

David, D. S., Sakai, S., Brennan, B. L., Riggio, R. A., Cheigh, J., Stenzel, K. H., Rubin, A. L., and Sherwood, L. M. (1973). Hypercalcemia after renal transplantation. *N. Engl. J. Med.* **289,** 398–401.

David, L., and Anast, C. S. (1974). Calcium metabolism in newborn infants. *J. Clin. Invest.* **54,** 287–296.

David, L., Chapuis, M.-C., Collombel, C., Racle, B., Racle, P., and François, R. (1975). Etudes du méchanisme pathogénique de l'hypocalcémie dans l'hypomagnésimie primitive. *Arch. Fr. Pédiatr.* **32,** 803–814.

Deftos, J., and Parthemore, J. G. (1974). Secretion of parathyroid hormone in patients with medullary carcinoma of the thyroid. *J. Clin. Invest.* **54,** 416–420.

Deftos, L. J., Lorenzi, M., Bohanon, N., Tsalakian, E., Schneider, V., and Gerich, J. E. (1976). Somatostatin does not suppress plasma parathyroid hormone. *J. Clin. Endocrinol. Metab.* **43,** 205–207.

Delmonico, F. L., Neer, R. M., Cosimi, A. B., Barnes, A. B., and Russell, P. S. (1976). Hyperparathyroidism during pregnancy. *Am. J. Surg.* **131,** 328–337.

DeLuca, H. F., Engstrom, G. W., and Rasmussen, H. (1962). The action of vitamin D and parathyroid hormone *in vitro* on calcium uptake and release by kidney mitochondria. *Proc. Natl. Acad. Sci. U.S.A.* **48,** 1604–1609.

Dempster, D. W., Born, W., Tobler, P. H., and Fischer, J. A. (1981). Effects of extracellular monovalent cation concentrations on dynamic secretory responses of parathyroid cells in vitro. *Calcif. Tissue Int.* **33,** 320 (abstr.).

Dent, C. E. (1964). Personal communication in Pyrah *et al.* (1966).

Dent, C. E., and Harter, C. M. (1962). Plasma alkaline phosphatase in normal adults and in patients with primary hyperparathyroidism. *Lancet* **1,** 559–563.

DeRubertis, F. R., and Craven, P. A. (1976). Hormonal modulation of cyclic adenosine 3′,5′-monophosphate-dependent protein kinase activity in rat renal cortex. *J. Clin. Invest.* **57,** 1442–1450.

Diaz-Buxo, J. A., and Knox, F. G. (1975). Effects of parathyroid hormone on renal function. *Mayo Clin. Proc.* **50,** 537–541.

Di Bella, F. P., Dousa, T. P., Miller, S. S., and Arnaud, C. D. (1974). Parathyroid hormone receptors of renal cortex: Specific binding of biologically active, ^{125}I-labeled hormone and relationship to adenylate cyclase activation. *Proc. Natl. Acad. Sci. U.S.A.* **71,** 723–726.

Di Bella, F. P., Gilkinson, J., Flueck, J., and Arnaud, C. D. (1978). Carboxyl terminal fragments of human parathyroid hormone in parathyroid tumors: Unique source of immunogens for the production of potentially useful antisera in the radioimmunoassay of parathyroid hormone in human serum. *J. Clin. Endocrinol. Metab.* **46,** 604–612.

Dietel, M., Altenähr, E., Montz, R., Hagemann, J., and Dorn, G. (1978). Correlation of electron microscopic and secretory response of human parathyroid adenomas with different calcium concentrations in organ culture. *Virchows Arch. A Pathol. Anat. Histol.* **378,** 229–246.

Dietrich, J. M., Canalis, E. M., Maina, D. M., and Raisz, L. G. (1976). Hormonal control of bone collagen synthesis *in vitro*: Effects of parathyroid hormone and calcitonin. *Endocrinology (Baltimore)* **98,** 943–949.

Di George, A. M., Lischner, H. W., Daccu, C., and Arey, J. B. (1967). Absence of the thymus. *Lancet* **1,** 1387.

Dominguez, J. H., Gray, R. W., and Lemann, J., Jr. (1976). Dietary phosphate deprivation in women and men: effects on mineral and acid balances, parathyroid hormone and the metabolism of 25-OH-vitamin D. *J. Clin. Endocrinol. Metab.* **43,** 1056–1068.

Doppman, J. L., Marx, S. J., Brennan, M. F., Beazley, R. M., Gelhoed, G., and Aurbach, G. D. (1977). The blood supply of mediastinal parathyroid adenomas. *Ann. Surg.* **185,** 488–490.

Doyle, F. H. (1972). Radiological patterns of bone disease associated with renal glomerular failure in adults. *Br. Med. Bull.* **28,** 220–224.

Drezner, M. K., Neelon, F. A., and Lebovitz, H. E. (1973). Pseudohypoparathyroidism type II: A possible defect in the reception of the cyclic AMP signal. *N. Engl. J. Med.* **289,** 1056–1060.

Drezner, M. K., Neelon, F. A., Curtis, H. B., and Lebovitz, H. E. (1976a). Renal cyclic adenosine monophosphate: An accurate index of parathyroid function. *Metab. Clin. Exp.* **25,** 1103–1112.

Drezner, M. K., Neelon, F. A., Haussler, M., McPherson, H. T., and Lebovitz, H. E. (1976b). 1,25-dihydroxycholecalciferol deficiency: The probable cause of hypocalcemia and metabolic bone disease in pseudohypoparathyroidism. *J. Clin. Endocrinol. Metab.* **42,** 621–628.

Drezner, M. K., and Burch, W. M., Jr. (1978). Altered activity of the nucleotide regulatory site in the parathyroid hormone-sensitive adenylate cyclase from the renal cortex of a patient with pseudohypoparathyroidism. *J. Clin. Invest.* **62,** 1222–1227.

Dufresne, L. R., and Gitelman, H. J. (1972). A possible role of adenyl cyclase in the regulation of parathyroid activity by calcium. *In* "Calcium, Parathyroid Hormone and the Calcitonins" (R. V. Talmage and P. L. Munson, eds.), pp. 202–206. Excerpta Medica, Amsterdam.

Eisenberg, H., Pallotta, J., and Sherwood, L. M. (1974). Selective arteriography, venography and venous hormone assay in diagnosis and localization of parathyroid lesions. *Am. J. Med.* **56,** 810–820.

Ellsworth, R., and Howard, J. E. (1934). Studies on the physiology of the parathyroid glands. VII. Some responses of normal kidney and blood intravenous parathyroid extract. *Bull. Johns Hopkins Hosp.* **55,** 296–308.

Estep, H., Shaw, W. A., Watlington, C., Hobe, R., Holland, W., and Tucker, S. G. (1969). Hypocalcemia due to hypomagnesemia and reversible parathyroid hormone unresponsiveness. *J. Clin. Endocrinol. Metab.* **29,** 842–848.

Evers, C., Murer, H., and Kinne, R. (1978). Effect of parathyrin on the transport properties of isolated renal brush-border vesicles. *Biochem. J.* **172,** 49–56.

Fairney, A. (1975). The role of parathyroid hormone in the etiology of neonatal hypocalcemia. *Postgrad. Med. J.* **51,** 18–24.

Fanconi, A., and Fischer, J. A. (1976). Parathyroid hormone in hereditary disease of mineral metabolism. *In* "Inborn Errors of Calcium and Bone Metabolism" (H. Bickel and J. Stern, eds.), pp. 52–62. MTP Press, Lancaster.

Fanconi, A., and Prader, A. (1967). Transient congenital idiopathic hypoparathyroidism. *Helv. Paediatr. Acta* **22,** 342–359.

Fanconi, A., Fischer, J. A., and Prader, A. (1974). Serum parathyroid hormone concentrations in hypophosphatemic vitamin D resistant rickets. *Helv. Paediatr. Acta* **29,** 187–194.

Fang, V. S., and Tashjian, A. H., Jr. (1972). Studies on the role of the liver in the metabolism of parathyroid hormone. I. Effects of partial hepatectomy and incubation of the hormone with tissue homogenates. *Endocrinology (Baltimore)* **90,** 1177–1184.

Farfel, Z., Brickman, A. S., Kaslow, H. R., Brothers, V. M., and Bourne, H. R. (1980). Defect of receptor-cyclase coupling protein in pseudohypoparathyroidism. *N. Engl. J. Med.* **303,** 237–242.

Feinblatt, J. D., Tai, L.-R., and Kenny, A. D. (1975). Avian parathyroid glands in organ culture: Secretion of parathyroid hormone and calcitonin. *Endocrinology (Baltimore)* **96,** 282–288.

Fetter, T. R., and McCuskey, B. M. (1960). Hyperparathyroidism and urolithiasis. *J. Urol.* **84,** 213–218.

Fischer, J. A., and Blum, J. W. (1980). Noncalcium control of parathyroid hormone secretion. *Mineral Electr. Metab.* **3,** 158–166.

Fischer, J. A., Oldham, S. B., Sizemore, G. W., and Arnaud, C. D. (1971). Calcitonin stimulation of parathyroid hormone secretion *in vitro*. *Horm. Metab. Res.* **3,** 223–224.

Fischer, J. A., Oldham, S. B., Sizemore, G. W., and Arnaud, C. D. (1972). Calcium-regulated parathyroid hormone peptidase. *Proc. Natl. Acad. Sci. U.S.A.* **69,** 2341–2345.

Fischer, J. A., Binswanger, U., and Blum, J. (1973a). The acute parathyroid hormone response to changes in ionized calcium during phosphate infusions in the cow. *Eur. J. Clin. Invest.* **3,** 151–155.

Fischer, J. A., Binswanger, U., Fanconi, A., Illig. R., Baerlocher, K., and Prader A. (1973b). Serum parathyroid hormone concentrations in vitamin D deficiency rickets of infancy: Effect of intravenous calcium and vitamin D. *Horm. Metab. Res.* **5,** 381–385.

Fischer, J. A., Blum, J. W., and Binswanger, U. (1973c). Acute parathyroid hormone response to epinephrine *in vivo*. *J. Clin. Invest.* **52,** 2434–2440.

Fischer, J. A., Binswanger, U., and Dietrich, F. M. (1974). Human parathyroid hormone: immunological characterization of antibodies against a glandular extract and the synthetic amino-terminal fragments 1–12 and 1–34 and their use in the determination of immunoreactive hormone in human sera. *J. Clin. Invest.* **54,** 1382–1394.

Fischer, J. A., Hunziker, W., Binswanger, U., Dambacher, M. A., and Dietrich, F. M. (1976). Circulating immunoreactive parathyroid hormone in man as evaluated by different radioimmunoassay systems. *In* "Renal Metabolism in Relation to Renal Function,' (U. Schmidt and U. C. Dubach, eds.), pp. 249–254. Huber, Bern.

Fischer, J. A., Dambacher, M. A., Born, W., and Binswanger, U. (1981). Circulating parathyroid hormone components and interpretation of radioimmunoassay results in normal subjects and in hyperparathyroid patients. *In* "Advances in Nephrology" (J. Hamburger, J. Crosnier, and J.-L. Funck-Brentano, eds.). Year Book Med. Publ., Chicago, Illinois.

Flueck, J. A., Di Bella, F. P., Edis, A. J., Kehrwald, J. M., and Arnaud, C. D. (1977). Immunoheterogeneity of parathyroid hormone in venous effluent serum from hyperfunctioning parathyroid glands. *J. Clin. Invest.* **60,** 1367–1375.

Forte, L. R., Nickols, G. A., and Anast, C. S. (1976). Renal adenylate cyclase and the interrelationship between parathyroid hormone and vitamin D in the regulation of urinary phosphate and adenosine cyclic 3′,5′-monophosphate excretion. *J. Clin. Invest.* **57,** 559–568.

Fournier, A. E., Arnaud, C. D., Johnson, W. J., Taylor W. F., and Godsmith, R. S. (1971). Etiology of hyperparathyroidism and bone disease during chronic hemodialysis. II. Factors affecting serum immunoreactive parathyroid hormone. *J. Clin. Invest.* **50,** 599–605.

Fraser, R., Harrison, N., and Ibbertson, K. (1960). The rate of calcium turnover in bone. *Q. J. Med.* [*N.S.*] **29,** 85–111.

Freitag, J., Martin, K. J., Hruska, K. A., Anderson, C., Conrades, M., Ladenson, J., Klahr, S., and Slatopolsky, E. (1978). Impaired parathyroid hormone metabolism in patients with chronic renal failure. *N. Engl. J. Med.* **298,** 29–32.

Freitag, J. J., Martin, K. J., Conrades, M. B., Bellorin-Font, E., Teitelbaum, S., Klahr, S., and Slatopolsky, E. (1979). Evidence for skeletal resistance to parathyroid hormone in magnesium deficiency. *J. Clin. Invest.* **64,** 1238–1244.

Fucik, R. F., Kukreja, S. C., Hargis, G. K., Bowser, E. N., Henderson, W. J., and Williams, G. A. (1975). Effect of glucocorticoids on function of the parathyroid gland in man. *J. Clin. Endocrinol. Metab.* **40,** 152–155.

Fujita, T., Okano, K., Orimo, H., Ohata, M., and Yoshikawa, M. (1972). A case of adult-onset vitamin-D-resistant osteomalacia with elevated plasma parathyroid hormone level. *J. Bone Jt. Surg. Am. Vol.* **54-A,** 181–188.

Fujita, T., Orimo, H., Ohata, M., Okano, K., and Yoshikawa, M. (1973a). Loss of immunoreactivity of human serum parathyroid hormone by the action of rat kidney enzyme, preferentially hydrolyzing parathyroid hormone. *Horm. Res.* **4,** 213–218.

Fujita, T., Orimo, H., Okano, K., and Yoshikawa, M. (1973b). Clinical application of parathyroid hormone radioimmunoassay. *In* "Clinical Aspects of Metabolic Bone Disease" (W. Frame, A. M. Parfitt, and H. Duncan, eds.), pp. 274–280. Excerpta Medica, Amsterdam.

Gaillard, P. J. (1961). Parathyroid and bone in tissue culture. *In* "The Parathyroids" (R. O. Greep and R. V. Talmage, eds.), pp. 20–48. Thomas, Springfield, Illinois.

Gaillard, P. J., Wassenaar, A. M., and Wijhe-Wheeler, M. E. (1977). Effects of parathyroid hormone and a synthetic fragment (PTH 1–34) on bone in vitro. *Proc. K. Ned. Akad. Wet., Ser. C* **80,** 267–280.

Garabedian, M., Holick, M. F., DeLuca, H. F., and Boyle, I. T. (1972). Control of 25-hydroxycholecalciferol metabolism by parathyroid glands. *Proc. Natl. Acad. Sci. U.S.A.* **69,** 1673–1676.

Garel, J.-M. (1972). Distribution of labeled parathyroid hormone in rat fetus. *Horm. Metab. Res.* **4,** 131–132.

Garner, A., and Ball, J. (1966). Quantitative observations on mineralised and unmineralised bone in chronic renal azotemia and intestinal malabsorption syndrome. *J. Pathol. Bacteriol.* **91,** 545–561.

Genant, H. K., Baron, J. M., Straus, F. H., Paloyan, E., and Jowsey, J. (1975). Osteosclerosis in primary hyperparathyroidism. *Am. J. Med.* **59,** 104–113.

Gerblich, A. A., Genuth, S. M., and Haddad, J. G., Jr. (1977). A case of idiopathic hypoparathyroidism and dietary vitamin D deficiency: The requirement for calcium and vitamin D for bone, but not renal responsiveness to PTH. *J. Clin. Endocrinol. Metab.* **44,** 507–513.

Gittes, R. F., and Raddé, I. C. (1966). Experimental hyperparathyroidism from multiple isologous parathyroid transplants: Homeostatic effect of simultaneous thyroid transplants. *Endocrinology (Baltimore)* **78,** 1015–1022.

Glorieux, F., and Scriver, C. R. (1972). Loss of a parathyroid hormone-sensitive component of phosphate transport in X-linked hypophosphatemia. *Science* **175,** 997–1000.

Goldberg, M. F., Tashjian, A. H., Jr., Order, S. E., and Dammin, G. J. (1964). Renal adenocarcinoma containing a parathyroid hormone-like substance and associated with marked hypercalcemia. *Am. J. Med.* **36,** 805–814.

Goldbloom, R. B., Gillis, D. A., and Prasad, M. (1972). Hereditary parathyroid hyperplasia: a surgical emergency of early infancy. *Pediatrics* **49,** 514–523.

Goldsmith, R. E., Sizemore, G. W., Chen, I.-W., Zalme, E., and Altemeier, W. A. (1976). Familial hyperparathyroidism. *Ann. Intern. Med.* **84,** 36–43.

Goldsmith, R. S., Furszyfer, J., Johnson, W. J., Fournier, A. E., Sizemore, G. W., and Arnaud, C. D. (1973). Etiology of hyperparathyroidism and bone disease during chronic hemodialysis. III. Evaluation of parathyroid suppressibility. *J. Clin. Invest.* **52,** 173–180.

Goltzman, D. (1978). Examination of the requirement for metabolism of parathyroid hormone in skeletal tissue before biological action. *Endocrinology (Baltimore)* **102,** 1555–1562.

Goltzman, D., Peytremann, A., Callahan, E., Tregear, G. W., and Potts, J. T., Jr. (1975). Analysis of the requirements for parathyroid hormone action in renal membranes with the use of inhibiting analogues. *J. Biol. Chem.* **250,** 3199–3202.

Goltzman, D., Callahan, E. N., Tregear, G. W., and Potts, J. T., Jr. (1976a). Conversion of proparathyroid hormone to parathyroid hormone. Studies *in vitro* with trypsin. *Biochemistry* **15,** 5076–5082.

Goltzman, D., Peytremann, A., Callahan, E. N., Segré, G. V., and Potts, J. T., Jr. (1976b). Metabolism and biological activity of parathyroid hormone in renal cortical membranes. *J. Clin. Invest.* **57,** 8–19.

Goltzman, D., Henderson, B., and Loveridge, N. (1980). Cytochemical bioassay of parathyroid hormone. Characteristics of the assay and analysis of circulating hormonal forms. *J. Clin. Invest.* **65,** 1309–1317.

Gonick, H. C., Lee, D. B. N., Drinkard, J. P., and Coulson, W. C. (1973). Interrelationship of acidosis, calcium balance, serum parathormone concentration, and bone morphology in type I renal tubular acidosis. *In* "Clinical Aspects of Metabolic Bone Disease" (B. Frame, A. Parfitt, and H. Duncan, eds.), pp. 403–408. Excerpta Medica, Amsterdam.

Gozariu, L., Forster, K., Faulhaber, J. D., Minne, H., and Ziegler, R. (1974). Parathyroid hormone and calcitonin: Influences upon lipolysis of human adipose tissue. *Horm. Metab. Res.* **6,** 243–245.

Gray, R. S., and Gillon, J. (1976). Normotensive pheochromocytoma with hypercalcemia: Correction after adrenalectomy. *Br. Med. J.* **1,** 378.

Gray, R. W., Wilz, D. R., Caldas, A. E., and Lemann, J., Jr. (1977). The importance of phosphate in regulating plasma 1,25-$(OH)_2$-vitamin D levels in humans: Studies in healthy subjects, in calcium-stone formers, and in patients with primary hyperparathyroidism. *J. Clin. Endocrinol. Metab.* **45,** 299–306.

Greenberg, P. B., Martin, T. J., and Sutcliffe, H. S. (1973). Synthesis and release of parathyroid hormone by a renal carcinoma in cell culture. *Clin. Sci.* **45,** 183–191.

Groth, C. G., Hammond, W. S., Iwatsuki, S., Popovtzer, M., Cascardo, S., Halgrimson, C. G., and Starzl, T. E. (1973). Survival of a homologous parathyroid implant in an immuno-suppressed patient. *Lancet* **1,** 1082–1085.

Grubenmann, W., Binswanger, U., and Fischer, J. A. (1978). Effect of calcium intake and renal function on plasma immunoreactive parathyroid hormone levels in rats. *Horm. Metab. Res.* **10,** 438–443.

Habener, J. F. (1978). Responsiveness of neoplastic and hyperplastic parathyroid tissues to calcium in vitro. *J. Clin. Invest.* **62,** 436–450.

Habener, J. F., and Potts, J. T., Jr. (1976). Relative effectiveness of magnesium and calcium on the secretion and biosynthesis of parathyroid hormones *in vitro*. *Endocrinology (Baltimore)* **98,** 197–202.

Habener, J. F., Powell, D., Murray, T. M., Mayer, G. P., and Potts, J. T., Jr. (1971). Parathyroid hormone: Secretion and metabolism in vivo. *Proc. Natl. Acad. Sci. U.S.A.* **68,** 2986–2991.

Habener, J. F., Tregear, G. W., Stevens, T. D., Dee, P. C., and Potts, J. T., Jr. (1974a). Radioimmunoassay for proparathyroid hormone. *Endocr. Res. Commun.* **1,** 1–17.

Habener, J. F., Kemper, B. W., Potts, J. T., Jr., and Rich, A. (1974b). Calcium-independent intracellular conversion of pro-parathyroid hormone to parathyroid hormone. *Endocr. Res. Commun.* **1,** 239–246.

Habener, J. F., Kemper, B. W., and Potts, J. T., Jr. (1975a). Calcium-dependent intracellular degradation of parathyroid hormone: A possible mechanism for the regulation of hormone stores. *Endocrinology (Baltimore)* **97,** 431–441.

Habener, J. F., Kemper, B., Potts, J. T., Jr., and Rich, A. (1975b). Pre-Pro-Parathyroid hormone identified by cell-free translation of messenger RNA from hyperplastic human parathyroid tissue. *J. Clin. Invest.* **56,** 1328–1333.

Habener, J. F., Stevens, T. D., Tregear, G. W., and Potts, J. T., Jr. (1976). Radioimmunoassay of human proparathyroid hormone: Analysis of hormone content in tissue extracts and in plasma. *J. Clin. Endocrinol. Metab.* **42,** 520–530.

Habener, J. F., Kemper, B. W., Rich, A., and Potts, J. T., Jr. (1977a). Biosynthesis of parathyroid hormone. *Recent Prog. Horm. Res.* **33,** 249–308.

Habener, J. F., Stevens, T. D., Ravazzola, M., Orci, L., and Potts, J. T., Jr. (1977b). Effects of calcium ionophores on the synthesis and release of parathyroid hormone. *Endocrinology (Baltimore)* **101,** 1524–1537.

Habener, J. F., Rosenblatt, M., Kemper, B., Kronenberg, H. M., Rich, A., and Potts, J. T., Jr. (1978). Pre-proparathyroid hormone: Amino acid sequence, chemical synthesis, and some biological studies of the precursor region. *Proc. Natl. Acad. Sci. U.S.A.* **75,** 2616–2620.

Habener, J. F., Amherdt, M., Ravazzola, M., and Orci, L. (1979). Parathyroid hormone biosynthesis: Correlation of conversion of biosynthetic precursors with intracellular protein migration as determined by electron microscope autoradiography. *J. Cell Biol.* **80,** 715–731.

Haddad, J. G., Walgate, J., Min, C., and Hahn, T. J. (1976). Vitamin D metabolite-binding proteins in human tissue. *Biochim. Biophys. Acta* **444,** 921–925.

Hahn, T. J., Scharp, C. R., Halstead, L. R., Haddad, J. G., Karl, D. M., and Avioli, L. V. (1975). Parathyroid hormone status and renal responsiveness in familial hypophosphatemic rickets. *J. Clin. Endocrinol. Metab.* **41,** 926–937.

Halver, B. (1967). The tubular transport of glucose as a measure of parathyroid function. *Acta Med. Scand.* **181,** 209–213.

Hamilton, J. W., Spierto, F. W., MacGregor, R. R., and Cohn, D. V. (1971). Studies of the biosynthesis *in vitro* of parathyroid hormone. II. The effect of calcium and magnesium on synthesis of parathyroid hormone isolated from bovine parathyroid tissue and incubation medium. *J. Biol. Chem.* **246,** 3224–3233.

Hamilton, J. W., Niall, H. D., Jacobs, J. W., Keutmann, H. T., Potts, J. T., Jr., and Cohn, D. V. (1974). The N-terminal amino acid sequence of bovine proparathyroid hormone. *Proc. Natl. Acad. Sci. U.S.A.* **71,** 653–656.

Hamilton, J. W., Hartman, C. R., McGregor, D. H., and Cohn, D. V. (1977). Synthesis of parathyroid hormone-like peptides by a human squamous cell carcinoma. *J. Clin. Endocrinol. Metab.* **45,** 1023–1030.

Hanley, D. A., Takatsuki, K., Sultan, J. M., Schneider, A. B., and Sherwood, L. M. (1978). Direct release of parathyroid hormone fragments from functioning bovine parathyroid glands *in vitro*. *J. Clin. Invest.* **62,** 1247–1254.

Hanley, D. A., Takatsuki, K., Birnbaumer, M. E., Schneider, A. B., and Sherwood, L. M. (1980). In vitro perifusion for the study of parathyroid hormone secretion: Effects of extracellular calcium concentration and beta-adrenergic regulation on bovine parathyroid hormone secretion in vitro. *Calcif. Tissue Int.* **32,** 19–27.

Hargis, G. K., Williams, G. A., Reynolds, W., Chertow, B. S., Kukreja, S. C., Bowser, E. N., and Henderson, W. J. (1978). Effect of somatostatin on parathyroid hormone and calcitonin secretion. *Endocrinology (Baltimore)* **102,** 745–749.

Harrison, A. R. (1960). The diagnosis of primary hyperparathyroidism in cases of renal lithiasis. *Br. J. Urol.* **32,** 383–388.

Harrison, A. R. (1964). Statistical report, St. Peter's, St. Paul's and St. Philip's Hospitals, London, 1961–1963, p. 14. Reviewed in Pyrah *et al.* (1966).

Harrison, H. C., Harrison, H. E., and Park, E. A. (1958). Vitamin D and citrate metabolism: Effect of vitamin D in rats fed diets adequate in both calcium and phosphorus. *Am. J. Physiol.* **192,** 432–436.

Harter, H. R., Mercado, A., Rutherford, W. E., Rodriguez, H., Slatopolsky, E., and Klahr, S. (1974). Effects of phosphate depletion and parathyroid hormone on renal glucose reabsorption. *Am. J. Physiol.* **227,** 1422–1427.

Haussler, M. R., Baylink, D. J., Hughes, M. R., Brumbaugh, P. F., Wergedahl, J. E., Shen, F. H., Nielsen, R. L., Counts, S. J., Bursac, K. M., and McCain, T. A. (1976). The assay of 1α,25-dihydroxyvitamin D_3: Physiologic and pathologic modulation of circulating hormone levels. *Clin. Endocrinol. (Oxford)* **5,** 151s–165s.

Heath, H., III, Sizemore, G. W., and Carney, J. A. (1976). Preoperative diagnosis of occult parathyroid hyperplasia by calcium infusion in patients with multiple endocrine neoplasia, type 2a. *J. Clin. Endocrinol. Metab.* **43,** 428–435.

Heath, H., III, Hodgson, S. F., and Kennedy, M. A. (1980). Primary hyperparathyroidism: Incidence, morbidity, and potential economic impact in a community. *N. Engl. J. Med.* **302,** 189–193.

Heersche, J. N. M., Marcus, R., and Aurbach, G. D. (1974). Calcitonin and the formation of 3′,5′-AMP in bone and kidney. *Endocrinology* **94,** 241–247.

Hellström, J., and Ivemark, B. I. (1962). Primary hyperparathyroidism. *Acta Chir. Scand., Suppl.* **294,** 1–112.

Hems, D. A., Harmon, C. S., and Whitton, P. D. (1975). Inhibition by parathyroid hormone of glycogen synthesis in the perfused rat liver. *FEBS Lett.* **58,** 167–169.

Hendy, G. N., Kronenberg, H. M., Potts, J. T., Jr., and Rich, A. (1981). Nucleotide sequence of cloned cDNAs encoding human preproparathyroid hormone. *Proc. Natl. Acad. Sci. U.S.A.,* in press.

Henry, H. L., and Norman, A. W. (1975). Studies on the mechanism of action of calciferol. VII. Localization of 1,25-dihydroxy-vitamin D_3 in chick parathyroid glands. *Biochem. Biophys. Res. Commun.* **62,** 781–788.

Henry, H. L., Taylor, A. N., and Norman, A. W. (1977). Response of chick parathyroid glands to the vitamin D metabolites, 1,25-dihydroxycholecalciferol and 24,25-dihydroxycholecalciferol. *J. Nutr.* **107,** 1919–1926.

Hohenwallner, W., and Wimmer, E. (1973). The malachite green micromethod for the determination of inorganic phosphate. *Clin. Chim. Acta* **45,** 169–175.

Horwitz, C. A., Myers, W. P. L., and Foote, F. W., Jr. (1972). Secondary malignant tumors of the parathyroid glands. *Am. J. Med.* **52,** 797–808.

Hruska, K. A., Kopelman, R., Rutherford, W. E., Klahr, S., and Slatopolsky, E. (1975). Metabolism of immunoreactive parathyroid hormone in the dog: The role of the kidney and the effects of chronic renal disease. *J. Clin. Invest.* **56,** 39–48.

Hruska, K. A., Martin, K., Mennes, P., Greenwalt, A., Anderson, C., Klahr, S., and Slatopolsky, E. (1977). Degradation of parathyroid hormone and fragment production by the isolated perfused dog kidney. *J. Clin. Invest.* **60,** 501–510.

Hruska, K. A., Korkor, A., Martin, K., and Slatopolsky, E. (1981). Peripheral metabolism of intact parathyroid hormone. *J. Clin. Invest.* **67,** 885–892.

Hughes, M. R., and Haussler, M. R. (1978). 1,25-dihydroxyvitamine D_3 receptors in parathyroid glands. *J. Biol. Chem.* **253,** 1065–1073.

Humes, H. D., Ichikawa, I., Troy, J. L., and Brenner, B. M. (1978). Evidence for a parathyroid hormone-dependent influence of calcium on the glomerular ultrafiltration coefficient. *J. Clin. Invest.* **61,** 32–40.

Hunziker, W. H., and Fischer, J. A. (1978). Characterization of circulating immunoreactive parathyroid hormone forms by gel filtration and affinity chromatography. *In* "Endocrinology of Calcium Metabolism" (D. H. Copp and R. V. Talmage, eds.), pp. 333–338. Excerpta Medica, Amsterdam.

Hunziker, W. H., Blum, J. W., and Fischer, J. A. (1977). Plasma kinetics of exogenous bovine parathyroid hormone in calves. *Pfluegers Arch.* **371,** 185–192.

Ichikawa, I., Humes, H. D., Dousa, T. P., and Brenner, B. M. (1978). Influence of parathyroid hormone on glomerular ultrafiltration in the rat. *Am. J. Physiol.* **234,** F393–F401.

Imbert, M., Chabardès, D., and Morel, F. (1974). Hormone-sensitive adenylate cyclase in isolated rabbit glomeruli. *Mol. Cell. Endocrinol.* **1,** 295–304.

Isaac, R., Merceron, R. E., Caillens, G., Raymond, J.-P., and Ardaillou, R. (1978). Effect of parathyroid hormone on plasma prolactin in man. *J. Clin. Endocr. Metab.* **47,** 18–23.

Jacobs, J. W., Kemper, B., Niall, H. D., Habener, J. F., and Potts, J. T., Jr. (1974). Structural analysis of human proparathyroid hormone by a new microsequencing approach. *Nature (London)* **249,** 155–157.

Joffe, B. J., Hackeng, W. H. L., Seftel, H. C., and Hartdegen, R. C. (1972). Parathyroid hormone concentrations in nutritional rickets. *Clin. Sci.* **42,** 113–116.

Johansson, H., Torén, L., and Werner, I. (1972). Hyperparathyroidism. *Upsala J. Med. Sci.* **77,** 41–46.

Jowsey, J. (1966). Quantitative microradiography. *Am. J. Med.* **40,** 485–491.

Jowsey, J., Riggs, B. L., Goldsmith, R. S., Kelly, P. J., and Arnaud, C. D. (1971). Effects of prolonged administration of porcine calcitonin in postmenopausal osteoporosis. *J. Clin. Endocrinol. Metab.* **33,** 752–758.

Jowsey, J., Reiss, E., and Canterbury, J. M. (1974). Long-term effects of high phosphate intake on parathyroid hormone levels and bone metabolism. *Acta Orthop. Scand.* **45,** 801–808.

Jubiz, W., Canterbury, J. M., Reiss, E., and Tyler, F. H. (1972). Circadian rhythm in serum parathyroid hormone concentration in human subjects: Correlation with serum calcium, phosphate, albumin, and growth hormone levels. *J. Clin. Invest.* **51,** 2040–2046.

Kalu, D. N., Doyle, F. H., Pennock, J., and Foster, G. V. (1970). Parathyroid hormone and experimental osteosclerosis. *Lancet* **1,** 1363–1366.

Kaplan, L., Katz, A. D., Ben-Isaac, C., and Massry, S. G. (1971). Malignant neoplasms and parathyroid adenoma. *Cancer* **28,** 401–407.

Karlinsky, M. L., Sager, D. S., Kurtzman, N. A., and Pillay, V. K. G. (1974). Effect of parathormone and cyclic adenosine monophosphate on renal bicarbonate reabsorption. *Am. J. Physiol.* **227,** 1226–1231.

Kather, H., and Simon, B. (1977). Adenylate cyclase of human fat cell ghosts. Stimulation of enzyme activity by parathyroid hormone. *J. Clin. Invest.* **59,** 730–733.

Kaye, M., Pritchard, J. E., Halpenny, G., and Light, W. (1960). Bone disease in chronic renal failure with particular reference to osteosclerosis. *Medicine (Baltimore)* **39,** 157–190.

Kaye, M., Chatterjee, G., Cohen, G. F., and Sagar, S. (1970). Arrest of hyperparathyroid bone disease with dihydrotachysterol in patients undergoing chronic hemodialysis. *Ann. Intern. Med.* **73,** 225–233.

Keating, F. R., Jr., Jones, J. D., Elveback, L. R., and Randall, R. V. (1969). The relation of age and sex to distribution of values in healthy adults of serum calcium, inorganic phosphorus, magnesium, alkaline phosphatase, total proteins, albumin and blood urea. *J. Lab. Clin. Med.* **73,** 825–834.

Kemper, B. (1976). Inactivation of parathyroid hormone mRNA by treatment with periodate and aniline. *Nature (London)* **262,** 321–323.

Kemper, B., Habener, J. F., Potts, J. T., Jr., and Rich, A. (1972). Proparathyroid hormone: Identification of a biosynthetic precursor to parathyroid hormone. *Proc. Natl. Acad. Sci. U.S.A.* **69,** 643–647.

Kemper, B., Habener, J. F., Mulligan, R. C., Potts, J. T., Jr., and Rich, A. (1974a). Preproparathyroid hormone: A direct translation product of parathyroid messenger RNA. *Proc. Natl. Acad. Sci. U.S.A.* **71,** 3731–3735.

Kemper, B., Habener, J. F., Rich, A., and Potts, J. T., Jr. (1974b). Parathyroid secretion: Discovery of a major calcium-dependent protein. *Science* **184,** 167–169.

Kemper, B., Habener, J. F., Rich, A., and Potts, J. T., Jr. (1975). Microtubules and the intracellular conversion of proparathyroid hormone to parathyroid hormone. *Endocrinology (Baltimore)* **96,** 903–912.

Kemper, B., Habener, J. F., Potts, J. T., Jr., and Rich, A. (1976b). Pre-Pro-Parathyroid hormone: Fidelity of the translation of parathyroid messenger RNA by extracts of wheat germ. *Biochemistry* **15,** 20–25.

Kempson, S. A., Colon-Otero, G., Ou, S.-Y. L., Turner, S. T., and Dousa, T. P. (1981). Possible role of nicotinamide adenine dinucleotide as an intracellular regulator of renal transport of phosphate in the rat. *J. Clin. Invest.* **67,** 1347–1360.

Keutmann, H. T., Aurbach, G. D., Dawson, B. F., Niall, H. D., Deftos, L. J., and Potts, J. T., Jr. (1971). Isolation and characterization of the bovine parathyroid isohormones. *Biochemistry* **10,** 2779–2787.

Keutmann, H. T., Dawson, B. F., Aurbach, G. D., and Potts, J. T., Jr. (1972). A biologically active amino-terminal fragment of bovine parathyroid hormone prepared by dilute acid hydrolysis. *Biochemistry* **11,** 1973–1979.

Keutmann, H. T., Barling, P. M., Hendy, G. N., Segré, G. V., Niall, H. D., Aurbach, G. D., Potts, J. T., Jr., and O'Riordan, J. L. H. (1974). Isolation of human parathyroid hormone. *Biochemistry* **13,** 1646–1652.

Keutmann, H. T., Sauer, M. M., Hendy, G. N., O'Riordan, J. L. H., and Potts, J. T., Jr. (1978). Complete amino acid sequence of human parathyroid hormone. *Biochemistry* **17,** 5723–5729.

Khairi, M. R. A., Dexter, R. N., Burzynski, N. J., and Johnston, C. C., Jr. (1975). Mucosal neuroma, pheochromocytoma and medullary thyroid carcinoma: Multiple endocrine neoplasia, type 3. *Medicine (Baltimore)* **54,** 89–112.

Kind, H. P., Parkinson, D. K., Suh, S. M., Fraser, D., and Kooh, S. W. (1973). Parathyroid hormone response and effects of vitamin D in hypoparathyroidism and pseudohypoparathyroidism. *Program 55th Annu. Meet. Endocr. Soc.* A-164 (abstr.).

Kind, H. P., Fischer, J. A., Rickham, P. T., Steinmann, B., Gnehm, H. P., Nüssli, R., and Prader, A. (1976). Hyperparathyroidism and alcaptonuria in a neonate. *Pediatr. Res.* **10,** 875 (abstr.).

Kinne, R., and Schwartz, I. L. (1977). Asymmetric distribution of renal epithelial cell membrane in the action of antidiuretic hormone and parathyroid hormone. *In* "Disturbances in Body Fluid Osmolality" (T. E. Andreoli, J. J. Grantham, and F. C. Rector, Jr., eds.), pp. 37–55. Am. Physiol. Soc., Bethesda, Maryland.

Kinne, R., Shlatz, L. J., Kinne-Saffran, E., and Schwartz, I. L. (1975). Distribution of membrane-bound cyclic AMP-dependent protein kinase in plasma membranes in cells of the kidney cortex. *J. Membr. Biol.* **24,** 145–159.

Kistler, H. J. (1976). Primärer Hyperparathyreoidismus. *Schweiz. Med. Wochenschr.* **106,** (suppl. 3), 1-61.

Kistler, H. J., Bonetti, A., Frey, P., and Fischer, J. A. (1976). Sporadische hypophosphataemische Vitamin-D-resistente Osteomalazie (Phosphatdiabetes) im Erwachsenenalter und Hyperparathyreoidismus. *Schweiz. Med. Wochenschr.* **106,** 1855-1862.

Kleerekoper, M., Basten, A., Penny, R., and Posen, S. (1974). Idiopathic hypoparathyroidism with primary ovarian failure. *Arch. Intern. Med.* **134,** 944-947.

Kleerekoper, M., Ibels, L. S., Ingham, J. P., McCarthy, S. W., Mahony, J. F., Stewart, J. H., and Posen, S. (1975). Hyperparathyroidism after renal transplantation *Br. Med. J.* **3,** 680-682.

Kleerekoper, M., Coffey, R., Greco, T., Nichols, S., Cooke, N., Murphy, W., and Avioli, L. V. (1977). Hypercalcemic hyperparathyroidism in hypophosphatemic rickets. *J. Clin. Endocrinol. Metab.* **45,** 86-94.

Knill-Jones, R. P., Buckle, R. M., Parsons, V., Calne, R. Y., and Williams, R. (1970). Hypercalcemia and increased parathyroid-hormone activity in a primary hepatoma. *N. Engl. J. Med.* **282,** 704-708.

Knox, F. G., Schneider, E. G., Willis, L. R., Strandhoy, J. W., and Ott, C. E. (1973). Site and control of phosphate reabsorption by the kidney. *Kidney Int.* **3,** 347-353.

Knox, F. G., Haas, J. A., and Lechene, C. P. (1976). Effect of parathyroid hormone on phosphate reabsorption in the presence of acetazolamide. *Kidney Int.* **10,** 216-220.

Kooh, S. W., Fraser, D., DeLuca, H. F., Holick, M. F., Belsey, R. D., Clark, M. B., and Murray, T. M. (1975). Treatment of hypoparathyroidism and pseudohypoparathyroidism with metabolites of vitamin D: Evidence for impaired conversion of 25-hydroxyvitamin D to 1α,25-dihydroxy-vitamin D. *N. Engl. J. Med.* **293,** 840-844.

Kooh, S. W., Fraser, D., Reilly, B. J., Hamilton, J. R., Gall, D. G., and Bell, L. (1977). Rickets due to calcium deficiency. *N. Engl. J. Med.* **297,** 1264-1266.

de Kretser, D. M., Martin, T. J., and Melick, R. A. (1970). The radioautographic localization of ^{125}I-labeled bovine parathyroid hormone. *J. Endocrinol.* **45,** 507-510.

Kripke, D. F., Lavie, P., Parker, D., Huey, L., and Deftos, L. J. (1978). Plasma parathyroid hormone and calcium are related to sleep stage cycles. *J. Clin. Endocrinol. Metab.* **47,** 1021-1027.

Kronenberg, H. M., Roberts, B. E., Habener, J. F., Potts, J. T., Jr., and Rich, A. (1977). DNA complementary to parathyroid mRNA directs synthesis of pre-proparathyroid hormone in a linked transcription-translation system. *Nature (London)* **267,** 804-807.

Kronenberg, H. M., McDevitt, B. E., Majzoub, J. A., Nathans, J., Sharp, P. A., Potts, J. T., Jr., and Rich, A. (1979). Cloning and nucleotide sequence of DNA coding for bovine preproparathyroid hormone. *Proc. Natl. Acad. Sci. U.S.A.* **76,** 4981-4985.

Kukreja, S. C., Hargis, G. K., Rosenthal, I. M., and Williams, G. A. (1973). Pheochromocytoma causing excessive parathyroid hormone production and hypercalcemia. *Ann. Intern. Med.* **79,** 838-840.

Kukreja, S. C., Hargis, G. K., Bowser, E. N., Henderson, W. J., Fisherman, E. W., and Williams, G. A. (1975). Role of adrenergic stimuli in parathyroid hormone secretion in man. *J. Clin. Endocrinol. Metab.* **40,** 478-481.

Kukreja, S. C., Bowser, E. N., Hargis, G. K., Henderson, W. J., and Williams, G. A. (1976a). Mechanism of glucocorticoid-induced osteopenia: Role of parathyroid glands. *Proc. Soc. Exp. Biol. Med.* **152,** 358-361.

Kukreja, S. C., Johnson, P. A., Ayala, G., Banerjee, P., Bowser, E. N., Hargis, G. K., and Williams, G. A. (1976b). Role of calcium and beta-adrenergic system in control of parathyroid hormone secretion. *Proc. Soc. Exp. Biol. Med.* **151,** 326-328.

Kunin, A. S., McKay, B. R., Burns, S. L., and Halberstam, M. J. (1963). The syndrome of hypoparathyroidism and adrenocortical insufficiency, a possible sequel of hepatitis. *Am. J. Med.* **34,** 856–866.

Lafferty, F. W., and Pearson, O. H. (1963). Skeletal and renal calcium dynamics in hyperparathyroidism. *J. Clin. Endocrinol. Metab.* **23,** 891–902.

Lahey, F. H., and Murphy, R. (1953). Primary hyperparathyroidism. *Surg. Clin. North Am.* **33,** 723–737.

Lancer, S. R., Bowser, E. N., Hargis, G. K., and Williams, G. A. (1976). The effect of growth hormone on parathyroid function in rats. *Endocrinology (Baltimore)* **98,** 1289–1293.

Lee, D. B. N., Drinkard, J. P., Gonick, H. C., Coulson, W. F., and Cracchiolo, A. (1976). Pathogenesis of renal calculi in distal renal tubular acidosis. *Clin. Orthop. Relat. Res.* **121,** 234–242.

Lee, J. B., Tashjian, A. H., Jr., Streeto, J. M., and Frantz, A. G. (1968). Familial pseudohypoparathyroidism. Role of parathyroid hormone and thyrocalcitonin. *N. Engl. J. Med.* **279,** 1179–1184.

Lee, M. J., and Roth, S. I. (1975). Effect of calcium and magnesium on deoxyribonucleic acid synthesis in rat parathyroid glands *in vitro*. *Lab. Invest.* **33,** 72–73.

Leonard, C. D., and Eichner, E. R. (1970). Acute renal failure and transient hypercalcemia in idiopathic rhabdomyolysis. *JAMA J. Am. Med. Assoc.* **211,** 1539–1540.

Lerman, S., Canterbury, J. M., and Reiss, E. (1977). Parathyroid hormone and the hypercalcemia of immobilization. *J. Clin. Endocrinol. Metab.* **45,** 425–428.

Levi, J., Massry, S. G., Coburn, J. W., Llach, F., and Kleeman, C. R. (1974). Hypocalcemia in magnesium-depleted dogs: Evidence for reduced responsiveness to parathyroid hormone and relative failure of parathyroid gland function. *Metab. Clin. Exp.* **23,** 323–325.

Levine, M. A., Downs, R. W., Jr., Singer, M., Marx, S. J., Aurbach, G. D., and Spiegel, A. M. (1980). Deficient activity of guanine nucleotide regulatory protein in erythrocytes from patients with pseudohypoparathyroidism. *Biochem. Biophys. Res. Commun.* **94,** 1319–1324.

Lewy, J. E., Cabana, E. C., Repetto, H. A., Canterbury, J. M., and Reiss, E. (1972). Serum parathyroid hormone in hypophosphatemic vitamin D-resistent rickets. *J. Pediatr.* **81,** 294–300.

Lifshitz, F., Harrison, H. C., and Harrison, H. E. (1969). Influence of parathyroid function upon the *in vitro* transport of calcium and phosphate by the rat intestine. *Endocrinology (Baltimore)* **84,** 912–917.

von Lilienfeld-Toal, H., Lambert, P. V., and Arnaud, C. D. (1976). Persistence of circulating carboxyl terminal fragments of parathyroid hormone during calcium infusion: the cause of the failure of hypercalcemia to suppress PTH in hyperparathyroidism. *Clin. Res.* **24,** 529A (abstr.).

Linarelli, L. G. (1972). Newborn urinary cyclic AMP and developmental renal responsiveness to parathyroid hormone. *Pediatrics* **50,** 14–23.

Lipsett, M. B. (1968). Hormonal syndromes associated with neoplasia. *Adv. Metab. Disord.* **3,** 111–152.

Littledike, E. T., and Hawker, C. D. (1967). Extraction, purification and partial characterization of porcine parathyroid hormone. *Endocrinology (Baltimore)* **81,** 261–266.

Llach, F., Massry, S. G., Singer, F. R., Kurokawa, K., Kaye, J. H., and Coburn, J. W. (1975). Skeletal resistance to endogenous parathyroid hormone in patients with early renal failure, a possible cause for secondary hyperparathyroidism. *J. Clin. Endocrinol. Metab.* **41,** 339–345.

Llach, F., Coburn, J. W., Brickman, A. S., Kurokawa, K., Norman, A. W., Canterbury, J. M., and Reiss, E. (1977). Acute actions of 1,25-dihydroxy-vitamin D_3 in normal man: Effect on calcium and parathyroid status. *J. Clin. Endocrinol. Metab.* **44,** 1054–1060.

Llach, F., Felsenfeld, A. J., and Haussler, M. R. (1981). Pathophysiology of altered calcium metabolism in rhabdomyolisis-induced acute renal failure. *N. Engl. J. Med.* **305,** 117–123.

Lockefeer, J. H., Hackeng, W. H. L., and Birkenhäger, J. C. (1974). Parathyroid hormone secretion in disorders of calcium metabolism studied by means of EDTA. *Acta Endocrinol. Copenhagen* **75,** 286–296.

Londos, C. D., and Bronner, F. (1973). Studies of parathyroid hormone enzymatic hydrolysis. *Proc. Eur. Symp. Calcif. Tissues, 9th, 1972* pp. 225–230.

Low, J. C., Schaaf, M., Earll, J. M., Piechocki, J. T., and Li, T. K. (1973). Ionic calcium determination in primary hyperparathyroidism. *JAMA, J. Am. Med. Assoc.* **223,** 152–155.

Luben, R. A., Goggins, J. F., and Raisz, L. G. (1974). Stimulation by parathyroid hormone of bone hyaluronate synthesis in organ culture. *Endocrinology (Baltimore)* **94,** 737–745.

Luben, R. A., Wong, G. L., and Cohn, D. V. (1976). Biochemical characterization with parathormone and calcitonin of isolated bone cells: Provisional identification of osteoclasts and osteoblasts. *Endocrinology (Baltimore)* **99,** 526–534.

Luben, R. A., Wong, G. L., and Cohn, D. V. (1977). Parathormone-stimulated resorption of devitalised bone by cultured osteoclast-type bone cells. *Nature (London)* **265,** 629–630.

Lund, B., Sorenson, O. H., Lund, Bi., Bishop, J. E., and Norman, A. W. (1980). Vitamin D metabolism in hypoparathyroidism. *J. Clin. Endocrinol. Metabol.* **51,** 606–610.

MacDonald, R. A., and Mallory, G. (1960). Hemochromatosis and hemosiderosis. *Arch. Intern. Med.* **105,** 686–700.

McGeown, M. G. (1960). Hyperparathyroidism amongst patients with renal calculi. *Br. J. Urol.* **32,** 389–391.

McGeown, M. G., and Morrison, E. (1959). Hyperparathyroidism. *Postgrad. Med. J.* **35,** 330–337.

MacGregor, R. R., Hamilton, J. W., and Cohn, D. V. (1975). The by-pass of tissue hormone stores during the secretion of newly synthetized parathyroid hormone. *Endocrinology (Baltimore)* **97,** 178–188.

MacGregor, R. R., Chu, L. L. H., and Cohn, D. V. (1976). Conversion of pro-parathyroid hormone to parathyroid hormone by a particulate enzyme of the parathyroid gland. *J. Biol. Chem.* **251,** 6711–6716.

McIntosh, H. W., Balfour, J. A., and Duffy, M. H. (1958). Recurrent renal calculi and hyperparathyroidism. *Br. J. Urol.* **30,** 292–296.

MacManus, J. P., and Whitfield, J. F. (1970). Inhibition by thyrocalcitonin of the mitogenic actions of parathyroid hormone and cyclic adenosine-3′,5′-monophosphate on rat thymocytes. *Endocrinology (Baltimore)* **86,** 934–939.

Marcus, R., and Aurbach, G. D. (1969). Bioassay of parathyroid hormone *in vitro* with a stable preparation of adenyl cyclase from rat kidney. *Endocrinology (Baltimore)* **85,** 801–810.

Martin, G. R., Mecca, C. E., Schiffmann, E., and Goldhaber, P. (1965). Alterations in bone metabolism induced by parathyroid extract. *In* "The Parathyroid Glands" (P. J. Gaillard, R. V. Talmage, and A. N. Budy, eds.), pp. 261–272. Univ. of Chicago Press, Chicago, Illinois.

Martin, K. J., Hruska, K., Greenwalt, A., Klahr, S., and Slatopolsky, E. (1976). Selective uptake of intact parathyroid hormone by the liver: Differences between hepatic and renal uptake. *J. Clin. Invest.* **58,** 781–788.

Martin, K. J., Hruska, K. A., Lewis, J., Anderson, C., and Slatopolsky, E. (1977). The renal handling of parathyroid hormone. Role of peritubular uptake and glomerular filtration. *J. Clin. Invest.* **60,** 808–814.

Martin, K. J., Freitag, J. J., Conrades, M. B., and Hruska, K. A. (1978). Selective uptake of the synthetic amino terminal fragment of bovine parathyroid hormone by isolated perfused bone. *J. Clin. Invest.* **62,** 256–261.

Martin, T. J., Melick, R. A., and DeLuise, M. (1969a). Metabolism of parathyroid hormone. Degradation of [^{125}I]-labeled hormone by a kidney enzyme. *Biochem. J.* **111,** 509–514.

Martin, T. J., Melick, R. A., and DeLuise, M. (1969b). The effect of nephrectomy on the metabolism of labeled parathyroid hormone. *Clin. Sci.* **37,** 137–142.

Martin, T. J., Greenberg, P. B., and Michelangeli, V. (1973). Synthesis of human parathyroid hormone by cultured cells: Evidence for release of prohormone by some adenomata. *Clin. Sci.* **44,** 1–8.

Martin, T. J., Vakakis, N., Eisman, J. A., Livesay, S. J., and Tregear, G. W. (1974). Chick kidney adenylate cyclase: Sensitivity to parathyroid hormone and synthetic human and bovine peptides. *J. Endocrinol.* **63,** 369–375.

Marx, S. J., Powell, D., Shimkin, P. M., Wells, S. A., Katcham, A. S., McGuigan, J. E., Bilezikian, J. P., and Aurbach, G. D. (1973). Familial hyperparathyroidism. *Ann. Intern. Med.* **78,** 371–377.

Marx, S. J., Spiegel, A. M., Brown, E. M., and Aurbach, G. D. (1977). Family studies in patients with primary parathyroid hyperplasia. *Am. J. Med.* **62,** 698–706.

Marx, S. J. (1980). Familial hypocalciuric hypercalcemia. *N. Engl. J. Med.* **303,** 810–811.

Massry, S. G., and Goldstein, D. A. (1978). Role of parathyroid hormone in uremic toxicity. *Kidney Int.* **13,** s39–s42.

Massry, S. G., Coburn, J. W., Lee, D. B. N., Jowsey, J., and Kleeman, C. R. (1973). Skeletal resistance to parathyroid hormone in renal failure. *Ann. Intern. Med.* **78,** 357–364.

Massry, S. G., Arieff, A. I., Coburn, J. W., Palmieri, G., and Kleeman, C. R. (1974). Divalent ion metabolism in patients with acute renal failure: Studies on the mechanism of hypocalcemia. *Kidney Int.* **5,** 437–445.

Matsuzaki, S., and Dumont, J. E. (1972). Effect of calcium ion on horse parathyroid gland adenyl cyclase. *Biochim. Biophys. Acta* **284,** 227–284.

Mavligit, G. M., Cohen, J. C., and Sherwood, L. M. (1971). Ectopic production of parathyroid hormone by carcinoma of the breast. *N. Engl. J. Med.* **285,** 154–156.

Mayer, G. P., and Hurst, J. G. (1978a). Sigmoidal relationship between parathyroid hormone secretion rate and plasma calcium concentration in calves. *Endocrinology (Baltimore)* **102,** 1036–1042.

Mayer, G. P., and Hurst, J. G. (1978b). Comparison of the effect of calcium and magnesium on parathyroid hormone secretion rate in calves. *Endocrinology (Baltimore)* **102,** 1803–1807.

Mayer, G. P., Habener, J. F., and Potts, J. T., Jr. (1976). Parathyroid hormone secretion *in vitro*: Demonstration of a calcium-independent nonsuppressible component of secretion. *J. Clin. Invest.* **57,** 678–683.

Mayer, G. P., Keaton, J. A., Hurst, J. G., and Habener, J. F. (1979). Effects of plasma calcium concentration on the relative proportion of hormone and carboxyl fragment in parathyroid venous blood. *Endocrinology (Baltimore)* **104,** 1778–1784.

Melick, R. A., and Henneman, P. H. (1958). Clinical and laboratory studies of 207 consecutive patients in a kidney-stone clinic. *N. Engl. J. Med.* **259,** 307–314.

Melick, R. A., and Martin, T. J. (1969). Parathyroid hormone metabolism in man: Effect of nephrectomy. *Clin. Sci.* **37,** 667–674.

Melick, R. A., Aurbach, G. D., and Potts, J. T., Jr. (1965). The distribution of half-life of [^{131}I]-labeled parathyroid hormone in the rat. *Endocrinology (Baltimore)* **77,** 198–202.

Melick, R. A., Gill, J. R., Jr., Berson, S. A., Yalow, R. S., Bartter, F. C., Potts, J. T., Jr., and Aurbach, G. D. (1967). Antibodies and clinical resistance to parathyroid hormone. *N. Engl. J. Med.* **276,** 144–147.

Meytes, D., Bogin, E., Ma, A., Dukes, P. P., and Massry, S. G. (1981). Effect of parathyroid hormone on erythropoiesis. *J. Clin. Invest.* **67,** 1263–1269.

Milhaud, G., and Bourichon, J. (1964). Etude du métabolisme du calcium chez l'homme à l'aide de calcium 45. L'hyperparathyroidie et l'hypoparathyroidie. *C. R. Holid. Séances Acad. Sci.* **258,** 3398–3401.

Miller, M. J., Frame, B., Poznanski, A. K., Jackson, C. E., and Bermudez, G. (1972). Branchial anomalies in idiopathic hypoparathyroidism: Branchial dysembryogenesis. *Henry Ford Hosp. Med. J.* **20,** 3–14.

Miller, S. S., Sizemore, G. W., Sheps, S. G., and Tyce, G. M. (1975). Parathyroid function in patients with pheochromocytoma. *Ann. Intern. Med.* **82,** 372–375.

Milne, J. (1954). Primary hyperparathyroidism. *N. Engl. J. Med.* **251,** 393–395.

Miravet, L., Matrait, H., Bordier, P. J., Tun-Chot, S., Gruson, M., and Hioco, D. (1969). Correlations between biochemical kinetic [^{45}Ca] and histological measurements in hyperparathyroidism. *Proc. R. Soc. Med.* **62,** 241–242.

Mitschke, H., Altenähr, E., Delling, G., and Weibel, J. (1973). Das pluriglanduläre Insuffizienzsyndrom. *Dtsch. Med. Wochenschr.* **98,** 1666–1669.

Monchick, J. M., Wray, H. L., Schaaf, M., and Earll, J. M. (1977). Nonautonomy of parathyroid hormone and urinary cyclic AMP in primary hyperparathyroidism. *Am. J. Surg.* **133,** 498–505.

Monteleone, J. A., Lee, J. B., Tashjian, A. H., Jr., and Cantor, H. E. (1975). Transient neonatal hypocalcemia, hypomagnesemia, and high serum parathyroid hormone with maternal hyperparathyroidism. *Ann. Intern. Med.* **82,** 670–672.

Moran, J. R., Born, W., Tuchschmid, C. R., and Fischer, J. A. (1981). Calcium-regulated biosynthesis of the parathyroid secretory protein, proparathyroid hormone, and parathyroid hormone in dispersed bovine parathyroid cells. *Endocrinology (Baltimore)* **108,** 2264–2268.

Morel, F., Chabardès, D., and Imbert, M. (1976). Functional segmentation of the rabbit distal tubule by microdetermination of hormone-dependent adenylate cyclase activity. *Kidney Int.* **9,** 264–277.

Morris, R. C., Jr. (1968). An experimental renal acidification defect in patients with hereditary fructose intolerance. *J. Clin. Invest.* **47,** 1648–1663.

Morris, R. C., Jr., McSherry, E., and Sebastian, A. (1971). Modulation of experimental renal dysfunction of hereditary fructose intolerance by circulating parathyroid hormone. *Proc. Natl. Acad. Sci. U.S.A.* **68,** 132–135.

Morrissey, J. J., and Cohn, D. V. (1978). The effects of calcium and magnesium on the secretion of parathormone and parathyroid secretory protein by isolated porcine parathyroid cells. *Endocrinology (Baltimore)* **103,** 2081–2090.

Morrissey, J. J., and Cohn, D. V. (1979). Regulation of secretion of parathormone and secretory protein-I from separate intracellular pools by calcium, dibutyryl cyclic AMP, and (1)-isoproterenol. *J. Cell Biology* **82,** 93–102.

Morrissey, J. J., Hamilton, J. W., and Cohn, D. V. (1978). The secretion of parathormone and glycosylated proteins by parathyroid cells in culture. *Biochem. Biophys. Res. Commun.* **82,** 1279–1286.

Morrissey, J. J., Hamilton, J. W., MacGregor, R. R., and Cohn, D. V. (1980). The secretion of parathormone fragments 34–84 and 37–84 by dispersed porcine parathyroid cells. *Endocrinology (Baltimore)* **107,** 164–171.

Moxley, M. A., Bell, N. H., Wagle, S. R., Allen, D. O., and Ashmore, J. (1974). Parathyroid hormone stimulation of glucose and urea production in isolated liver cells. *Am. J. Physiol.* **227,** 1058–1061.

Muldowney, F. P., McKenna, T. J., Kyle, L. H., Freaney, R., and Swan, M. (1970). Parathormone-like effect of magnesium replenishment in steatorrhea. *N. Engl. J. Med.* **282,** 61–68.

Muldowney, F. P., O'Donohoe, J. F., Carroll, D. V., Powell, D., and Freaney, R. (1972). Parathyroid acidosis in uremia. *Q. J. Med.* [*N.S.*] **46,** 321–342.

Muldowney, F. P., Freaney, R., McMullin, J. P., Towers, R. P., Spillane, A., O'Connor, P., O'Donohoe, P., and Moloney, M. (1976). Serum ionized calcium and parathyroid hormone in renal stone disease. *Q. J. Med.* [*N.S.*] **45,** 75–86.

Munson, P. L. (1961). Biological assay of parathyroid hormone. *In* "The Parathyroids" (R. O. Greep and R. V. Talmage, eds.), pp. 94–118. Thomas, Springfield, Illinois.

Murray, T. M., Peacock, M., Powell, D., Monchik, J. M., and Potts, J. T., Jr. (1972). Non-autonomy of hormone secretion in primary hyperparathyroidism. *Clin. Endocrinol. (Oxford)* **1,** 235–246.

Murray, T. M., Muzaffar, S. A., Parsons, J. A., and Keutmann, H. T. (1975). A biologically active hormonal fragment isolated from bovine parathyroid glands (BPTH-(1–65)). *Biochemistry* **14,** 2705–2711.

Myers, W. P. L. (1973). Hypercalcemia associated with malignant diseases. *In* "Endocrine and Non-endocrine Hormone-producing Tumors," pp. 147–171. Year Book Med. Publ., Chicago, Illinois.

Nagant de Deuxchaisnes, C., and Krane, S. M. (1978). Hypoparathyroidism. *In* "Metabolic Bone Disease" (L. V. Avioli and S. M. Krane, eds.), Vol. 2, pp. 217–445. Academic Press, New York.

Nagant de Deuxchaisnes, C., Fischer, J. A., Dambacher, M. A., Devogelaer, J.-P., Arber, C. E., Zanelli, J. M., Parsons, J. A., Loveridge, N., Bitensky, L., and Chayen, J. (1981). Dissociation of bioactive and immunoreactive parathyroid hormone in pseudohypoparathyroidism type I. *J. Clin. Endocrinol. Metab.* (in press).

Nagata, N., and Rasmussen, H. (1970). Parathyroid hormone, 3′,5′-AMP, Ca^{++}, and renal gluconeogenesis. *Proc. Natl. Acad. Sci. U.S.A.* **65,** 368–374.

Nagata, N., Kimura, N., Sasaki, M., Nakane, K., and Tanaka, Y. (1976). Localization of cell groups sensitive to parathyroid hormone and calcitonin in rat skeletal tissue. *Biochim. Biophys. Acta* **421,** 218–227.

Neer, R. M., Tregear, G. W., and Potts, J. T., Jr. (1977). Renal effects of native parathyroid hormone and synthetic biologically active fragments in pseudohypoparathyroidism and hypoparathyroidism. *J. Clin. Endocrinol. Metab.* **38,** 420–423.

Nemere, I., and Szego, C. M. (1981). Early actions of parathyroid hormone and 1,25-dihydroxycholecalciferol on isolated epithelial cells from rat intestine: I. Limited lysosomal enzyme release and calcium uptake. *Endocrinology (Baltimore)* **108,** 1450–1462.

Neuman, M. W., Neuman, W. F., and Lane, K. (1975). The metabolism of labeled parathyroid hormone. VII. Attempts to modify hormone deposition. *Calcif. Tissue Res.* **19,** 169–178.

Neuman, W. F., Neuman, M. W., Sammon, P. J., and Casarett, G. W. (1975a). The metabolism of labeled parathyroid hormone. IV. Autoradiographic studies. *Calcif. Tissue Res.* **18,** 263–270.

Neuman, W. F., Neuman, M. W., Lane, K., Miller, L., and Sammon, P. J. (1975b). The metabolism of labeled parathyroid hormone. V. Collected biological studies. *Calcif. Tissue Res.* **18,** 271–287.

Nezelof, C., Satge, P., Lavaud, J., and Le Sec, G. (1975). L'agénésie thymique et parathyroidienne (syndrome de Di George). *Arch. Fr. Pediatr.* **32,** 161–176.

Niall, H. D., Keutmann, H., Sauer, R., Hogan, N., Dawson, B., Aurbach, G., and Potts, J. T., Jr. (1970). The amino acid sequence of bovine parathyroid hormone. *Hoppe-Seyler's Z. Physiol. Chem.* **351,** 1586–1588.

Niall, H. D., Sauer, R. T., Jacobs, J. W., Keutmann, H. T., Segré, G. V., O'Riordan, J. L. H., Aurbach, G. D., and Potts, J. T., Jr. (1974). The amino-acid sequence of the amino-terminal 37 residues of human parathyroid hormone. *Proc. Natl. Acad. Sci. U.S.A.* **71,** 384–388.

Nissenson, R. A., and Arnaud, C. D. (1979). Properties of the parathyroid hormone receptor-adenylate cyclase system in chicken renal plasma membranes. *J. Biol. Chem.* **254,** 1469–1475.

Nissenson, R. A., Abbott, S. R., Teitelbaum, A. P., Clark, O. H., and Arnaud, C. D. (1981). Endogenous biologically active human parathyroid hormone: Measurement by a guanyl nucleotide-amplified renal adenylate cyclase assay. *J. Clin. Endocrinol. Metab.* **52,** 840–846.

Norberg, K.-A., Persson, B., and Granberg, P.-O. (1975). Adrenergic innervation of the human parathyroid glands. *Acta Chir. Scand.* **141,** 319–322.

Nordin, B. E. C., and Bulusu, L. (1968). A modified index of phosphate excretion. *Postgrad. Med. J.* **44,** 93–97.

Nordin, B. E. C., and Peacock, M. (1969). The role of the kidney in the regulation of plasma-calcium. *Lancet* **2,** 1280–1283.

Nordquist, R. E., and Palmieri, G. M. A. (1974). Intracellular localization of parathyroid hormone in the kidney. *Endocrinology (Baltimore)* **95,** 229–237.

Norris, E. H. (1947). Parathyroid adenoma: Study of 322 cases. *Int. Abstr. Surg.* **84,** 1–41.

Northcutt, R. C., Levinson, J. D., and Ernest, J. B. (1969). Hypocalcemia resulting from infraction of a parathyroid adenoma. *Ann. Intern. Med.* **70,** 353–356.

Northrop, G., Misenheimer, H. P., and Becker, F. O. (1977). Failure of parathyroid hormone to cross the nonhuman primate placenta. *Am. J. Obstet. Gynecol.* **129,** 449–453.

Nusynowitz, M. L., and Klein, M. H. (1973). Pseudoidiopathic hypoparathyroidism. Hypoparathyroidism with ineffective parathyroid hormone. *Am. J. Med.* **55,** 677–686.

Oldham, S. B., Fischer, J. A., Capen, C., and Arnaud, C. D. (1971). Dynamics of parathyroid hormone secretion *in vitro*. *Am. J. Med.* **50,** 650–657.

Oldham, S. B., Fischer, J. A., Shen, L. H., and Arnaud, C. D. (1974). Isolation and properties of a calcium-binding protein from porcine parathyroid glands. *Biochemistry* **13,** 4790–4796.

Oldham, S. B., Finck, E. J., and Singer, F. R. (1978). Parathyroid hormone clearance in man. *Metabolism Clin. Exp.* **27,** 993–1001.

Omenn, G. S., Roth, S. I., and Baker, W. H. (1969). Hyperparathyroidism associated with malignant tumors of non-parathyroid origin. *Cancer* **24,** 1004–1012.

O'Riordan, J. L. H., Woodhead, J. S., Hendy, G. N., Parsons, J. A., Robinson, C. J., Keutmann, H. T., Dawson, B. F., and Potts, J. T., Jr. (1974). Effect of oxidation on biological and immunological activity of parcine parathyroid hormone. *J. Endocrinol.* **63,** 117–124.

Pak, C. Y. C., Ohata, M., Lawrence, E. C., and Snyder, W. (1974). The hypercalciurias: causes, parathyroid functions, and diagnostic criteria. *J. Clin. Invest.* **54,** 384–400.

Palmieri, G. M. A., Nordquist, R. E., and Omenn, G. S. (1974). Immunochemical localization of parathyroid hormone in cancer tissue from patients with ectopic hyperparathyroidism. *J. Clin. Invest.* **53,** 1726–1735.

Papapoulos, S. E., Tomlinson, H. S., Lewin, I. G., and O'Riordan, J. L. H. (1977). Clearance of exogenous parathyroid hormone in normal and uraemic man. *Clin. Endocrinol. (Oxford)* **7,** 211–225.

Papapoulos, S. E., Fraher, L. J., Sandler, L. M., Clemens, T. L., Lewin, I. G., O'Riordan, J. L. H. (1979). 1,25-dihydroxycholecalciferol in the pathogenesis of the hypercalcaemia of sarcoidosis. *Lancet* **1,** 627–630.

Parfitt, A. M., and Dent, C. E. (1970). Hyperparathyroidism and hypercalcemia *Q. J. Med.* [*N.S.*] **39,** 171–187.

Park, H. Z., and Talmage, R. V. (1968). Comparison of the effect of calcium and endogenous parathyroid hormone on RNA synthesis in rat bone. *In* "Parathyroid Hormone and Thyrocalcitonin (Calcitonin)" (R. V. Talmage, and L. F. Bélanger, eds.), pp. 203–215. Excerpta Medica, Amsterdam.

Parsons, J. A. (1976). Parathyroid physiology and the skeleton. *In* "Biochemistry and Physiology of the Bone" (G. H. Bourne, ed.), 2nd ed., Vol. 4, pp. 159–225. Academic Press, New York.

Parsons, J. A., Reit, W., and Robinson, C. J. (1973). A bioassay for parathyroid hormone using chicks. *Endocrinology (Baltimore)* **92,** 454–462.

Parthemore, J. G., and Deftos, L. J. (1979). Calcitonin secretion in primary hyperparathyroidism. *J. Clin. Endocrinol. Metab.* **49,** 223–226.

Paunier, L., Radde, I. C., Kooh, S. W., Cohen, P. E., and Fraser, D. (1968). Primary hypomagnesia with secondary hypocalcemia in an infant. *Pediatrics* **41,** 384–402.

Pearse, A. G. E., and Takor, T. T. (1976). Neuroendocrine embryology and the APUD concept. *J. Clin. Endocrinol. Metab.* **5,** 229s–244s.

Peck, W. A., Carpenter, J., Messinger, K., and de Bra, D. (1973). Cyclic 3′,5′-adenosine monophosphate in isolated bone cells: Response to low concentrations of parathyroid hormone. *Endocrinology (Baltimore)* **92,** 692–697.

Perris, A. D., and Whitfield, J. F. (1971). Calcium homeostasis and erythropoietic control in the rat. *Can. J. Physiol. Pharmacol.* **49,** 22–35.

Pietrek, J., Kokot, F., and Kuska, J. (1978). Serum 25-hydroxyvitamin D and parathyroid hormone in patients with acute renal failure. *Kidney Int.* **13,** 178–185.

Pletka, P., Bernstein, D. S., Hampers, C. L., Merrill, J. P., and Sherwood, L. M. (1974). Relationship between magnesium and secondary hyperparathyroidism during long-term hemodialysis. *Metab. Clin. Exp.* **23,** 619–630.

Pletka, P. G., Strom, T. B., Hampers, C. L., Griffith, H., Wilson, R. E., Bernstein, D. S., Sherwood, L. M., and Merrill, J. P. (1976). Secondary hyperparathyroidism in human kidney transplant recipients. *Nephron* **17,** 371–381.

Potter, D. E., Wilson, C. J., and Ozonoff, M. B. (1974). Hyperparathyroid bone disease in children undergoing long-term hemodialysis: Treatment with vitamin D. *J. Pediatr.* **85,** 60–66.

Potts, J. T., Jr., Tregear, G. W., Keutmann, H. T., Niall, H. D., Sauer, R., Deftos, L. J., Dawson, B. F., Hogan, M. L., and Aurbach, G. D. (1971). Synthesis of a biologically active N-terminal tetratriacontapeptide of parathyroid hormone. *Proc Natl. Acad. Sci. U.S.A.* **68,** 63–76.

Purnell, D. C., Scholz, D. A., Smith, L. H., Sizemore, G. W., Black, B. M., Goldsmith, R. S., and Arnaud, C. D. (1974). Treatment of primary hyperparathyroidism *Am. J. Med.* **56,** 800–809.

Pyrah, L. N., Hodgkinson, A., and Anderson, C. K. (1966). Primary hyperparathyroidism *Br. J. Surg.* **53,** 245–316.

Raisz, L. G. (1963a). Stimulation of bone resorption by parathyroid hormone in tissue culture. *Nature (London)* **197,** 1015–1016.

Raisz, L. G. (1963b). Regulation by calcium of parathyroid growth and secretion *in vitro*. *Nature (London)* **197,** 1115–1116.

Raisz, L. G. (1965). Bone resorption in tissue culture. Factors influencing the response to parathyroid hormone. *J. Clin. Invest.* **44,** 103–116.

Raisz, L. G. (1967). Effects of calcium on uptake and incorporation of amino acids in the parathyroid glands. *Biochim. Biophys. Acta* **148,** 460–468.

Ramp, W. K., Cooper, C. W., Ross III, A. J., and Wells, S. A., Jr. (1979). Effects of calcium and cyclic nucleotides on rat calcitonin and parathyroid hormone secretion. *Mol. Cell. Endocrinol.* **14,** 205–215.

Rasmussen, H. (1970). Cell communication, calcium ion, and cyclic adenosine monophosphate. *Science* **170,** 404–412.

Rasmussen, H., and Bordier, P. (1974). "The Physiological and Cellular Basis of Metabolic Bone Disease." Williams & Wilkins, Baltimore, Maryland.

Rasmussen, H., and Craig, L. C. (1959). Purification of parathyroid hormone by use of countercurrent distribution. *J. Am. Chem. Soc.* **81,** 5003.

Rasmussen, H., and Craig, L. C. (1961). Isolation and characterization of bovine parathyroid hormone. *J. Biol. Chem.* **236,** 759–764.

Rasmussen, H., and DeLuca, H. F. (1963). Calcium homeostasis. *Ergeb. Physiol. Biol. Chem. Exp. Pharmakol.* **53,** 108–173.

Rasmussen, H., DeLuca, H. F., Arnaud, C. D., Hawker, C., and Stedingk, M. (1963). The relationship between vitamin D and parathyroid hormone. *J. Clin. Invest.* **42,** 1940–1946.

Rasmussen, H., Arnaud, C. D., and Hawker, C. (1964a). Actinomycin D and the response to parathyroid hormone. *Science* **144,** 1019–1021.

Rasmussen, H., Fischer, J. A., and Arnaud, C. D. (1964b). Parathyroid hormone, ion exchange, and mitochondrial swelling. *Proc. Natl. Acad. Sci. U.S.A.* **52,** 1198–1203.

Rasmussen, H., Sze, Y. L., and Young, R. (1964c). Further studies on the isolation and characterization of parathyroid polypeptides. *J. Biol. Chem.* **239,** 2852–2857.

Rasmussen, H., Pechet, M., and Fast, D. (1968). Effect of dibutyryl cyclic adenosine 3′,5′-monophosphate, theophylline, and other nucleotides upon calcium and phosphate metabolism. *J. Clin. Invest.* **47,** 1843–1850.

Rasmussen, H., Wong, M., Bikle, D., and Goodman, D. B. P. (1972). Hormonal control of the renal conversion of 25-hydroxycholecalciferol to 1,25-dihydroxycholecalciferol. *J. Clin. Invest.* **51,** 2502–2504.

Reeve, J., Tregear, G. W., and Parsons, J. A. (1976a). Preliminary trial of low doses of human parathyroid hormone 1–34 peptide in treatment of osteoporosis. *Calcif. Tissue Res.* **21,** 469–477.

Reeve, J., Williams, D., Hesp, R., Hulme, P., Klenerman, L., Zanelli, J. M., Darby, A. J., Tregear, G. W., and Parsons, J. A. (1976b). Anabolic effect of low doses of a fragment of human parathyroid hormone on the skeleton in postmenopausal osteoporosis. *Lancet* **1,** 1035–1038.

Reiss, E., and Canterbury, J. M. (1968). A radioimmunoassay for parathyroid hormone in man. *Proc. Soc. Exp. Biol. Med.* **128,** 501–504.

Reiss, E., and Canterbury, J. M. (1969). Primary hyperparathyroidism: Application of radioimmunoassay to differentiation of adenoma and hyperplasia in the preoperative localization of hyperfunctioning parathyroid glands. *N. Engl. J. Med.* **280,** 1381–1385.

Reiss, E., Canterbury, J. M., Bercovitz, M. A., and Kaplan, E. L. (1970). The role of phosphate in the secretion of parathyroid hormone in man. *J. Clin. Invest.* **49,** 2146–2150.

Reitz, R. E., and Weinstein, R. L. (1973). Parathyroid hormone secretion in familial vitamin-D resistant rickets. *N. Engl. J. Med.* **289,** 941–945.

Rhone, D. P. (1975). Primary neonatal hyperparathyroidism. *Am. J. Clin. Pathol.* **64,** 488–499.

Richardson, J. E. (1953). The early renal symptoms of hyperparathyroidism. *Ann. R. Coll. Surg. Engl.* **13,** 100–126.

Rienhoff, W. F. (1950). The surgical treatment of hyperparathyroidism. *Ann. Surg.* **131,** 917–944.

Riggs, B. L., Arnaud, C. D., Goldsmith, R. S., Taylor, W. F., McCall, T., and Sessler, A. D. (1971a). Plasma kinetics and acute effects of pharmacologic doses of porcine calcitonin in man. *J. Clin. Endocrinol. Metab.* **33,** 115–127.

Riggs, B. L., Arnaud, C. D., Reynolds, J. C., and Smith, L. H. (1971b). Immunologic differentiation of primary hyperparathyroidism from hyperparathyroidism due to nonparathyroid cancer. *J. Clin. Invest.* **50,** 2079–2083.

Riggs, B. L., Arnaud, C. D., Jowsey, J., Goldsmith, R. S., and Kelly, P. J. (1973). Parathyroid function in primary osteoporosis. *J. Clin. Invest.* **52,** 181–184.

Riggs, B. L., Jowsey, J., Kelly, P. J., Hoffman, D. L., and Arnaud, C. D. (1976). Effects of oral therapy with calcium and vitamin D in primary osteoporosis. *J. Clin. Endocrinol. Metab.* **42,** 1139–1144.

Rixon, R. H., and Whitfield, J. F. (1976). The control of liver regeneration by parathyroid hormone and calcium. *J. Cell. Physiol.* **87,** 147–156.

Robertson, G. M., Moore, E. W., Switz, D. M., and Estep, H. L. (1976). Inadequate parathyroid response in acute pancreatitis. *N. Engl. J. Med.* **294,** 512–516.

Robertson, W. G., Peacock, M., Atkins, D., and Webster, L. A. (1972). The effect of parathyroid hormone on the uptake and release of calcium by bone in tissue culture. *Clin. Sci.* **43,** 715–718.

Rodan, S. B., and Rodan, G. A. (1974). The effect of parathyroid hormone and thyrocalcitonin on the accumulation of cyclic adenosine 3′,5′-monophosphate in freshly isolated bone cells. *J. Biol. Chem.* **249,** 3068–3074.

Rodriguez, H. J., Villareal, H., Jr., Klahr, S., and Slatopolsky, E. (1974). Pseudohypoparathyroidism type II: Restoration of normal renal responsiveness to parathyroid hormone by calcium administration. *J. Clin. Endocrinol. Metab.* **39,** 693–701.

Roof, B. S., Carpenter, B., Fink, D. J., and Gordan, G. S. (1971). Some thoughts on the nature of ectopic parathyroid hormones. *Am. J. Med.* **50,** 686–691.

Root, A., Gruskin, A., Reber, R. M., Stopa, A., and Duckett, G. (1974). Serum concentrations of parathyroid hormone in infants, children, and adolescents. *J. Pediatr.* **85,** 329–336.

Rosenblatt, M., Goltzman, D., Keutmann, H. T., Tregear, G. W., and Potts, J. T., Jr. (1976). Chemical and biological properties of synthetic, sulfur-free analogues of parathyroid hormones. *J. Biol. Chem.* **451,** 159–164.

Rosenblatt, M., Segre, G. V., and Potts, J. T., Jr. (1977). Synthesis of a fragment of parathyroid hormone, bPTH-(28–48): An inhibitor of hormone cleavage in vivo. *Biochemistry* **16,** 2811–2816.

Roth, S. I. (1971). Recent advances in parathyroid gland pathology. *Am. J. Med.* **50,** 612–622.

Roth, S. I., and Capen, C. C. (1974). Ultrastructural and functional correlations of the parathyroid gland. *Int. Rev. Exp. Pathol.* **13,** 161–221.

Roth, S. I., and Raisz, L. G. (1966). The course and reversibility of the calcium effect on the ultrastructure of the rat parathyroid gland in organ culture. *Lab. Invest.* **15,** 1187–1211.

Rude, R. K., Oldham, S. B., and Singer, F. R. (1976). Functional hypoparathyroidism and parathyroid hormone end-organ resistance in human magnesium deficiency. *Clin. Endocrinol. (Oxford)* **5,** 209–224.

Rude, R. K., Sharp, C. F., Jr., Fredericks, R. S., Oldham, S. B., Elbaum, N., Link, J., Irwin, L., and Singer, F. R. (1981). Urinary and nephrogenous adenosine 3′,5′-monophosphate in the hypercalcemia of malignancy. *J. Clin. Endocrinol. Metab.* **52,** 765–771.

Russell, R. G. G., Casey, P. A., and Fleisch, H. (1968). Stimulation of phosphate excretion by renal arterial infusion of 3′,5′-AMP. A possible mechanism of action of parathyroid hormone. *Calcif. Tissue Res.* **2,** Suppl. 54.

Rutherford, W. E., Bordier, P., Marie, P., Hruska, K., Harter, H., Greenwalt, A., Blondin, J., Haddad, J., Bricker, N., and Slatopolsky, E. (1977). Phosphate control and 25-hydroxycholecalciferol administration in preventing experimental renal osteodystrophy in the dog. *J. Clin. Invest.* **60,** 332–341.

St. Goar, W. T. (1963). Discussion, case record 29–1963, Massachusetts General Hospital. *N. Engl. J. Med.* **268,** 949.

Sakai, M., Matsushita, S., Nakano, T., Kimura, N., Araki, N., and Nagata, N. (1976). Effects of parathyroid hormone *in vivo* on the protein kinase activity in rat kidney. *Endocrinology (Baltimore)* **98,** 1443–1450.

Sakamoto, S., Sakamoto, M., Goldhaber, P., and Glimcher, M. (1975). Collagenase and bone resorption: Isolation of collagenase from culture medium containing serum after stimulation of bone resorption by addition of parathyroid hormone extracts. *Biochem. Biophys. Res. Commun.* **63,** 172–178.

Sammon, P. J., Stacey, R. E., and Bronner, F. (1970). Role of parathyroid hormone in calcium homeostasis and metabolism. *Am. J. Physiol.* **218,** 479–485.

Sauer, R. T., Niall, H. D., Hogan, M. L., Keutmann, H. T., O'Riordan, J. L. H., and Potts, J. T., Jr. (1974). The amino acid sequence of porcine parathyroid hormone. *Biochemistry* **13,** 1994–1999.

Schantz, A., and Castleman, B. (1973). Parathyroid carcinoma: A study of 70 cases. *Cancer* **31,** 600–615.

Schenk, R. K., Olah, A. J., and Merz, W. A. (1973). Bone cell counts. *In* "Clinical Aspects of Metabolic Bone Disease" (B. Frame, A. M. Parfitt, and H. Duncan, eds.), pp. 103–113. Excerpta Medica, Amsterdam.

Schmidt-Gayk, H., Stengel, R., Haueisen, H., Hüfner, M., Ritz, E., and Jakobs, K. H. (1977). Hyperparathyroidism: Influence of glomerular filtration rate on urinary excretion of cyclic AMP. *Klin. Wochenschr.* **55,** 275–281.

Schneider, P., Paunier, L., Sizonenko, P. C., and Wyss, M. (1977). Effects of parathyroid hormone on total protein, calcium, magnesium, phosphorus, sodium and potassium concentrations of normal human parotid saliva. *Eur. J. Clin. Invest.* **7,** 121–126.

Schwartz, G. H., David, D. S., Riggio, R. R., Saville, P. D., Whitsell, J. C., Stenzel, K. H., and Rubin, A. L. (1970). Hypercalcemia after renal transplantation. *Am. J. Med.* **49,** 42–51.

Segre, G. V. Habener, J. F., Powell, D., Tregear, G. W., and Potts, J. T., Jr. (1972). Parathyroid hormone in human plasma. Immunochemical characterization and biological implication. *J. Clin. Invest.* **51,** 3163–3172.

Segre, G. V., Niall, H. D., Habener, J. F., and Potts, J. T., Jr. (1974). Metabolism of parathyroid hormone. Physiologic and clinical significance. *Am. J. Med.* **56,** 774–784.

Segre, G. V., D'Amour, P., and Potts, J. T., Jr. (1976). Metabolism of radioiodinated bovine parathyroid hormone in rat. *Endocrinology (Baltimore)* **99,** 1645–1652.

Segre, G. V., Niall, H. D., Sauer, P. T., and Potts, J. T., Jr. (1977). Edman degradation of radioiodinated parathyroid hormone: Application to sequence analysis and hormone metabolism in vivo. *Biochemistry* **16,** 2417–2427.

Segre, G. V., D'Amour, P., Hultman, A., and Potts, J. T., Jr. (1981a). Effects of hepatectomy, nephrectomy, and nephrectomy/uremia on the metabolism of parathyroid hormone in the rat. *J. Clin. Invest.* **67,** 439–448.

Segre, G. V., Perkins, A. S., Witters, L. A., and Potts, J. T., Jr. (1981b). Metabolism of parathyroid hormone by isolated rat Kupffer cells and hepatocytes. *J. Clin. Invest.* **67,** 449–457.

Shah, J. H., Motto, G. S., Kukreja, S. C., Hargis, G. K., and Williams, G. A. (1975). Stimulation of the secretion of parathyroid hormone during hypoglycemic stress. *J. Clin. Endocrinol. Metab.* **41,** 692–696.

Shannon, W. A., Jr., and Roth, S. I. (1974). An ultrastructural study of acid phosphatase activity in normal, adenomatous and hyperplastic (chief cell type) human parathyroid glands. *Am. J. Pathol.* **77,** 493–506.

Shaw, J. W., Oldham, S. B., Bethune, J. E., and Fichman, M. P. (1974). Parathyroid hormone-mediated rise in urinary cyclic AMP during acute extracellular fluid expansion natiuresis. *J. Clin. Endocrinol. Metab.* **39,** 311–315.

Sherman, L. A., Pfefferbaum, A., and Brown, E. B., Jr. (1970). Hypoparathyroidism in a patient with longstanding iron storage disease. *Ann. Intern. Med.* **73,** 259–261.

Sherwood, L. M., and Abe, M. (1972a). Magnesium ion, parathyroid hormone secretion and cyclic 3′,5′-AMP. *Clin. Res.* **20,** 756 (abstr.).

Sherwood, L. M., and Abe, M. (1972b). Adrenergic receptors and the release of parathyroid hormone. *J. Clin. Invest.* **51,** 88A (abstr.).

Sherwood, L. M., Potts, J. T., Jr., Care, A. D., Mayer, G. P., and Aurbach, G. D. (1966). Evaluation by radioimmunoassay of factors controlling the secretion of parathyroid hormone. Intravenous infusions of calcium and ethylene-diamine tetraacetic acid in the cow and goat. *Nature (London)* **209,** 52–55.

Sherwood ,L. M., Mayer, G. P., Ramberg, C. F., Jr., Kronfeld, D. S., Aurbach, G. D., and Potts, J. T., Jr. (1968). Regulation of parathyroid hormone secretion: Proportional control by calcium, lack of effect of phosphate. *Endocrinology (Baltimore)* **83,** 1043–1051.

Sherwood, L. M., Herrmann, I., and Bassett, C. A. (1970a). Parathyroid hormone secretion in vitro: Regulation by calcium and magnesium ions. *Nature (London)* **225,** 1056–1058.

Sherwood, L. M., Rodman, J. S., and Lundberg, W. B. (1970b). Evidence for a precursor to circulating parathyroid hormone. *Proc. Natl. Acad. Sci. U.S.A.* **67,** 1631–1638.

Shimkin, P. M., and Powell, D. (1973). Parathyroid hormone levels in thyroid-vein blood of patients without abnormalities of calcium metabolism. *Ann. Intern. Med.* **78,** 714–716.

Shlatz, L. J., Schwartz, J. L., Kinne-Saffran, E., and Kinne, R. (1975). Distribution of parathyroid hormone-stimulated adenylate cyclase in plasma membrane cells of the kidney cortex. *J. Membr. Biol.* **24,** 131–144.

Short, E. M., Elsass, L. J., and Rosenberg, L. E. (1974). Effect of parathyroid hormone on renal tubular reabsorption of amino acids. *Metab. Clin. Exp.* **23,** 715–727.

Short, E. M., Morris, R. C., Jr., Sebastian, A., and Spencer, M. (1976). Exaggerated phosphaturic response to circulating parathyroid hormone in patients with familial X-linked hypophosphatemic rickets. *J. Clin. Invest.* **58,** 152–163.

Signer, E., Brechbühler, T., and Fischer, J. A. (1975). Primäre magnesium-malabsorption und hypoparathyreoidismus. *Jahresversamml. Schweiz. Ges. Paediatr.* p. 17 (abstr.).

Silverman, R., and Yalow, R. S. (1973). Heterogeneity of parathyroid hormone. Clinical and physiological implications. *J. Clin. Invest.* **52,** 1958–1971.

Singer, F. R., Segré, G. V., Habener, J. F., and Potts, J. T., Jr. (1975). Peripheral metabolism of bovine parathyroid hormone in the dog. *Metab. Clin. Exp.* **24,** 139–144.

Sinha, T. K., Miller, S., Fleming, J., Khairi, R., Edmondson, J., Johnston, C. C., Jr., and Bell, N. H. (1975). Demonstration of a diurnal variation in serum parathyroid hormone in primary and secondary hyperparathyroidism. *J. Clin. Endocrinol. Metab.* **41,** 1009–1013.

Sinha, T. K., Thajchayapong, P., Queener, S. F., Allen, D. O., and Bell, N. H. (1976). On the lipolytic action of parathyroid hormone in man. *Metab. Clin. Exp.* **25,** 251–260.

Slatopolsky, E., Caglar, S., Pennell, J. P., Taggart, D. D., Canterbury, J. M., Reiss, E., and Bricker, N. S. (1971). On the pathogenesis of hyperparathyroidism in chronic experimental renal insufficiency in the dog. *J. Clin. Invest.* **50,** 492–499.

Smith, D. M., and Johnston, C. C., Jr. (1975). Cyclic 3′,5′-adenosine monophosphate levels in separated bone cells. *Endocrinology (Baltimore)* **96,** 1261–1269.

Sraer, J., Ardaillou, R., Loreau, N., and Sraer, J.-D. (1974). Evidence for parathyroid hormone sensitive adenylate cyclase in rat glomeruli. *Mol. Cell. Endocrinol.* **1,** 285–294.

Stanbury, S. W., and Lumb, G. A. (1966). Parathyroid function in chronic renal failure. *Q. J. Med.* [*N.S.*] **35,** 1–23.

Steele, T. H. (1976). Renal resistance to parathyroid hormone during phosphorous deprivation. *J. Clin. Invest.* **58,** 1461–1464.

Steiner, A. L., Goodman, A. D., and Powers, S. R. (1968). Study of a kindred with pheochromacytoma medullary thyroid carcinoma, hyperparathyroidism and Cushing's disease: Multiple endocrine neoplasia, type 2. *Medicine (Baltimore)* **47,** 371–409.

Stern, P. H., De Olazabal, J., and Bell, N. H. (1980). Evidence for abnormal regulation of circulating 1α,25-dihydroxyvitamin D in patients with sarcoidosis and normal calcium metabolism. *J. Clin. Invest.* **66,** 852–855.

Stewart, A. F., Horst, R., Deftos, L. J., Cadman, E. C., Lang, R., and Broadus, A. E. (1980). Biochemical evaluation of patients with cancer-associated hypercalcemia: evidence for humoral and nonhumoral groups. *N. Engl. J. Med.* **303,** 1377–1383.

Stögmann, W., and Fischer, J. A. (1975). Pseudohypoparathyroidism: Disappearance of the resistance to exogenous parathyroid extract during treatment with vitamin D. *Am. J. Med.* **58,** 140–144.

Takatsuki, K., Hanley, D. A., and Sherwood, L. M. (1980). Effects of magnesium ion on parathyroid hormone secretion in vitro. *Calcif. Tissue Int.* **32,** 201–206.

Takatsuki, K., Schneider, A. B., Shin, K. Y., and Sherwood, L. M. (1981). Extraction, purification and partial characterization of bovine parathyroid secretory protein. *J. Biol. Chem.* **256,** 2342–2345.

Suh, S. M., Fraser, D., and Kooh, S. W. (1970). Pseudohypoparathyroidism: Responsiveness to parathyroid extract induced by vitamin D therapy. *J. Clin. Endocrinol. Metab.* **30,** 609–614.

Suh, S. M., Tashjian, A. H., Jr., Matsuo, N., Parkinson, D. K., and Fraser, D. (1973). Pathogenesis of hypocalcemia in primary hypomagnesemia: Normal end-organ responsiveness to parathyroid hormone, impaired parathyroid gland function. *J. Clin. Invest.* **52,** 153–160.

Sutcliffe, H. S., Martin, T. J., Eisman, J. A., and Pilczyk, R. (1973). Binding of parathyroid hormone to bovine kidney-cortex plasma membranes. *Biochem. J.* **134,** 913–921.

Swinton, N. W., Jr., Clerkin, E. P., and Flint, L. D. (1972). Hypercalcemia and familial pheochromocytoma. Correction after adrenectomy. *Ann. Intern. Med.* **76,** 455–457.

Talmage, R. V., Taft, R. J., and Davis, R. (1960). Parathyroid activity in nephrectomized rats. *Tex. Rep. Biol. Med.* **18,** 298–308.

Talwalker, J. B., Musgrave, J. E., Buist, N. R. M., Campbell, R. A., and Campbell, J. R. (1974). Vitamin D-resistant rickets and parathyroid adenomas. *Am. J. Dis. Child.* **128,** 704–708.

Tashjian, A. H., Jr., Levine, L., and Munson, P. L. (1964a). Immunochemical identification of parathyroid hormone in non parathyroid neoplasms associated with hypercalcemia. *J. Exp. Med.* **119,** 467–484.

Tashjian, A. H., Jr., Ontjes. D. A., and Munson, D. L. (1964b). Alkylation and oxidation of methionine in bovine parathyroid hormone: Effects on hormonal activity and antigenicity. *Biochemistry* **3,** 1175–1182.

Tavill, A. S., Evanson, J. M., de C. Baker, S. B., and Hewitt, V. (1964). Idiopathic paroxysmal myoglobinuria with acute renal failure and hypercalcemia. *N. Engl. J. Med.* **271,** 283–287.

Tenenhouse, A., Meier, R., and Rasmussen, H. (1966). Parathyroid hormone and bone mobilization in vitro. *J. Biol. Chem.* **241,** 1314–1318.

Thajchayapong, P., Queener, S. F., McClintock, R., Allen, D. O., and Bell, N. H. (1976). Demonstration that cyclic adenosine 3′,5′-monophosphate mediates the lipolytic action of parathyroid hormone. *Horm. Metab. Res.* **8,** 190–195.

Tisell, L.-E., Hansson, G., Lindberg, S., and Ragnhult, I. (1978). Occurrence of previous neck radiotherapy among patients with associated non-medullary thyroid carcinoma and parathyroid adenoma or hyperplasia. *Acta Chir. Scand.* **144,** 7–11.

Tregear, G. W., and Potts, J. T., Jr. (1975). Synthetic analogues of residues 1–34 of human parathyroid hormone: Influence of residue number 1 on biological potency *in vitro*. *Endocr. Res. Commun.* **2,** 561–570.

Tregear, G. W., van Rietschoten, J., Greene, E., Keutmann, H. T., Niall, H. D., Reit, B., Parsons, J. A., and Potts, J. T., Jr. (1973). Bovine parathyroid hormone: Minimum chain length of synthetic peptide required for biological activity. *Endocrinology (Baltimore)* **93,** 1349–1353.

Tregear, G. W., van Rietschoten, J., Greene, E., Niall, H. D., Keutmann, H. T., Parsons, J. A., O'Riordan, J. L. H., and Potts, J. T., Jr. (1974). Solid-phase synthesis of the biologically active N-terminal 1–34 peptide of human parathyroid hormone. *Hoppe-Seyler's Z. Physiol. Chem.* **355,** 415–421.

Tsang, R. C., Chen, I.-W., Friedman, M. A., and Chen, I. (1973). Neonatal parathyroid function: Role of gestational age and postnatal age. *J. Pediatr.* **83,** 728–738.

Tsang, R. C., Chen, I.-W., Friedman, M. A., Gigger, M., Steichen, J., Koffler, H., Fenton, L., Brown, D., Pramanik, A., Keenan, W., Strub, R., and Joyce, T. (1975). Parathyroid function in infants of diabetic mothers. *J. Pediatr.* **86,** 399–404.

Vaes, G. (1967). "La résorption osseuse et l'hormone parathyroidienne." Visscher, Bruxelles.

Van Arsdel, P. P., Jr. (1955). Maternal hyperparathyroidism as a cause of neonatal tetany. *J. Clin. Endocrinol. Metab.* **15,** 680–684.

Vegt, G. B., and De Ruijter, M. (1977). The effect of parathyroid hormone on the uptake of calcium by fetal rat intestinal tissue and by isolated intestinal epithelial cells. *Proc. K. Ned. Akad. Wet., Series C* **80,** 48–71.

Wallach, S., Baker, R. K., and Nicastri, A. (1972). Primary renal tubular acidosis and secondary hyperparathyroidism. *Am. J. Med.* **52,** 809–816.

Webster, G. D., Mann, J. B., and Hills, A. G. (1967). The effect of phosphate infusions upon renal phosphate clearance in man. Evidence for tubular phosphate secretion. *Metab. Clin. Exp.* **16,** 797–814.

Webster, L. A., Atkins, D., and Peacock, M. (1974). A bioassay for parathyroid hormone using whole mouse calvaria in tissue culture. *J. Endocrinol.* **62,** 631–637.

Weisbrode, S. E., Capen, C. C., and Nagode, L. A. (1974). Effects of parathyroid hormone on bone of parathyroidectomized rats. *Am. J. Pathol.* **75,** 529–536.

Wells, S. A., Gunnells, J. C., Shelbourne, J. D., Schneider, A. E., and Sherwood, L. M. (1975). Transplantation of the parathyroid glands in man: Clinical indications and results. *Surgery* **78,** 34–44.

Wells, S. A., Ellis, G. J., Gunnells, J. C., Schneider, A. E., and Sherwood, L. M. (1976). Parathyroid autotransplantation in primary parathyroid hyperplasia. *N. Engl. J. Med.* **295,** 57–62.

Werder, E. A., Illig. R., Bernasconi, S., Kind, H.-P., Prader, A., Fischer, J. A., and Fanconi, A. (1975). Excessive thyrotropin response to thyrotropin-releasing hormone in pseudohypoparathyroidism. *Pediatr. Res.* **9,** 12–16.

Werder, E. A., Fischer, J. A., Illig. R., Bernasconi, S., Fanconi, A., and Prader, A. (1978). Pseudohypoparathyroidism and idiopathic hypoparathyroidism: Relationships between serum calcium and parathyroid hormone levels and the urinary cyclic adenosine3′,5′-monophosphate response to parathyroid extract. *J. Clin. Endocrinol. Metab.* **46,** 872–879.

Werner, S. H., and Löw, H. (1973). Stimulation of lipolysis and calcium accumulation by parathyroid hormone in rat adipose tissue *in vitro* after adrenalectomy and administration of high doses of cortisone acetate. *Horm. Metab. Res.* **5,** 292–296.

Whitfield, J. F., MacManus, J. P., Youdale, T., and Franks, D. J. (1971). The roles of calcium and cyclic AMP in the stimulatory action of parathyroid hormone on thymic lymphocyte proliferation. *J. Cell. Physiol.* **78,** 355–368.

Wieland, P., Fischer, J. A., Binswanger, U., and Duc, G. (1979). Parathyroid hormone response in newborn infants during exchange transfusion with blood supplemented with citrate and phosphate: Effect of iv calcium. *Pediatr. Res.* **13,** 963–968.

Wieland, P., Fischer, J. A., Trechsel, U., Roth, H.-R., Vetter, K., Schneider, H., and Huch, A. (1980). Perinatal parathyroid hormone, vitamin D metabolites, and calcitonin in man. *Am. J. Physiol.* **239,** E385–E390.

Willgoss, D., Jacobi, J. M., de Jersey, J., Bartley, P. C., and Lloyd, H. M. (1980). Effect of calcium on cyclic nucleotide phosphodiesterase in parathyroid tissue. *Biochem. Biophys. Res. Commun.* **94,** 763–768.

Williams, G. A., Hargis, G. K., Bowser, E. N., Henderson, W. J., and Martinez, N. J. (1973). Evidence for a role of adenosine 3′,5′-monophosphate in parathyroid hormone release. *Endocrinology (Baltimore)* **92,** 687–691.

Williams, G. A., Peterson, W. C., Bowser, E. N., Henderson, W. J., Hargis, G. K., and Martinez, N. J. (1974). Interrelationship of parathyroid and adrenocortical function in calcium homeostasis in the rat. *Endocrinology (Baltimore)* **95,** 707–712.

Wolinsky, J., and Cohn, D. V. (1969). Oxygen uptake and $^{14}CO_2$ production from citrate and isocitrate by control and parathyroid hormone-treated bone maintained in tissue culture. *Endocrinology (Baltimore)* **84,** 28–35.

Wong, G. L., and Cohn, D. V. (1974). Separation of parathyroid hormone and calcitonin-sensitive cells from non-responsive bone cells. *Nature (London)* **252,** 713–715.

Wong, G. L., and Cohn, D. V. (1975). Target cells in bone for parathormone and calcitonin are different: Enrichment for each cell type by sequential digestion of mouse calvaria and selective adhesion to polymeric surfaces. *Proc. Natl. Acad. Sci. U.S.A.* **72,** 3167–3171.

Woodhead, J. S., O'Riordan, J. L. H., Keutmann, H. T., Stoltz, M. L., Dawson, B. F., Niall, H. D., Robinson, C. J., and Potts, J. T., Jr. (1971). Isolation and chemical properties of porcine parathyroid hormone. *Biochemistry* **10,** 2787–2792.

Woodhouse, N. J. Y., Doyle, F. H., and Joplin, G. F. (1971). Vitamin D deficiency and primary hyperparathyroidism. *Lancet* **2,** 283–287.

Woodward, J. E., Webster, P. D., and Carr, A. A. (1972). Primary hypomagnesemia with secondary hypocalcemia, diarrhea and insensitivity to parathyroid hormone. *Am. J. Dig. Dis.* **17,** 612–618.

Wu, B. C., Pillay, V. K. G., Hawker, C. D., Armbruster, K. F. W., Shapiro, H. S., and Ing, T. S. (1972). Hypercalcemia in acute renal failure of acute alcoholic rhabdomyolysis. *S. Afr. Med. J.* **46,** 1631–1633.

Yeghiayan, E., Rojo-Ortega, J. M., and Genest, J. (1972). Parathyroid vessel innervation: An ultrastructural study. *J. Anat.* **112,** 137–142.

Zanelli, J. M., Lea, D. J., and Nisbet, J. A. (1969). A bioassay method *in vitro* for parathyroid hormone. *J. Endocrinol.* **43,** 33–46.

Zull, J. E., Malbon, C. C., and Chuang, J. (1977). Binding of tritiated bovine parathyroid hormone to plasma membranes from bovine kidney cortex. *J. Biol. Chem.* **252,** 1071–1078.

7

Vitamin D: Metabolism, Actions, and Disease States

Mark R. Haussler and Arnold S. Brickman

Disorders of Mineral Metabolism, Vol. II

ISBN 0-12-135302-8

I. INTRODUCTION

During the last decade there have been dramatic advances in our understanding of the hormonal principles involved in the homeostatic control of calcium and phosphorus metabolism and the modulation of growth and remodeling of bone. Detailed studies have delineated the metabolic pathway for the bioactivation of vitamin D, which involves the photobiogenesis of the pro-hormone in the skin, subsequent metabolism in the liver, and final enzymatic conversion to the active hormone in the kidney. It is now apparent that in various animal species, biologically active metabolites may also be formed in other organs; the physiologic significance of these latter metabolic events is unclear. The renal metabolite, 1,25-dihydroxyvitamin D ($1,25(OH)_2D$)[1], has emerged as a major regulator of mineral metabolism in various animal species, including man. It is produced from vitamin D in response to situations of calcium and phosphorus needs and functions at several target organs, including the intestine, bone, and possibly the kidney, to mediate calcium and phosphorus homeostasis. The interplay between activation of vitamin D and other hormones, such as parathyroid hormone (PTH) and calcitonin is currently being clarified. The elucidation of this intricate pathway has led to avid investigation of the physiologic regulation of vitamin D metabolism as well as an attempt to define the molecular mechanism whereby $1,25(OH)_2D$ operates in target cells. In the latter case, it has been shown that $1,25(OH)_2D$ appears to act in a biochemical fashion like other steroid hormones. Although much attention has centered on the physiologic functions of $1,25(OH)_2D$, several other vitamin D metabolites also display biologic activities in bone and muscle. The concept that other specific hormonal forms of vitamin D exist with distinctive biological functions remains a possibility.

The discovery that the metabolic steps of vitamin D metabolism occur in

[1]Abbreviations used: $1,25(OH)_2D$, 1,25-dihydroxyvitamin D; 25(OH)D, 25-hydroxyvitamin D; $24,25(OH)_2D$, 24,25-dihydroxyvitamin D; $1,24,25(OH)_3D$, 1,24,25-trihydroxyvitamin D; 1α-(OH)D, 1α-hydroxyvitamin D [For the D vitamins, all cholecalciferol forms are designated as D_3 and ergocalciferol forms as D_2; when no subscript is present after the D, both D_2 and D_3 forms are implied]; 25-OHase, vitamin D-25-hydroxylase; 1α-OHase, 25-hydroxyvitamin D-1α-hydroxylase; 24-OHase, 25-hydroxyvitamin D-24-hydroxylase; PTH; parathyroid hormone; mRNA, messenger RNA; PTX, parathyroidectomized; HPLC, high pressure liquid chromatography.

different organs such as the liver and kidney has helped to clarify our understanding of the disorders of mineral metabolism related to vitamin D. Syndromes previously attributed to antagonism, resistance, or hypersensitivity to vitamin D have been further defined in terms of particular alterations of vitamin D metabolism and/or target organ responsiveness. Particularly important in this regard has been the development of sensitive competitive binding assays for the measurement of circulating levels of vitamin D metabolites. Moreover, as a result of the structural characterization of the various metabolities of vitamin D and their synthetic analogs, it has been possible to synthesize adequate quantities of these compounds and to employ them therapeutically with remarkable success. One example is the beneficial use of $1,25(OH)_2D$ and its analogs in the management of patients with end-stage renal failure.

This chapter will review current knowledge about the metabolism and the proposed mechanism of action of vitamin D, the available assays for measurement of vitamin D metabolites, and the functions of vitamin D. This will be followed by a discussion of the pathophysiology of various disorders of vitamin D. Since some of the diseases constitute topics in other chapters in this treatise, discussion will be restricted to those aspects of pathophysiology that directly relate to altered vitamin D metabolism. As is true for any field where new information is accumulating rapidly, opinions based on current knowledge are likely to be modified or supplanted by new information that may become available tomorrow. Nevertheless, knowledge already available concerning the role of vitamin D in calcium and phosphorus homeostasis has provided substantial insights into normal and abnormal mineral function is in mammals and birds.

II. PHYSIOLOGIC EFFECTS OF VITAMIN D

The primary physiologic function of vitamin D is to facilitate maintenance of calcium and phosphorus homeostasis by modulating ionic transport processes at target tissues such as intestine, bone, and kidney. In so doing, the vitamin permits normal bone mineralization to occur. The calcemic action of vitamin D (in conjunction with PTH) contributes to the maintenance of serum calcium within normal boundaries on the one hand and, because of its paramount role in stimulating the assimilation of dietary calcium, ensures maintenance of the skeletal calcium reserve. Calcitonin and possibly other hormones may aid vitamin D in this latter function by their direct action on the skeleton to prevent demineralization. It is not known whether a form of vitamin D acts directly on the bone cells to promote mineralization, but recent data imply that a vitamin D metabolite other than $1,25(OH)_2D$ may be involved in mediating this process. There is also some indication that vitamin D may stimulate the maturation of the collagen macromolecular matrix that constitutes the organic phase of bone. An additional function of vitamin D involves muscle metabolism. Clinically it has long been known that muscle weakness is present in vitamin D deficiency, whether nutritional in origin in the form of rickets or osteomalacia, or whether osteomalacia due to malabsorption or that associated with chronic renal insufficiency. The immediate effect of vitamin D to improve muscle strength could be direct or indirect, involving a rise in plasma calcium and/or phosphorus. We shall detail the functions of vitamin D by discussing individual tissues where it acts on mineral transport.

A. Intestine

The best-documented effect of vitamin D is to facilitate calcium absorption from the intestine. Vitamin D also stimulates a sodium-dependent phosphate transport system in the intestine that is distinct from the calcium transport process (Wasserman and Taylor, 1973). Enhanced absorption of both minerals by the intestine occurs with physiologic levels of $1,25(OH)_2D_3$ (Haussler *et al.*, 1971; Walling, 1977). The movement of calcium is against an electropotential gradient and requires metabolic energy, features consistent with an active transport process (Adams and Norman, 1970).

Calcium is also absorbed by a nonsaturable mechanism that is vitamin D-dependent and resembles diffusional transfer. Several models have been proposed for the transport of calcium across the intestine (Wasserman, 1981). Calcium is thought to diffuse from the intestinal lumen into the cytoplasm where it is then transiently accumulated by mitochondria or other intracellular vesicles and then released at the basal-lateral region of the cell. The ion is actively extruded into blood by a Ca-ATPase pump or by calcium–sodium exchange. Alternatively, calcium could traverse the intestinal wall via endocytotic vesicles, which ultimately fuse with the basal lateral portion of the cell, or calcium could possibly travel through a paracellular (shunt) path (Wasserman, 1981). In any event, the ultimate expression of vitamin D action is thought to be at the intestinal brush-border membrane, where the vitamin in some way alters the properties of the microvillar surface to allow the entry of these ions into the cell. The net result of the action of vitamin D on the gut is the raising of serum calcium and phosphorus to permit normal skeletal mineralization and other physiologic functions of these minerals.

B. Bone

Bone is a second tissue which vitamin D acts upon to mobilize calcium for the circulation. The process of calcium resorption from bone has been investigated *in vivo* (Holick *et al.*, 1972) and in organ culture (Reynolds *et al.*, 1974), with all findings pointing to $1,25(OH)_2D_3$ as the active metabolite. Although it is thought that PTH is required for the action of $1,25(OH)_2D_3$ to mobilize bone calcium *in vivo* (DeLuca, 1978), Reynolds *et al.* (1976) found that PTH was not necessary for this effect in mice. Also, vitamin D metabolites do not require the presence of PTH to resorb bone calcium in organ culture. Thus, it is not certain whether $1,25(OH)_2D_3$ and PTH function independently or synergistically to mobilize skeletal calcium. Whether $1,25(OH)_2D_3$ produces phosphorus mobilization from bone under normal physiologic conditions remains to be demonstrated.

A subject that has been debated for some time but is only now being approached experimentally is whether vitamin D directly influences bone mineralization, independent of its action to raise the calcium phosphate ion product. Recently, $1,25(OH)_2D_3$ receptors have been found in osteoblast-like bone cells (Manolagas *et al.*, 1980). Also, $1,25(OH)_2D_3$ has been shown to act synergistically with 24,25-dihydroxyvitamin D_3 ($24,25(OH)_2D_3$) to promote mineralization of chick femora in organ culture (Endo *et al.*, 1980). Therefore, it is likely that vitamin D not only functions to mobilize bone calcium, but also directly stimulates bone-forming cells, possibly to elicit mineral deposition.

C. Kidney

The question of a direct action of vitamin D on renal handling of calcium or phosphorus has long been controversial. The availability of synthetic analogs of vitamin D_3 has made it possible to investigate this question. However, these studies have been plagued with a number of difficulties; these include (1) the need to investigate the actions of the metabolites under conditions of vitamin D deficiency; (2) the relatively slow onset of the action of some vitamin D analogs in bone and intestine raised the possibility that a delayed response in the kidney may preclude the use of clearance techniques; (3) elaborate experimental protocols that involve nonphysiologic conditions might be required to demonstrate renal actions of vitamin D sterols. In spite of these limitations, evidence suggests that one or more metabolites of vitamin D appear to act directly on the renal handling of calcium and phosphorus. Puschett *et al.* (1972b) have found that $25(OH)D_3$ and vitamin D_3 decrease the fractional excretion of phosphorus within 2–3 hr after the metabolites were administered to the thyroparathyroidectomized dog, but only if the animal received large doses of antidiuretic hormone. The effect was reversible with large amounts of parathyroid hormone. Similar but quantitatively smaller effects were observed with $1,25(OH)_2D_3$ (Puschett *et al.*, 1972a). However, Sutton *et al.* (1975) found no effect of $25(OH)D_3$ or $1,25(OH)_2D_3$ on renal phosphate handling in the anesthetized, parathyroidectomized (PTX) dog.

Popovtzer *et al.* (1974, 1977) found an antiphosphaturic effect of $25(OH)D_3$ when it was given concurrently with parathyroid hormone or calcitonin. They also observed that the sterol could block the effect of either calcitonin or PTH to increase the urinary excretion of cyclic AMP. Similar observations were made by Puschett *et al.* (1975) in vitamin D-deficient parathyroidectomized rats. Burnatowsky *et al.* (1977) found that 1,25(OH)D_3 was capable of reducing the fractional excretion of phosphorus in the hamster, but only in the presence of PTH.

In contrast Bonjour *et al.* (1977) observed that what appear to have been physiological quantities of 1,25$(OH)_2D_3$, when administered to thyroparathyroidectomized rats, restored the capacity of the kidney to vary phosphate excretion with phosphate intake. Garabedian *et al.* (1976) also observed that 1,25$(OH)_2D_3$ was capable of lowering the serum phosphorus in hyperphosphatemic PTX rats. These observations suggest that both 25(OH)D_3 and 1,25$(OH)_2D_3$ act to augment tubular reabsorption of phosphorus during phosphate deprivation or vitamin D deficiency, whereas animals with normal phosphate stores or with hyperphosphatemia may exhibit phosphaturia in response to the administration of vitamin D sterols.

Less information is available concerning the actions of vitamin D sterols on the renal handling of calcium. Studies in man have demonstrated that treatment with several vitamin D analogs, including 1,25$(OH)_2D_3$, augment the urinary excretion of calcium. However, with such studies it is not possible to exclude an effect of the sterol to augment intestinal absorption of calcium and increase the filtered load of calcium. This would augment urinary calcium by suppression of parathyroid hormone. When there is significant osteomalacia, an increased skeletal avidity for calcium may decrease urinary excretion of calcium. Ney *et al.* (1968) and Gran (1960) observed a decrease in the urinary excretion of calcium following the administration of pharmacologic doses of vitamin D_3 to rachitic dogs. Puschett *et al.* (1972b) noted a decrease in the fractional excretion of calcium following administration of large doses of 25(OH)D_3 to the thyroparathyroidectomized dog; these observations were again dependent on the presence of pharmacologic doses of antidiuretic hormone and of small amounts of parathyroid hormone. It thus appears that 25(OH)D_3 can enhance the distal tubular reabsorption of calcium (see also Sutton *et al.*, 1975).

D. Other Target Tissues

The myopathy of vitamin D deficiency (Schott and Wills, 1976) can respond to treatment with vitamin D or one of its metabolites independent of any measured effect on serum calcium and phosphate concentrations (Rodman and Baker, 1978), indicating that muscle may be a vitamin D target organ. Another site of vitamin D action is the parathyroid gland. It has been demonstrated that PTH is a positive tropic modulator of the renal production of 1,25$(OH)_2D_3$ (Garabedian et al., 1972). By analogy with other endocrine systems, such as corticotropin-cortisol, 1,25$(OH)_2D_3$ was thought to act on the parathyroid gland by negative feedback. The data, however, are contradictory. Inhibition of PTH secretion by 1,25$(OH)_2D_3$ has been demonstrated *in vitro* (Chertow *et al.*, 1975; Au and Bukowski, 1976). *In vivo,* PTH levels have been shown to be suppressed independently of the calcemic action of 1,25$(OH)_2D_3$ (Chertow *et al.*, 1975), but other studies (Coburn *et al.*, 1975; Care *et al.*, 1976) have not confirmed this observation. 1,25$(OH)_2D_3$ may not act to alter PTH secretion *in vivo,* but may inhibit the development and/or activity of secretory cells for parathyroid hormone. The localization of labeled 1,25$(OH)_2D_3$ in parathyroid gland (Henry and Norman, 1975) and the existence of specific macromolecular receptors for the sterol (Brumbaugh *et al.*, 1975) are consistent with a direct molecular effect of 1,25$(OH)_2D_3$ on parathyroid cells. In fact, employing long term organ cultures of parathyroid glands, Dietel *et al.* (1979) have recently shown that 1,25$(OH)_2D_3$ elicits both ultrastructural changes in the parathyroid and inhibits the biosynthesis and secretion of PTH *in vitro*.

Of interest is the recent observation of specific 1,25$(OH)_2D_3$ receptors in presumed new target organs for vitamin D. The 3–3.7S cytosolic receptor for 1,25$(OH)_2D_3$ is found in endocrine organs besides the parathyroid, namely, the pituitary and pancreas (Pike *et al.*, 1980). Receptors for the vitamin D hormone also are present in certain specialized tissues involved in mineral transport like placenta (Pike *et al.*, 1980), mammary gland (Eisman *et al.*, 1980), and avian shell gland (Coty, 1980). It is therefore possible that 1,25$(OH)_2D_3$ plays several roles in the body with respect to mineral transport. By acting on gut, bone, and kidney, it mediates systemic calcium and phosphate homeostasis. Fine regulation of mineral balance and modulation during growth and reproduction might be accomplished by feedback effects of 1,25$(OH)_2D_3$ on the endocrine glands that influence calcium and vitamin D metabolism. Finally, the 1,25$(OH)_2D_3$ hormone likely functions at unique local sites of calcium transport such as placenta and breast.

III. METABOLISM OF VITAMIN D

A. Sources of Vitamin D

Most foods are not very good sources of vitamin D. In the Western World, therefore, an adequate dietary supply requires fortified foods or supplementation with fish liver oils. Much of man's body stores of vitamin D arise in the skin when 7-dehydrocholesterol is converted to previtamin D_3 under the influence of ultraviolet light (280–300 nm wave length). The previtamin D_3 is then further converted by a thermal reaction to native vitamin D_3, the storage form (Holick *et al.*, 1977a). Vitamin D_3 may be termed a prohormone since it must be further metabolized before it functions at the target tissues. Since food supplementation is usually with vitamin D_2, it is possible to assess the relative contribution of the nutritional (vitamin D_2) and sunlight-produced (vitamin D_3) forms. By assaying circulating 25(OH)D_2 and 25(OH)D_3 separately in human serum, it has been found that 85–90% of the vitamin D pool probably is derived from solar irradiation (Haddad and Hahn, 1973; Hughes *et al.*, 1976). Only at higher latitudes in the winter months is this dramatic predominance of the vitamin D_3 forms reduced, and even then dietarily derived vitamin D_2 still only accounts for 33% of the total vitamin D pool (Arnaud *et al.*, 1977). Thus, as is discussed in more detail below under the topic of nutritional rickets, sunlight is the key determinant of vitamin D status in most instances.

B. Metabolic Pathway for Vitamin D Activation; Chemistry and Functions of the Metabolites

The liver and kidney are the organs in which vitamin D is transformed. Figure 1 pictures the chemical structures of many metabolites of vitamin D_3 that have been characterized. These sterols are arranged according to the sequence of generation from native vitamin D_3, with the most important pathways shown in bold arrows. The initial transformation is catalyzed by a vitamin D_3-25-hydroxylase enzyme (25-OHase) present in the liver microsomal fraction of all

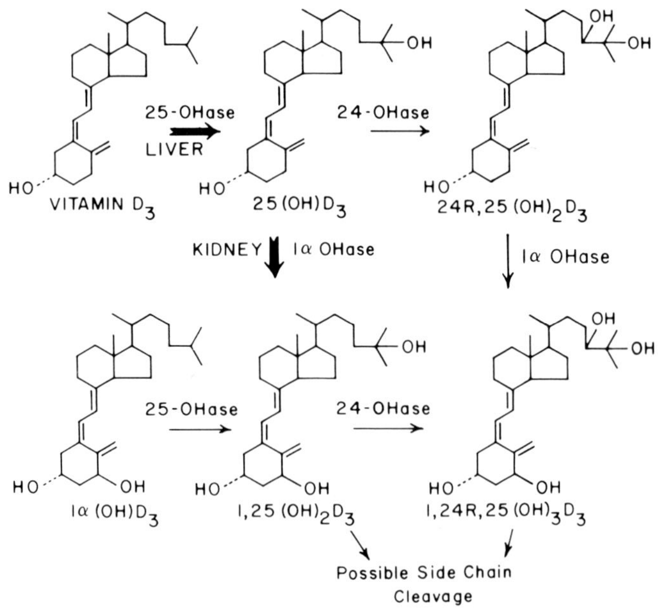

Fig. 1. Metabolism of Vitamin D_3. (From Haussler and McCain, 1977. Reprinted, by permission, from *The New England Journal of Medicine,* **297,** 974–983.)

species studied (Bhattacharyya and DeLuca, 1974). In the chicken, the 25-OHase exists in extrahepatic sites, such as intestine and kidney (Tucker *et al.*, 1973), but the liver is the predominant site of vitamin D_3-25-hydroxylation in mammals (Olson *et al.*, 1976). The product of the reaction, 25-hydroxyvitamin D_3 (25(OH)D_3), is the most abundant form of vitamin D_3 found in the circulation and is intermediate in the biosynthesis of a more potent sterol.

The crucial hydroxylation in the activation of vitamin D_3 is catalyzed by the renal 25-hydroxyvitamin D_3-lα-hydroxylase (lα-OHase) that produces 1,25(OH)$_2D_3$, the hormonal form of vitamin D_3. This rate-limiting enzyme is found exclusively in the mitochondria of kidney tissue (Fraser and Kodicek, 1970) and is composed of a flavoprotein, renal ferredoxin, and cytochrome P_{450} (DeLuca, 1976) and requires the presence of NADPH and molecular oxygen. 1,25(OH)$_2D_3$ was originally detected in chick intestinal chromatin (Haussler *et al.*, 1968) and proposed as the active form of vitamin D_3. The metabolite was isolated from incubations of 25(OH)D_3 in renal homogenates (Lawson *et al.*, 1971) and independently purified from the chick gut (Holick *et al.*, 1971) and was identified as 1,25(OH)$_2D_3$. This metabolite satisfies numerous criteria for being the functional form of vitamin D_3. When chronically administered to animals that receive a vitamin D-deficient diet, it prevents rickets and maintains normal mineral metabolism (McNutt and Haussler, 1973). 1,25(OH)$_2D_3$ is at least five times as biologically active as vitamin D_3 or 25(OH)D_3 and it functions three times faster than either of its precursors in promoting calcium absorption (Haussler *et al.*, 1971). When assayed for bone calcium resportion activity, *in vitro,* 1,25(OH)$_2D_3$ is at least 100 times as active as 25(OH)D_3 (Raisz *et al.*, 1972). Nephrectomy prevents the response of intestinal calcium transport (Wong *et al.*, 1972) and bone calcium mobilization (Holick *et al.*, 1972) to 25(OH)D_3 but not to 1,25(OH)$_2D_3$, when their compounds are given in physiologic amounts. These findings provide compelling evidence that 1,25(OH)$_2D_3$ is the active form of vitamin D.

Several observations indicate that 25(OH)D_3 may have a biologic function other than to serve as an intermediate in the formation of 1,25(OH)$_2D_3$. Bordier *et al.* (1973) reported that anephric patients, who cannot form 1,25(OH)$_2D_3$, may not exhibit histologic evidence of osteomalacia. Since bone mineralization may occur normally in patients lacking kidneys and since 25(OH)D_3 is effective in reversing renal osteodystrophy when given in moderate doses (Recker *et al.*, 1978), 25(OH)D_3 may directly affect bone remodeling. Interestingly, when vitamin D-deficient chicks are given a physiologic dose of radioactive vitamin D_3, the major metabolite present in bone is 25(OH)D_3, rather than 1,25(OH)$_2D_3$, which predominates in the intestine (Haussler and Rasmussen, 1972). Wezeman (1976) has found by autoradiographic means that 25(OH)D_3 is localized in areas of active mineralization. In addition, 25(OH)D_3 also acts in muscle (Birge and Haddad, 1975) and kidney (Puschett *et al.*, 1972b). Even though these findings indicate that $25(OH)D_3$ (or a metabolite of $25(OH)D_3$ other than $1,25(OH)_2D_3$) could act in some tissues, the data can also be explained with $25(OH)D_3$ acting as a $1,25(OH)_2D_3$ analog at high concentrations—particularly since its circulating (half-life) is much greater than that of $1,25(OH)_2D_3$.

Another enzyme that metabolizes $25(OH)D_3$ is the 25-hydroxyvitamin D_3-24-hydroxylase (24-OHase). This enzyme is present in kidney mitochondria, although there is evidence for the extrarenal production of the 24,25-dihydroxylated metabolite in rats (Kumar *et al.*, 1978) and man (Haddad *et al.*, 1977; Shepard *et al.*, 1979). Both epimeric forms, 24*R*,25-dihydroxyvitamin D_3 [$24,25(OH)_2D_3$] and 24*S*,25-dihydroxyvitamin D_3 have been chemically synthesized, and the *R*-epimer has been identified as the natural form (DeLuca, 1976). The significance of 24-hydroxylation remains a mystery; suggestions have ranged from degradation to synthesis of another functional metabolite. Kanis *et al.* (1978) have reported that small doses of $24,25(OH)_2D_3$ augment intestinal absorption of calcium in uremic patients. Llach *et al.* (1978) also have shown that $24,25(OH)_2D_3$ increases calcium absorption in uremic patients, but only at doses of 20 μg or greater. The metabolite can suppress PTH secretion (Canterbury *et al.*, 1978) and may stimulate the synthesis of proteoglycans in chondrocytes (Corvol *et al.*, 1978). Thus, $24,25(OH)_2D_3$ has been proposed as the "bone mineralizating" form of vitamin D. However, 24-hydroxylation of vitamin D uniformly diminishes biologic potency. Examples include the failure of $24,25(OH)_2D_3$ to equal the potency of $1,25(OH)_2D_3$ in increasing bone ash (Boris *et al.*, 1977) and its lower ability to stimulate intestinal calcium and phosphate absorption (Walling, 1977) or bone calcium resorption (Mahgoub and Sheppard, 1977). 24-Hydroxylation may therefore constitute an early step in the degradation of 25(OH)D. Indeed, the true "mission" of the 24-OHase may be to inactivate $1,25(OH)_2D_3$ by producing 1,24,25-trihydroxyvitamin D_3 [$1,24,25(OH)_3D_3$], and $24,25(OH)_2D_3$ may simply exist as by-product of the nonspecific 24-OHase enzyme.

$1,24,25(OH)_3D_3$ is the only trihydroxylated derivative of vitamin D_3 discovered to date. This metabolite has been detected primarily following incubations *in vitro*. Some controversy exists concerning its existence *in vivo* (Friedlander and Norman, 1975). $1,24,25(OH)_3D_3$ apparently can arise from 1α-hydroxylation of $24,25(OH)_2D_3$ or from 24-hydroxylation of $1,25(OH)_2D_3$ (Figure 1). This reduces the biopotency of $1,25(OH)_2D_3$ (Boris *et al.*, 1977) and may be an initial step in the catabolism of the hormone. In fact, the presence of vicinal hydroxyl groups in $1,24,25(OH)_3D_3$ is conducive to carbon–carbon bond cleavage between C-24 and C-25, resulting in side chain scission. Experiments with $1,25(OH)_2D_3$ labeled with ^{14}C at C-26 and C-27 have revealed that side chain oxidation of the hormone is a rapid occurrence (Kumar *et al.*, 1976), but it is not known whether $1,25(OH)_2D_3$ is 24-hydroxylated prior to the loss of C-26 and C-27 as CO_2.

C. Analogs and Derivatives of Vitamin D

The structure of 1α-hydroxyvitamin D_3 (1α(OH)D_3), a major synthetic vitamin D_3 analog in terms of clinical application, is also shown in Fig. 1. Although it probably does not occur naturally, this sterol was originally noted to have high biological activity (Haussler *et al.*, 1973). Zerwekh *et al.* (1974a) used radioreceptor assay techniques to demonstrate that 1α(OH)D_3 functions by rapid metabolism to 1,25$(OH)_2D_3$. Subsequent work with radioactive 1α(OH)D_3 has confirmed that it can be an effective precursor of the natural hormone in rats (Holick *et al.*, 1976) and humans (Holick *et al.*, 1977b). Thus, the high biological activity and clinical efficacy of 1α(OH)D_3 derive from its conversion to 1,25$(OH)_2D_3$ via a route circumventing the rate-limiting step of 1α-hydroxylation in the kidney.

Dihydrotachysterol, a chemical reduction product of vitamin D, has long been used clinically to treat vitamin D-resistant forms of rickets and hypocalcemia. This synthetic sterol contains a hydroxyl group in the pseudo-1α position; this is the reason why it displays clinical efficacy in vitamin D-refractory maladies and constitutes an effective analog of 1,25$(OH)_2D_3$ (Kaye and Sagar, 1972). Other vitamin analogs with a hydroxyl group functioning as if in the 1α-position, such as 5,6-*trans*-25-hydroxyvitamin D_3, have also been synthesized (DeLuca and Schnoes, 1976). These analogs, along with 25(OH)D_3 and 1,25$(OH)_2D_3$, have provided clinicians with potent therapeutic tools for the treatment of vitamin D-resistant disorders. In addition, Johnson *et al.* (1975) have presented preliminary evidence for antivitamin D sterols that may be useful in treating hypervitaminosis D or diseases characterized by hypersensitivity to vitamin D, such as sarcoidosis.

Several derivatives of 1,25$(OH)_2D_3$ have been found in certain plants. Glycosides of 1,25$(OH)_2D_3$ have been identified in the calcinogenic plants *Solanum malacoxylon* (Wasserman *et al.*, 1976) and *Cestrum diurnum* (Hughes *et al.*, 1977a). When ingested, these plants cause calcinosis in grazing animals, probably because the glycosides are cleaved *in vivo* to produce 1,25$(OH)_2D_3$, which causes hypercalcemia, because the normal regulation of the biosynthesis of the hormone is circumvented. Also an extract of *S. malacoxylon* has been used in the treatment of uremic bone disease (von Herrath *et al.*, 1975).

D. Regulation of Vitamin D. Metabolism

For 1,25$(OH)_2D$ to function as a hormone, its production from the parent vitamin must be modulated according to the needs of the organism for calcium and phosphorus. This modulation could be effected by the hepatic 25-OHase or the renal 1α-OHase. Although the regulation of the 25-OHase has been debated, initial reports of a "feedback control" of this enzyme (DeLuca, 1971) were not supported by later findings (Tucker *et al.*, 1973). In addition neither calcium nor phosphorus status influences the activity of chick liver 25-OHase. Moreover, the administration of large doses of vitamin D_3 leads to marked increases in circulating 25(OH)D, an indication that the 25-OHase catalyzed reaction is not tightly controlled (Hughes *et al.*, 1976, 1977b). Thus, while 25(OH)D was elevated as much as 30-fold in the plasma, $1,25(OH)_2D$ was normal or depressed. This indicates stringent control of the production of $1,25(OH)_2D$ from 25-(OH)D.

In the past 5 years, much information concerning factors that regulate the biosynthesis of $1,25(OH)_2D_3$ has become available. Experimental approaches have included the use of intact animals, of homogenates from renal tissue, of isolated renal tubules, and of kidney cells maintained in culture. As a result, there has emerged a general scheme concerning the control of the renal 1α-OHase, which primarily involves PTH, phosphate, and $1,25(OH)_2D_3$ itself. Moreover, other hormones known to influence growth and reproduction may also modulate the renal enzyme.

A major factor influencing the biosynthesis of $1,25(OH)_2D_3$ is the the organism's need for calcium. Dietary calcium intake has been shown to affect the rate of conversion of $25(OH)D_3$ to $1,25(OH)D_3$ (Boyle *et al.*, 1971), with conversion stimulated at low dietary calcium levels. Inasmuch as the parathyroid gland is the chief "calcium sensing" organ in the body, PTH may mediate the response of the renal 1α-OHase. Garabedian *et al.* (1972) demonstrated that removal of the parathyroid glands eliminated the enhanced production of $1,25(OH)_2D_3$, the animals instead synthesizing primarily $24,25(OH)_2D_3$. Administration of PTH restored this response; in fact, PTH injection into normal animals stimulates the biosynthesis of $1,25(OH)_2D_3$ (Tanaka *et al.*, 1976). Measurements of circulating levels of $1,25(OH)_2D_3$ in intact and thyroparathyroidectomized (TPTX) rats maintained on a low calcium diet have provided additional proof that circulating $1,25(OH)_2D_3$ increases strikingly during adaptation to calcium restriction, and that this response is dependent (for the most part) on intact parathyroid glands (Hughes *et al.*, 1975).

Parathyroidectomy in chicks does not diminish the renal 1-OHase unless there is a concomitant elevation in plasma phosphate (Galante *et al.*, 1973; Booth *et al.*, 1977). TPTX rats placed on a low-phosphate diet can amplify their production of $1,25(OH)_2D_3$ (Tanaka and DeLuca, 1973) and achieve a fivefold augmentation of circulating $1,25(OH)_2D_3$ (Hughes *et al.*, 1975). Therefore, low serum phosphate appears to stimulate the 1α-OHase independent of PTH, whereas high serum phosphate has the opposite effect. Although one study of the renal 1α-OHase (measured *in vitro*) in chicks following phosphate deprivation confirmed this notion (Baxter and DeLuca, 1976), Henry *et al.* (1974) report that phosphate depletion does not stimulate the 1α-OHase in chicks. Phosphate-depleted intact rats and pigs (Haussler *et al.*, 1977a) show markedly elevated circulating levels of $1,25(OH)_2D$. The increase in circulating $1,25(OH)_2D_3$ could be caused in part by decreased degradation of the hormone. Phosphate depletion also could influence $1,25(OH)_2D_3$ retention in the intestine or directly alter calcium absorption by the gut (Ribovich and DeLuca, 1975).

Another important regulator of the renal 1α-OHase is $1,25(OH)_2D_3$. The administration of $1,25(OH)_2D_3$ to vitamin D-deficient animals, whose 1α-OHase enzyme activity is markedly increased, leads to a disappearance of this renal enzyme and the appearance of 24-OHase activity (Cork *et al.*, 1974; Tanaka and DeLuca, 1974). Similar effects have also been observed in cultures of renal cells (Henry, 1977). Since treatment with inhibitors of transcription can block this effect of $1,25(OH)_2D_3$ *in vivo* (Colston *et al.*, 1977), it may be concluded that processes other than product feedback by $1,25(OH)_2D_3$ are involved such as alterations in enzyme biosynthesis. Because $1,25(OH)_2D_3$ induces 24-OHase activity and, as discussed above, 24-hydroxylation can diminish biologic activity, it is tempting to speculate that the $1,25(OH)_2D_3$ functions to stimulate degradation, thereby shortening the hormone's half-life. In addition, $1,25(OH)_2D_3$ may suppress endogenous PTH secretion, thereby bringing into play an additional feedback mechanism.

Aside from perturbations in dietary intake of calcium, phosphate, or vitamin D, there exist several normal physiologic conditions in which the production of $1,25(OH)_2D_3$ might be expected to be altered. In physiologic states of increased calcium need, such as, growth, pregnancy, lactation, and egg production, $1,25(OH)_2D_3$ levels may also be increased. This is the case in growing animals and children (Pike *et al.*, 1977), in human pregnancy near the end of gestation (Pike *et al.*, 1977), in pregnant and lactating rats (Boass *et al.*, 1977 Pike *et al.*, 1979), and in the laying hen (Spanos *et al.*, 1976a). Experimental studies of the effect of reproductive hormones on the 1α-OHase activity have also been done. Spanos *et al.* (1976b) reported that prolactin stimulates the renal 1α-OHase in chicks. In birds estrogen can ehance the formation of $1,25(OH)_2D_3$ (Tanaka *et al.*, 1976; Baksi and Kenny, 1977); this appears also true for rats (Baksi and Kenny, 1978). Moreover, circulating $1,25(OH)_2D_3$ is lowered in hypophysectomized rats and restored to normal by growth hormone administration (Spanos *et al.*, 1978). Rats with streptozotocin-induced diabetes possess a block in vitamin D metabolism at the renal 1α-OHase step; this can be corrected with insulin (Schneider *et al.*, 1977a). Insulin may therefore also act as a trophic hormone for $1,25(OH)_2D_3$ production. Although other hormones, particularly those of the pituitary and gonads may function to make calcium available by enhancing $1,25(OH)_2D_3$ production, experiments are needed to demonstrate direct action on 1α-hydroxylation. Otherwise, an intermediate effect of PTH cannot be excluded.

Figure 2 summarizes the complex interplay of hormones and other humoral factors that are postulated to regulate 1α-hydroxylation of $25(OH)D_3$ in the kidney. The primary stimuli of the renal 1α-OHase appear to be low serum phosphate and low serum calcium. Low phosphate may act directly at the kidney,

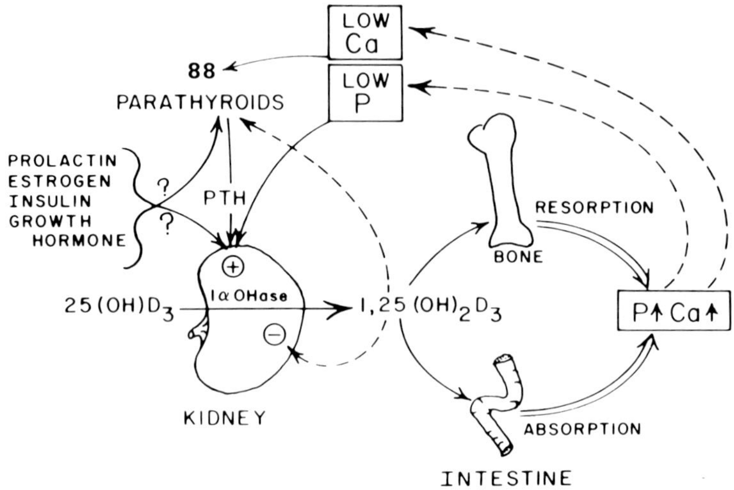

Fig. 2. Model for the regulation of $1,25(OH)_2D_3$ biosynthesis. Solid arrows indicate a positive effect; dashed arrows refer to negative feedback.

while the low calcium signal acts through the parathyroid glands, with PTH the mediator of the low calcium response. Once the levels of $1,25(OH)_2D_3$ are enhanced in blood, the hormone acts on intestine and bone to mobilize phosphate and calcium. This corrects hypophosphatemia and hypocalcemia. In the course of the response to the low serum calcium, excess phosphate can be eliminated in the urine by way of PTH-induced inhibition of the renal reabsorption of phosphate. When hypophosphatemia is corrected by the action of $1,25(OH)_2D_3$, extra calcium can be passed into the urine because PTH is suppressed with reduced renal calcium reabsorption. In addition, $1,25(OH)_2D_3$ may govern its own synthesis by acting as a feedback regulator both in the parathyroid glands and/or in the kidney. Finally, other hormonal regulators of $1,25(OH)_2D_3$ production may function during states of mineral need.

E. Transport and Binding Proteins for Vitamin D and Its Metabolites

Vitamin D and its metabolities are transported in the blood, bound to a specific plasma protein that has been isolated from animals and humans (Haddad and Walgate, 1976a; Bouillon *et al.*, 1976; Imawari *et al.*, 1976). The purified human protein is an α-globulin with a sedimentation coefficient of approximately 4 S and a molecular weight between 50,000 and 60,000. The protein binds $25(OH)D_3$ with an affinity ($K_d = 6 \times 10^{-8}$ M), greater than for either vitamin D_3 or $1,25(OH)_2D_3$. An antibody to this protein has been prepared and immunoprecipitation studies suggested that the human binding protein is identical to a serum factor known as group-specific component. When a variety of ligands were tested for binding to the group specific component, a family of genetic variants of an α-globulin originally discovered in 1959, only labeled $25(OH)D_3$ was found to bind specifically (Haddad, 1979). Electrophoretic comigration of radioactive $25(OH)D_3$ and immunoreactive group specific component provided final proof of the identity of vitamin D-binding protein and group specific component.

Moreover, immunoprecipitation completely neutralized binding of vitamin D_3, $25\text{-}(OH)D_3$ and $1,25(OH)_2D_3$, indicating a common transport protein for all these sterols in human plasma; but the circulating form is only 1–3% saturated with vitamin D or its metabolites (Haddad and Walgate, 1976b). There is no change in the amount of the binding protein in diseases of calcium or phosphorus metabolism. However, in pregnancy, the protein is increased.

Several intracellular binding proteins for vitamin D metabolites have been discovered. Notable among these is the 3–3.7S cytosol receptor for $1,25(OH)_2D_3$ obtained from chick intestine (Brumbaugh and Haussler, 1975; Kream *et al.*, 1976). As discussed in detail in the next section, this protein binds $1,25(OH)_2D_3$ preferentially as compared to $25(OH)D_3$ and other vitamin D sterols and acts as a receptor protein in target cells. A second binding protein has been reported as occurring in the cytosol of all nucleated cells. It binds $25(OH)D_3$ with high affinity and selectivity. Originally thought to be a 6S binding protein (Haddad and Birge, 1975), its binding unit is actually the 4S plasma protein that transports $25(OH)D_3$ (Van Baelen *et al.*, 1977). This 4S unit may originate from serum during tissue homogenization and combine with an intracellular peptide to create the 6S conjugate found in the cytosol fraction. Thus, the 6S unit could be an artifact of the cytosol preparation or be involved in the internalization of bound $25(OH)D_3$ prior to its utilization by target cells.

IV. BIOCHEMICAL MECHANISM OF ACTION IN TARGET TISSUES

A. Intestine

Studies of the cellular mode of action of $1,25(OH)_2D_3$ have focused on its role in intestinal calcium absorption. As with other steroid hormones, there is a 2-hr latent period between the administration of $1,25(OH)_2D_3$ (or its $1\alpha\text{-}(OH)D_3$ analog) and the first detectable increase in intestinal calcium transport (Haussler *et al.*, 1973); alteration in gene expression and the induction of new proteins are thought to occur in this period. The induction process is the hallmark of the currently accepted molecular mechanism whereby steroid hormones, such as estradiol-17β and progesterone, alter cell function (O'Malley and Schrader, 1976). The key features of this mechanism are the binding of the steroid to a high affinity receptor in the cytoplasm, migration of the hormone-receptor complex into the nucleus where association to the genome occurs, activation of selected genes, and the biosynthesis of new messenger RNAs (mRNA) which code for proteins capable of changing cellular activity. The bulk of the evidence indicates that 1,25$(OH)_2D_3$ functions in a manner similar to steroid hormones.

Experiments utilizing inhibitors of mRNA and protein synthesis, *in vivo,* have suggested that 1,25$(OH)_2D_3$ action depends on a message synthesis followed by protein synthesis. Actinomycin D blocks the effects of 1,25$(OH)_2D_3$ on calcium absorption in the rachitic chick but not in the vitamin D-deficient rat (DeLuca, 1978). 1,25$(OH)_2D_3$ action on vitamin D-replete animals, however, is not blocked by actinomycin D (F. Bronner, personal communication). In organ culture of chick intestine, where vitamin D-depletion is attained with certainty and optimal inhibitor levels can be achieved, Corradino (1973) has shown that mRNA synthesis inhibitors, such as α-amanitin and actinomycin D, interfere with the action of 1,25$(OH)_2D_3$ in causing calcium uptake to increase. Cycloheximide, an inhibitor of protein synthesis, readily blocks chick intestinal response to 1,25$(OH)_2D_3$ *in vivo*. Complementing these studies and pointing to a transcriptional site of action of 1,25$(OH)_2D_3$ are biochemical localization studies that reveal that after injection of either vitamin D_3 or 1,25-$(OH)_2D_3$ into D-deficient animals, the hormonal sterol is localized in the nucleus of the intestinal cell (Haussler *et al.*, 1968; Tsai *et al.*, 1972). To verify that the observed nuclear localization is not an artifact of the subcellular fractionation procedure, Zile *et al.* (1978) and Jones and Haussler (1979) recently employed autoradiography. Figure 3 illustrates such experiments. Two hours after intracardial administration of a physiologic dose of 1,25$(OH)_2D_3$ to vitamin D-deficient chicks, there occurred a distinct concentration of the hormone in the nuclei of the intestinal crypt cells (Fig. 3A). When a 100-fold excess of nonradioactive 1,25$(OH)_2D_3$ was used, localization was abolished (Fig. 3B). Additional studies have indicated that 1,25$(OH)_2D_3$ is bound to the chromatin fraction of the nucleus and that this binding is rapid and saturable. Therefore, 1,25$(OH)_2D_3$ rapidly associates with the transcriptional machinery of the intestinal cell—a fact consistent with its proposed influence on mRNA biosynthesis.

Moreover, a receptor system for 1,25$(OH)_2D_3$ has been identified in the chick intestine (Brumbaugh and Haussler, 1974a,b, 1975). The receptor apparently serves the purpose of translocating the hormone to the nucleus. When whole intestine or intestinal homogenates were incubated with labeled 1,25$(OH)_2D_3$ at 0°C, the hormone remained bound to the cytosol fraction of the cell. When the mixture was warmed to 37°C, the hormone migrated to the nuclear chromatin fraction, with concomitant reduction of the radioactive hormone in the cytosol.

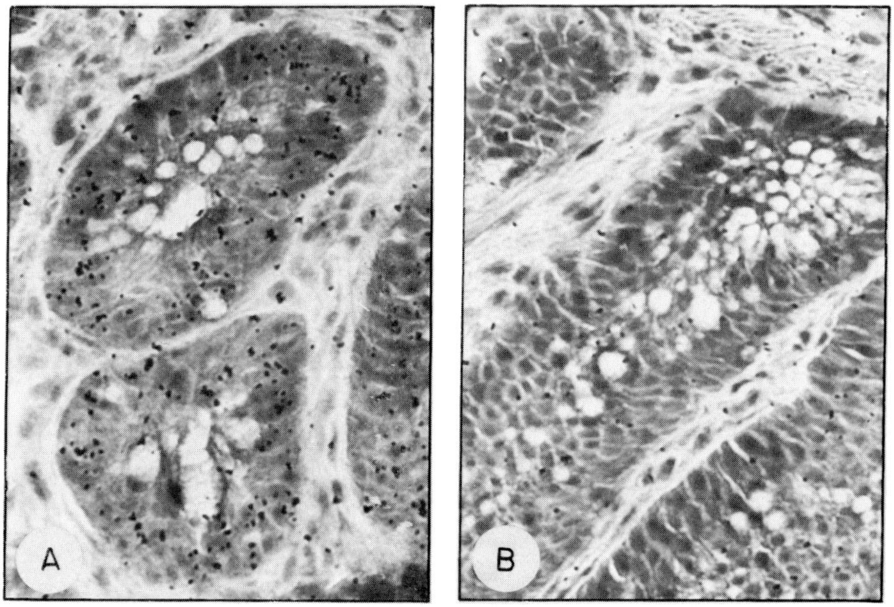

Fig. 3. Scintillation autoradiographic localization (× 400) of 1,25$(OH)_2$[^{3}H]D_3 in chick intestinal nuclei. After an intracardial injection of 0.52 nmol of 1,25$(OH)_2$[^{3}H]D_3 (11.2 Ci/mmol), chick duodena were flash-frozen in isopentane immersed in liquid nitrogen. Four-μm cross sections of the frozen tissues were cut at −20°C on a cryostat and, in complete darkness, the tissue sections were mounted on emulsion precoated slides and exposed at −20°C. The emulsion precoated slides were prepared by dipping a microscope slide into Kodak NTB_3 nuclear track emulsion at 42°C in a darkroom, drying overnight, dipping again in standard liquid scintillation solution, and drying again. After approximately 6 months the slides were developed and stained with hematoxylin and eosin. The concentration of 1,25$(OH)_2$[^{3}H]D_3 over the darker staining nuclei of intestinal crypt of Lieberkühn cells (A) is evident. A 100-fold excess dose of unlabeled 1,25$(OH)_2D_3$ given in addition to 1,25$(OH)_2$-[^{3}H]D_3 diminishes nuclear localization in intestinal crypt of Lieberkühn cells (B).

The temperature-dependent distribution of the hormone permits investigation of the cytosol-binding component, presumed to be the first binding site for the hormone. This cytosolic protein had an apparent molecular weight of 47,000 and sedimented at 3.7S in high-salt sucrose gradients (Brumbaugh and Haussler, 1975). The high binding affinity of the receptor protein for 1,25$(OH)_2D_3$ ($K_d = 10^{-10}\,M$) and its specificity have led to its use both in a radioreceptor assay (Brumbaugh *et al.*, 1974a; Eisman *et al.*, 1976) to assess circulating 1,25$(OH)_2D_3$ levels and for a binding assay for "vitamin D activity" at the molecular level (Brumbaugh and Haussler, 1973; Proscal *et al.*, 1975). In terms of mechanism, the 1,25$(OH)_2D_3$ compound may by itself be unable to affect gene transcription;

rather, it appears to be the hormone-receptor complex that stimulates mRNA biosynthesis (Tsai and Norman, 1973; Zerwekh *et al.*, 1974b, 1976).

If new species of mRNA are formed in response to the binding of $1,25(OH)_2D_3$ to the nucleus, these would lead to the synthesis of proteins present in normal and absent in vitamin D-deficient intestine. Two such proteins have been reported. The first is a phosphatase enzyme, alternatively described as an alkaline phosphatase (Haussler *et al.*, 1970) or a calcium-dependent ATPase (Melancon and DeLuca, 1970). The rate at which this protein appears after administration of $1,25(OH)_2D_3$ is slower than the rate at which calcium absorption increases (Norman and Henry, 1974). This protein may therefore not be involved in calcium transport, but could of course mediate later vitamin D effects, e.g., phosphate transport.

The second specific protein is the duodenal calcium-binding protein (CaBP), first described in the chick by Wasserman and associates (1968). This protein is dependent upon the presence of vitamin D and its concentration appears to correlate with the degree of calcium absorption under a variety of conditions (Wasserman, 1981). The chicken protein has a molecular weight of 28,000, whereas mammalian intestinal CaBPs are small (MW = 9000–12,000), and each has two calcium binding sites with an apparent association constant of $10^6\ M^{-1}$. The amino acid sequence of porcine CaBP has been determined (Hofmann *et al.*, 1979) and it has been shown that CaBP belongs to the troponin C superfamily of calcium binding proteins. CaBP is essentially a soluble or cytosolic protein, with the exception of 5–10%, which may be an intrinsic membrane protein because detergent is required for its solubilization.

Intestinal CaBP is enhanced in animals placed on a low calcium diet (Freund and Bronner, 1975a) and is increased by treatment of rachitic chicks and normal rats with $1,25(OH)_2D_3$ (Spencer *et al.*, 1976b; Buckley and Bronner, 1980). However, a careful examination via immunoelectrophoresis of its time course of appearance after $1,25(OH)_2D_3$ administration (Spencer *et al.*, 1976b), reveals that CaBP appears in 4–6 hr, laging behind increased calcium absorption, which is first seen at 2 hr. Moreover, transport was found to decay more rapidly than CaBP after a single dose of $1,25(OH)_2D_3$ (Thomasset *et al.*, 1979). These data suggest that CaBP may not be involved directly in calcium transport, but may instead be induced by increased intracellular calcium as a consequence of $1,25(OH)_2D_3$ action. Alternatively, CaBP might be one of several vitamin D-dependent proteins that comprise the overall transport of calcium. In this context, Kowarski and Schachter (1980) have provided evidence for a calcium binding protein integral to the intestinal microvillar membrane which is distinct from CaBP; and Wilson and Lawson (1977) reported the identification of two brush border membrane proteins which are synthesized more rapidly than CaBP in response to $1,25(OH)_2D_3$. The catalytic properties of these macromolecules are not known.

Further biochemical experiments have supported the significance of CaBP as a molecular expression of 1,25$(OH)_2D_3$ action. Freund and Bronner (1975b) showed that 1,25$(OH)_2D_3$ rapidly stimulates both CaBP and calcium uptake when added to isolated intestinal cells *in vitro*. The CaBP and calcium transport responses to 1,25$(OH)_2D_3$ of cultured duodena are coordinately blocked by actinomycin D (Corradino, 1973), and the hormone has been shown to enhance the level of polysomal CaBP-mRNA levels in chicks (Spencer *et al.*, 1976a). Finally, purifed CaBP has been reconstituted with 1,25$(OH)_2D_3$-deficient duodena in culture, with a subsequent increase in calcium uptake by the tissue (Corradino *et al.*, 1976). Although none of these experiments prove that CaBP is directly involved in transmembrane calcium movement, they do show that CaBP is a critical part of the intestinal response to 1,25$(OH)_2D_3$.

In summary, Fig. 4 schematizes the current working model for the molecular mechanism of 1,25$(OH)_2D_3$ action. The salient features of this mechanism are the binding of the hormone to the cytosol receptor protein, migration to the nuclear chromatin where nonhistone proteins are postulated to specify the binding site(s) of the receptor on DNA (Pike and Haussler, 1979), presumed exposure

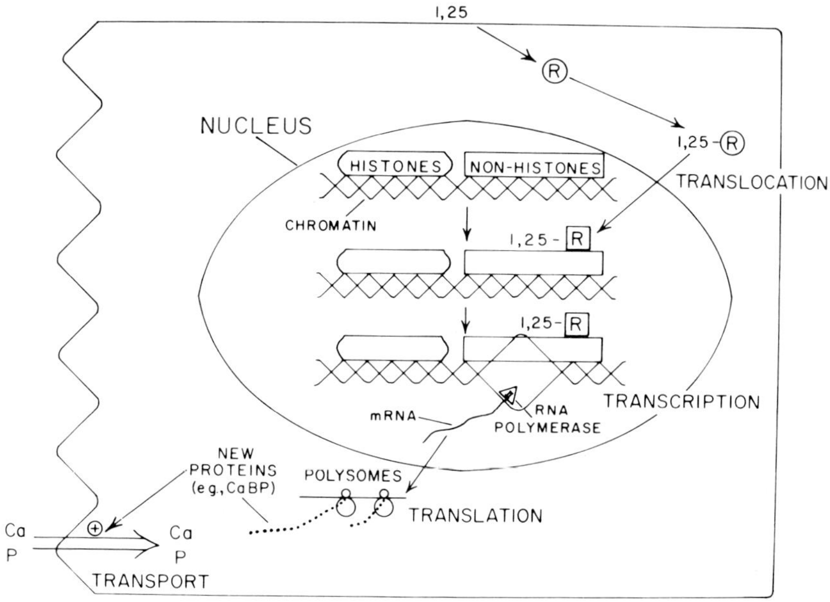

Fig. 4. Proposed molecular mechanism of action of 1,25$(OH)_2D_3$ (1,25) in the intestinal mucosa cell. Ⓡ represents receptor protein in the cytosol and [R] equals nuclear receptor protein. (From Haussler and McCain, 1977. Reprinted, by permission, from *The New England Journal of Medicine* **297,** 974–983.)

of a unique gene or set of genes which are transcribed into new mRNAs by RNA polymerase II, translation in the polysomes of the new messages into functional proteins (such as CaBP), and ultimate participation of induced proteins in the alteration of cell function, which is expressed primarily as enhanced calcium and phosphate translocation. This model will of course be tested and modified as more experiments are completed in this active research area of the molecular biology of $1,25(OH)_2D_3$ action.

B. Bone, Kidney, and Other Organs

Other tissues in which the mechanism of $1,25(OH)_2D_3$ action has been probed include bone, kidney, and parathyroid gland. Bone has been studied only in terms of the sterol's action to resorb calcium. This response to the hormone is inhibited by prior administration of actinomycin D (Tanaka and DeLuca, 1971), suggesting that $1,25(OH)_2D_3$ requires RNA synthesis to mobilize bone calcium. Based upon this finding it is probable that $1,25(OH)_2D_3$ performs in the bone cell in the same molecular fashion as described for the intestine, and evidence indicates that a specific cytosol receptor for $1,25(OH)_2D_3$ exists in bone (Kream *et al.*, 1977). Also, data on ^{45}Ca release from bone incubated in culture with a series of vitamin D analogs of differing biological potencies (Stern *et al.*, 1976) show that the relative abilities of these sterols to liberate ^{45}Ca correlates with the relative binding affinities for the sterols to the intestinal receptor protein. Assuming the identity of the bone and intestinal receptors, a mechanism of action of $1,25(OH)_2D_3$ in bone can be proposed which is analogous to that outlined for intestine (Fig. 4), with the exception that calcium may be moved from bone fluid to the plasma compartment.

With regard to the kidney, Chen and DeLuca (1973) reported that $1,25(OH)_2D_3$ rapidly stimlulates renal biosynthesis of RNA, and a vitamin D-dependent calcium binding protein has been detected in chick kidney (Taylor and Wasserman, 1972). Further molecular insight awaits a better understanding of the physiologic function of vitamin D or its metabolites in this tissue, although recent discovery of the $1,25(OH)_2D_3$ receptor in rat kidney (Chandler *et al.*, 1979) is indicative of an important role for the $1,25(OH)_2D_3$ hormone in the kidney. The possible action of $1,25(OH)_2D_3$ in parathyroid gland, although controversial, has been the subject of some mechanistic probing. There is direct evidence for the existence of specific, high affinity receptors for $1,25(OH)_2D_3$ in chick parathyroid glands (Brumbaugh *et al.*, 1975), porcine glands (Cloix *et al.*, 1976), and in human parathyroid adenoma (Haddad *et al.*, 1976a; Hughes and Haussler, 1978). Detailed study of this receptor system in the chick parathyroid gland indicates that it is strikingly similar to that found in the chick intestine (Brumbaugh *et al.*, 1975). The cytoplasmic receptor protein migrates at 3–3.7S in high-salt sucrose gradients, and apparently transports $1,25(OH)_2D_3$

to the parathyroid chromatin fraction via a temperature-dependent process. If one assumes that $1,25(OH)_2D_3$ operates through an alteration of genetic expression, it is possible that new gene products either assist calcium in its well known feedback effect on PTH secretion or that they somehow directly modulate the biosynthesis of PTH and/or its secretion at the membrane level.

V. CLINICALLY RELEVANT ASSAYS FOR VITAMIN D METABOLITES

The basic advances in our understanding of the metabolism and mechanism of action of vitamin D recorded above have been applied to the pathophysiology of a myriad of metabolic bone disorders. Developments that have helped bridge the gap between biochemical experiments and clinical reality have been the advent of assay procedures for accurately measuring vitamin D metabolites in the circulation. To date, three biologically important vitamin D metabolites have been quantitated in human plasma. In normal man, plasma concentrations of 25(OH)D, $24,25(OH)_2D$, and $1,25(OH)_2D$ are approximately 30 ng/ml (75n*M*), 3 ng/ml (7.5 n*M*), and 30 pg/ml (75p*M*), respectively. The methodology most often employed to assay these metabolites is that of competitive protein binding, with a variety of high affinity binding proteins such as plasma carriers and intracellular receptors. Other methods include physical measurements and radioimmunoassays. Data obtained from the assay of each metabolite in question are summarized below. How this information may apply to an understanding of diseases due to a defect in vitamin D metabolism is discussed in the last section of this chapter.

A. 25-Hydroxyvitamin D

Several types of assays for 25(OH)D have been devised. Haddad and Chyu (1971) originally employed kidney cytosol from rachitic rats to develop a competitive binding radioassay for 25(OH)D; this assay does not discriminate between $25(OH)D_2$ and $25(OH)D_3$. The normal range of 25(OH)D in humans as determined by this assay is 15–40 ng/ml plasma. In subsequent work the assay was combined with chromatographic resolution into cholecaliciferol (D_3) and ergocalciferol (D_2) forms. This showed that over 80% of total 25(OH)D in normal individuals exists as $25(OH)D_3$ (Haddad and Hahn, 1973). Belsey and associates, who had developed a similar assay (1971), subsequently proposed one in which the sterol was not isolated chromatographically from plasma (Belsey *et al.*, 1974). However, the plasma $24,25(OH)_2D$ concentration is appreciable and it also binds effectively to 25(OH)D binding proteins; thus, the nonchromatographic method probably overestimates serum 25(OH)D (Haddad *et al.*, 1976b).

Numerous workers have modified these two basic procedures, and a considerable amount of data has been accumulated on circulating levels of 25(OH)D in man. Most assays have yielded normal plasma concentrations of 25(OH)D ranging from 10–80 ng/ml, although the normal level in the United Kingdom (5–20 ng/ml) is approximately one-fourth that seen in sun-rich areas of the United States. These values are dependent upon diet and sunlight exposure. Humans display a seasonal variation in circulating levels of 25(OH)D_3, with highest levels occurring during the late summer months and lowest during the late winter months (McLaughlin *et al.*, 1974; Arnaud *et al.*, 1977; Poskitt *et al.*, 1979; Lund and Sorensen, 1979).

In addition to the competitive binding radioassay techniques, several other methods are currently available for directly measuring the appreciable levels of 25(OH)D_3 in the circulation. Thus, gas chromatography (Sklan *et al.*, 1973) and mass fragmentographic analysis (Björkhem and Holmberg, 1976) have been employed. Perhaps the most popular new technique is the direct quantitation of 25(OH)D by its ultraviolet absorbance at 254 nm as it emerges from a high pressure liquid chromatographic (HPLC) apparatus (Schaefer and Goldsmith, 1978). In such a procedure, 1–2 ml of plasma is extracted with organic solvents, and the lipid extract prepurified on a small Sephadex LH-20 column (Holick and DeLuca, 1971). The 25(OH)D region from the first column is then applied to HPLC. Figure 5 illustrates a typical trace obtained in our laboratory when 2 ml of human plasma extract is utilized. 25(OH)D_3, which is the predominant form of the metabolite in Arizona normal volunteers (Hughes *et al.*, 1976), elutes as an unambiguous peak in 13.5 min; absolute identification is made by exact comigration with a tritiated 25(OH)D_3 internal standard. By similarly chromatographing crystaline 25(OH)D_3 of known concentrations and taking into account the yield of tritium internal standard, one can calculate the endogenous level of the sterol in the patient. Since the HPLC method provides simultaneous purification and quantitation, it offers distinct advantages over binding assays. Thus, HPLC has become the technique of choice for the isolation and monitoring of a wide range of drugs and biologically important small molecules.

Plasma 25(OH)D levels have been measured in a variety of diseases. In general, the circulating levels are normal unless there is either a deficiency of vitamin D intake and/or sunlight or a disturbance in the small intestine, liver, or gallbladder. These three tissues participate in the absorption, 25-hydroxylation, and enterohepatic circulation of vitamin D as 25(OH)D (Arnaud *et al.*, 1975). Table I lists some observations concerning plasma levels of 25(OH)D in a number of disease states.

Many of the situations in which low plasma 25(OH)D exists, notably vitamin D-deficiency rickets, gastrointestinal disorders, chronic liver disease, and anticonvulsant drug therapy, are characterized by osteopenia. Presumably the relative lack of 25(OH)D itself, or more probably its active metabolites, contributes

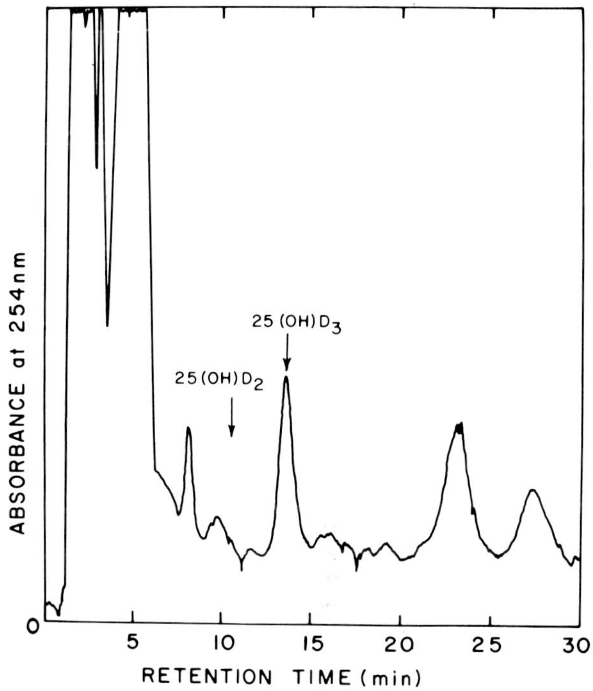

Fig. 5. Combined HPLC purification and quantitation of 25(OH)D_3 extracted from human plasma. Two ml of normal human plasma were extracted with organic solvents and the combined extract purified on a Sephadex LH-20 pre-column eluted with 65% chloroform in hexane. The 25(OH)D peak was then injected onto a tandem of two 2.1 mm × 25 cm Zorbax-sil (DuPont) columns and eluted with 2.5% isopropanol in hexane at a pressure of 3000 psi (flow rate was 0.8 ml/min). Yield of 25(OH)D_3 was 70% as determined by introducing 2000 dpm of authentic 25(OH)[^{3}H]D_3 (94 Ci/mmol) into the plasma prior to extraction and chromatography. No detectable 25(OH)D_2 was found in the plasma of this volunteer and the other UV absorbing peaks were not identified.

to the bone disease. In other cases, such as neonatal hypocalcemia and nephrotic syndrome, a deficiency of 25(OH)D may cause symptoms such as hypocalcemia. In the case of the nephrotic syndrome, 25(OH)D, bound to its binding protein, appears to be lost in the urine (Schmidt-Gayk *et al.*, 1977; Barragry *et al.*, 1977; Goldstein *et al.*, 1977).

On the other hand, many metabolic disorders of bone and mineral metabolism, such as renal osteodystrophy, parathyroid related bone disease, renal stone formation, and osteoporosis do not seem to involve aberrations in circulating 25(OH)D. In these cases we must look to other steps in vitamin D metabolism or to other factors mediating bone mineral homeostasis. One clinical syndrome in which abnormally high levels of 25(OH)D appears to be pathogenic is hyper-

TABLE I

Circulating 25(OH)D in Diseases of Mineral Metabolism

Low	Normal	High
Vitamin D-deficiency osteomalacia[a]	Chronic renal failure[i]	Hypervitaminosis D[n]
Gastrointestinal malabsorption[b]	Parathyroid disease[j]	
Chronic liver disease[c]	Idiopathic hypercalciuria[j]	
Biliary disease[d]	Familial hypophosphatemic rickets[k]	
Anticonvulsant therapy[e]	Postmenopausal osteoporosis[l]	
Neonatal hypocalcemia[f]	Corticosteroid therapy[m]	
Nephrotic syndrome[g]		
Thyrotoxicosis[h]		

[a] Preece *et al.* (1973); [b] Arnaud *et al.* (1976a); [c] Long *et al.* (1976); [d] Compston and Thompson (1977); [e] Stamp *et al.* (1972); [f] Rosen *et al.* (1974); [g] Goldstein *et al.* (1977); [h] Valentzas *et al.* (1977); [i] Shen *et al.* (1975); [j] M. R. Haussler and C. Y. C. Pak, unpublished observation; [k] Haddad *et al.* (1973); [l] DeLuca (1978); [m] Hahn *et al.* (1977); [n] Hughes *et al.* (1976).

vitaminosis D. Because 25-hydroxylation is not stringently regulated, excessive doses of exogenous vitamin D are metabolized to massive levels of 25(OH)D; this then simulates elevated 1,25$(OH)_2$D at target tissue receptors, which causes hypercalcemia and other symptoms of vitamin D intoxication.

B. 1,25-Dihydroxyvitamin D

The 25(OH)D content of in human blood is an excellent index of vitamin D status and serves as a useful adjunct to other methods for detecting vitamin D deficiency. As will be discussed subsequently, in certain disease states it is the circulating levels of 1,25$(OH)_2$D that are altered rather than those of 25(OH)D. Development of assay methods for 1,25$(OH)_2$D proved to be difficult because of its extremely low concentration in blood, which is less than 1/500 that of 25(OH)D. While the 3–3.7S receptor protein for 1,25$(OH)_2$D from chick intestinal cytosol might be used in a competitive protein binding assay, it is extremely labile. Moreover, it was difficult to separate the bound from the free ligand by standard procedures and tedious to purify the 1,25$(OH)_2$D hormone extensively so as to eliminate substances that interfere with the assay.

In the process of developing an assay for 1,25$(OH)_2D_3$, Brumbaugh *et al.* (1974b) employed a procedure that utilized an isolated receptor binding system prepared from chick intestinal mucosa. The method involved initial association of the hormone with the high-affinity cytoplasmic receptor and subsequent binding of the hormone-receptor complex to chromatin. It is the association of the hormone-receptor complex with chromatin which stabilizes it and allows for the separation of bound from free hormone using filtration techniques. Figure 6 depicts the steps comprising the radioreceptor assay of $1,25(OH)_2D$, as modified from the original assay of Brumbaugh *et al*. (1974b). The primary refinement in the current assay is the use of very high specific activity tracer $1,25(OH)_2D_3$ (94 Ci/mmol), allowing the utilization of less receptor system per assay tube and correspondingly greater sensitivity. As shown in Fig. 7 (insert), the receptor system saturates at about 16 pg of added tracer $1,25(OH)_2D_3$; when this amount of tracer is added to each tube, the assay is capable of detecting 1–2 pg of nonradioactive $1,25(OH)_2D_3$ (Fig. 7), with a useful range of 2–12 pg. This permits assaying of 1–2ml of plasma, but the endogenous $1,25(OH)_2D$ must still be purified from plasma by a 2–3 step chromatographic procedure prior to radioreceptor assay (Brumbaugh *et al*., 1974b).

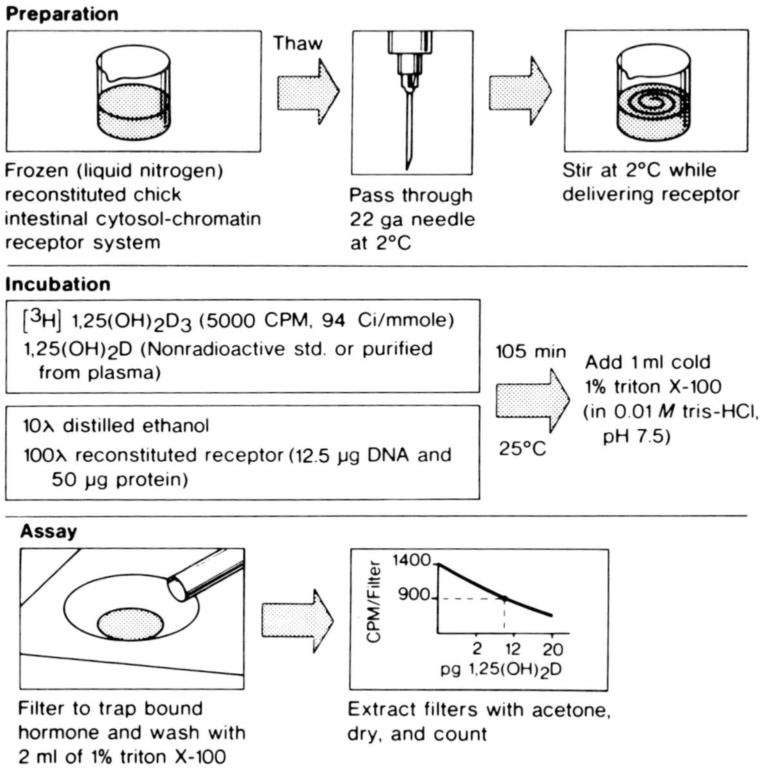

Fig. 6. Description of the methodology involved in the radioreceptor assay of $1,25(OH)_2D$.

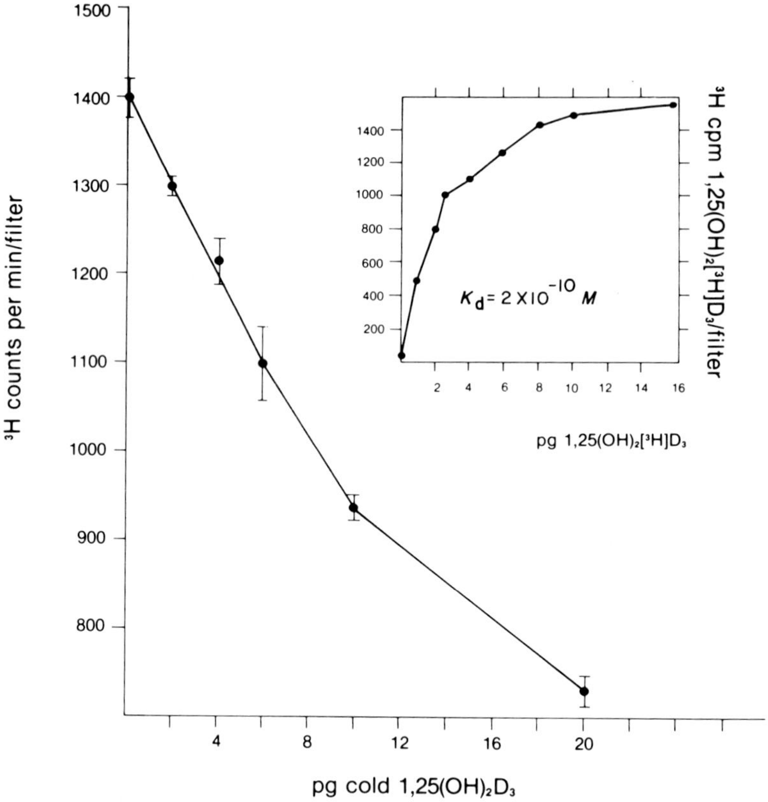

Fig. 7. Standard curve for the quantitation of $1,25(OH)_2D$ purified from human plasma. The curve is generated with 0–20 pg of nonradioactive, crystalline $1,25(OH)_2D_3$ exactly as depicted in Fig. 6. Minimum significant sensitivity of the assay is actually 1 pg of $1,25(OH)_2D_3$ although the lowest amount pictured is 2 pg. As discussed in the text, the inset shows that the receptor system saturates at 16 pg of added tracer, which corresponds to a dissociation constant of 2×10^{-10} *M* when the data from the inset are plotted by the method of Scatchard.

When determined by this technique, normal plasma $1,25(OH)_2D$ levels range from 20–45 pg/ml (Haussler *et al.*, 1976). As also true for 25(OH)D, more than 90% of the hormone is in the D_3 form (Hughes *et al.*, 1976). $1,25(OH)_2D$ plasma levels are not subject to seasonal variations as a result of changes in exposure to sunlight (Haussler, 1980). They also do not vary with vitamin D intake except under conditions of extreme deprivation or overdose of the vitamin. One physiologic modulation in $1,25(OH)_2D$ is a doubling of the hormone in plasma near the end of the third trimester of pregnancy, and children under 10 years old display a somewhat elevated level of the hormone, possibly due to increased calcium requirement during the growing period (Pike *et al.*, 1977).

Several other competitive binding radioassays utilizing the same binding protein from chick intestinal cytosol have been reported recently. Eisman *et al.* (1976) introduced the novel method of polyethylene glycol precipitation for separating bound from free hormone and first applied HPLC to the purification of plasma 1,25(OH)$_2$D in preparation for assay. Norman *et al.* (1978) employed hydroxylapatite to separate bound from free hormone. The following average normal values for circulating 1,25(OH)$_2$D have been reported: 29 pg/ml (Eisman *et al.*, 1976), 36 pg/ml (Gray *et al.*, 1977), 35 pg/ml (Lambert *et al.*, 1977), and 32 pg/ml (Norman *et al.*, 1978). These concentrations confirm the average level of 33 pg/ml originally reported by Haussler *et al.* (1976). Unfortunately, the radioreceptor assay of 1,25(OH)$_2$D is still not a routine laboratory procedure for two reasons: First, because the intestinal binding protein is extremely labile, and, although it has been partially purified (McCain *et al.*, 1978; Pike and Haussler, 1979), it has not been stabilized successfully. Second, the isolation of 1,25(OH)$_2$D requires one of several separation procedures with column chromatography followed by use of HPLC. Clemens *et al.* (1978) have recently raised a specific antibody to 1,25(OH)$_2$D and devised a radioimmunoassay for the hormone (normal level—35 pg/ml). The use of this antiserum obviates the problems with the intestinal cytosol receptor mentioned above, but interfering substances must still be removed by HPLC prior to the radioimmunoassay. Finally, an elegant bioassay has been developed by Stern *et al.* (1977), who applied ^{45}Ca resorption from bone in culture to the quantitation of 1,25(OH)$_2$D. The assay is exceedingly sensitive to a level of 1 pg of 1,25(OH)$_2$D. As with the competitive binding radioreceptor assay, a somewhat laborious purification procedure for the hormone, including high pressure liquid chromatography, is coupled with the biological assay in culture. The disadvantages of this assay are that it requires the highly specialized technique of fetal bone organ culture and suffers from inherently large variations characteristic of bioassays.

A number of disorders of mineral metabolism have been probed for aberrations in the plasma level of 1,25(OH)$_2$D. Figure 8 illustrates data from Haussler *et al.* (1977b) that show the striking reduction in circulating 1,25(OH)$_2$D in end-stage renal failure and the restoration of hormone levels to normal that follows successful renal transplantation. Also, shown in Fig. 8 are results of 1,25(OH)$_2$D assays in patients with primary hyperparathyroidism and idiopathic hypercalciuria, two disorders in which circulating levels of 1,25(OH)$_2$D are frequently elevated (Kaplan *et al.*, 1977; Shen *et al.*, 1977a; Gray *et al.*, 1977). As discussed in the last part of this chapter, the lack of 1,25(OH)$_2$D in uremic patients is undoubtedly one cause of renal osteodystrophy; excess hormone must contribute to the hyperabsorption of calcium and the resulting nephrolithiasis of primary hyperparathyroidism and idiopathic hypercalciuria.

Table II summarizes the diseases in which 1,25(OH)$_2$D measurements have been made. In addition to the disorders already described, other clinical entities

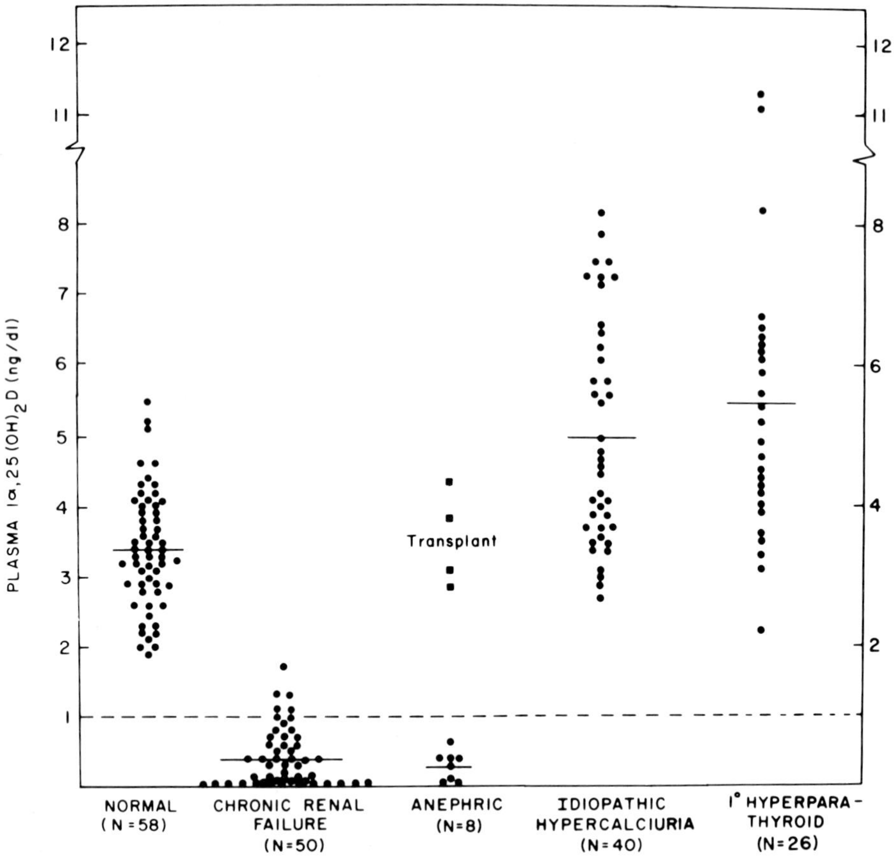

Fig. 8. Circulating $1,25(OH)_2D$ as determined via radioreceptor assay in patients with various disorders of mineral metabolism. Shown as closed squares are observations in four anephric subjects who underwent successful renal transplantation and were subsequently reassayed for $1,25(OH)_2D$. The dashed line indicates the minimum sensitivity of the assay. All assays were carried out at the University of Arizona, Department of Biochemistry.

include vitamin D-dependent rickets, an inherited defect in the renal 1α-OHase enzyme (Fraser *et al.*, 1973; DeLuca, 1978) and postmenopausal osteoporosis, where $1,25(OH)_2D_3$ may be reduced because of estrogen deficiency (DeLuca, 1978; Gallagher *et al.*, 1978). Since PTH is a positive modulator of the 1α-OHase (Garabedian *et al.*, 1972) and plasma $1,25(OH)_2D$ is increased in primary hyperparathyroidism (Fig. 8), the observation that $1,25(OH)_2D$ is subnormal in hypoparathyroidism and pseudohypoparathyroidism (Drezner *et al.*, 1976; Metz *et al.*, 1977) is not surprising. One curious set of disorders is the variety of

TABLE II

Circulating $1,25(OH)_2D$ in Diseases of Mineral Metabolism

Low	Normal	High
Nutritional osteomalacia[a]	Hypervitaminosis D[e]	1°Hyperparathyroidism[h]
Chronic renal failure[b]	Anticonvulsant therapy[f]	Idiopathic hypercalciuria[i]
Hypoparathyroidism[b]	Familial hypophosphatemic rickets[g]	
Pseudohypoparathyroidism[b]	Neoplastic hypercalcemia[b]	
Vitamin D-dependent rickets[c]	Sarcoidosis[a]	
Postmenopausal osteoporosis[c]		
Osteomalacia and mesenchymal tumor[d]		

[a] Haussler *et al.* (1977b); [b] Haussler *et al.* (1976); [c] DeLuca (1978); [d] Drezner and Feinglos (1977); [e] Hughes *et al.* (1976); [f] Jubiz *et al.* (1977); [g] Haussler *et al.* (1977a); [h] Kaplan *et al.* (1977); [i] Shen *et al.* (1977a).

osteomalacic syndromes caused by severe hypophosphatemia. Thus, tumor-induced hypophosphatemic osteomalacia seems to be associated with low $1,25(OH)_2D$, while patients with the classic X-linked familial form of hypophosphatemic rickets may have normal plasma levels of $1,25(OH)_2D$. Some forms of vitamin D-resistant rickets and states characterized by hyperabsorption of calcium in the face of normal $1,25(OH)_2D$ concentrations, e.g., some patients with idiopathic hypercalciuria, could represent, respectively, conditions in which there is either hypo- or hyper-responsiveness to $1,25(OH)_2D$ at the site of the target organ.

C. 24,25-Dihydroxyvitamin D

Although the function of $24,25(OH)_2D$ is not understood, it was apparent that the development of assays for this metabolite in human blood might assist in assigning a role for this sterol. Several competitive binding radioassays for $24,25(OH)_2D$ have been reported (Taylor *et al.*, 1976; Haddad *et al.*, 1977; Kremer and Guillemant, 1978). All apply binding proteins originally used to assay 25(OH)D and take advantage of the fact that the two sterols bind with similar affinities to these proteins. Taylor *et al.* (1976) used rachitic rat kidney cytosol as a source of binding protein, while the other two methods employ serum binding proteins. All methods essentially involve displacement of labeled

$25(OH)D_3$, and separate bound from free hormone with the aid of dextran-coated charcoal; chromatography is employed to isolate $24,25(OH)_2D$ for assay. Normal subjects in the United Kingdom have circulating levels of $24,25(OH)_2D$ of 1–2 ng/ml or one-tenth the plasma 25(OH)D concentration. Mendelsohn *et al.* (1976), assaying normal individuals in St. Louis, found levels of about 8 ng/ml. More recent binding assay values of $24,25(OH)_2D$ in healthy adults fall in the range of 2–5 ng/ml (Caldas *et al.*, 1978); Norman *et al.*, 1978; Horst *et al.*, 1979), and one report of direct HPLC quantitation has yielded a level of 2 ng/ml (Lambert *et al.*, 1977). In general, the levels of circulating $24,25(OH)_2D$ are about one-tenth of those of its precursor 25(OH)D and the plasma concentrations of the two metabolites are positively correlated. This would be consistent with unregulated conversion of 25(OH)D to its 24-hydroxylated derivative, constituting perhaps a step in the inactivation of 25(OH)D. Although plasma levels of $24,25(OH)_2D$ may vary simply as a function of the pool size of 25(OH)D and $1,25(OH)_2D$, there is some evidence that modulation occurs in relation to mineral homeostasis. This is suggested by the observed decrease in $24,25(OH)_2D$ in rats deprived of either dietary calcium or phosphorus (Whyte *et al.*, 1978).

Somewhat more controversial are possible alterations of $24,25(OH)_2D$ in various disease states of bone and calcium metabolism. Haddad *et al.* (1977) have reported normal serum $24,25(OH)_2D$ concentrations in anephric patients, while Taylor (1977a) was unable to detect the metabolite in such subjects. Most workers agree that plasma $24,25(OH)_2D$ levels are decreased in patients with chronic renal failure who have retained their diseased kidneys. In primary hyperparathyroidism, Taylor (1977b) found that $24,25(OH)_2D$ was elevated, but the metabolite is apparently unchanged in calcium stone formers without hyperparathyroidism (Caldas *et al.*, 1978).

It may be interesting to assay $24,25(OH)_2D$ in various osteopenic states to determine if $24,25(OH)_2D$ is indeed a "mineralization" metabolite of vitamin D. 24,25-Dihydroxyvitamin D_3, when administered orally, appears to have unique effects. Thus, in both normal and uremic subjects, this metabolite may cause slight but definite decreases in serum calcium, although there is considerable individual variation (Llach *et al.*, 1979). Moreover, in individuals with normal renal function, an increase in calcium absorption does not appear to be accompanied by changes in urinary calcium, e.g., urinary calcium may remain unchanged or decrease slightly, even though intestinal calcium absorption has increased (Brickman *et al.*, 1979). These observations provide support for the view that $24,25(OH)_2D_3$ may promote deposition of calcium in bone matrix. Bordier *et al.* (1978) reported that combined treatment with both $24,25(OH)_2D_3$ and $1,25(OH)_2D_3$ was more effective in healing the skeletal lesions of nutritional osteomalacia than was treatment with either metabolite alone. Additional studies are required to elucidate these interesting properties of $24,25(OH)_2D_3$.

VI. DISORDERS OF CALCIUM AND PHOSPHORUS METABOLISM RELATED TO ABERRATIONS IN THE AVAILABILITY, METABOLISM, OR EXPRESSION OF VITAMIN D

A. Vitamin D Deficiency Diseases

1. *Nutritional Rickets and Osteomalacia*

The terms rickets and osteomalacia encompass a group of diseases that have similar histologic findings but that arise from diverse causes. Inadequate mineralization of bone matrix is the unifying pathophysiologic feature. The prevention of rickets involves the maintenance of the ion product of calcium and phosphate in the blood at a level that is adequate for normal bone mineraliztion. Sufficient exposure to the sun prevents rickets in individuals who maintain a diet adequate in calcium and phosphorus. Rickets appears in environmental settings of sunlight deprivation, such as occurred during the Industrial Revolution when air pollution filtered out ultraviolet light. Supplementation of food products in the United States has virtually eliminated classical vitamin D-deficiency rickets. However, on a world-wide basis deficiency rickets and osteomalacia still represent a health problem. Reports from the United Kingdom indicate that rickets is a significant problem among the migrant Asian population (Preece *et al.*, 1973); in Glasgow, 9% of young children demonstrate radiographic characteristics of rickets (Richards *et al.*, 1968). Rickets also occurs in sun-rich areas where it is usually related to diets high in phytate or to social customs, such as the practice of purdah or the use of veils and clothing that limit skin exposure to sunlight.

The clinical manifestations of rickets or osteomalacia include bone pain, skeletal deformities, pathologic fractures, and muscle weakness due to a poorly defined myopathy. Radiographs of patients with rickets or osteomalacia often show a decreased density of bone and may reveal characteristic pseudofractures. Some cases also display radiographic changes typical of hyperparathyroidism, such as subperiosteal resorption and loss of *lamina dura*. However, because of the insensitivity of skeletal X rays, bone may appear normal in many patients with osteomalacia. Bone biopsy provides the most unequivocal diagnostic procedure for establishing the presence of osteomalacia, with demonstration of excessive amounts of unmineralized osteoid tissue in a histologic section of bone. The width and number of osteoid seams and the extent to which osteoid covers bone provide an index of the degree of osteomalacia.

The classic biochemical abnormalities of vitamin D-deficiency rickets are hypocalcemia, hypophosphatemia, elevated serum alkaline phosphatase, and depressed serum 25(OH)D levels. During the course of development of rickets, the initial hypocalcemia resulting from inadequate intestinal calcium absorption is thought to elicit secondary hyperparathyroidism. Excess PTH may temporarily correct the hypocalcemia but causes hypophosphatemia and, if vitamin D deficiency persists, serum 25(OH)D (and presumably $1,25(OH)_2D$) levels fall, resulting in severe malabsorption of calcium. Moreover, low levels of these sterols may impair the action(s) of PTH to mobilize stores of calcium. Thus, hypocalcemia eventually returns and is superimposed upon long-standing hypophosphatemia, with the inevitable result being florid rickets. The degree of hypophosphatemia often correlates with the severity of skeletal lesions; this suggests that hypophosphatemia per se is an important component in the development of rickets or osteomalacia. This is true also of other types of rickets, such as familial hypophosphatemic rickets.

Although the pathogenesis of nutritional rickets or osteomalacia is well understood, some details remain to be clarified as to the relative contributions of various sources of vitamin D and the degree of vitamin D deficiency required to elicit rickets. Since natural foods contain very little vitamin D, direct exposure to outdoor sunlight is the most important source of vitamin D in countries where vitamin D_2 or D_3 is not added as a food supplement. Neer *et al.* (1977) have summarized the environmental factors that affect photoactivation of vitamin D precursor in the skin. Using plasma 25(OH)D levels as an index, they report that the major determinants of vitamin D production in adult males are geography (latitude), occupational sunlight exposure, and the season of the year. These findings correlate with clinical reports that rickets has a higher incidence in northern latitudes and that femoral neck fractures in the United Kingdom increase in late winter and early spring (Aaron *et al.*, 1974).

Even in countries such as the United States where milk products are supplemented with vitamin D (often vitamin D_2), more than 85% of the vitamin D that ends up as $25(OH)D_3$ and $1,25(OH)_2D_3$ (Hughes *et al.*, 1976) is derived from sterols that have been converted in the skin by photochemical action. However, in the northern portions of the United States, especially during the winter months, dietary vitamin D_2 must contribute significantly to the vitamin D pool because up to one-third of the circulating 25(OH)D has been found to exist in the form of $25(OH)D_2$ (Arnaud *et al.*, 1977). It is difficult to document whether vitamin D deficiency, insufficient sunlight exposure, or both, are the actual causes of rickets or osteomalacia. Plasma 25(OH)D rises after increased intake of vitamin D (Stamp *et al.*, 1977) and the level of 25(OH)D in the plasma is at present the best guide as to whether an individual's intake of vitamin D should be increased. The need to fortify the diet with vitamin D probably differs in various latitudes. Also, the plasma level of 25(OH)D at which vitamin D action is insufficient and rickets is initiated is not precisely defined. Thus, Preece *et al.* (1975) found that 25(OH)D levels were virtually all below the normal range in patients with rickets; yet Arnaud *et al.* (1976b) reported rickets in several children with circulating 25(OH)D concentrations within the low range of normal. However, the critical concentration of 25(OH)D in blood is that required to provide a substrate for the formation of adequate amounts of its active metabolities, $1,25(OH)_2D$, and possibly $24,25(OH)_2D$. This concentration of 25(OH)D could be as low as 5 ng/ml (M. R. Haussler, unpublished observation), but it seems advisable and safe to maintain plasma 25(OH)D at levels of 20–30 ng/ml under normal conditions and during vitamin D therapy for nutritional rickets. Haussler *et al.* (1977b) found that $1,25(OH)_2D$ levels were very low in a small number of patients with rickets. Similar data have been obtained by Taylor *et al.* (1979) and Papapoulous *et al.* (1980). In contrast, Eastwood *et al.* (1979) found normal plasma levels of $1,25(OH)_2D$ as did Rasmussen *et al.* (1980) in a proportion of their cases of osteomalacia. Therefore, there is no universal correlation between low plasma $1,25(OH)_2D$ and the occurrence of osteomalacia, and factors such as mineral ion product and possibly other vitamin D metabolites may come into play (Rasmussen *et al.*, 1980).

2. *Gastrointestional Diseases Impairing Vitamin D Absorption*

Intestinal malabsorption syndromes resulting in inefficient assimilation of orally administered vitamin D and/or calcium are a cause of deficiency rickets and osteomalacia in the northern latitudes of United States and Western Europe. Circulating 25(OH)D is approximately half-normal in nontropical sprue (Arnaud *et al.*, 1976c) and is also depressed in some cases of diarrhea and/or steatorrhea (Hodgson *et al.*, 1976). In celiac disease, therapy with $1\alpha(OH)D_3$ has been reported to have led to a reversal of hypocalcemia and a reduction of fecal calcium losses (Bordier *et al.*, 1974). Also, simple exposure to ultraviolet light of subjects with osteomalacia of malabsorption can result in healing of the bone disease within several months (Jung *et al.*, 1978). Taken together, the above findings suggest that abnormal vitamin D absorption in association with fat malabsorption plus a lack of sunlight play important roles in the pathogenesis of rickets or osteomalacia in such patients.

Intestinal bypass surgery for severe obesity also alters vitamin D status and may be a cause of osteomalacia. In one study, histologically defined osteomalacia was found in 36% of patients with resection of the small intestine (Compston *et al.*, 1978a). In another study, serum 25(OH)D was dramatically subnormal in 61% of the jejunal-ileal bypass cases. However, some adaptive normalization of the vitamin D metabolities apparently occurs with time (Teitelbaum *et al.*, 1977). Serum $1,25(OH)_2D$ is also depressed in these patients (Lund *et al.*, 1978), although neither the circulating level of $1,25(OH)_2D$ (Lund *et al.*,

1978) nor 25(OH)D (Compston *et al.*, 1978b) correlated with the degree of bone disease as monitored by either photon absorptiometry or bone histology. Nevertheless, there is little doubt that suboptimal vitamin D metabolite levels are a part of the etiology of this type of osteomalacia and that intestinal shunt surgery may have an adverse effect on bone (Teitelbaum *et al.*, 1979).

Arnaud *et al.* (1975) have shown that 25(OH)D undergoes enterohepatic circulation. Following intravenous injection of radioactive 25(OH)D_3, one-third of the sterol was secreted into the duodenum during 24 hr, and 85% of this was subsequently reabsorbed by the ileum. A failure to resorb 25(OH)D which is secreted in bile may explain the osteomalacia that develops in some patients who have adequate exposure to sunlight. An interruption of the enterohepatic circulation may therefore be considered a common denominator in vitamin D deficiency associated with gastrointestinal and hepatobiliary disease (discussed below).

B. Excess Vitamin D Intake—Hypervitaminosis D

Acute vitamin D toxicity occurs in humans when very large doses of vitamin D are administered, usually to patients with various ("vitamin D-resistant") hypocalcemic conditions. The symptoms and signs are essentially those of hypercalcemia. The deleterious consequences of chronic hypervitaminosis D include soft tissue calcification in vital organs. If the conversion of vitamin D to its active metabolities is carefully regulated by calcium needs, why is the native vitamin toxic when ingested in pharmacologic quantities? The answer to this question apparently lies in the fact that control of all steps in vitamin D metabolism is not absolute. An important observation concerning the etiology of vitamin D intoxication is the finding that 25(OH)D_3, when present in excessive amounts, can simulate 1,25$(OH)_2D_3$ at the intestinal receptor (Brumbaugh and Haussler, 1973). Raisz *et al.* (1972) found that concentrations of 25(OH)D_3 100- to 500-fold greater than 1,25$(OH)_2D_3$ were capable of mobilizing bone calcium *in vitro*. These observations, coupled with the relative absence of regulation of the liver 25-OHase enzyme (Tucker *et al.*, 1973), suggested that 25(OH)D, rather than 1,25$(OH)_2$D, was responsible for the symptoms of hypervitaminosis D. This hypothesis (Brumbaugh and Haussler, 1973) was verified by the demonstration that anephric patients, incapable of biosynthesizing 1,25$(OH)_2$D, can become intoxicated with vitamin D (Counts *et al.*, 1975). Moreover, intoxicated patients with intact kidneys have normal or low circulating levels of 1,25$(OH)_2$D and strikingly enhanced levels of 25(OH)D (Hughes *et al.*, 1976). Figure 9 depicts the metabolite profile in normal individuals and a patient with hypervitaminosis D_2 (Hughes *et al.*, 1976). The average circulating level of 25(OH)D in normal individuals was 32 ng/ml and 3.5 ng/dl in the case of 1,25$(OH)_2D_3$. In

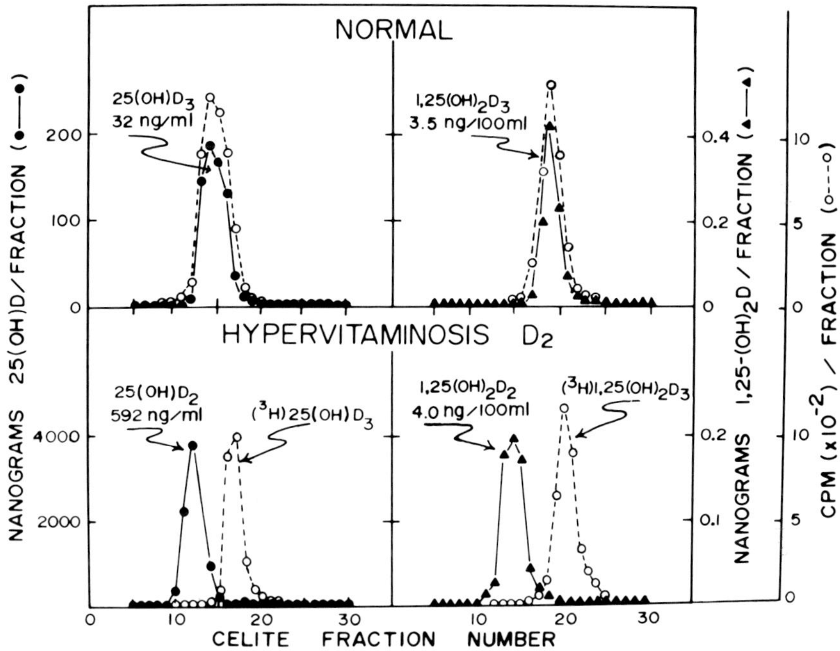

Fig. 9. Celite column chromatographic resolution and radioreceptor assay of vitamin D metabolities in normal subjects and in a patient with hypervitaminosis D_2. At the time of this study, the intoxicated patient was receiving 250,000 IU vitamin D_2 per day and had a serum calcium level of 14 mg/dl. Further experimental details are available in Hughes *et al.* (1976).

addition, all metabolities were in the vitamin D_3 form. In contrast, a typical case of hypervitaminosis D_2 exhibited an 18-fold increase in plasma 25(OH)D concentration with virtually all metabolites existing in the vitamin D_2 form. Unlike 25(OH)D, the level of 1,25$(OH)_2$D was not substantially increased as a result of vitamin D intoxification. These data suggest that the level of 25(OH)D is not or cannot be tightly regulated and point to 25(OH)D as the causative agent in hypervitaminosis D.

Mason and Posen (1979), in their assessment of patients treated with ergocalciferol, have found that serum calcium and plasma 25(OH)D correlated well with hypercalcemia occurring when serum levels of 25(OH)D exceeded 280 ng/ml.

After cessation of vitamin D input, 25(OH)D levels decrease with a $T_{\frac{1}{2}}$ of $\sim$10 days (Counts *et al.*, 1975). However, in acute cases of vitamin D poisoning, more aggressive measures may have to be instituted, such as therapy with large doses of glucocorticoids and the use of plasmaphoresis. Administration of adrenal steroids, which are thought to antagonize 25(OH)D action, usually reduces serum calcium rapidly.

C. Diseases Influencing Circulating 25-Hydroxyvitamin D

1. *Hepatobiliary Abnormalities*

Metabolic bone disease may occur in conjunction with severe chronic liver diseases. Skeletal disease resembling or identical to osteomalacia occurs more commonly in association with cholestatic liver disease, e.g., primary biliary cirrhosis or biliary atresia, than with hepatocellular diseases such as those associated with chronic alcoholism (Hepner, 1977). The latter may be more commonly associated with osteoporosis (Meunier *et al.*, 1973).

The liver plays a major role in vitamin D homeostasis. Thus, alterations in the role of the liver in metabolizing vitamin D to 25(OH)D, the formation of bile salts, which play an important role in the absorption and enterohepatic circulation of 25(OH)D and its metabolites and the hepatic synthesis of vitamin D-binding protein, may each alone or in combination contribute to vitamin D deficiency. Several reports have indicated that 25(OH)D levels are low in patients with primary biliary cirrhosis (Wagonfeld *et al.*, 1976; Reed *et al.*, 1977). In general, the presence of a low level of 25(OH)D has been found to correlate with a histologic diagnosis of osteomalacia when bone biopsies are performed (Reed *et al.*, 1977; Long *et al.*, 1978). However, osteomalacia may be present even when plasma levels of 25(OH)D are normal; other factors may therefore be involved in the development of the osteomalacia of primary biliary cirrhosis.

The pathogenesis of low levels of 25(OH)D in primary biliary cirrhosis is apparently multifactorial. Decreased availability of vitamin D may occur as a consequence of malabsorption. Thus, Compston and Thompson (1977) found impaired absorption of an acute oral dose of 25(OH)D_3 in patients with primary biliary cirrhosis. This may be attributable to altered synthesis of bile salts and may contribute to the disruption of the enterohepatic circulation of several vitamin D metabolities (Arnaud *et al.*, 1975; Kumar *et al.*, 1980). Wagonfeld *et al.* (1976) found that neither parenterally nor orally administered vitamin D raised circulating levels of 25(OH)D, observations consistent with both impaired 25-hydroxylation in the liver and intestinal malabsorption of the precursor. However, Skinner *et al.* (1977) found that parenteral administration of pharmacologic doses of vitamin D_2 resulted in a rise in circulating levels of 25(OH)D_2; this suggests that there may be considerable interpatient variation in terms of capacity for hepatic 25-hydroxylation. In addition to impaired absorption and 25-hydroxylation of vitamin D, increased urinary excretion of vitamin D metabolites has been reported in patients with biliary cirrhosis (Krawitt *et al.*, 1977). The significance of this finding is uncertain since increased urinary excretion may simply reflect an alternate excretory pathway when excretion in the bile is impaired. Finally, the levels of the vitamin D binding protein in the plasma may be reduced in primary biliary cirrhosis; however, it is unlikely that this contributes significantly since the transport protein is relatively unsaturated.

Long *et al.* (1978) have reported that treatment with parenteral $1,25(OH)_2D_3$ was effective in improving the osteomalacia in four patients with biliary cirrhosis who had failed to respond to treatment with parenteral vitamin D_2. Similarly, Reed *et al.* (1977) found that treatment with oral $25(OH)D_3$ resulted in histologic improvement or healing in five patients with this disorder. Thus, treatment with either of these analogs of vitamin D_3 may be clinically effective, whereas treatment with $1\alpha(OH)D_3$, which requires hepatic-25-hydroxylation prior to exerting a biological action, would be less effective, particularly in patients who have severe hepatic parenchymal disease or who receive drugs that alter the activity of the hepatic microsomal 25-hydroxylases.

Serum levels of 25(OH)D may also be decreased in other predominantly parenchymal liver disorders. Thus, a wide range of levels of 25(OH)D have been reported in groups of patients with various etiologies for hepatic disease or cirrhosis, including alcoholic hepatitis, chronic active hepatitis, lupoid hepatitis, and so-called cryptogenic cirrhosis (Hepner *et al.*, 1975; Long *et al.*, 1976). Alcoholic liver disease of a mild degree and alcoholism per se are not necessarily associated with low 25(OH)D levels. However, with advanced liver disease and cirrhosis, there is a greater likelihood of vitamin D deficiency. Hepner *et al.* (1975) found that plasma 25(OH)D levels correlated closely with results of an aminopyrine breath test that reflects parenchymal cell function through microsomal metabolic activity. As in the case for biliary cirrhosis, a number of factors may contribute to developing deranged vitamin D regulation in patients with hepatocellular disorders. These include lack of adequate solar exposure, nutritional deprivation of vitamin D fortified foods, malabsorption of vitamin D, and impairment of hepatic 25-hydroxylation capacities.

2. *Rickets Associated with Anticonvulsant Drug Therapy*

Anticonvulsant drugs, particularly diphenylhydantoin and phenobarbital, are thought to affect calcium metabolism and to cause rickets or osteomalacia (Hahn and Avioli, 1975). However, this view is not universally accepted, and Livingston *et al.* (1973) claimed that cases of rickets in 15,000 patients on anticonvulsant medication represent merely coincidental occurrences. Nevertheless, osteomalacia associated with anticonvulsant therapy has still received attention. Hypocalcemia has been reported in approximately 30% of institutionalized children and adults receiving long-term anticonvulsant drug treatment for epilepsy (Hunter *et al.*, 1971). Tolman *et al.* (1975) found osteomalacia in 67 of 289 institutionalized, retarded children, and all cases of osteomalacia were associated with anticonvulsant therapy; a comparison of children with and without osteomalacia revealed no differences in activity, sunlight exposure, or vitamin D intake. Bone mineral mass, as measured by photon absorptiometry, may be significantly depressed in epileptic children receiving phenobarbital, diphenylhydantoin, or both (Hahn *et al.,* 1975).

Perhaps most striking is the depression of circulating levels of 25(OH)D seen in most but not all patients on anticonvulsants (Stamp *et al.,* 1972; Hahn *et al.,* 1975; Jubiz *et al.,* 1977). The prevailing theory is that subnormal 25(OH)D occurs secondary to the induction of hepatic microsomal enzymes that degrade vitamin D, 25(OH)D, or both. However, diminished hepatic production of 25(OH)D via inhibition of the 25-hydroxylase enzyme may also be a factor (Roginski and Faminini, 1978). Successful treatment of anticonvulsant osteomalacia can be achieved with moderate doses of 1000–4000 IU of vitamin D per day (Peterson *et al.,* 1976; Liakakos *et al.,* 1975) and with small doses of 25(OH)D_3 (Stamp *et al.,* 1972). Thus, as with deficiency rickets, the osteomalacia of malabsorption and hepatobiliary disorders, the rickets of anticonvulsant therapy seems to be caused by inefficient maintenance of serum levels of 25(OH)D, either because of inadequate precursor availability or because of accelerated disappearance of 25(OH)D from plasma. Initially, it was assumed that depressed circulating 25(OH)D led to a concomitant reduction in the plasma levels of its more active metabolites, notably 1,25$(OH)_2$D. However, the serum 25(OH)D levels are apparently not sufficiently low to preclude the normal synthesis of the 1,25$(OH)_2$D hormone, because Jubiz *et al.* (1977) report that 1,25$(OH)_2$D levels were normal or even increased in patients on anticonvulsant drugs. Figure 10 illustrates that, in the patients studied by Jubiz *et al.* (1977), 25(OH)D can be suppressed by anticonvulsant drugs, while 1,25$(OH)_2$D is normal or even elevated in patients receiving phenobarbital alone. These data are somewhat surprising and indicate that low levels of 25(OH)D do not necessarily lead to reduced levels of 1,25$(OH)_2$D. Although assay measurements were not correlated with histologic evidence of osteomalacia in this study, the patients were the same as those reported in the earlier study by Tolman *et al.* (1975). Therefore, the bone and serum biochemical alterations occurring with anticonvulsant therapy cannot be explained by postulated subnormal levels of 1,25$(OH)_2$D. One possibility is that 25(OH)D itself is required for normal bone mineralization, or that 24,25$(OH)_2D_3$ is the missing "mineralization factor" in these patients; levels of the latter metabolite have recently been reported to be subnormal in individuals receiving anticonvulsant therapy (Weisman *et al.,* 1979).

Another mechanism may explain anticonvulsant-induced osteomalacia. Studies in rats (Harrison and Harrison, 1976) and in chick duodena in organ culture (Corradino, 1976) indicate that anticonvulsant drugs may act on the gastrointestinal tract, the primary effect being a decrease in calcium absorption.

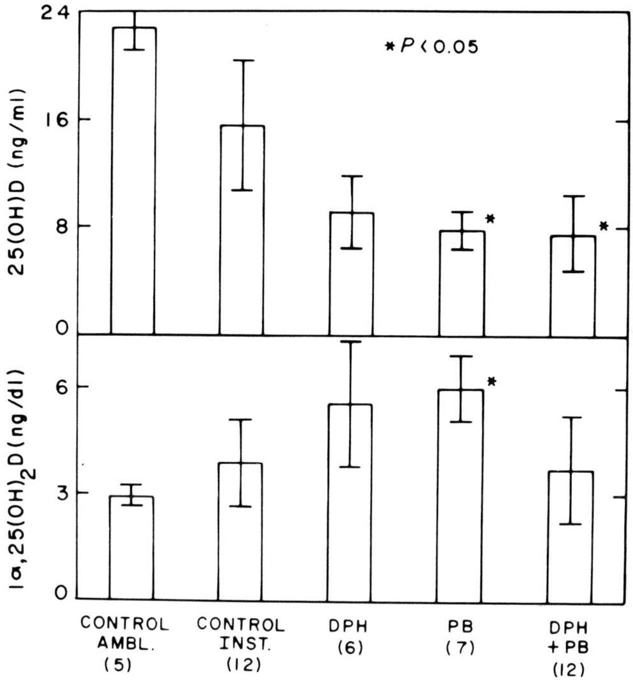

Fig. 10. Circulating vitamin D metabolites in patients receiving anticonvulsants. Number of cases is shown in parentheses and bars represent standard error of mean. Patients were age-matched, with ambulatory (ambl.) or institutionalized (inst.) controls. DPH = diphenylhydantoin, PB = phenobarbital.

Another tissue possibly affected by anticonvulsants is bone itself, and diphenylhydantoin has been shown to inhibit PTH- and 25(OH)D_3-induced calcium resorption in organ-cultured mouse calvaria (Jenkins *et al.*, 1974). More recently, Hahn *et al.* (1978) have demonstrated that 1,25$(OH)_2$D-induced bone resorption in fetal rat bones can be blocked by both diphenylhydantoin and phenobarbital. Thus, it is conceivable that there is a drug-elicited hyporesponsiveness to 1,25$(OH)_2$D in the gut and bone, a phenomenon ultimately manifested as classic osteomalacia. However, the fact that administration of vitamin D or 25(OH)D_3 corrects symptoms of osteomalacia in patients on anticonvulsant drugs leaves open the question of the pathogenesis of anticonvulsant-induced osteomalacia.

D. Disorders with a Deficiency of 1,25-Dihydroxyvitamin D

The diseases detailed in this section include both proved lesions in the 1α-hydroxylase system and a number of syndromes where a deficiency in

$1,25(OH)_2D$ is inferred or where $1\alpha(OH)D_3$ or $1,25(OH)_2D_3$ has been found therapeutically effective. In these disorders both vitamin D intake and circulating 25(OH)D are generally normal.

1. Uremic Osteodystrophy

Altered bone and mineral homeostasis is a frequent accompaniment of varieties of advanced renal failure. The pathogenesis of renal osteodystrophy is complex, and multifactorial alterations in vitamin D metabolism appear to play a central role. The skeletal lesions are diverse and may take the form of rickets, osteomalacia, osteitis fibrosa, osteopenia, or a combination thereof. A hallmark of advanced renal failure is an increase in the fecal excretion of calcium, i.e., malabsorption of calcium, which leads to negative calcium balance—a classic finding of vitamin D deficiency. By direct measurements, calcium absorption has been demonstrated to be reduced in chronic renal failure (Coburn *et al.*, 1973). Renal osteodystrophy is frequently refractory to treatment with physiologic doses of vitamin D. Although the pathogenesis of uremic bone disease remains incompletely explained, two main mechanisms acting in concert are probably responsible: abnormalities in metabolism of vitamin D and secondary hyperparathyroidism.

Brickman *et al.* (1972) first successfully treated the hypocalcemia and negative calcium balance of chronic renal failure with $1,25(OH)_2D_3$. Later, Mawer *et al.* (1973), utilizing double label techniques with $[^3H]$- and $[^{14}C]$-vitamin D_3 in vitamin D-deficient patients with and without chronic renal insufficiency, showed that the subjects with kidney failure could not biosynthesize $1,25(OH)_2D_3$. Utilizing a radioreceptor assay, Brumbaugh *et al.* (1974a) obtained data indicating that total circulating levels of $1,25(OH)_2D_3$ were reduced in chronic renal failure.

Subsequent work has confirmed that circulating levels of $1,25(OH)_2D$ in patients with end stage renal failure are very low and undetectable in nephrectomized patients (Haussler *et al.*, 1976) (Fig. 8). Moreover, successul renal transplantation restores plasma $1,25(OH)_2D$ levels to normal. These data suggest that deficiency of $1,25(OH)_2D$ may be a major factor contributing to the development of skeletal disease in patients with chronic renal failure.

Deficiency of other vitamin D metabolites may also be implicated in the pathogenesis of uremic bone disease. Thus, Eastwood *et al.* (1976) observed a correlation between low levels of 25(OH)D and the presence of osteomalacia in uremic patients. Treatment with small doses of $25(OH)D_3$, which resulted in an elevation of plasma levels of the sterol to slightly above normal, produced healing of the skeletal lesions. This suggested that this form of osteomalacia results from a relative lack of 25(OH)D superimposed on an existing deficiency of $1,25(OH)_2D$, rather than from a deficiency of $1,25(OH)_2D$ alone. In general, however, plasma levels of 25(OH)D are normal or slightly increased in patients with chronic renal failure.

Recent observations indicate that levels of $24,25(OH)_2D$ are also depressed in patients with chronic renal failure (Taylor, 1977a). Since $24,25(OH)_2D_3$ may have biologic actions in patients with renal failure, e.g., it may promote calcium absorption, lower serum calcium and stimulate alkaline phosphatase activity, deficiency of this sterol has been postulated to play a role in the pathogenesis of uremic osteodystrophy (Kanis *et al.*, 1978; Llach *et al.*, 1979). At present, the general consensus is that the serum level of $24,25(OH)_2D$ is either undetectable or very low in nephrectomized patients.

The above findings indicate that a low level of $1,25\text{-}(OH)_2D$ is not necessarily the cause of all forms of metabolic bone disease encountered in renal failure. Bordier *et al.* (1973) have reported for example, the absence of histologic evidence of osteomalacia in several anephric patients who had been treated with hemodialysis for several years.

A rapidly growing number of studies attest to the clinical usefulness of vitamin D_3 analogs including $25(OH)D_3$, $1\alpha(OH)D_3$, and $1,25(OH)_2D_3$ in managing different forms of uremic bone disease. Dramatic results have been reported with all three sterols. What sort of mechanism accounts for the unexpected functioning of $25(OH)D_3$ in renal patients incapable of biosynthesis of $1,25(OH)_2D_3$? Most likely, superphysiologic circulating levels of $25(OH)D_3$ are caused by the therapy, which in turn simulate $1,25(OH)_2D_3$ at target organs to cause calcium mobilization. Therapeutic trials with both $1\alpha(OH)D_3$ and $1,25(OH)_2D_3$ have been particularly impressive in the management of skeletal lesions of secondary hyperparathyroidism, e.g., osteitis fibrosa. Histologic improvement has paralleled correction of hypocalcemia and suppression of high circulating levels of PTH (Davie *et al.*, 1976; Catto *et al.*, 1975; Tougaard *et al.*, 1976; Hirooka *et al.*, 1975; Naik *et al.*, 1976; Brickman *et al.*, 1972, 1974, 1976; Henderson *et al.*, 1974). The initial results concerning improvement in the osteomalacic component of uremic bone disease during treatment with the 1α-hydroxylated compounds were less impressive, an observation which may have several causes. The long mineralization lag found in many uremic patients indicates that significant histologic response to treatment may require a minimum of 1–2 years. In addition, several subtypes of "osteomalacia" have been described, and those patients who have skeletal lesions most closely resembling simple nutritional osteomalacia (e.g., a mixed histologic lesion with both defective mineralization and osteitis fibrosa), frequently show excellent clinical, chemical, and histologic response to treatment with either $1\alpha(OH)D_3$ or $1,25(OH)_2D_3$. Patients may also show excellent responses to treatment with $25(OH)D_3$ (Teitelbaum *et al.*, 1976; Eastwood *et al.*, 1977). Other patients who appear histologically to have little evidence of osteitis fibrosa and in addition have low levels of PTH do not tend to improve very much when treated with any of the vitamin D analogs. Such patients frequently exhibit hypersensitivity to vitamin D analogs and rapidly develop hypercalcemia and may not suffer from disordered vitamin D metabolism (Brickman *et al.*, 1979; Coburn *et al.*, 1979; Sherrard *et al.*, 1979).

Frequently, clinical improvement occurs even though therapy with $1,25(OH)_2D_3$ or $1\alpha(OH)D_3$ fails to produce dramatic evidence of histologic or radiologic healing. The latter may be due to the relief of hypocalcemia and variable suppression of PTH hypersection. PTH has been considered to be a general uremic toxin, and suppression of high endogeneous levels appear to correlate with improvement in such conditions as anemia, neuropathy, and impaired sexual function, all of which are encountered in chronic renal failure. Moreover, amelioration of the myopathy (muscle weakness) of uremia occurs with startling rapidity following institution of treatment with either $25(OH)D_3$ or 1α-hydroxylated vitamin D_3 compounds (Davie *et al.*, 1976; Henderson *et al.*, 1974; Coburn, 1980).

Although successful therapy has been achieved in some cases of renal osteodystrophy, several issues remain unsettled regarding the relationship between $1,25(OH)_2D$ and the pathophysiology of this disease. In order to comprehend the influence of impaired production of $1,25(OH)_2D$ on the pathogenesis of renal bone disease, it is necessary to monitor $1,25(OH)_2D$ throughout the disease. Bone disease generally appears when the GFR falls below 30 ml/min, and calcium malabsorption also develops as a function of degree of renal impairment (Werner *et al.*, 1976). Figure 11 depicts preliminary data on the circulating level of $1,25(OH)_2D$ as a function of GFR. Although data are limited in the critical region, it appears that $1,25(OH)_2D$ may fall below normal at a GFR of approximately 20–30 ml/min; this corresponds to the observations on intestinal calcium absorption. These data suggest a fairly direct relation between renal impairment and altered vitamin D metabolism. However, more subtle disturbances in renal function may also influence $1,25(OH)_2D$ production. Animal studies have given rise to controversy whether uremia per se can inhibit $1,25(OH)_2D$ biosynthesis or whether the only mechanism for such a block is a loss of renal mass. Most

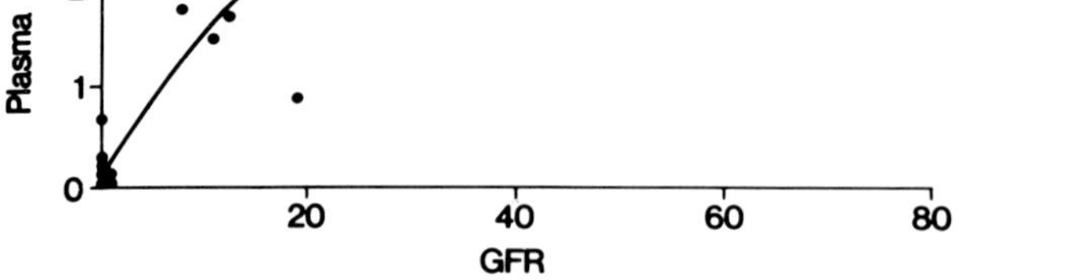

Fig. 11. Circulating $1,25(OH)_2D$ versus degree of renal impairment in humans. GFR is glomerular filtration rate expressed by creatinine clearance.

patients on hemodialysis, some of whom may still have significant amounts of functioning renal tissue, have undetectable levels of $1,25(OH)_2D$ in the plasma (Fig. 8). Acidosis and hyperphosphatemia would be two possible mechanisms for inhibition of $1,25(OH)_2D$ biosynthesis; both of these are relatively independent of renal mass.

2. *Renal Tubular Disorders*

A variety of renal tubular abnormalities are associated with clinical rickets or osteomalacia. These dysfunctions range from conditions in which phosphate wasting is present, as in X-linked hypophosphatemia, to those with more complex defects in renal tubular handling of phosphate, glucose, amino acids, bicarbonate, and hydrogen ion (Fanconi syndrome). The hallmark of these disorders is renal phosphate wasting, which can lead to florid rickets or osteomalacia.

a. X-linked Hypophosphatemia Familial hypophosphatemic rickets is transmitted via an X-linked dominant gene and is characterized by low plasma phosphate, high clearance of phosphate by the kidney, and normal serum levels of PTH (Arnaud *et al.*, 1971). Although it has been suggested that this disease involves the inability to absorb calcium normally from the intestine or that it is due to a defect in vitamin D metabolism, the bulk of the evidence points to a primary renal tubular and intestinal defect in phosphate transport (Glorieux *et al.*, 1972; Short *et al.*, 1973). Consistent with this is the report that short-term therapy with $1,25(OH)_2D_3$ is ineffectual in reversing the renal phosphate wasting of this disorder (Brickman *et al.*, 1973; Offermann *et al.*, 1978). Yet, a combination of vitamin D (Glorieux *et al.*, 1972) or $1\alpha(OH)D_3$ (Rasmussen *et al.*, 1976) and phosphate supplements is apparently effective in healing the rickets in children with X-linked hypophosphatemia. These findings do not necessarily contradict the theory that the fundamental defect is in phosphate reabsorption by the kidney, but do intimate that there still may exist a subtle aberration in vitamin D metabolism. Serum concentrations of 25(OH)D have been found to be normal (Haddad *et al.*, 1973), and $1,25(OH)_2D$ is also normal in most patients (see Fig. 12 and Haussler *et al.*, 1979; Drezner *et al.*, 1980). Thus, there is no absolute lack in an ability of these patients to biosynthesize $1,25(OH)_2D$. However, the degree of hypophosphatemia would produce a striking enhancement in circulating levels of $1,25(OH)_2D_3$ in normal individuals (Gray *et al.*, 1977); hence, an unresponsive renal 1α-OHase enzyme is suggested.

Thus, there may be three different end-organ expressions of the single genetic lesion in hypophosphatemic rickets: intestinal malabsorption of phosphorus, renal phosphorus wasting, and, a relative impairment of $1,25(OH)_2D$ production. As indicated above, defective intestinal absorption of inorganic phosphate has been reported in X-linked hypophosphatemia (Short *et al.*, 1973). Although administration of $1,25(OH)_2D_3$ to patients with this disorder reduces fecal phos-

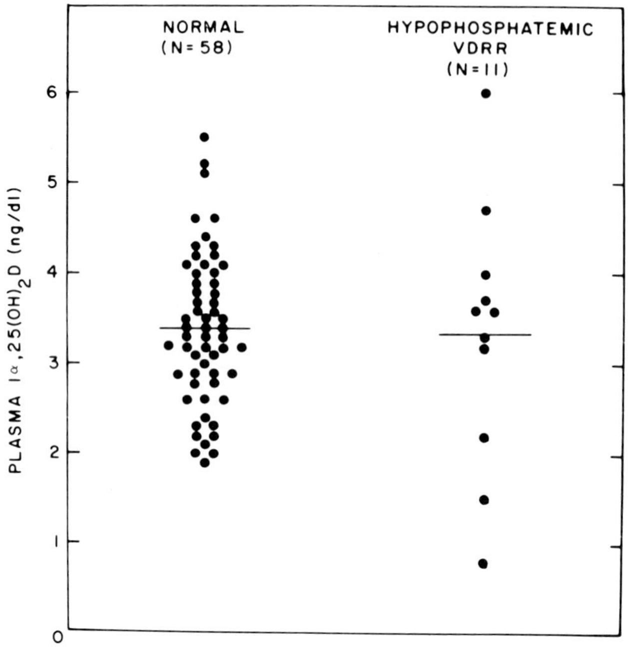

Fig. 12. Circulating $1,25(OH)_2D$ in familial hypophosphatemic vitamin D-resistant rickets (VDRR). (From Haussler *et al.*, 1977a, by courtesy of Plenum Press.)

phorus excretion, it is unknown at present if $1,25(OH)_2D_3$ is acting at the site of defective intestinal phosphorus transport. However, a mouse model of the human condition exhibits defective intestinal phosphate absorption that is not corrected by the administration of $1,25(OH)_2D_3$ (O'Doherty and DeLuca, 1976). At the kidney, there may be dual manifestations of the genetic error, including both a lack of phosphate conservation and absence of transmission of the hypophosphatemic signal to the 1αOHase. Theoretically, these expressions together may be accounted for by a single defective phosphate transport protein. Its absence in gut and kidney precludes the normal movement of phosphate, and intracellular phosphate concentration may be maintained in such a way as to deceive the renal 1αOHase.

b. Fanconi Syndrome The Fanconi syndrome is characterized by dysfunction of the proximal renal tubule with impaired reabsorption of amino acids, glucose, bicarbonate, and phosphate. Patients have hypophosphatemia and a high incidence of skeletal disease—rickets or osteomalacia. Pharmacological doses of vitamin D are required to control osteopenia, and skeletal improvement may occur without an increase in serum phosphate levels. Brewer *et al.* (1977a) have studied vitamin D metabolism in an animal model of Fanconi syndrome produced by the administration of maleic acid. These rats exhibit markedly diminished production of $1,25(OH)_2D_3$ from injected $25(OH)[^3H]D_3$. In other studies, Brewer *et al.* (1976) found that labeled $25(OH)D_3$ was not converted to $1,25(OH)_2D_3$ in children with the Fanconi syndrome and that total circulating $1,25(OH)_2D$ was depressed in afflicted children as compared to controls of the same age (Brewer *et al.*, 1977b). Thus, $1,25(OH)_2D$ biosynthesis appears to be altered in Fanconi syndrome and may be affected similarly but to varying degrees in the spectrum of renal tubular disorders seen in man. The effects on $1,25(OH)_2D$ probably explain, at least in part, the occurrence of bone disease in such cases.

3. *Vitamin D-Dependent Rickets*

This disorder is believed to be inherited as an autosomal recessive trait and is characterized by hypocalcemia, hypophosphatemia, elevated serum alkaline phosphatase, and severe rachitic bone lesions. It differs from X-linked hypophosphatemic rickets in that afflicted children are regularly hypocalcemic and differs from nutritional rickets in that pharmacologic doses of vitamin D or 25(OH)D are necessary to alleviate the skeletal disease. Fraser *et al.* (1973) studied five patients and observed that 1 μg/day of $1,25(OH)_2D_3$ promptly initiated healing. These data suggest that this genetic disease is characterized by either a complete lack of the renal lαOHase enzyme or a congenital defect in its regulation. However, Balsan *et al.* (1975) found that children with nutritional rickets responded promptly to 0.5 μg/day, while patients with vitamin D-dependent rickets were only partially improved by this dose of $1,25(OH)_2D_3$.

Recent measurements of circulating vitamin D metabolites in cases of vitamin D-dependent rickets strongly support the concept that this disorder is an inborn error in the renal lαOHase enzyme (Haussler *et al.*, 1979). DeLuca (1978) has reported that low serum levels of $1,25(OH)_2D$ coexist with normal concentrations of 25(OH)D and that children cured with very large doses of vitamin D or 25(OH)D show no improvement in serum $1,25(OH)_2D$ levels. However, in cases successfully treated with exogenous $1,25(OH)_2D_3$, serum $1,25(OH)_2D$ returned to normal values. These data also indicate that 25(OH)D is the pharmacologically active agent when high doses of vitamin D are administered, as in renal patients treated with 25(OH)D or in hypervitaminosis D.

4. *Abnormalities of the Parathyroid Glands*

a. Hypoparathyroidism Hypoparathyroidism, either idiopathic or resulting from thyroid–parathyroid surgery, has hypocalcemia as a major clinical consequence. The absence of PTH reduces skeletal calcium mobilization and renal calcium reabsorption; the hypocalcemia of this disease is aggravated by a partial deficiency of 1,25(OH)$_2$D production. As a result patients may exhibit mildly depressed intestinal absorption of calcium, and the radioreceptor assay of circulating 1,25(OH)$_2$D indicates subnormal levels in most cases of hypoparathyroidism (Haussler *et al.*, 1976). Although the hyperphosphatemia characteristic of this disorder may suppress 1,25(OH)$_2$D formation, the lack of PTH, which normally exerts a positive influence on biosynthesis of 1,25(OH)$_2$D, is probably more important in this context. Thus, when either animals (Hughes *et al.*, 1975) or humans (Bilezikian *et al.*, 1978) with intact parathyroid glands were made hypocalcemic by dietary or drug maneuvers, the circulating level of 1,25(OH)$_2$D$_3$ rose at least 3-fold. Hypocalcemia, per se, may also stimulate 1,25(OH)$_2$D$_3$ production in the absence of PTH in the rat (Hughes *et al.*, 1975; Trechsel *et al.*, 1980). It is unclear what role hypocalcemia may have in stimulating 1,25(OH)$_2$D$_3$, even to a small degree, in patients with hypoparathyroidism. It is possible that reduced 1,25(OH)$_2$D$_3$ biosynthesis may be attributable, at least in part, to impaired responsiveness of the renal 1αOHase in hypocalcemia.

Very large doses of vitamin D, i.e., 1.25 to 2.5 mg/day or greater, are frequently required to correct the hypocalcemia of hypoparathyroidism, while 1–2 μg/day of 1,25(OH)$_2$D$_3$ is necessary to restore serum calcium to normal in some cases (Russell *et al.*, 1974; Kooh *et al.*, 1975; Haussler, 1978). However, Chesney *et al.* (1977) reported that 2–6 μg of the sterol were ineffective in one subject with idiopathic hypoparathyroidism. Supplemental oral calcium may be required in conjunction with the 1,25-(OH)$_2$D$_3$ therapy. In most patients, the deficiency of 1,25(OH)$_2$D is less marked than in nutritional or renal rickets, and in most cases the hyperphosphatemia, normal 25(OH)D and low rate of bone turnover probably prevent the development of osteomalacia. However, Drezner *et al.* (1977) have reported a case of long-standing hypoparathyroidism in which circulating 1,25(OH)$_2$D was reduced to 4 pg/ml (normal = 20–45 pg/ml), and the patient had incapacitating bone pain and histological osteomalacia. They postulate that the hypocalcemia and 1,25(OH)$_2$D deficiency may combine to limit calcium available for bone mineralization and perhaps cause a lesion in synthesis of bone matrix.

b. Pseudohypoparathyroidism Pseudohypoparathyroidism is a pleiotropic, genetic disease of variable expression. As originally described by Albright *et al.* (1942), the disorder is a state of resistance to parathyroid hormone associated with characteristic somatic features, such as short metacarpals, diminished height, and a round face. In adults, the biochemical abnormalities of the complete syndrome are hypocalcemia, hyperphosphatemia, elevated serum concentration of endogenous PTH, and deficient calcemic and phosphaturic responses to exogenous PTH.

The characteristic failure of exogenously administered PTH to enhance urinary cyclic 3′,5′-adenosine monophosphate (cyclic AMP) excretion in patients with this disorder suggests that the renal refractoriness is secondary to a genetic defect manifested by defective activation of renal PTH-dependent adenylate cyclase activity (Chase *et al.*, 1969). In contrast, recent observations (Haussler *et al.*, 1976; Drezner *et al.*, 1976; Sinha *et al.*, 1977) indicate that the hypocalcemia and the bone cell unresponsiveness to PTH are acquired in some patients and may be related to impaired production of $1,25(OH)_2D$. Thus, Drezner *et al.* (1976) found reduced plasma levels of $1,25(OH)_2D$ in three cases of Type 1 pseudohypoparathyroidism and Haussler *et al.* (1976, 1977b) reported that circulating $1,25(OH)_2D$ in a number of cases of pseudohypoparathyroidism resembled those found in hypoparathyroidism, with low or occasionally "normal" levels being associated with hypocalcemia. Like hypoparathyroidism, the hypocalcemia in most patients with pseudohypoparathyroidism is correctable with small doses of either $1\alpha(OH)D_3$ or $1,25(OH)_2D_3$ (Kooh *et al.*, 1975) and with large doses of vitamin D (Drezner *et al.*, 1976).

Although long-term treatment with vitamin D may restore the calcemic response to exogenous parathyroid hormone, it has not been demonstrated that this is attributable to normalization of plasma $1,25(OH)_2D$. Indeed, Brickman *et al.* (1977) were unable to show an improved calcemic response in three patients with pseudohypoparathyroidism following 2–3 weeks of therapy with $1,25(OH)_2D_3$, 2 μg/day. Of interest is the report of Metz *et al.* (1977) of a patient with hypocalcemia and osteomalacia who had a normalization of the calcemic response to exogenous PTH after 5 days of treatment with $1,25(OH)_2D_3$. This response must be attributed to correction of low levels of $1,25(OH)_2D_3$, since it is far too rapid to be attributable to skeletal healing. Restoration of the calcemic response to PTH could also be the result of increased serum calcium level elicited by $1,25(OH)_2D_3$.

The blunted phosphaturic response to exogenous PTH may also be restored to normal in pseudohypoparathyroidism during long-term treatment with vitamin D or treatment with $1,25(OH)_2D_3$ (2.0 μg/day) for only 7 days (Brickman *et al.*, 1977). The latter occurs without a change in urinary excretion of cyclic AMP. The molecular lesion associated with the altered phosphaturic response to PTH in pseudohypoparathyroidism could occur at one of several biochemical steps in the kidney; the relationship between this defect and altered biosynthesis of $1,25(OH)_2D$ is not completely understood. As previously discussed, Bonjour *et al.* (1977) have shown that in the thyroparathyroidectomized rat $1,25(OH)_2D_3$ restores the normal capacity of the kidney to adapt to differing dietary loads of phosphorus. Recently, Lambert *et al.* (1980) have provided preliminary evidence that PTH stimulated production of $1,25(OH)_2D_3$ is impaired in pseudohypoparthyroidism. It may be postulated that this may involve an abnormality in a step in cyclic AMP metabolism which involves $1,25(OH)_2D_3$ biosynthesis.

Finally, although pseudohypoparathyroidism is often a hypocalcemic disorder, an incompletely expressed form, with normocalcemia, has been recognized (Mann *et al.*, 1962). The presence of normal serum calcium suggests that production of 1,25$(OH)_2$D may be normal, and Drezner and Haussler (1978) have recently confirmed this notion by showing that such a patient had a normal circulating 1,25$(OH)_2$D concentration. Based upon the contrast between 1,25$(OH)_2$D levels in hypocalcemic and normocalcemic pseudohypoparathyroidism, it is possible that variable penetrance of disordered vitamin D_3 metabolism may underlie the hypocalcemia and bone refractoriness to PTH in pseudohypoparathyroidism.

5. *Neonatal Hypocalcemia*

Infantile hypocalcemia is the most common cause of seizures in human neonates, and its pathogenesis is poorly understood. This disorder occurs infrequently in term infants, but has a higher incidence in premature infants and offspring of diabetic and hyperparathyroid mothers (Monteleone *et al.*, 1975). It usually lasts about 1–3 days, and one explanation is that it involves both a transient hypoparathyroidism and insufficient renal tubular response to PTH (David and Anast, 1974). This "first day" hypocalcemia is also seen in low birth weight infants and in those born of mothers with complications at the time of delivery. A second variety of neonatal hypocalcemia usually appears between the fifth and tenth days of life in babies fed cow's milk instead of being breast fed. The hypocalcemia is thought to be caused by the high phosphorus load in the cow's milk, although delayed PTH secretion is another possible cause.

That premature babies are prone to develop rickets has been known for many years. The conventional explanation has been that the rapid growth rate of premature infants leads to an increased requirement of vitamin D, but rates of vitamin D utilization have not, in fact, been measured in these babies. At birth the serum concentrations of 25(OH)D mainly reflect maternal levels and are independent of gestational age. During the first month of life, the mature baby can maintain normal serum levels of 25(OH)D, but the premature baby cannot (Hillman and Haddad, 1975). Furthermore, oral or even intravenous supplements of vitamin D do not appreciably increase serum 25(OH)D concentrations in premature infants; this suggests that the conversion of vitamin D to 25(OH)D in the liver is impaired in the premature infant. Indeed, Rosen *et al.* (1974) have found low plasma 25(OH)D levels in 11 of 15 pairs of mothers and premature infants with the children's serum calcium less than 7.5 mg% during the first 48 hr of life. Thus, 25(OH)D deficiency in the premature newborn, which may be secondary to maternal vitamin D deficiency and sustained by a possible inadequacy of hepatic 25-hydroxylation in the premature infant, may be an important factor in the pathogenesis of neonatal tetany and infantile rickets.

Although most cases of neonatal hypocalcemia last no more than 2–3 days, the hypocalcemia may be protracted, lasting up to several weeks in a small number of cases. To overcome this condition may require continuous intravenous calcium therapy, which in turn may lead to serious problems. Kooh *et al.* (1976)

have shown that the intravenous administration of $1,25(OH)_2D_3$ corrected the hypocalcemia of six infants even though they were being fed low phosphate formula. Four of the infants remained normocalcemic after $1,25(OH)_2D_3$ was discontinued. These data do not prove that vitamin D metabolism is altered in neonatal hypocalcemia, but suggest that the normal metabolism of vitamin D may be impaired.

6. *Osteoporosis (see Chapter 2, Vol. III)*

Osteoporosis is a common generalized disorder of bone. It is characterized by too little calcified bone and is apparently the end result of a number of disease states that affect the skeleton. Of necessity osteoporosis results when bone mineral resorption exceeds new bone mineral deposition. There are probably many causes, and the putative role of vitamin D in either pathogenesis or therapy remains open to question. The disease is rarely encountered in young adults; its incidence rises sharply in the sixth decade in women and the seventh in men. It is especially prevalent in postmenopausal women. One appealing hypothesis is that blood levels of estrogen are diminished in the postmenopausal state and cause hypersensitivity of the skeleton to the resorbing action of PTH (Heaney, 1974). Riggs *et al.* (1976) further suggest that this increased sensitivity of the skeleton leads to transient hypercalcemia which in turn elicits suppression of PTH; mild hypoparathyroidism has been reported in one study (Riggs *et al.*, 1976) but is not a universal finding. This reduction in PTH secretion is thought to lessen renal calcium conservation and curtail $1,25(OH)_2D$ biosynthesis. In at least in one population of patients with postmenopausal osteoporosis, the triad of increased skeletal resorption, hypercalciuria, and calcium malabsorption could occur and account for the bone disease. Gallagher *et al.* (1976), found plasma $1,25(OH)_2D$ to be significantly reduced by only about 10% from normal, age-matched controls. On the other hand, in another study of 26 women with crush fractures and postmenopausal osteoporosis, the circulating level of $1,25(OH)_2D$ was shown to be normal (Haussler *et al.*, 1979). These findings suggest that osteoporosis is not caused by a simple deficiency in the hormonal form of vitamin D but rather must result from a complex imbalance of the factors regulating bone metabolism. There may be a subtle aberration in vitamin D metabolism, and a recent report by Gallagher *et al.* (1978) indicates that estrogen therapy in postmenopausal osteoporosis can return the circulating level of $1,25(OH)_2D$ from mildly depressed to normal value.

Lund *et al.* (1975) reported an improvement in skeletal mineralization in elderly osteoporotic patients treated with $1\alpha(OH)D_3$. These investigations also found that $1,25(OH)_2D_3$ treatment increases calcium absorption in patients with osteoporosis. However, the fact that $1\alpha(OH)D_3$ or $1,25(OH)_2D_3$ increases urinary calcium excretion as well as absorption suggests that these metabolites may not be ideal therapy when used alone. The increase in intestinal calcium absorption without an increase in urinary calcium observed by Kanis *et al.* (1978) in normal subjects given 24,25$(OH)_2D_3$ raises the possibility that this latter sterol may be useful in osteoporosis.

7. *Diabetes*

Osteopenia was first described in association with diabetes mellitus by Albright and Reifenstein (1948). Later, diabetes was shown to coexist with osteoporosis (Berney, 1952), and this bone disease was judged to be clinically significant by the demonstration of a 22% incidence of hip fractures in a group of diabetic patients (Menczel *et al.*, 1972). Two recent studies using photon absorption (Levin *et al.*, 1976) and measures of cortical bone thickness (Santiago *et al.*, 1977) have confirmed and extended earlier conclusions. Levin *et al.* (1976) showed a significant loss of bone mass in both juvenile- and adult-onset diabetic patients and the decrease was already present in patients with diabetes of less

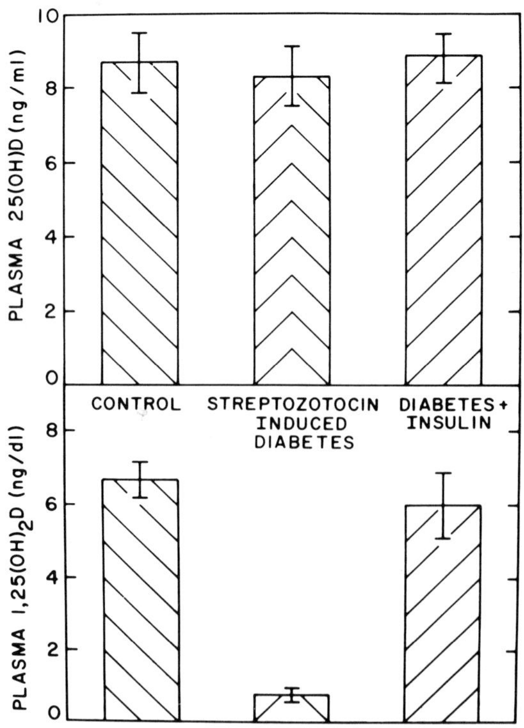

Fig. 13. Vitamin D metabolite levels in diabetic rats. Plasma 25(OH)D is unchanged by diabetes, but 1,25$(OH)_2D$ is strikingly suppressed in streptozotocin-induced diabetes. Insulin injection restores 1,25$(OH)_2D$ to normal in rats treated with streptozotocin. See Schneider *et al.* (1977a) for details. (From Haussler *et al.*, 1977c.)

than 5 years duration; osteopenia had a prevalence rate approaching 60%. In a study of 107 diabetic children, Santiago *et al.* (1977) reported that 25% of the cases displayed abnormally decreased cortical bone thickness. McNair *et al.* (1979) have recently shown a correlation between increased urinary calcium excretion and the incidence of mineral loss in diabetes mellitus. Urinary calcium and phosphorus loss correlated positively with both degree of hyperglycemia and glycosuria. Thus, osteopenia seems to be a common clinical finding in diabetic patients, but the cause of this derangement in bone metabolism is unknown. As detailed below, one likely possibility is that there exists an interference in vitamin D metabolism in diabetes.

Experiments in rats with streptozotocin-induced diabetes indicate that duodenal calcium absorption is depressed (Schneider *et al.*, 1977b), as is the level of intestinal CaBP (Schneider *et al.*, 1973). Correction of this defect in absorption can be achieved with exogenous 1,25$(OH)_2D_3$ but not with vitamin D_3 or 25$(OH)D_3$ (Schneider *et al.*, 1976). Of interest, as illustrated in Fig. 13, are direct measurements of circulating levels of 25(OH)D and 1,25$(OH)_2$D in diabetic rats that have shown that serum 1,25$(OH)_2$D is dramatically reduced in diabetic animals, while 25(OH)D remains normal (Schneider *et al.*, 1977a). Moreover, the depression in serum 1,25$(OH)_2$D (Fig. 13) and the observed decrease in intestinal calcium transport are completely reversible with insulin (Schneider *et al.*, 1977b). These data strongly suggest that renal 1α-

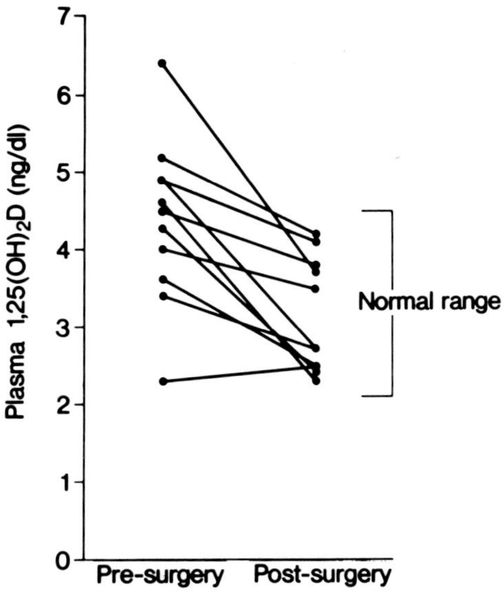

Fig. 14. Reduction of circulating 1,25$(OH)_2$D after surgical removal of adenoma in primary hyperparathyroidism. Post-surgery assays were performed 3–12 months after removal of the adenoma.

hydroxylation of 25(OH)D is impaired in diabetes and that a resulting deficiency in $1,25(OH)_2D$ may cause subnormal calcium absorption and inadequate bone mineralization. However, preliminary measurements of circulating $1,25(OH)_2D$ in human diabetics have failed to detect any significant depression in this hormone (Heath *et al.*, 1979; Haussler *et al.*, 1979).

8. *Osteomalacia and Mesenchymal Tumor*

Severe unexplained osteomalacia which remits after resection of an osseous or soft tissue tumor has been reported by a number of investigators (Salassa *et al.*, 1970; Olefsky *et al.*, 1972; Drezner and Feinglos, 1977). Giant cell tumors of bone have been present in 46% of the reported cases and a variety of mesenchymal tumors in the remainder. Biochemical features include marked hypophosphatemia and normal or slightly reduced serum calcium. Drezner and Feinglos (1977) recently showed that low serum $1,25(OH)_2D$ existed in one patient with a giant cell tumor of bone and with osteomalacia proved by biopsy. Since 25(OH)D was normal, it was suggested that the tumor or some factor elaborated by the neoplasm inhibited the renal formation of $1,25(OH)_2D$. Consistent with this notion is the fact that this patient responded to 1–3 μg/day of $1,25(OH)_2D_3$ by a resolution of the biochemical abnormalities and a healing of osteomalacia. Later excision of the tumor elicited effects similar to those produced by therapy with the vitamin D metabolite. Low circulating $1,25(OH)_2D$ has also recently been detected in hypophosphatemic osteomalacia associated with prostatic carcinoma (Lyles *et al.*, 1980). These findings raise the possibility that other adult cases of sporadic, hypophosphatemic rickets may be caused by interference in the 1α-hydroxylation of 25(OH)D in a fashion analogous to that noted in oncogenic osteomalacia.

E. Diseases with Excess 1,25-Dihydroxyvitamin D

1. *Primary Hyperparathyroidism*

As detailed earlier in this chapter, PTH has a profound positive influence on the renal activation of vitamin D. Patients with primary hyperparathyroidism frequently display enhanced intestinal calcium absorption (Kaplan *et al.*, 1977). Several laboratories (Haussler *et al.*, 1976; Kaplan *et al.*, 1977; Gray *et al.*, 1977) have demonstrated that plasma levels of $1,25(OH)_2D$ are above normal in most patients with primary hyperparathyroidism (Fig. 8). Additional results in primary hyperparathyroidism (Kaplan *et al.*, 1977) indicate that increased levels of $1,25(OH)_2D$ are correlated with increased calcium absorption. Moreover, in a recent study of ten patients with primary hyperparathyroidism (Bone *et al.*, 1979), it was found that circulating $1,25(OH)_2D$ fell in nine of the ten cases following surgery, and only the patient with the lowest level of $1,25(OH)_2D$

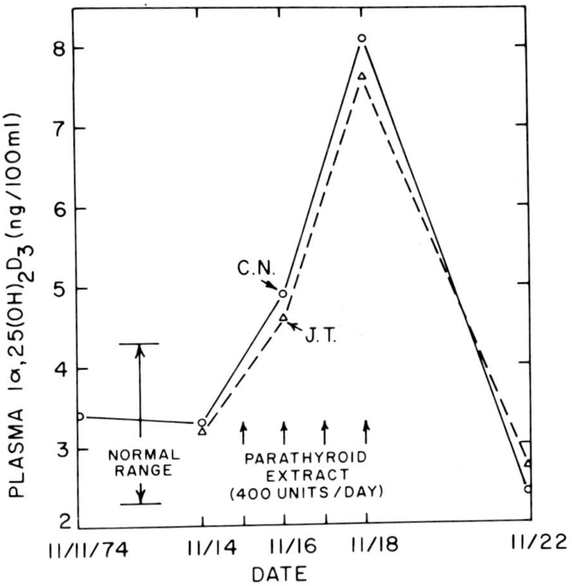

Fig. 15. Enhancement of plasma 1,25(OH)$_2$D in two normal humans given 400 units of parathyroid extract (Lily) for 4 days. Note the sharp increase in 1,25(OH)$_2$D after administration of parathyroid extract and the rapid return to normal after cessation of dosing. Experiments were carried out by C. Y. C. Pak and M. R. Haussler (From Haussler *et al.,* 1975.)

failed to show a reduction in the sterol (Fig. 14). Conversely, Fig. 15 shows results in two normal humans given PTH. There is a clear increase plasma 1,25(OH)$_2$D within 24 hr and two- to threefold enhancement in 1,25(OH)$_2$D by 72 hr. These data confirm that PTH elevates 1,25(OH)$_2$D in humans as it does in experimental animals and provide a model to approximate primary hyperparathyroidism. The exact clinical significance of elevated 1,25(OH)$_2$D in primary hyperparathyroidism is not known, but it is probable that intestinal hyperabsorption of calcium contributes to the hypercalcemia, hypercalciuria, and nephrolithiasis occurring in this disorder.

Hypophosphatemia is frequently observed in primary hyperparathyroidism, and the relative roles of low serum phosphorus and elevated levels of PTH in stimulating the production of 1,25(OH)$_2$D$_3$ are unclear. Most reports suggest that plasma 25(OH)D levels are normal, while levels of 24,25(OH)$_2$D are elevated, perhaps attributable to the effect of elevated levels of 1,25(OH)$_2$D on 24-OHase activity. It is intriguing to speculate that the vitamin D status of a patient may play a role in the clinical expression of primary hyperparathyroidism, possibly explaining why some patients tend to have metabolic bone disease (osteitis fibrosa cystica) while others manifest nephrolithiasis. Indeed, in patients with osteomalacia accompanying primary normocalcemic hyperparathyroidism treatment with vitamin D has been reported to lead to overt hypercalcemia; this may constitute a provocative test for this disorder.

2. *Idiopathic Hypercalciuria*

Thirty percent of all patients with recurrent renal calcium stones have excessive urinary calcium excretion (Rose and Harrision, 1944). Primary hyperparathyroidism accounts for only a small number of these patients. Because no other causes have been identified, the disease has been termed "idiopathic hypercalciuria." Two important early observations in this disease state were the presence of intestinal hyperabsorption of calcium and of hypophosphatemia (Albright *et al.,* 1953; Pak *et al.,* 1974). The role of disordered PTH metabolism in this disorder has been controversial. Coe and Kavalach (1974) found that PTH was elevated in 27 out of 40 patients studied, but others have reported that PTH is low or normal in most cases (Pak *et al.,* 1974; Shen *et al.,* 1977a).

This conflict can be partially resolved by dividing idiopathic hypercalciuria into two categories, and a simple test for the differential diagnosis of the hypercalciurias has been described (Pak *et al.,* 1975). The first of these, termed renal hypercalciuria, involves a primary leak of calcium into the urine, secondary hyperparathyroidism, and, at least in preliminary measurements (Kaplan *et al.,* 1977), elevated circulating 1,25$(OH)_2$D. The cause of calcium wasting by the kidney is unknown. The second kind of idiopathic hypercalciuria, designated absorptive hypercalciuria, is characterized by normal or low PTH, accompanied by a striking enhancement of intestinal calcium absorption. Hyperabsorption of calcium may result from either increased circulating 1,25$(OH)_2$D or from an intestinal lesion, per se. From recent measurements of 1,25$(OH)_2$D in 40 cases of absorptive hypercalciuria (Fig. 8), it is evident that the entire population of patients displays a significant elevation of circulating 1,25-$(OH)_2$D; but two subpopulations can be distinguished, one having a range coincident with the normal subjects and the other having 1,25$(OH)_2$D level above 5 ng/dl in all cases. The former group, having normal circulating 1,25$(OH)_2$D but enhanced calcium absorption, probably have a defect at the level of the intestine which is manifested as hyperabsorption of calcium. The second group has strikingly increased 1,25$(OH)_2$D concentrations, which account for their hyperabsorption of calcium. The cause of the 1,25$(OH)_2$D increase in this subpopulation is unknown, but it does not appear to be elevated PTH. One clue is their hypophosphatemia, a known stimulator of 1,25$(OH)_2$D production in experimental animals. A current hypothesis for the etiology of this type of idiopathic hypercalciuria is that the primary lesion is an unexplained phosphate leak at the kidney (Shen *et al.,* 1977b; Gray *et al.,* 1977). The resulting hypophosphatemia then stimulates the production of 1,25$(OH)_2$D and an augmented intestinal calcium absorption occurs. Either a transient increase in blood calcium or enhanced circulating 1,25$(OH)_2$D, or both, may then feedback inhibit the secretion of PTH to cause relative hypoparathyroidism. The combination of aberrantly high plasma 1,25$(OH)_2$D, and low PTH creates an ideal situation for stimulated absorption of calcium from the intestine and decreased renal tubular reabsorption of calcium—all of which may result in hypercalciuria and renal stone disease. The data of Gray *et al.* (1977), showing increased 1,25$(OH)_2$D in hypophosphatemic patients with idiopathic hypercalciuria, plus a correlation between serum phosphate and 1,25$(OH)_2$D, provide excellent support for the above theory. Furthermore, the concept has been substantiated by Shen *et al.* (1977b) and Van Den Berg *et al.* (1980), who reported that oral phosphate therapy, which would be expected to counteract the original hypophosphatemic signal, reduces urinary calcium excretion and circulating 1,25$(OH)_2$D while enhancing PTH. Therefore, therapeutic measures to reduce circulating 1,25$(OH)_2$D may be one approach to treatment of this type of idopathic hypercalciuria.

However, alternate views of the pathogenesis of idopathic hypercalciuria have been presented by Barilla *et al.* (1979), who favor the primacy of intestinal hyperabsorption of calcium over any effect of hypophosphatemia and increased 1,25$(OH)_2$D, and by Maggio *et al.* (1979), who provide an excellent summary of the various possible causes of this disorder.

F. Possible End-Organ Defects in the Expression of Vitamin D

Theoretically, end-organ aberrations in the response to vitamin D or 1,25$(OH)_2$D could be either in the form of under-responsiveness or abnormal sensitivity. In terms of phosphate metabolism, X-linked hypophosphatemia could be classified as an end-organ defect because of the proposed deletion of a phosphate transport system which may be thought to respond normally to 1,25$(OH)_2$D. Other hyporesponsive states could be anticonvulsant-induced osteomalacia or steroid-induced osteopenia, where intestine and bone calcium translocation are affected by the drugs and where this is not corrected by endogenous 1,25$(OH)_2$D. Several patients with an end-organ defect in the response to 1,25$(OH)_2$D have been identified (Brooks *et al.*, 1978; Marx *et al.*, 1978). Brooks *et al.* (1978) have named this disease "vitamin D-dependent rickets, Type II." A 22-year-old woman was found with hypocalcemia, osteomalacia, and secondary hyperparathyroidism, with accompanying osteitis fibrosa, all despite the presence of elevated serum levels of 1,25$(OH)_2$D (Brooks *et al.*, 1978). The administration of a large dose of vitamin D corrected the hypocalcemia, but the circulating 1,25$(OH)_2$D rose to a value almost 10 times normal. Thus, unlike classic vitamin D-dependent rickets (Type I), where the defect lies in the renal production of 1,25$(OH)_2$D, in type II disease there appears to be an abnormality in the end-organ responsiveness to 1,25$(OH)_2$D.

A number of yet uncharacterized hypercalcemic maladies could involve an exaggerated sensitivity of the gut and/or bone to vitamin D metabolites. As discussed above, one type of absorptive hypercalciuria, where the serum level of 1,25$(OH)_2D$ is normal, might be such a lesion. Patients with sarcoidosis often display hyperabsorption of calcium, hypercalciuria and (sometimes) hypercalcemia. Although hypersensitivity to vitamin D has been implicated in this condition, Bell *et al.* (1979) have now shown elevated circulating levels of 1,25$(OH)_2D_3$ in some patients with sarcoidosis. Other end-organ aberrations in the action of vitamin D are not known at present, but when *in vitro* receptor measurements and cell culture assays become commonplace, more target organ defects in the vitamin D system are likely to be identified.

VII. CONCLUSIONS

Vitamin D is now known to be metabolized to a number of hydroxylated derivatives. Of paramount importance is the production of 1,25$(OH)_2D$, the hormonal form of vitamin D. In the kidney there occurs an interplay between PTH and phosphate and possibly other factors to adjust the output of 1,25$(OH)_2D$. Once in the blood, the 1,25$(OH)_2D$ hormone travels to target organs, such as intestine and bone, where it acts to induce the biosynthesis of new proteins that in turn alter cellular function.

Identification of binding and receptor proteins has led to the development of clinically important assays for vitamin D metabolities. An understanding of the metabolism of vitamin D and its regulation has yielded exciting new insights into diseases of mineral metabolism. A number of clinical syndromes in which aberrations in the metabolism or action of vitamin D are implicated, have been identified. Various vitamin D sterols have been applied therapeutically. Native vitamin D still represents the therapy of choice in simple vitamin D-deficiency rickets, because its subsequent activation is exquisitely regulated. We now understand several of the vitamin D-resistant osteopenic states, and synthetically produced metabolites appropriate to the inferred enzyme block in vitamin D metabolism have been administered with substantial success.

REFERENCES

Aaron, J. E., Gallagher, J. C., and Nordin, B. E. C. (1974). Seasonal variation of histological osteomalacia in femoral-neck fractures. *Lancet* **2,** 84–85.

Adams, T. H., and Norman, A. W. (1970). Studies on the mechanism of action of calciferol. *J. Biol. Chem.* **245,** 4421–4431.

Albright, F., and Reifenstein, E. C. (1948). "Parathyroid Gland and Metabolic Bone Disease," p. 150. Williams & Wilkins, Baltimore, Maryland.

Albright, F., Burnett, C. H., Smith, P. S., and Parson, W. (1942). Pseudo-hypoparathyroidism—an example of 'Seabright-Bantam Syndrome.' *Endocrinology (Baltimore)* **30,** 922–932.

Albright, F., Henneman, P. H., Benedict, P. H., and Forbes, A. P. (1953). Idiopathic hypercalciuria. *Proc. R. Soc. Med.* **46,** 1077–1081.

Arnaud, C., Glorieux, F., and Scriver, C. R. (1971). Serum parathyroid hormone in X-linked hypophosphatemia. *Science* **173,** 845–847.

Arnaud, S. B., Goldsmith, R. S., Lambert, P. W., and Go, V. L. W. (1975). 25-hydroxyvitamin D_3: Evidence of an enterohepatic circulation in man (38853). *Proc. Soc. Exp. Biol. Med.* **149,** 570–572.

Arnaud, S. B., Newcomer, A. D., and Go, V. L. W. (1976a). Hypomagnesemia (↓ Mg) and vitamin D deficiency (−D) in patients with nontropical sprue (NTS). *Clin. Res.* **24,** 564A.

Arnaud, S. B., Stickler, G. B., and Haworth, J. C. (1976b). Serum 25-hydroxyvitamin D in infantile rickets. *Pediatrics* **57,** 221–225.

Arnaud, S. B., Newcomer, A. D., Dickson, E. R., Arnaud, C. D., and Go, V. L. W. (1976c). Altered mineral metabolism in patients with gastrointestinal diseases. *Gastroenterology* **70,** 860.

Arnaud, S. B., Matthusen, M., Gilkinson, J. B., and Goldsmith, R. S. (1977). Components of 25-hydroxyvitamin D in serum of young children in upper midwestern United States. *Am. J. Clin. Nutr.* **30,** 1082–1086.

Au, W. Y. W., and Bukowski, A. (1976). Inhibition of PTH secretion by vitamin D metabolites in organ cultures of rat parathyroids. *Fed. Proc., Fed. Am. Soc. Exp. Biol.* **35,** 301.

Baksi, S. N., and Kenny, A. D. (1977). Vitamin D_3 metabolism in immature Japanese quail: Effects of ovarian hormones. *Endocrinology (Baltimore)* **101,** 1216–1220.

Baksi, S. N., and Kenny, A. D. (1978). Does estradiol simulate in vivo production of 1,25-dihydroxyvitamin D_3 in the rat? *Life Sci.* **22,** 787–792.

Balsan, S., Garabedian, M., Sorgniard, R., Holick, M. F., and DeLuca, H. F. (1975). 1,25-Dihydroxyvitamin D_3 and 1α-hydroxyvitamin D_3 in children: Biologic and therapeutic effects in nutritional rickets and different types of vitamin D resistance. *Pediatr. Res.* **9,** 586–593.

Barilla, D. E., Zerwekh, J. E., and Pak, C. Y. C. (1979). A critical evaluation of the role of phosphate in the pathogenesis of absorptive hypercalciuria. *Miner. Electrolyte Metab.* **2,** 302–309.

Barragry, J. M., Carter, N. D., Beer, M., France, M. W., Auton, J. A., and Boucher, B. J. (1977). Vitamin D metabolism in nephrotic syndrome. *Lancet* **2,** 629–632.

Baxter, L. A., and DeLuca, H. F. (1976). Stimulation of 25-hydroxyvitamin D_3-1α-hydroxylase by phosphate depletion. *J. Biol. Chem.* **251,** 3158–3161.

Bell, N. H., Stern, P. H., Pantzer, E., Sinha, T. K., and DeLuca, H. F. (1979). Evidence that increased circulating 1,25-dihydroxyvitamin D is the probable cause for abnormal calcium metabolism in sarcoidosis. *J. Clin. Invest.* **64,** 218–225.

Belsey, R. E., DeLuca, H. F., and Potts, J. T., Jr. (1971). Competitive binding assay for vitamin D and 25-OH vitamin D. *J. Clin. Endocrinol. Metab.* **33,** 554–557.

Belsey, R. E., DeLuca, H. F., and Potts, J. T., Jr. (1974). A rapid assay for 25-OH-vitamin D_3 without preparative chromatography. *J. Clin. Endocrinol. Metab.* **38,** 1046–1051.

Berney, P. W. (1952). Osteoporosis and diabetes mellitus. *J. Iowa Med. Soc.* **42,** 10–12.

Bhattacharyya, M. H., and DeLuca, H. F. (1974). Subcellular location of rat liver calciferol-25-hydroxylase. *Arch. Biochem. Biophys.* **160,** 58–62.

Bilezikian, J. P., Canfield, R. E., Jacobs, T. P., Polay, J. S., D'Adams, A. P., Eisman, J. A. and DeLuca, H. F. (1978). Response of 1α-25-dihydroxyvitamin D_3 to hypocalcemia in human subjects. *N. Engl. J. Med.* **299,** 437–441.

Birge, S. J., and Haddad, J. G. (1975). 25-hydroxycholecalciferol stimulation of muscle metabolism. *J. Clin. Invest.* **56,** 1100–1107.

Björkhem, I., and Holmberg, I. (1976). A novel specific assay of 25-hydroxyvitamin D_3. *Clin. Chim. Acta* **68,** 215–221.

Boass, A., Toverud, S. U., McCain, T. A., Pike, J. W., and Haussler, M. R. (1977). Elevated serum levels of 1α,25-dihydroxycholecalciferol in lactating rats. *Nature (London)* **267,** 630–632.

Bone, H. G., Zerwekh, J. E., Haussler, M. R., and Pak, C. Y. C. (1979). Effect of parathyroidectomy on serum 1,25-dihydroxyvitamin D and intestinal calcium absorption in primary hyperparathyroidism. *J. Clin. Endocrinol. Metab.* **48,** 877–879.

Bonjour, J. P., Preston, C., and Fleisch, H. (1977). Effects of 1,25-dihydroxyvitamin D_3 on the renal handling of Pi in thyroparathyroidectomized rats. *J. Clin. Invest.* **60,** 1419–1428.

Booth, B. E., Tsai, H. C., and Morris, R. C., Jr. (1977). Parathyroidectomy reduces 25-hydroxyvitamin D_3-1α-hydroxylase activity in the hypocalcemic vitamin D-deficient chick. *J. Clin. Invest.* **60,** 1314–1320.

Bordier, P. J., Chot, S. Tun, Eastwood, J. B., Fournier, A., and de Wardener, H. E. (1973). Lack of histological evidence of vitamin D abnormality in the bones of anephric patients *Clin. Sci.* **44,** 33–41.

Bordier, P. J., Pechet, M. M., Hesse, R., Marie, P., and Rasmussen, H. (1974). Response of adult patients with osteomalacia to treatment with crystalline 1α-hydroxyvitamin D_3. *N. Engl. J. Med.* **291,** 866–871.

Bordier, P. J., Rasmussen, H., Marie, P., Miravet, L., Guéris, J., and Ryckwaert, A. (1978). Vitamin D metabolites and bone mineralization in man. *J. Clin. Endocrinol. Metab.* **46,** 284–294.

Boris, A., Hurley, J. F., and Trmal, T. (1977). Relative activities of some metabolites and analogs of cholecalciferol in stimulation of tibia ash weight in chicks otherwise deprived of vitamin D. *J. Nutr.* **107,** 194–198.

Bouillon, R., van Baelen, H., Bombauts, W., and de Moor, P. (1976). The purification and characterization of the human-serum binding protein for the 25-hydroxycholecalciferol (transcalciferin). *Eur. J. Biochem.* **66,** 285–291.

Boyle, I. T., Gray, R. W., and DeLuca, H. F. (1971). Regulation by calcium of *in vivo* synthesis of 1,25-dihydroxycholecalciferol and 21,25-dihydroxycholecalciferol. *Proc. Natl. Acad. Sci. U.S.A.* **68,** 2131–2134.

Brewer, E. D., Tsai, H. C., and Morris, R. C. (1976). Evidence for impairment of metabolism of 25-hydroxyvitamin D_3 in children with Fanconi syndrome. *Clin. Res.* **24,** 154A.

Brewer, E. D., Tsai, H. C., Szeto, K.-S., and Morris, R. C., Jr. (1977a). Maleic acid impaired conversion of $25(OH)D_3$ to $1,25\text{-}(OH)_2D_3$: implications for Fanconi's syndrome. *Kidney Int.* **12,** 244–252.

Brewer, E. D., Tsai, H., and Morris, R. C. (1977b). Fanconi syndrome and its relationship to vitamin D. *In* "Vitamin D: Biochemical, Chemical and Clinical Aspects Related to Calcium Metabolism" (A. W. Norman, K. Schaefer, J. W. Coburn, H. F. DeLuca, D. Fraser, H. G. Grigoleit, and D. von Herrath, eds.), pp. 937–949. de Gruyter, Berlin.

Brickman, A. S., Coburn, J. W., and Norman, A. W. (1972). Action of 1,25-dihydroxycholecalciferol, a potent kidney-produced metabolite of vitamin D_3, in uremic man. *N. Engl. J. Med.* **287,** 891–895.

Brickman, A. S., Coburn, J. W., Kurokawa, K., Bethune, J. E., Harrison, H. E., and Norman, A. W. (1973). Action of 1,25-dihydroxycholecalciferol in patients with hypophosphatemic, vitamin D-resistant rickets. *N. Engl. J. Med.* **289,** 495–498.

Brickman, A. S., Sherrard, D. J., Jowsey, J., Singer, F. R., Baylink, D. J., Malone, N., Massry, S. G., Norman, A. W., and Coburn, J. W. (1974). 1,25-Dihydroxycholecalciferol, effect on skeletal lesions and plasma parathyroid hormone levels in uremic osteodystrophy. *Arch. Intern. Med.* **134,** 883–888.

Brickman, A. S., Coburn, J. W., Friedman, G. R., Okamura, W. H., Massry, S. G., and Norman, A. W. (1976). Comparison of effects of 1α-hydroxy-vitamin D_3 and 1,25-dihydroxy-vitamin D_3 in man. *J. Clin. Invest.* **57,** 1540–1547.

Brickman, A. S., Norman, A. W., and Coburn, J. W. (1977). Vitamin D and pseudohypoparathyroidism. *In* "Vitamin D: Biochemical, Chemical and Clinical Aspects Related to Calcium Metabolism" (A. W. Norman, K. Schaefer, J. W. Coburn, H. F. DeLuca, D. Fraser, H. G. Grigoleit, and D. von Herrath, eds.), pp. 867–876. de Gruyter, Berlin.

Brickman, A. S., Coburn, J. W., Sherrard, D. J., Wong, E. G. C., Norman, A. W., and Singer, F. R. (1980). Clinical effects of 1,25-dihydroxy-vitamin D_3 in uremic patients with overt osteodystrophy. *In* "Contributions to Nephrology" (J. W. Coburn and S. G. Massry, eds.), Vol. 18, pp. 29–41. Karger, Basel.

Brooks, M. H., Bell, N. H., Love, L., Stern, P. H., Orfei, E., Queener, S. F., Hamstra, A. J., and DeLuca, H. F. (1978). Vitamin D-dependent rickets type II-resistance of target organs to 1,25-dihydroxyvitamin D. *N. Engl. J. Med.* **298,** 996–999.

Brumbaugh, P. F., and Haussler, M. R. (1973). 1α-25-dihydroxyvitamin D_3 receptor: Competitive binding of vitamin D analogs. *Life Sci.* **13,** 1737–1746.

Brumbaugh, P. F., and Haussler, M. R. (1974a). 1α,25-dihydroxycholecalciferol receptors in intestine (I) Association of 1α,25-dihydroxycholecalciferol with intestinal mucosa chromatin. *J. Biol. Chem.* **249,** 1251–1257.

Brumbaugh, P. F., and Haussler, M. R. (1974b). 1α,25-dihydroxycholecalciferol receptors in intestine (II) Temperature dependent transfer of the hormone to chromatin via a specific cytosol receptor. *J. Biol. Chem.* **249,** 1258–1262.

Brumbaugh, P. F., and Haussler, M. R. (1975). Specific binding of 1α-25-dihydroxycholecalciferol to nuclear components of chick intestine. *J Biol. Chem.* **250,** 1588–1594.

Brumbaugh, P. F., Haussler, D. H., Bressler, R., and Haussler, M. R. (1974a). Radioreceptor assay for 1α,25-dihydroxyvitamin D_3. *Science* **183,** 1089–1091.

Brumbaugh, P. F., Haussler, D. H., Bursac, K. M., and Haussler, M. R. (1974b). Filter assay for 1α,25-dihydroxyvitamin D_3. Utilization of the hormone's target tissue chromatin receptor. *Biochemistry* **13,** 4091–4097.

Brumbaugh, P. F., Hughes, M. R., and Haussler, M. R. (1975). Cytoplasmic and nuclear binding components for 1α,25-dihydroxyvitamin D_3 in chick parathyroid glands. *Proc. Natl. Acad. Sci. U.S.A.* **72,** 4871–4875.

Buckley, M., and Bronner, F. (1980). Calcium-binding protein biosynthesis in the rat: Regulation by calcium and 1,25-dihydroxyvitamin D_3. *Arch. Biochem. Biophys.* **202,** 235–241.

Burnatowsky, M. A., Harris, C. A., Sutton, R. A. L., and Seely, J. F. (1977). Effects of $1,25(OH)_2D_3$ on Ca, Mg and Pi excretion in the hamster. *Abstr. Book Am. Soc. Nephrol.* p. 2A.

Caldas, A. E., Gray, R. W., and Lemann, J., Jr. (1978). The simultaneous measurement of vitamin D metabolites in plasma: Studies in healthy adults and in patients with calcium nephrolithiasis. *J. Lab. Clin. Med.* **91,** 840–849.

Canterbury, J. M., Lerman, S., Claflin, A. J., Henry, H., Norman, A., and Reiss, E. (1978). Inhibition of parathyroid hormone secretion by 25-hydroxycholecalciferol and 24,25-dihydroxycholecalciferol in the dog. *J. Clin. Invest.* **61,** 1375–1383.

Care, A. D., Bates, R. F. L., Pickard, D. W., Peacock, M., Tomlinson, S., O'Riordan, J. L. H., Mawer, E. B., Taylor, C. M., DeLuca, H. F., and Norman, A. W. (1976). The effects of vitamin D metabolites and their analogues on the secretion of parathyroid hormone. *Calcif. Tissue Res.* **21,** Suppl., 142–146.

Catto, G. R. D., MacLeod, M., Pelc, B., and Kodicek, E. (1975). 1α-Hydroxycholecalciferol: a treatment for renal bone disease. *Br. Med. J.* **1,** 12–14.

Chandler, J. S., Pike, J. W., and Haussler, M. R. (1979). 1,25-Dihydroxyvitamin D_3 receptors in rat kidney cytosol. *Biochem. Biophys. Res. Commun.* **90,** 1057–1063.

Chase, L. R., Melson, G. L., and Aurbach, G. D. (1969). Pseudohypoparathyroidism: Defective excretion of 3′,5′-AMP in response to parathyroid hormone. *J. Clin. Invest.* **48,** 1832–1844.

Chen, T. C., and DeLuca, H. F. (1973). Stimulation of [^{3}H]uridine incorporation into nuclear RNA of rat kidney by vitamin D metabolities. *Arch. Biochem. Biophys.* **156,** 321–327.

Chertow, B. S., Baylink, D. J., Wergedal, J. E., Su, M. H. H., and Norman, A. W. (1975). Decrease in serum immunoreactive parathyroid hormone in rats and in parathyroid hormone secretion in vitro by 1,25-dihydroxycholecalciferol. *J. Clin. Invest.* **56,** 668–678.

Chesney, R. W., Horowitz, S. D., Kream, B. E., Eisman, J. A., Hong, R., and DeLuca, H. F. (1977). Failure of conventional doses of 1α-25-dihydroxycholecalciferol to correct hypocalcemia in a girl with idiopathic hypoparathyroidism. *N. Engl. J. Med.* **297,** 1272–1275.

Clemens, T. L., Hendy, G. N., Graham, R. F., Baggiolini, E. G., Uskoković, M. R., and O'Riordan, J. L. H. (1978). A radioimmunoassay for 1,25-dihydroxycholecalciferol. *Clin. Sci. Mol. Med.* **54,** 329–332.

Cloix, J. F., Ulmann, A., Bachelet, M., and Funck-Brentano, J. L. (1976). Cholecalciferol metabolites binding in porcine parathyroid glands. *Steroids* **28,** 743–749.

Coburn, J. W. (1980). Renal osteodystrophy. *Kidney Int.* **17,** 677–693.

Coburn, J. W., Koppel, M. H., Brinkman, A. S., and Massry, S. G. (1973). Study of intestinal absorption of calcium in patients with renal failure. *Kidney Int.* **3,** 264–272.

Coburn, J. W., Brickman, A. S., Llach, F., Kurokawa, K., Canterbury, J., Riess, E., and Norman, A. W. (1975). Acute actions of 1,25-dihydroxyvitamin D_3 on calcium and parathyroid hormone in normal man. *Clin. Res.* **23,** 134a.

Coburn, J. W., Sherrard, D. J., Brickman, A. S., Wong, E. G. C., Norman, A. W., and Singer, F. R. (1979). A skeletal mineralizing defect in dialysis patients; a syndrome resembling osteomalacia but unrelated to vitamin D. *In* "Contribution to Nephrology" (J. W. Coburn and S. G. Massry, eds.), Vol. 18, pp. 172–183. Karger, Basel.

Coe, F. L., and Kavalach, A. G. (1974). Hypercalciuria and hyperuricosuria in patients with calcium nephrolithiasis. *N. Engl. J. Med.* **291,** 1344–1350.

Colston, K. W., Evans, I. M. A., Spelsberg, T. C., and MacIntyre, I. (1977). Feedback regulation of vitamin D metabolism by 1,25-dihydroxycholecalciferol. *Biochem. J.* **164,** 83–89.

Compston, J. E., and Thompson, R. P. H. (1977). Intestinal absorption of 25-hydroxyvitamin D and osteomalacia in primary biliary cirrhosis. *Lancet* **1,** 721–724.

Compston, J. E., Ayers, A. B., Horton, L. W. L., Tighe, J. R., and Creamer, B. (1978a). Osteomalacia after small intestinal resection. *Lancet* **1,** 9–12.

Compston, J. E., Horton, L. W. L., Laker, M. F., Ayers, A. B., Woodhead, J. S., Bull, H. J., Gazet, J. C., and Pilkington, T. R. E. (1978b). Bone disease after jejuno-ileal bypass for obesity. *Lancet* **2,** 1–7.

Cork, D. J., Haussler, M. R., Pitt, M. J., Rizzardo, E., Hesse, R. H., and Pechet, M. M. (1974). 1α-hydroxyvitamin D_3: A synthetic sterol which is highly active in preventing rickets in the chick. *Endocrinology (Baltimore)* **94,** 1337–1345.

Corradino, R. A. (1973). 1,25-dihydroxycholecalciferol: Inhibition of action in organ-cultured intestine by actinomycin D and α-amanitin. *Nature (London)* **243,** 41–43.

Corradino, R. A. (1976). Diphenylhydantoin: Direct inhibition of the vitamin D_3-mediated calcium absorptive mechanism in organ-cultured duodenum. *Biochem. Pharmacol.* **25,** 863–864.

Corradino, R. A., Fullmer, C. S., and Wasserman, R. H. (1976). Embryonic chick intestine in organ culture: Stimulation of calcium transport by exogenous vitamin D-induced calcium-binding protein. *Arch. Biochem. Biophys.* **174,** 738–743.

Corvol, M. T., Dumontier, M. F., Garabedian, M., and Rappaport, R. (1978). Vitamin D and cartilage. II. Biological activity of 25-hydroxycholecalciferol and 24,25- and 1,25-

dihydroxycholecalciferol on cultured growth plate chondrocytes. *Endocrinology (Baltimore)* **102,** 1269–1274.

Coty, W. A. (1980). A specific, high affinity binding protein for 1,25-dihydroxy vitamin D in the chick oviduct shell gland. *Biochem. Biophys. Res. Commun.* **93,** 285–292.

Counts, S. J., Baylink, D. J., Shen, F.-H., Sherrard, D. J., and Hickman, R. O. (1975). Vitamin D intoxication in an anephric child. *Ann. Intern. Med.* **82,** 196–200.

David, L., and Anast, C. (1974). Calcium metabolism in newborn infants. *J. Clin. Invest.* **54,** 287–296.

Davie, M. W. J., Chalmers, T. M., Hunter, J. O., Pelc, B., and Kodicek, E. (1976). 1-Alpha-hydroxycholecalciferol in chronic renal failure. *Ann. Intern. Med.* **84,** 281–285.

DeLuca, H. F. (1971). The role of vitamin D and its relationship to parathyroid hormone and calcitonin. *Recent Prog. Horm. Res.* **27,** 479–516.

DeLuca, H. F. (1976). Recent advances in our understanding of the metabolism of vitamin D and its regulation. *Clin. Endocrinol. (Oxford)* **5,** Suppl., 97s–108s.

DeLuca, H. F. (1978). Vitamin D metabolism and function. *Arch. Intern. Med.* **138,** 836–847.

DeLuca, H. F., and Schnoes, H. K. (1976). Metabolism and mechanism of action of vitamin D. *Annu. Rev. Biochem.* **45,** 631–666.

Dietel, M., Dorn, G., Montz, R., and Altenahr, E. (1979). Influence of vitamin D_3, 1,25-dihydroxyvitamin D_3, and 24,25-dihydroxyvitamin D_3 on parathyroid hormone secretion, adenosine 3′,5′-monophosphate release, and ultrastructure of parathyroid glands in organ culture. *Endocrinology (Baltimore)* **105,** 237–245.

Drezner, M. K., and Feinglos, M. N. (1977). Osteomalacia due to 1α-25-dihydroxycholecalciferol deficiency. *J. Clin. Invest.* **60,** 1046–1053.

Drezner, M. K., and Haussler, M. R. (1978). Normocalcemic pseudohypoparathyroidism: association with normal vitamin D_3 metabolism. *Am. J. Med.* **66,** 503–508.

Drezner, M. K., Neelon, F. A., Haussler, M. R., McPherson, H. T., and Lebovitz, H. E. (1976). 1,25-dihydroxycholecalciferol deficiency: The probable cause of hypocalcemia and metabolic bone disease in pseudohypoparathyroidism. *Clin. Endocrinol. Metab.* **42,** 621–628.

Drezner, M. K., Neelon, F. A., Jowsey, J., and Lebovitz, H. E. (1977). Hypoparathyroidism: a possible cause of osteomalacia. *J. Clin. Endocrinol. Metab.* **45,** 114–122.

Drezner, M. K., Lyles, K. W., Haussler, M. R., and Harrelson, J. M. (1980). Evaluation of a role of 1-25-dihydroxyvitamin D_3 in the pathogenesis and treatment of X-linked hypophosphatemic rickets and osteomalacia. *J. Clin. Invest.* **66,** 1020–1032.

Eastwood, J. B., Harris, E., Stamp, T. C. B., and deWardener, H. E. (1976). Vitamin D-deficiency in the osteomalacia of chronic renal failure. *Lancet* **2,** 1209–1211.

Eastwood, J. B., Stamp, T. C. B., de Wardener, H. E., Bordier, P. J., and Arnaud, C. D. (1977). The effect of 25-hydroxy vitamin D_3 in the osteomalacia of chronic renal failure. *Clin. Sci. Mol. Med.* **52,** 499–508.

Eastwood, J. B., de Wardener, H. E., Gray, R. W., and Lemann, J. L., Jr. (1979). Normal plasma $1,25(OH)_2$ vitamin D concentrations in nutritional osteomalacia. *Lancet* **1,** 1377–1378.

Eisman, J. A., Hamstra, A. J., Kream, B. A., and DeLuca, H. F. (1976). A sensitive precise and convenient method for determination of 1,25-dihydroxyvitamin D in human plasma. *Arch. Biochem. Biophys.* **176,** 235–243.

Eisman, J. A., MacIntyre, I., Martin, T. J., Frampton, R. M., and King, R. J. B. (1980). Normal and malignant breast tissue is a target organ for $1,25\text{-}(OH)_2$ vitamin D_3. *Clin. Endocrinol. (Oxford)* **13,** 267–272.

Endo, H., Kiyoki, M., Kawashima, K., Naruchi, T., and Hashimoto, Y. (1980). Vitamin D_3 metabolites and PTH synergistically stimulate bone formation of chick embryonic femur *in vitro*. *Nature (London)* **286,** 262–264.

Fraser, D. R., and Kodicek, E. (1970). Unique biosynthesis by kidney of a biologically active vitamin D metabolite. *Nature (London)* **228,** 764–766.

Fraser, D., Kooh, S. W., Kind, H. P., Holick, M. F., Tanaka, Y., and DeLuca, H. F. (1973). Pathogenesis of hereditary vitamin D-dependent rickets. *N. Engl. J. Med.* **289,** 817–822.

Freund, T., and Bronner, F. (1975a). Regulation of intestinal calcium-binding protein by calcium intake in the rat. *Am. J. Physiol.* **228,** 861–869.

Freund, T., and Bronner, F. (1975b). Stimulation in vitro by 1,25-dihydroxyvitamin D_3 of intestinal cell calcium uptake and calcium-binding protein. *Science* **190,** 1300–1302.

Friedlander, E. J., and Norman, A. W. (1975). Studies on the metabolism of Calciferol XII. Production *in vitro* of 1,24,25-$(OH)_3$-vitamin D_3 and a search for its occurrence *in vivo*. *Arch. Biochem. Biophys.* **170,** 731–738.

Galante, L., Colston, K. W., Evans, I. M. A., Byfield, P. G. H., Matthews, E. W., and MacIntyre, I. (1973). The regulation of vitamin D metabolism. *Nature (London)* **244,** 438–440.

Gallagher, J. C., Riggs, B. L., Eisman, J., Arnaud, S. B., and DeLuca, H. F. (1976). Impaired production of 1,25-dihydroxyvitamin D in postmenopausal osteoporosis. *Clin. Res.* **24,** 580A.

Gallagher, J. C., Riggs, B. L., Hamstra, A., and DeLuca, H. F. (1978). Effect of estrogen therapy on calcium absorption and vitamin D metabolism in postmenopausal osteoporosis. *Clin. Res.* **26,** 32A.

Garabedian, M., Holick, M. F., DeLuca, H. F., and Boyle, I. T. (1972). Control of 25-hydroxycholecalciferol metabolism by parathyroid glands. *Proc. Natl. Acad. Sci. U.S.A.* **69,** 1673–1676.

Garabedian, M., Pezant, E., Miravet, L., Fellot, C., and Balsan, S. (1976). 1,25-Dihydroxycholecalciferol effect on serum phosphorus homeostasis in rats. *Endocrinology* **98,** 794–799.

Glorieux, F. H., Scriver, C. R., Reade, T. M., Goldman, H., and Roseborough, A. (1972). Use of phosphate and vitamin D to prevent dwarfism and rickets in X-linked hypophosphatemia. *N. Engl. J. Med.* **287,** 481–487.

Goldstein, D. A., Oda, Y., Kurokawa, K., and Massry, S. G. (1977). Blood levels of 25-hydroxyvitamin D in nephrotic syndrome. *Ann. Intern. Med.* **87,** 664–667.

Gran, F. L. (1960). The retention of parenterally injected calcium in rachitic dogs. *Acta Physiol. Scand.* **50,** 132–135.

Gray, R. W., Wilz, D. R., Caldas, A. E., and Lemann, J., Jr. (1977). The importance of phosphate in regulating plasma 1,25-$(OH)_2$-vitamin D levels in humans: Studies in healthy subjects, in calcium-stone formers and in patients with primary hyperparathyroidism. *J. Clin. Endocrinol. Metab.* **45,** 299–306.

Haddad, J. G. (1979). Transport of vitamin D metabolities. *Clin. Orthop. Relat. Res.* **142,** 249–261.

Haddad, J. G., and Birge, S. J. (1975). Widespread, specific binding of 25-hydroxycholecalciferol in rat tissues. *J. Biol. Chem.* **250,** 299–303.

Haddad, J. G., and Chyu, K. J. (1971). Competitive protein-binding radioassay for 25-hydroxycholecalciferol. *J. Clin. Endocrinol. Metab.* **33,** 992–995.

Haddad J. G., and Hahn, T. J. (1973). Natural and synthetic sources of circulating 25-hydroxyvitamin D in man. *Nature (London)* **244,** 515–517.

Haddad, J. G., and Walgate, J. (1976a). 25-hydroxyvitamin D transport in human plasma. *J. Biol. Chem.* **251,** 4803–4809.

Haddad, J. G., and Walgate, J. (1976b). Radioimmunoassay of the binding protein for vitamin D and its metabolites in human serum. *J. Clin. Invest.* **58,** 1217–1222.

Haddad, J. G., Chyu, K. J., Hahn, T. J., and Stamp, T. C. B. (1973). Serum concentrations of 25-hydroxyvitamin D in sex-linked hypophosphatemic vitamin D-resistant rickets. *J. Lab. Clin. Med.* **81,** 22–27.

Haddad, J. G., Walgate, J., Min, C., and Hahn, T. J. (1976a). Vitamin D metabolite-binding proteins in human tissue. *Biochim. Biophys. Acta* **444,** 921–925.

Haddad, J. G., Min, C., Walgate, J., and Hahn, T. (1976b). Competition by 24,25-dihydroxycholecalciferol in the competitive protein binding radioassay of 25-hydroxycalciferol. *J. Clin. Endocrinol. Metab.* **43,** 712–714.

Haddad, J. G., Min, C., Mendelsohn, M., Slatopolsky, E., and Hahn, T. J. (1977). Competitive protein-binding radioassay of 24,25-dihydroxyvitamin D in sera from normal and anephric subjects. *Arch. Biochem. Biophys.* **182,** 390–395.

Hahn, T. J., and Avioli, L. V. (1975). Anticonvulsant osteomalacia. *Arch. Intern. Med.* **135,** 997–1000.

Hahn, T. J., Hendin, B. A., Scharp, C. R., Boisseau, V. C., and Haddad, J. G., Jr. (1975). Serum 25-hydroxycalciferol levels and bone mass in children on chronic anticonvulsant therapy. *N. Engl. J. Med.* **292,** 550–554.

Hahn, T. J., Halstead, L. R., and Haddad, J. G. (1977). Serum 25-hydroxyvitamin D concentrations in patients receiving chronic corticosteroid therapy. *J. Lab. Clin. Med.* **90,** 399–404.

Hahn, T. J., Scharp, C. R., Richardson, C. A., Halstead, L. R., Kahn, A. J., and Teitelbaum, S. L. (1978). Interaction of diphenylhydantoin. (Phenytoin) and phenobarbital with hormonal mediation of fetal rat bone resorption *in vitro*. *J. Clin. Invest.* **61,** 406–414.

Harrison, H. C., and Harrison, H. E. (1976). Inhibition of vitamin D-stimulated active transport of calcium of rat intestine by diphenylhydantoin-phenobarbital treatment. *Proc. Soc. Exp. Biol. Med.* **153,** 220–224.

Haussler, M. R. (1978). Vitamin D: Metabolism, drug interactions and therapeutic applications in humans. *In* "Nutrition and Drug Interrelations" (J. N. Hathcock and J. Coon, eds.), pp. 717–750. Academic Press, New York.

Haussler, M. R. (1980). Radioreceptor assay for 1α,25-dihydroxyvitamin D: clinical defects in vitamin D metabolism. *In* "Vitamin D: Molecular Biology and Clinical Nutrition" (A. W. Norman, ed.), pp. 603–634, 699–708. Dekker, New York.

Haussler, M. R., and McCain, T. A. (1977). Basic and clinical concepts related to vitamin D metabolism and action. *N. Engl. J. Med.* **297,** 974–983, 1041–1050.

Haussler, M. R., and Rasmussen, H. (1972). The metabolism of vitamin D_3 in the chick. *J. Biol. Chem.* **247,** 2328–2335.

Haussler, M. R., Myrtle, J. F., and Norman, A. W. (1968). The association of a metabolite of vitamin D_3 with intestinal mucosa chromatin *in vivo*. *J. Biol. Chem.* **243,** 4055–4064.

Haussler, M. R., Nagode, L. A., and Rasmussen, H. (1970). Induction of intestinal brush border alkaline phosphatase by vitamin D and identity with Ca-ATPase. *Nature (London)* **228,** 1199–1201.

Haussler, M. R., Boyce, D. W., Littledike, E. T., and Rasmussen, H. (1971). A rapidly acting metabolite of vitamin D_3. *Proc. Natl. Acad. Sci. U.S.A.* **68,** 177–181.

Haussler, M. R., Zerwekh, J. E., Hesse, R. H., Rizzardo, E., and Pechet, M. M. (1973). Biological activity of 1α-hydroxycholecalciferol, a synthetic analog of the hormonal form of vitamin D_3. *Proc. Natl. Acad. Sci. U.S.A.* **70,** 2248–2252.

Haussler, M. R., Bursac, K. M., Bone, H., and Pak, C. Y. C. (1975). Increased circulating 1,25-dihydroxyvitamin D_3 in patients with primary hyperparathyroidism. *Clin. Res.* **23,** 322A.

Haussler, M. R., Baylink, D. J., Hughes, M. R., Brumbaugh, P. F., Wergedal, J. E., Shen, F. H., Nielsen, R. L., Counts, S. J., Bursac, K. M., and McCain, T. A. (1976). The assay of 1α,25-dihydroxyvitamin D_3: Physiologic and pathologic modulation of circulating hormone levels. *Clin. Endocrinol. (Oxford)* **5,** 151s–165s.

Haussler, M. R., Hughes, M., Baylink, D., Littledike, E. T., Cork, D., and Pitt, M. (1977a). Influence of phosphate depletion on the biosynthesis and circulating level of 1α,25-dihydroxyvitamin D. *In* "Phosphate Metabolism" (S. G. Massry and E. Ritz, eds.), pp. 233–250. Plenum, New York.

Haussler, M. R., Hughes, M. R., Pike, J. W., and McCain, T. A. (1977b). Radioligand receptor assay for 1,25-dihydroxyvitamin D: Biochemical, physiologic and clinical applications. *In* "Vitamin D: Biochemical, Chemical and Clinical Aspects Related to Calcium Metabolism" (A. W. Norman, K. Schaefer, J. W. Coburn, H. F. DeLuca, D. Fraser, H. G. Grigoleit, and D. von Herrath, eds.), pp. 473–482. de Gruyter, Berlin.

Haussler, M. R., Hughes, M. R., McCain, T. A., and Pike, J. W. (1977c). 1,25-Dihydroxyvitamin D: molecular mechanism, physiologic regulation and clinical implications. *In* "Molecular Endocrinology" (I. MacIntyre and M. Szelke, eds.), pp. 101–116. Elsevier/North Holland, Amsterdam.

Haussler, M. R., Drezner, M. K., Pike, J. W., Chandler, J. S., and Hagan, L. A. (1979). Assay of 1,25-dihydroxyvitamin D and other active vitamin D metabolites in serum: Application to animals and humans. *In* "Vitamin D, Basic Research and its Clinical Application" (A. W. Norman, K. Schaefer, D. V. Herrath, H. G. Grigoleit, J. W. Coburn, H. F. DeLuca, E. B. Mawer, and T. Suda, eds.), pp. 189–196. de Gruyter, Berlin.

Heaney, R. P. (1974). Pathophysiology of osteoporosis: Implications for treatment. *Tex. Med.* **70,** 37–45.

Heath, H., III, Lambert, P. W., Service, F. J., and Arnaud, S. B. (1979). Calcium homeostasis in diabetes mellitus. *J. Clin. Endocrinol. Metab.* **49,** 462–466.

Henderson, R. G., Russell, R. G. G., Ledingham, J. G. G., Smith, R., Oliver, D. O., Walton, R. J., Small, D. G., Preston, C., Warner, G. T., and Norman, A. W. (1974). Effects of 1,25-dihydroxycholecalciferol on calcium absorption, muscle weakness, and bone disease in chronic renal failure. *Lancet* **1,** 379–394.

Henry, H. L. (1977). Metabolism of 25-hydroxyvitamin D_3 by primary culture of chick kidney cells. *Biochem. Biophys. Res. Commun.* **74,** 768–774.

Henry, H. L., and Norman, A. W. (1975). Studies on the mechanism of action of calciferol VII. Localization of 1,25-dihydroxyvitamin D_3 in chick parathyroid glands. *Biochem. Biophys. Res. Commun.* **62,** 781–788.

Henry, H. L., Midgett, R. J., and Norman, A. W. (1974). Regulation of 25-hydroxyvitamin D_3-1-hydroxylase in vivo. *J. Biol. Chem.* **249,** 7584–7592.

Hepner, G. W. (1977). Vitamin D in primary biliary cirrhosis. *Lancet* **2,** 792–796.

Hepner, G. W. Roginsky, M., and Moo, H. F. (1975). Low serum 25-hydroxyvitamin D levels in patients with hepatic dysfunctions. *In* "Vitamin D and Problems Related to Uremic Bone Disease" (A. W. Norman, K. Schaefer, H. G. Grigoleit, and D. von Herrath, eds.), pp. 325–330. de Gruyter, Berlin.

Hillman, L., and Haddad, J. G., Jr. (1975). Perinatal vitamin D metabolism. *J. Pediatr.* **86,** 928–935.

Hirooka, M., Wako, H., Kaneko, C., Ishikawa, M., Sasaki, S., and Suda, T. (1975). Curative effects of 1α-hydroxycholecalciferol on calcium metabolism and bone disease in patients with chronic renal failure. *J. Nutr. Sci. Vitaminol.* **21,** 277–285.

Hodgson, S. F., Arnaud, S. B., Newcomer, A. D., and Jowsey, J. O. (1976). The relationship of bone morphology to serum calcium and calcitiropic hormones in patients with diarrhea and/or steatorrhea. *Clin. Res.* **24,** 565A.

Hofmann, T., Kawakami, M., Hitchman, A. J. W., Harrison, J. E., and Dorrington, K. J. (1979) The amino acid sequence of porcine intestinal calcium-binding protein. *Can. J. Biochem.* **57,** 737–748.

Holick, M. F., and DeLuca, H. F. (1971). A new chromatographic system for vitamin D_3 and its metabolites: Resolution of a new vitamin D_3 metabolite. *J. Lipid Res.* **12,** 460–465.

Holick, M. F., Schnoes, H. K., DeLuca, H. F., Suda, T., and Cousins, R. J. (1971). Isolation and identification of 1,25-dihydroxycholecalciferol. A metabolite of vitamin D active in intestine. *Biochemistry* **10,** 2799–2804.

Holick, M. F., Garabedian, M., and DeLuca, H. F. (1972). 1,25-dihyroxycholecalciferol: Metabolite of vitamin D_3 active on bone in anephric rats. *Science* **176,** 1146–1147.

Holick, M. F., Tavela, T. E., Holick, S. A., Schnoes, H. K., DeLuca, H. F., and Gallagher, B. M. (1976). Synthesis of 1α-hydroxy[6-^{3}H]vitamin D_3 and its metabolism to 1α-dihydroxy[6-^{3}H]vitamin D_3 in the rat. *J. Biol. Chem.* **251,** 1020–1024.

Holick, M. F., Frommer, J. E., McNeill, S. B., Richtand, N. M., Henley, J. W., and Potts, J. T. (1977a). Photometabolism of 7-dehydrocholesterol to previtamin D_3 in skin. *Biochem. Biophys. Res. Commun.* **76,** 107–114.

Holick, M. F., de Blanco, M. C., Clark, M. B., Henley, J. W., Neer, R. M., DeLuca, H. F., and Potts, J. T. (1977b). The metabolism of [6-^{3}H]1α hydroxycholecalciferol to [6-^{3}H]1α,25-dihydroxycholecalciferol in a patient with renal insufficiency. *J. Clin. Endocrinol. Metab.* **44,** 595–598.

Horst, R. L., Shepard, R. M., Jorgensen, N. A., and DeLuca, H. F. (1979). The determination of 24,25-dihydroxyvitamin D and 25,26-dihydroxyvitamin D in plasma for normal and nephrectomized man. *J. Lab. Clin. Med.* **93,** 277–285.

Hughes, M. R., and Haussler, M. R. (1978). 1,25-dihydroxyvitamin D_3 receptors in parathyroid glands. *J. Biol. Chem.* **253,** 1065–1073.

Hughes, M. R., Brumbaugh, P. F., Haussler, M. R., Wergedal, J. E., and Baylink, D. J. (1975). Regulation of serum 1α,25-dihydroxyvitamin D_3 by calcium and phosphate in the rat. *Science* **190,** 578–580.

Hughes, M. R., Baylink, D. J., Jones, P. G., and Haussler, M. R. (1976). Radioligand receptor assay for 25-hydroxyvitamin D_2/D_3 and 1α,25-dihydroxyvitamin D_2/D_3. Application to hypervitaminosis D. *J. Clin. Invest.* **58,** 61–70.

Hughes, M. R., McCain, T. A., Chang, S. Y., Haussler, M. R., Villareale, M., and Wasserman, R. H. (1977a). Presence of 1,25-dihydroxyvitamin D_3-glycoside in the calcinogenic plant *Cestrum diurnum. Nature (London)* **268,** 347–349.

Hughes, M. R., Baylink, D. J., Gonnerman, W. A., Toverud, S. U., Ramp, W. K., and Haussler, M. R. (1977b). Influence of dietary vitamin D_3 on the circulating concentration of its active metabolites in the chick and rat. *Endocrinology (Baltimore)* **100,** 799–806.

Hunter, J., Maxwell, J. D., Steward, D. A., Parsons, V., and Williams, R. (1971). Altered calcium metabolism in epileptic children on anticonvulsants. *Br. Med. J.* **4,** 202–204.

Imawari, M., Kida, K., and Goodman, D. S. (1976). The transport of vitamin D and its 25-hydroxy metabolite in human plasma. *J. Clin. Invest.* **58,** 514–523.

Jenkins, M. V., Harris, M., and Wills, M. R. (1974). The effect of Phenytoin on parathyroid extract and 25-hydroxycholecalciferol-induced bone resorption: Adenosine 3′,5′-cyclic monophosphate production. *Calcif. Tissue Res.* **16,** 163–167.

Johnson, R. L., Okamura, W. H., and Norman, A. W. (1975). Studies on the mode of action of calciferol X. 24-nor-25-hydroxyvitamin D_3, and anolog of 25-hydroxyvitamin D_3 having "anti-vitamin" activity. *Biochem. Biophys. Res. Commun.* **67,** 797–802.

Jones, P. G., and Haussler, M. R. (1979). Scintillation autoradiographic localization of 1,25-dihydroxyvitamin D_3 in chick intestine. *Endocrinology (Baltimore)* **104,** 313–321.

Jubiz, W., Haussler, M. R., McCain, T. A., and Tolman, K. G. (1977). Plasma 1,25-dihydroxyvitamin D levels in patients receiving anticonvulsant drugs. *J. Clin. Endocrinol. Metab.* **44,** 617–621.

Jung, R. T., Davie, M., Hunter, J. O., and Chalmers, T. M. (1978). Ultraviolet light: An effective treatment of osteomalacia in malabsorption. *Br. Med. J.* **1,** 1668–1669.

Kanis, J. A., Cundy, T., Bartlett, M., Smith, R., Heynen, G., Warner, G. T., and Russell, R. G. G. (1978). Is 24,25-dihydroxycholecalciferol a calcium-regulating hormone in man? *Br. Med. J.* **1,** 1382–1386.

Kaplan, R. A., Haussler, M. R., Deftos, L. J., Bone, H., and Pak, C. Y. C. (1977). The role of 1α,25-dihydroxyvitamin D in the mediation of intestinal hyperabsorption of calcium in primary hyperparathyroidism and absorptive hypercalciuria. *J. Clin. Invest.* **59,** 756–760.

Kaye, M., and Sagar, S. (1972). Effect of a dihydrotachysterol on calcium absorption in uremia. *Metab. Clin. Exp.* **21,** 815–824.

Kooh, S. W., Fraser, D., DeLuca, H. F., Holick, M. F., Belsey, R. E., Clark, M. B., and Murray, T. M. (1975). Treatment of hypoparathyroidism and pseudohypoparathyroidism with metabolites of vitamin D: Evidence for impaired conversion of 25-hydroxyvitamin D to 1α,25-dihydroxyvitamin D. *N. Engl. J. Med.* **293,** 840–844.

Kooh, S. W., Fraser, D., Toon, R., and DeLuca, H. F. (1976). Response of protracted neonatal hypocalcaemia to 1α,25-dihydroxyvitamin D_3. *Lancet* **2,** 1105–1107.

Kowarski, S., and Schachter, D. (1980). Intestinal membrane calcium-binding protein. *J. Biol. Chem.* **255,** 10834–10840.

Krawitt, E. L., Grundman, M. J., and Mawer, E. B. (1977). Absorption, hydroxylation, and excretion of viatmin D_3 in primary biliary cirrhosis. *Lancet* **2,** 1246–1249.

Kream, B. E., Reynolds, R. D., Knutson, J. C., Eisman, J. A., and DeLuca, H. F. (1976). Intestinal cytosol binders of 1,25-dihydroxyvitamin D_3 and 25-hydroxyvitamin D_3. *Arch. Biochem. Biophys.* **176,** 779–787.

Kream, B. E., Jose, M., Yamada, S., and DeLuca, H. F. (1977). A specific high-affinity binding macromolecule for 1,25-dihydroxyvitamin D_3 in fetal bone. *Science* **197,** 1036–1088.

Kremer, R., and Guillemant, S. (1978). A simple and specific competitive protein binding assay for 24,25-dihydroxyvitamin D in human serum. *Clin. Chim. Acta* **86,** 187–194.

Kumar, R., Harnden, D., and DeLuca, H. F. (1976). Metabolism of 1,25-dihydroxyvitamin D_3: Evidence for side-chain oxidation. *Biochemistry* **15,** 2420–2423.

Kumar, R., Schnoes, H. K., and DeLuca, H. F. (1978). Rat intestinal 25-hydroxyvitamin D_3- and 1α,25-dihydroxyvitamin D_3-24-hydroxylase. *J. Biol. Chem.* **253,** 3804–3809.

Kumar, R., Nagubandi, S., and Londowski, J. M. (1980). The enterohepatic physiology of 24,25-dihydroxyvitamin D_3. *J. Lab. Clin. Med.* **96,** 278–284.

Lambert, P., Hollis, B., Bell, N. H., and Epstein, S. (1980). Lack of change in serum 1α, 25-dihydroxyvitamin D in response to parathyroid extract in pseudohypoparathyroidism. *Calcif. Tissue Int.* **31,** 80.

Lambert, P. W., Syverson, B. J., Arnaud, C. D., and Spelsberg, T. C. (1977). Isolation and quantitation of endogenous vitamin D and its physiologically important metabolites in human plasma by high pressure liquid chromatography. *J. Steroid Biochem.* **8,** 929–937.

Lawson, D. E., Fraswer, D. R., Kodicek, E., Morris, H. R., and Williams, D. H. (1971). Identification of 1,25-dihydroxycholecalciferol, a new kidney hormone controlling calcium metabolism. *Nature (London)* **230,** 228–230.

Levin, M. W., Boisseau, V. C., and Avioli, L. V. (1976). Effects of diabetes mellitus on bone mass in juvenile and adult-onset diabetes. *N. Engl. J. Med.* **294,** 241–245.

Liakakos, D., Papadopoulos, Z., Vlachos, P., Boviatsi, E., and Varonos, D. D. (1975). Serum alkaline phosphatase and urinary hydroxyproline values in children receiving phenobarbital with and without vitamin D. *J. Pediatr.* **87,** 291–296.

Livingston, S., Berman, W., and Pauli, L. L. (1973). Anticonvulsant drugs and vitamin D metabolism. *JAMA, J. Am. Med. Assoc.* **224,** 1634–1635.

Llach, F., Brickman, A. S., Gerszi, K., Norman, A. W., and Coburn, J. W. (1978). Actions of 24,25-dihydroxyvitamin D_3 in uremic man. *Clin. Res.* **26,** 543A.

Llach, F., Brickman, A. S., Singer, F. R., and Coburn, J. W. (1979). 24,25-Dihydroxycholecalciferol, a vitamin D sterol with qualitatively unique effects in uremic man. *Metab. Bone Dis. Relat. Res.* **2,** 11–16.

Long, R. G., Wills, M. R., Skinner, R. K., and Sherlock, S. (1976). Serum-25-hydroxyvitamin D in untreated parenchymal and cholestatic liver disease. *Lancet* **2,** 650–652.

Long, R. G., Varghese, Z., Meinhard, E. A., Skinner, R. K., Wills, M. R., and Sherlock, S. (1978). Parenteral 1,25-dihydroxycholecalciferol in hepatic osteomalacia. *Br. Med. J.* **1,** 75–77.

Lund, B., and Sorensen, O. H. (1979). Measurement of 25-hydroxyvitamin D in serum and its relation to sunshine, age and vitamin D intake in the Danish population. *Scand. J. Clin. Lab. Invest.* **39,** 23–30.

Lund, B., Hjorth, L., Kjaer, I., Friis, T., Reimann, I., Anderson, R. B., and Sorensen, O. H. (1975). Treatment of osteoporosis of ageing with 1α-hydroxycholecalciferol. *Lancet* **2,** 1168–1171.

Lund, B., Hey, H., Lund, B., Sorensen, O. H., and Christensen, M. S. (1978). Vitamin D and jejunal-ileal bypass. *Lancet* **2,** 264–265.

Lyles, K. W., Berry, W. R., Haussler, M., Harrelson, J. M., and Drezner, M. K. (1980). Hypophosphatemic osteomalacia: Association with prostatic carcinoma. *Ann. Intern. Med.* **93,** 275–278.

McCain, T. A., Haussler, M. R., Okrent, D., and Hughes, M. R. (1978). Partial purification of the chick intestinal receptor for 1,25-dihydroxyvitamin D by ion exchange and blue dextran-Sepharose chromatography. *FEBS Lett.* **86,** 65–70.

McLaughlin, M., Fairney, A., Lester, E., Raggatt, P. R., Brown, D. J., and Wills, M. R. (1974). Seasonal variations in serum 25-hydroxycholecalciferol in healthy people. *Lancet* **1,** 536–538.

McNair, P., Madsbad, S., Christensen, M. S., Christiansen, C., Faber, O. K., Binder, C., and Transbol, I. (1979). Bone mineral loss in insulin-treated diabetes mellitus: Studies on pathogenesis. *Acta Endocrinol. (Copenhagen)* **90,** 463–472.

McNutt, K. W., and Haussler, M. R. (1973). Nutritional effectiveness of 1,25-dihydroxycholecalciferol in preventing rickets in chicks. *J. Nutr.* **103,** 681–689.

Maggio, A. J., Jr., Coburn, J. W., Brosman, S. A., and Das, S. (1979). The role of vitamin D in idiopathic hypercalciuria. *J. Urol.* **122,** 147–151.

Mahgoub, A., and Sheppard, H. (1977). Effect of hydroxyvitamin D_3 derivatives on ^{45}Ca release from rat fetal bones *in vitro*. *Endocrinology (Baltimore)* **100,** 629–634.

Mann, J. B., Alterman, S., and Hills, A. G. (1962). Albright's hereditary osteodystrophy comprising pseudohypoparathyroidism and pseudopseudohypoparathyroidism. *Ann. Intern. Med.* **56,** 315–342.

Manolagas, S. C., Haussler, M. R., and Deftos, L. J. (1980). 1,25-Dihydroxyvitamin D_3 receptor-like macromolecule in rat osteogenic sarcoma cell lines. *J. Biol. Chem.* **255,** 4414–4417.

Marx, S. J., Spiegel, A. M., Brown, E. M., Gardner, D. G., Downs, R. W., Jr., Attie, M., Hamstra, A. J., and DeLuca, H. F. (1978). A familial syndrome of decrease in sensitivity to 1,25-dihydroxyvitamin D. *J. Clin. Endocrinol. Metab.* **47,** 1303–1310.

Mason, R. S., and Posen, S. (1979). The relevance of 25-hydroxycalciferol measurements in the treatment of hypoparathyroidism. *Clin. Endocrinol. (Oxford)* **10,** 265–269.

Mawer, E. B., Backhouse, J., Taylor, C. M., Lumb, G. A., and Stanbury, S. W. (1973). Failure of formation of 1,25-dihydroxycholecalciferol in chronic renal insufficiency. *Lancet* **1,** 626–628.

Melancon, M. J., and DeLuca, H. F. (1970). Vitamin D stimulation of calcium-dependent adenosine triphosphatase in chick intestinal brush borders. *Biochemistry* **9,** 1658–1664.

Menczel, J., Makin, M., Robin, G., Jaye, I., and Naor, E. (1972). Prevalence of diabetes in Jerusalem. *Isr. J. Med. Sci.* **8,** 918–919.

Mendelsohn, M., Min, C., Haddad, J., Hahn, T., and Slatopolsky, E. (1976). Assay of 24,25-dihydroxyvitamin D in serum. *Clin. Res.* **24,** 582A.

Metz, S. A., Baylink, D. J., Hughes, M. R., Haussler, M. R., and Robertson, R. P. (1977). Selective deficiency of 1,25-dihydroxycholecalciferol. *N. Engl. J. Med.* **297,** 1084–1090.

Meunier, P., Dechavanne, M., and Prost, G. (1973). Bone in cirrhosis-quantitative osseous biopsy study [Translated title]. *Lyon Med.* **229,** 1089–1095.

Monteleone, J. A., Lee, J. B., Tashjian, A. H., and Cantor, H. E. (1975). Transient neonatal hypocalcemia, hypomagnesemia, and high serum parathyroid hormone with maternal hyperparathyroidism. *Ann. Intern. Med.* **82,** 670–672.

Naik, R. B., Gosling, P., Price, C. P., Robinson, B. H. B., Dabek, J. T., Heath, D. A., James, H. M., Kanis, J. A., and Smith, R. (1976). Whole-body *in vivo* neutron activation analysis in assessing treatment of renal osteodystrophy with 1-alpha-hydroxycholecalciferol. *Br. Med. J.* **2,** 79–83.

Neer, R., Clark, M., Friedman, V., Belsey, R., Sweeney, M., Buonchristiani, J., and Potts, J., Jr. (1977). Environmental and nutritional influences on plasma 25-hydroxyvitamin D concentration and calcium metabolism in man. *In* "Vitamin D: Biochemical, Chemical and Clinical Aspects Related to Calcium Metabolism" (A. W. Norman, K. Schaefer, J. W. Coburn, H. F. DeLuca, D. Fraser, H. G. Grigoleit, and D. von Herrath, eds.), pp. 595–606. de Gruyter, Berlin.

Ney, R. L., Kelly, G., and Bartter, F. C. (1968). Actions of vitamin D independent of the parathyroid glands. *Endocrinology (Baltimore)* **82,** 760–766.

Norman, A. W., and Henry, H. (1974). 1,25-dihydroxycholecalciferol—a hormonally active form of vitamin D_3. *Recent Prog. Horm. Res.* **30,** 431–473.

Norman, A. W., Henry, H., Bishop, J. E., and Coburn, J. W. (1978). Simultaneous measurement of 25-(OH)D, 24,25-$(OH)_2D$ and 1,25$(OH)_2D$ in plasma samples by steroid competition assay. *Clin. Res.* **26,** 423A.

O'Doherty, P. J. A., and DeLuca, H. F. (1976). Intestinal calcium and phosphate transport in genetic hypophosphatemic mice. *Biochem. Biophys. Res. Commun.* **71,** 617–621.

Offermann, G., Delling, G., and Haussler, M. R. (1978). 1,25-Dihydroxycholecalciferol in hypophosphatemic osteomalacia presenting in adults. *Acta Endocrinol. (Copenhagen)* **88,** 408–416.

Olefsky, J., Kempson, R., Jones, H., and Reaven, G. (1972). "Tertiary" hyperparathyroidism and apparent "cure" of vitamin D-resistant rickets after removal of an ossifying mesenchymal tumor of the pharynx. *N. Engl. J. Med.* **286,** 740–745.

Olson, E. G., Knutson, J. C., Bhattacharyya, M. H., and DeLuca, H. F. (1976). The effect of hepatectomy on the synthesis of 25-hydroxyvitamin D_3. *J. Clin. Invest.* **57,** 1213–1220.

O'Malley, B. W., and Schrader, W. T. (1976). The receptors of steroid hormones. *Sci. Am.* **234,** 32–43.

Pak, C. Y. C., Ohata, M., Lawrence, E. C., and Snyder, W. (1974). The hypercalciurias. *J. Clin. Invest.* **54,** 387–400.

Pak, C. Y. C., Kaplan, R., Bone, H., Townsend, J., and Waters, O. (1975). A simple test for the diagnosis of absorptive, resorptive, and renal hypercalciurias. *N. Engl. J. Med.* **292,** 497–500.

Papapoulos, S. E., Fraher, L. J., Clemens, T. L., Gleed, J., and O'Riordan, J. L. H. (1980). Metabolites of vitamin D in human vitamin-D deficiency: Effect of vitamin D_3 or 1,25-dihydroxycholecalciferol. *Lancet* **2,** 612–615.

Peterson, P., Gray, P., and Tolman, K. G. (1976). Calcium balance in drug-induced osteomalacia: Response to vitamin D. *Clin. Pharmacol. Ther.* **18,** 63–67.

Pike, J. W., and Haussler, M. R. (1979). Purification of chicken intestinal receptor for 1,25-dihydroxyvitamin D. *Proc. Natl. Acad. Sci. U.S.A.* **76,** 5485–5489.

Pike, J. W., Toverud, S., Boass, A., McCain, T., and Haussler, M. R. (1977). Circulating 1α,25-$(OH)_2D$ during physiological states of calcium stress. *In* "Vitamin D: Biochemical, Chemical and Clinical Aspects Related to Calcium and Metabolism'' (A. W. Norman, K. Schaefer, J. W. Coburn, H. F. DeLuca, D. Fraser, H. G. Grigoleit, and D. von Herrath, eds.), pp. 187–189. de Gruyter, Berlin.

Pike, J. W., Parker, J. B., Haussler, M. R., Boass, A., and Toverud, S. U. (1979). Dynamic changes in circulating 1,25-dihydroxyvitamin D during reproduction in rats. *Science* **204,** 1427–1429.

Pike, J. W., Gooze, L. L., and Haussler, M. R. (1980). Biochemical evidence for 1,25-dihydroxyvitamin D receptor macromolecules in parathyroid, pancreatic, pituitary, and placental tissues. *Life Sci.* **26,** 407–414.

Popovtzer, M. M., Robinette, J. B., DeLuca, H. F., and Holick, M. F. (1974). The acute effects of 25-dihydroxycholecalciferol on renal hanlding of phosphorus. Evidence for a parathyroid-dependent mechanism. *J. Clin. Invest.* **53,** 913–924.

Popovtzer, M. M., Blum, M. S., and Flis, R. S. (1977). Evidence for interference of 25(OH)vitamin D_3 with phosphaturic action of calcitonin. *Am. J. Physiol.* **232,** E515–E521.

Poskitt, E. E. M., Cole, T. J., and Lawson, D. E. M. (1979). Diet, sunlight, and 25-hydroxy vitamin D in healthy children and adults. *Br. Med. J.* **1,** 221–223.

Preece, M. A., McIntosh, W. B., Tomlinson, S., Ford, J. A., Dunnigan, M. G., and O'Riordan, J. L. H. (1973). Vitamin D-deficiency among Asian immigrants to Britain. *Lancet* **1,** 907–910.

Preece, M. A., Tomlinson, S., Ribot, C. A., Pietrek, J., Korn, H. T., Davies, D. M., Ford, J. A., Dunnigan, M. G., and O'Riordan, J. L. H. (1975). Studies of vitamin D deficiency in man. *Q. J. Med.* [N.S.] **44,** 575–598.

Procsal, D. A., Okamura, W. H., and Norman, A. W. (1975). Structural requirements for the interaction of $1\alpha,25\text{-(OH)}_2$-vitamin D_3 with its chick intestinal receptor system *J. Biol. Chem.* **250,** 8382–8388.

Puschett, J. B., Fernandez, P. C., Boyle, I. T., Gray, R. W., Omdahl, J. L., and DeLuca, H. F. (1972a). The acute renal tubular effects of 1,25-dihydroxycholecalciferol (36781). *Proc. Soc. Exp. Biol. Med.* **141,** 379–384.

Puschett, J. B., Moranz, J., and Kurnick, W. S. (1972b). Evidence for a direct action of cholecalciferol and 25-hydroxycholecalciferol on the renal transport of phosphate, sodium and calcium. *J. Clin. Invest.* **51,** 373–385.

Puschett, J. B., Beck, W. S., and Jelonek, A. (1975). Parathyroid hormone and 25-hydroxy-vitamin D_3. Synergistic and antagonistic effects on renal phosphate transport. *Science* **190,** 473–475.

Raisz, L. G., Trummel, C. L., Holick, M. F., and DeLuca, H. F. (1972). 1,25-dihydroxycholecalciferol: A potent stimulator of bone resorption in tissue culture. *Science* **175,** 768–769.

Rasmussen, H., Anast, C., Parks, J., Haussler, M., Lane, J., and Pechet, M. (1976). $1\alpha(OH)D_3$ in treatment of hypophosphatemic rickets. *Clin. Res.* **24,** 486A.

Rasmussen, H., Baron, R., Broadus, A., DeFronzo, R., Lang, R., and Horst, R. (1980). $1,25(OH)_2D_3$ is not the only D metabolite involved in the pathogenesis of osteomalacia. *Am. J. Med.* **69,** 360–368.

Recker, R., Schoenfeld, P., Letteri, J., Slatopolsky. E., Goldsmith, R., and Brickman, A. (1978). The efficacy of calcifediol in renal osteodystrophy. *Arch. Intern. Med.* **138,** 857–863.

Reed, J. S., Meredith, S. C., Nemchausky, B. A., Rosenberg, I. H., and Boyer, J. L. (1977). Assessment of morphologic response to 25-OH vitamin D (25-OH D) therapy in patients with primary biliary cirrhosis (PBC). *Gastroenterology* **72,** 1181 (abstr.).

Reynolds, J. J., Holick, M. F. and DeLuca, H. F. (1974). The effects of vitamin D analogues on bone resorption. *Calcif. Tissue Res.* **15,** 333–339.

Reynolds, J. J., Pavlovitch, H., and Balsan, S. (1976). 1,25-dihydroxycholecalciferol increases bone resorption in thyroparathyroidectomized mice. *Calcif. Tissue Res.* **21,** 207–212.

Ribovich, M. L., and DeLuca, H. F. (1975). The influence of dietary calcium and phosphorus on intestinal calcium transport in rats given vitamin D metabolites. Arch. *Biochem. Biophys.* **170,** 529–535.

Richards, I. D. G., Sweet, E. M. and Arneil, G. C. (1968). Infantile rickets persists in Glasgow. *Lancet* **1,** 803–805.

Riggs, B. L., Jowsey, J., Kelly, P. J., and Arnaud, C. D. (1976). Role of hormonal factors in the pathogenesis of postmenopausal osteoporosis. *Isr. J. Med. Sci.* **12,** 615–619.

Rodman, J. S., and Baker, T. (1978). Changes in the kinetics of muscle contraction in vitamin D-depleted rats. *Kidney Int.* **13,** 189–193.

Roginsky, M. S., and Faminini, M. (1978). Mechanism of the low serum 25-hydroxycholecalciferol in epileptics receiving anticonvulsants. *Clin. Res.* **26,** 426A.

Rose, C. A., and Harrison, A. R. (1944). The incidence, investigation and treatment of idiopathic hypercalciuria. *Br. J. Urol.* **46,** 261–274.

Rosen, J. F., Roginsky, M., Nathenson, G., and Finberg, L. (1974). 25-hydroxyvitamin D plasma levels in mothers and their premature infants with neonatal hypocalcemia. *Am. J. Dis. Child.* **127,** 220–223.

Russell, R. G. G., Walton, R. J., Smith, R., Preston, C., Basson, R., Henderson, R. G. and Norman, A. W. (1974). 1,25-Dihydroxycholecalciferol and 1α-hydroxycholecalciferol in hypoparathyroidism. *Lancet* **2,** 14–17.

Salassa, R. M., Jowsey, J., and Arnaud, C. D. (1970). Hypophosphatemic osteomalacia associated with "nonendocrine" tumors. *N. Engl. J. Med.* **283,** 65–70.

Santiago, J. V., McAlister, W. H., Ratzon, S. K., Bussman, Y., Haymond, M. W., Shackelford, G., and Weldon, V. V. (1977). Decreased cortical thickness and osteopenia in children with diabetes mellitus. *J. Clin. Endocrinol. Metab.* **45,** 845–848.

Schaefer, P. C., and Goldsmith, R. S. (1978). Quantitation of 25-hydroxycholecalciferol in human serum by high-pressure liquid chromatography. *J. Lab. Clin. Med.* **91,** 104–108.

Schmidt-Gayk, H., Schmitt, W., Grawunder, C., Ritz, E., Tschope, N., and Piersch, V. (1977). 25-Hydroxy-vitamin-D in nephrotic syndrome. *Lancet* **2,** 105–108.

Schneider, L. E., Wilson, H. D., and Schedl, H. P. (1973). Intestinal calcium binding protein in the diabetic rat. *Nature (London)* **245,** 327–328.

Schneider, L. E., Omdahl, J., and Schedl, H. P. (1976). Effects of vitamin D and its metabolites on calcium transport in the diabetic rat. *Endocrinology (Baltimore)* **99,** 793–799.

Schneider, L. E., Schedl, H. P., McCain, T., and Haussler, M. R. (1977a). Experimental diabetes reduces circulating 1,25-dihydroxyvitamin D in the rat. *Science* **196,** 1452–1454.

Schneider, L. E., Nowosielski, L. M., and Schedl, H. P. (1977b). Insulin treatment of diabetic rats: Effects on duodenal calcium absorption. *Endocrinology (Baltimore)* **100,** 67–73.

Schott, G. D., and Wills, M. R. (1976). Muscle weakness in osteomalacia. *Lancet* **1,** 626–629.

Shen, F. H., Baylink, D. J., Sherrard, D. J., Shen, L., Maloney, N. A., and Wergedal, J. E. (1975). Serum immunoreactive parathyroid hormone and 25-hydroxyvitamin D in patients with uremic bone disease. *J. Clin. Endocrinol. Metab.* **40,** 1009–1017.

Shen, F. H., Baylink, D. J., Nielsen, R. L., Sherrard, D. J., Ivey, J. L., and Haussler, M. R. (1977a). Increased serum 1,25-dihydroxyvitamin D in idiopathic hypercalciuria. *J. Lab. Clin. Med.* **90,** 955–962.

Shen, F. H., Baylink, D. J., Sherrard, D. J., and Haussler, M. R. (1977b). Idiopathic hypercalciuria: The "phosphate leak" hypothesis and effects of oral phosphate supplement. *Clin. Res.* **25,** 129A.

Shepard, R. M., Horst, R. L., Hamstra, A. J., and DeLuca, H. F. (1979). Determination of vitamin D and its metabolites in plasma from normal and anephric man. *Biochem. J.* **182,** 55–69.

Sherrard, D. J., Coburn, J. W., Brickman, A. S., Singer, F. R., and Maloney, N. (1980). Skeletal response to treatment with 1,25-dihydroxy-vitamin D in renal failure. *In* "Contributions to Nephrology" (J. W. Coburn and S. G. Massry, eds.), Vol. 18, pp. 92–97. Karger, Basel.

Short, E. M., Binder, H. J., and Rosenberg, L. E. (1973). Familial hypophosphatemic rickets: Defective transport of inorganic phosphate by intestinal mucosa. *Science* **179,** 700–702.

Sinha, T. K., DeLuca, H. F., and Bell, N. H. (1977). Evidence for a defect in the formation of 1α,25-dihydroxyvitamin D in pseudohypoparathyroidism. *Metab., Clin. Exp.* **26,** 731–738.

Skinner, R. K., Long, R. G., Sherlock, S., and Wills, M. R. (1977). 25-Hydroxylation of vitamin D in primary biliary cirrhosis. *Lancet* **1,** 720–721.

Sklan, D., Budowksi, P., and Katz, M. (1973). Determination of 25-hydroxycholecalciferol by combined thin layer and gas chromatography. *Anal. Biochem.* **56,** 606–609.

Spanos, E., Pike, J. W., Haussler, M. R., Colston, K. W., Evans, I. M. A., Goldner, A. M., McCain, T. A., and MacIntyre, I. (1976a). Circulating 1α,25-dihydorxyvitamin D in the chicken: Enhancement by injection of prolactin and during egg laying. *Life Sci.* **19,** 1751–1756.

Spanos, E., Colston, K. W., Evans, I. M. A., Galante, L. S., MacAuley, S. J., and MacIntyre, I. (1976b). Effect of prolactin on vitamin D metabolism. *Mol. Cell. Endocrinol.* **5,** 163–167.

Spanos, E., Barrett, D., MacIntyre, I., Pike, J. W., Safilian, E. F., and Haussler, M. R. (1978). Effect of growth hormone on vitamin D metabolism. *Nature (London)* **273,** 246–247.

Spencer, R., Charman, M., Emtage, J. S., and Lawson, D. E. M. (1976a). Production and properties of vitamin D-induced mRNA for chick calcium-binding protein. *Eur. J. Biochem.* **71,** 399–409.

Spencer, R., Charman, M., Wilson, P., and Lawson, D. E. M. (1976b). Vitamin D-stimulated intestinal calcium absorption may not involve calcium-binding protein directly. *Nature (London)* **263,** 161–163.

Stamp, T. C. B., Round, J. M., Rowe, D. J. F., and Haddad, J. G. (1972). Plasma levels and therapeutic effect of 25-hydroxycholecalciferol in epileptic patients taking anticonvulsant drugs. *Br. Med. J.* **4,** 9–12.

Stamp, T. C. B., Haddad, J. G., Jr., and Twigg, C. A. (1977). Potency of natural and artificial ultraviolet irradiation as determinants of plasma 25-hydroxyvitamin D in man. *In* "Vitamin D: Biochemical, Chemical and Clinical Aspects Related to Calcium Metabolism" (A. W. Norman, K. Schaefer, J. W. Coburn, H. F. DeLuca, D. Fraser, H. G. Grigoleit, and D. von Herrath, eds.), pp. 615–617. de Gruyter, Berlin.

Stern, P. H., Mavreas, T., Trummel, C. L., Schnoes, H. K., and DeLuca, H. F. (1976). Bone-resorbing activity of analogues of 25-hydroxycholecalciferol and 1,25-dihydroxycholecalciferol: Effects of side chain modificaiton and stereoisomerization on responses of fetal rat bones in vitro. *Mol. Pharmacol.* **12,** 879–886.

Stern, P. H., Phillips, T. E., Lucas, S. V., Hamstra, A. J., DeLuca, H. F., and Bell, N. H. (1977). Bone organ culture bioassay for determination of 1,25-$(OH)_2D$. *In* "Biochemical, Chemical and Clinical Aspects Related to Calcium Metabolism" (A. W. Norman, K. Schaefer, J. W. Coburn, H. F. DeLuca, D. Fraser, H. G. Grigoleit, and D. von Herrath, eds.), pp. 531–540. de Gruyter, Berlin.

Sutton, R. A. L., Wong, N. L. M., and Dirks, J. H. (1975). 25-Hydroxy vitamin D_3. Enhancement of distal tubular calcium reabsorption in the dog. *Abstr. Book Am. Soc. Nephrol.* p. 8.

Tanaka, Y., and DeLuca, H. F. (1971). Bone mineral mobilization activity of 1,25-dihydroxycholecalciferol, a metabolite of vitamin D. *Arch. Biochem. Biophys.* **146,** 574–578.

Tanaka, Y., and DeLuca, H. F. (1973). The control of 25-hydroxyvitamin D metabolism by inorganic phosphorus. *Arch. Biochem. Biophys.* **154,** 566–574.

Tanaka, Y., and DeLuca, H. F. (1974). Stimulation of 24,25-dihydroxyvitamin D_3 production by 1,25-dihydroxyvitamin D_3. *Science* **183,** 1198–1200.

Tanaka, Y., Castillo, L., and DeLuca, H. F. (1976). Control of renal vitamin D hydroxylases in birds by sex hormones. *Proc. Natl. Acad. Sci. U.S.A.* **73,** 2701–2705.

Taylor, A. N., and Wasserman, R. H. (1972). Vitamin D-induced calcium-binding protein: comparative aspects in kidney and intestine. *Am. J. Physiol.* **223,** 110–114.

Taylor, C. M. (1977a). The measurement of 24,25-dihydroxycholecalciferol in human serum. *In* "Vitamin D: Biochemical, Chemical and Clinical Aspects Related to Calcium Metabolism" (A. W. Norman, K. Schaefer, J. W. Coburn, H. F. DeLuca, D. Fraser, H. G. Grigoleit, and D. von Herrath, eds.), pp. 541–543. de Gruyter, Berlin.

Taylor, C. M. (1977b). Serum 24,25-dihydroxycholecalciferol levels in primary hyperparathyroidism. *Clin. Sci. Mol. Med.* **52,** 29p–30p.

Taylor, C. M., Hughes, S. E., and de Silva, P. (1976). Competitive protein binding assay for 24,25-dihydroxycholecalciferol. *Biochem. Biophys. Res. Commun.* **70,** 1243–1249.

Taylor, C. M., Hann, H., St. John, J., Wallace, J. E., and Mawer, E. B. (1979). 1,25-Dihydroxycholecalciferol in human serum and its relationship with other metabolites of vitamin D-3. *Clin. Chim. Acta* **96,** 1–8.

Teitelbaum, S. L., Bone, J. M., Stein, P. M., Gilden, J. J., Bates, M., Boisseau, V. C. and Avioli, L. V. (1976). Calcifediol in chronic renal insufficiency, skeletal response. *JAMA J. Am. Med. Assoc.* **235,** 164–167.

Teitelbaum, S. L., Halverson, J. D., Bates, M., Wise, L., and Haddad, J. G. (1977). Abnormalities of circulating 25-OH-vitamin D after jejunal-ileal bypass for obesity. *Ann. Intern. Med.* **86,** 289–293.

Thomasset, M., Cuisinier-Gleizes, P., and Mathieu, H. (1979). 1,25-Dihydroxycholecaliferol: Dynamics of the stimulation of duodenal calcium-binding protein, calcium transport and bone calcium mobilization in vitamin D and calcium-deficient rats. *FEBS Lett.* **107,** 91–94.

Tolman, K. G., Jubiz, W., Sannella, J. J., Madsen, J. A., Belsey, R. E., Goldsmith, R. S., and Freston, J. W. (1975). Osteomalacia associated with anticonvulsant drug therapy in mentally retarded children. *Pediatrics* **56,** 45–51.

Tougaard, L., Christensen, M. S., Rodbro, P., and Sorensen, A. W. S. (1976). Controlled trial of 1α-hydroxycholecalciferol in chronic renal failure. *Lancet* **1,** 1044–1047.

Trechsel, U., Eisman, J. A., Fischer, J. A., Bonjour, J.-P., and Fleisch, H. (1980). Calcium-dependent parathyroid hormone-independent regulation of 1,25-dihyroxyvitamin D. *Am. J. Physiol.* **239,** E119–E124.

Tsai, H. C. and Norman, A. W. (1973). Studies on the mode of action of calciferol VI: Effect of 1,25-dihydroxyvitamin D_3 on RNA synthesis in the intestinal mucosa. *Biochem. Biophys. Res. Commun.* **54,** 622–627.

Tsai, H. C., Wong, R. G., and Norman, A. W. (1972). Studies on Calciferol Metabolism IV. Subcellular localization of 1,25-dihydroxyvitamin D_3 in intestinal mucosa and correlation with increased calcium transport. *J. Biol. Chem.* **247,** 5511–5519.

Tucker, G., Gagnon, R. E., and Haussler, M. R. (1973). Vitamin D_3-25-hydroxylase: Tissue occurrence and apparent lack of regulation. *Arch. Biochem. Biophys.* **155,** 47–57.

Valentzas, C., Oreopoulos, D. G., From, G., Porret, B., and Rapoport, A. (1977). Vitamin D levels in thyrotoxicosis. *Lancet* **1,** 370–371.

Van Baelen, H., Bouillon, R., and de Moor, P. (1977). Binding of 25-hydroxycholecalciferol in tissues. *J. Biol. Chem.* **252,** 2515–2518.

Van Den Berg, C. J., Kumar, R., Wilson, D. M., Heath, H., III, and Smith, L. H. (1980). Orthophosphate therapy decreases urinary calcium excretion and serum 1,25-dihydroxyvitamin D concentrations in idiopathic hypercalciuria. *J. Clin Endocrinol. Metab.* **51,** 998–1001.

von Herrath, D., Schaeffer, K., Kraft, D., and Offermann, G. (1975). Effect of *Solanum malacoxylon* on calcium metabolism in experimental uremia and uremic patients. *In* "Vitamin D and Problems Related to Uremic Bone Disease" (A. W. Norman, K. Schaefer, H. G. Grigoleit, D. von Herrath, and E. Ritz, eds.), pp. 703–708. de Gruyter, Berlin.

Wagonfeld, J. B., Nemchausky, B. A., Bolt, M., Horst, J. V., Boyer, J. L., and Rosenberg, I. H. (1976). Comparison of vitamin D and 25-hydroxyvitamin D in the therapy of primary biliary cirrhosis. *Lancet* **2,** 391–394.

Walling, M. W. (1977). Intestinal Ca and phosphate transport: Differential response to vitamin D_3 metabolites. *Am. J. Physiol.* **233,** E488–E494.

Wasserman, R. H. (1981). Intestinal absorption of calcium and phosphorus. *Fed. Proc. Fed. Am. Soc. Exp. Biol.* **40,** 68–72.

Wasserman, R. H., and Taylor, A. N. (1973). Intestinal absorption of phosphate in the chick: Effect of vitamin D_3 and other parameters. *J. Nutr.* **103,** 586–599.

Wasserman, R. H., Corradino, R. A., and Taylor, A. N. (1968). Vitamin D-dependent calcium-binding protein. *J. Biol. Chem.* **243,** 3978–3986.

Wasserman, R. H., Henion, J. D., Haussler, M. R., and McCain, T. A. (1976). Calcinogenic factor in *Solanum malacoxylon:* Evidence that it is 1,25-dihydroxyvitamin D_3-glycoside. *Science* **194,** 853–855.

Weisman, Y., Fattal, A., Eisenberg, Z., Harel, S., Spirer, Z., and Harell, A. (1979). Decreased serum 24,25-dihydroxy vitamin D concentrations in children receiving chronic anticonvulsant therapy. *Br. Med. J.* **2,** 521–523.

Werner, E., Malluche, H. H., Kutschera, J., Hodgson, M., and Schoeppe, W. (1976). Intestinal calcium absorption and whole-body calcium retention in various stages of renal insufficiency. *Calcif. Tissue Res.* **21,** Suppl., 210–215.

Wezeman, F. H. (1976). 25-hydroxyvitamin D_3: Autoradiographic evidence of sites of action in epiphyseal cartilage and bone. *Science* **194,** 1069–1071.

Whyte, M. P., Min, C., and Haddad, J. G. (1978). Dietary, substrate, and hormonal regulation of rat serum 24,25-dihydroxyvitamin D (24,25). *Clin. Res.* **26,** 430A.

Wilson, P. W., and Lawson, D. E. M. (1977). 1,25-dihydroxyvitamin D stimulation of specific membrane proteins in chick intestine. *Biochim. Biophys. Acta* **497,** 805–811.

Wong, R. G., Norman, A. W., Reddy, C. R., and Coburn, J. W. (1972). Biologic effects of 1,25-dihydroxycholecalciferol (a highly active vitamin D metabolite) in acutely uremic rats. *J. Clin. Invest.* **51,** 1287–1291.

Zerwekh, J. E., Brumbaugh, P. F., Haussler, D. H., Cork, D. J., and Haussler, M. R. (1974a). 1α-hydroxyvitamin D_3. An analog of vitamin D which apparently acts by metabolism to 1α,25-dihydroxyvitamin D_3. *Biochemistry* **13,** 4097–4102.

Zerwekh, J. E., Haussler, M. R., and Lindell, T. J. (1974b). Rapid enhancement of chick intestinal DNA-dependent RNA polymerase II activity by 1α,25-dihydroxyvitamin D_3, *in vivo*. *Proc. Natl. Acad. Sci. U.S.A.* **71,** 2337–2341.

Zerwekh, J. E., Lindell, T. J., and Haussler, M. R. (1976). Increased intestinal chromatin template activity. Influence of 1α,25-dihydroxyvitamin D_3 and hormone receptor complexes. *J. Biol. Chem.* **251,** 2388–2394.

Zile, M., Bunge, E. C., Barsness, L., Yamada, S., Schnoes, H. K., and DeLuca, H. F. (1978). Localization of 1,25-dihydroxyvitamin D_3 in intestinal nuclei *in vivo*. *Arch. Biochem. Biophys.* **186,** 15–24.

8

Calcitonin Secretion

Leonard J. Deftos

I. CALCITONIN

In 1962, Copp and his colleagues observed that perfusion of the thyroid–parathyroid gland complex of the dog with blood high in calcium caused a greater decline in systemic blood calcium than that produced by parathyroidectomy. Since the hypocalcemia could not be ascribed to inhibition of parathyroid hormone secretion by the hypocalcemic perfusion, Copp proposed the existence of a

Disorders of Mineral Metabolism, Vol. II

ISBN 0-12-135302-8

hypocalcemic hormone that was secreted by the parathyroid gland and named it "calcitonin." In the course of studies in parathyroidectomized rats, Hirsch *et al.* (1963) made the astute observation that parathyroidectomy by electrocautery produced a greater fall in calcium than did surgical parathyroidectomy. They concluded that cautery of the adjacent thyroid gland released a calcium-lowering factor from the thyroid gland. A hypocalcemic factor was extracted from the thyroid gland, and it was named "thyrocalcitonin" to distinguish it from calcitonin (Hirsch *et al.,* 1964). The initial controversy regarding the source of this hormone was resolved in 1964 by Foster and his colleagues (1964a), who demonstrated its thyroid origin and suggested that the source of calcitonin in the dog was the cell population corresponding to the parafollicular cells of Nonidez (1932) and the parenchymatous cells of Baber (1876). Further histochemical studies (Foster *et al.,* 1964b; Pearse, 1966; Solcia and Sampietro, 1968; Wetzel and Gittes, 1966) and more specific immunohistochemical studies (Bussolati and Pearse, 1967; Kalina *et al.,* 1970; Kracht *et al.,* 1968; McMillan *et al.,* 1974; Wolfe, *et al.,* 1974) established a discrete population of cells—the C cells—of the thyroid gland as the source of calcitonin in man and other mammals. In submammals, calcitonin was found to be produced by the ultimobranchial glands (Copp *et al.,* 1967; Tauber, 1967).

A. Biochemistry

Although rat thyroid glands provided the first crude extracts of calcitonin (Hirsch *et al.*, 1963), sufficient hormone for biochemical studies came from the porcine thyroid. The amino acid composition (Putter *et al.*, 1968) and sequence (Neher *et al.,* 1968a; Potts *et al.,* 1968) of porcine calcitonin revealed a 32-amino-acid peptide that was subsequently synthesized (Guttman *et al.,* 1968; Rittel *et al.,* 1968). Human calcitonin was isolated from a medullary thyroid carcinoma (Riniker *et al.,* 1968), its sequence determined (Neher *et al.,* 1968b), and synthesis accomplished (Sieber *et al.* 1968). The structure of bovine (Brewer and Ronan, 1969), ovine (Sauer *et al.,* 1970), salmon (Keutmann *et al.,* 1970, 1972; Niall *et al.,* 1969), rat (Byfield *et al.,* 1976; Raulais *et al.,* 1974), and eel (Noda and Narita, 1976; Otani *et al.,* 1976) calcitonin have also been determined (Fig. 1).

Examination of the naturally occurring calcitonins reveals certain common features, together with a considerable amount of apparent variability. The common features include the 1,7-amino-terminal disulfide bridge and the carboxyl-terminal prolinamide residue. Seven of the amino-terminal 9 residues are identical in all calcitonins. Residues 28 (glycine) and 32 (prolinamide) are the only other sequence positions completely conserved. In general, there is also considerable homology in the 10–27 region among porcine, bovine, and ovine calcitonin, between human and rat calcitonin, and between salmon and eel calcitonin,

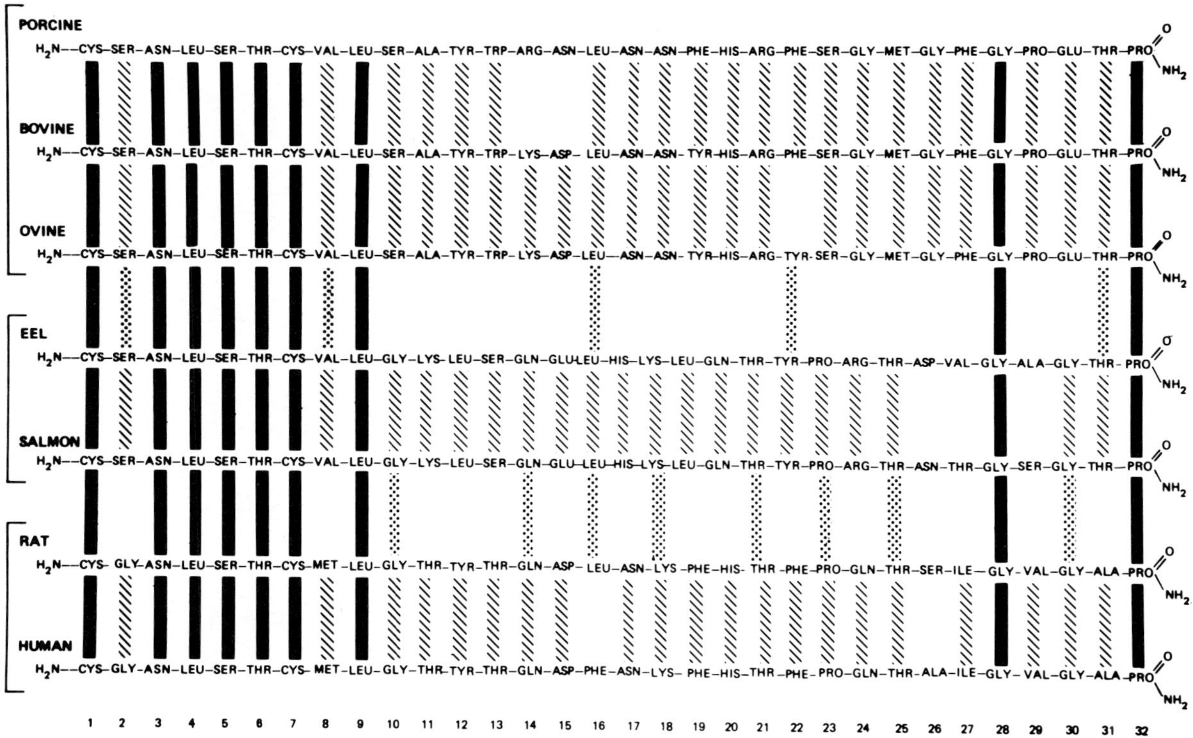

Fig. 1. Amino acid sequence of seven species of calcitonin. The molecules are bracketed on the left according to similarities of amino acid structure into three groups: the artiodactyl calcitonins—porcine, bovine, and ovine; eel and salmon calcitonin; and rat and human calcitonin. The solid bars indicate amino acids that are invariable. The striped bars indicate amino acid similarities within each of the three groups. The dotted bars indicate amino acid similarities between members of each of the three groups.

respectively. It is interesting to note that human calcitonin differs more from porcine (18 of 32 amino acids) than salmon calcitonin (15 of 32 amino acids). [It is also likely that there is considerable homology between salmon and chicken calcitonin, since radioimmunoassays based on the former can be used to measure the latter (Cutler *et al.*, 1974a,b).]

Calcitonins from ultimobranchial glands isolated from chum, sockeye, pink, and coho salmon species reveal microheterogeneity in that each species secretes two forms of calcitonin, designated salmon calcitonin I and either II or III. Salmon II calcitonin differs from Salmon I calcitonin in positions 15, 22, 29, and 31. Salmon III calcitonin is identical to Salmon II calcitonin in these positions but differs from that of Salmon I calcitonin in an additional position (residue 8), where methionine replaces valine (Keutmann *et al.*, 1972).

The sequence variability of the middle region of calcitonin (residues 10–27 inclusive) is perhaps more apparent than real. Many differences can be explained by a single base exchange (mutation). Though no single amino acid in this region is constant in all seven calcitonins, there is considerable similarity when the comparison is based on the chemical properties of the amino acid side chains. Acidic residues (aspartic or glutamic acid) are found only at position 15. (The only other acidic residue is found at position 30 in porcine, bovine, and ovine calcitonins.) Basic residues are also confined to a relatively few positions. Where substitutions are found for basic residues, asparagine or glutamine is the most common replacement. This is a conservative change since the amides are regarded as possessing weakly basic properties and the basic amino acid–amide exchange is extremely common in other groups of related proteins and peptides. Hydrophobic residues (leucine, phenylalanine, or tyrosine) are distributed almost regularly along the peptide chain, occupying positions 4, 9, 12, 16, 19, and 22.

All calcitonins contain at least one acidic residue at positions 15 and/or 30. Moderate conservation regarding the distribution of basic residues has been observed, as discussed above. Postions 14, 17, 18, and 20 are occupied by either a basic residue (arginine, lysine, or histidine) or an amide. All calcitonins contain at least two basic residues. Methionine is found at two positions in the calcitonins, 8 and 25. Methionine is not required, however, for biological activity, since salmon and eel calcitonin lack methionine. Tryptophan is present in porcine, bovine, and ovine calcitonins at position 13, but salmon, human, rat, and eel calcitonins lack tryptophan. The number of tyrosines present in the calcitonins varies from zero (in salmon II and III) to three (in ovine calcitonin). When present, tyrosines occupy positions 12, 19, and/or 22. Though tyrosine is plainly not essential for biological activity, it is always replaced by a hydrophobic residue at these positions, as mentioned above.

In general, the ultimobranchial calcitonins, which have more basic amino acids, are more potent than the thyroidal calcitonins. Amino acid substitutions in human calcitonin, which make its structure more similar to salmon calcitonin, result in an increase in potency (Maier *et al.*, 1975). The potency of human and porcine calcitonin can be decreased by deletion of the C-terminal amide, shortening of the length at the C terminus, and opening the disulfide ring; potency is unaffected or even enhanced by N-terminal modifications (Rittel *et al.*, 1976; Sieber *et al.*, 1970). The stability of calcitonin to plasma enzymes also appears to play a role in the potency of the hormone with salmon calcitonin being more stable than mammalian calcitonin (Habener *et al.*, 1971). The search for "active fragments" of calcitonin has not been rewarding. This suggests that the whole peptide chain is involved in the biological activity of the hormone, with the overall size and chain length and the chemical groupings at either end of the chain being particularly critical for binding to receptor sites (Potts *et al.*, 1971b).

B. Biological Effects

Calcitonin exerts its biologic effects by acting on three primary target organs—bone, kidney, and the gastrointestinal (GI) tract. Like many other peptide hormones, calcitonin seems to mediate its effects via adenylate cyclase (Care *et al.*, 1970; Heersche *et al.*, 1974; Marx and Aurbach, 1975). The effect of calcitonin in blood—to decrease plasma calcium and phosphate concentration—is the summation of these multiple actions of the hormone.

1. *Bone*

The major biologic effect of calcitonin is to decrease bone resorption by inhibiting the activity of osteoclasts and osteocysts. This is reflected by the decrease in alkaline phosphatase produced by calcitonin. It has also been suggested that calcitonin promotes bone formation but this has been difficult to establish conclusively. Calcitonin acts on both the mineral and organic phases of bone. By inhibiting the resorption of the mineral phase, calcitonin prevents the translocation of calcium and phosphorus from bone. Thus, in those situations in which bone turnover is sufficiently high, calcitonin will produce hypocalcemia and hypophosphatemia. By inhibiting the resorption of the organic phase of bone, calcitonin decreases the excretion of urinary hydroxyproline (Hirsch and Munson, 1969).

2. *Kidney*

Calcitonin increases the urinary excretion of calicum and phosphorus (Ardaillou *et al.*, 1967). Calcitonin also promotes the renal excretion of sodium and chloride and, to a lesser extent, potassium (Bijvoet *et al.*, 1971). The physiologic significance of these renal effects of calcitonin is not understood (Ardaillou, 1975).

3. Gastrointestinal Tract

Studies in animals by several investigators have produced apparently conflicting results. In a study of intact rats, Milhaud and Moukhtar (1966) found that administration of calcitonin produced an increase in intestinal calcium absorption and a decrease in endogenous fecal calcium excretion. The study did not exclude parathyroid hormone as the mediator of this effect. Olson *et al.* (1972) studied the effect of calcitonin on isolated rat intestinal segments perfused with an artificial blood supply. They found that small doses of calcitonin produced a marked and rapid increase in calcium absorption that occurred more rapidly than the rise observed after administration of parathyroid hormone; this suggested that parathyroid hormone did not mediate the calcitonin effect. Cramer and his colleagues (1969) found no effect of hog or chicken calcitonin on calcium absorption by isolated gut loops in dogs. Cramer also found no effects of salmon calcitonin on calcium absorption in rats injected repeatedly with salmon calcitonin over several hours (Cramer, 1973).

Studies in humans have been equally inconclusive. Hioco and his colleagues (1970) found that when porcine calcitonin was given to human patients with poor calcium absorption associated with osteoporosis, true intestinal absorption increased as did urinary calcium excretion; serum calcium did not change. Pak found that administration of calcitonin to patients who were surgically hypoparathyroid produced an increase in gut absorption of calcium in two of three cases (G. Y. C. Pak, personal communications). Swaminathan and his colleagues (1974) found that in pigs infused with porcine calcitonin over several days there was initially a rise in calcium absorption, followed by a fall to levels below those observed in the basal state. Gray and his colleagues (1973) and Hirsch and his colleagues (1974) and others have studied the effects of calcitonin on human intestinal function using a triple-lumen jejunal tube technique. Using salmon calcitonin, they noted marked effects on secretion of water and electrolytes but observed no direct effect on calcium absorption or secretion.

In summary, several studies can be cited indicating that calcitonin increases, decreases, or does not directly affect the absorption of calcium by the intestine in man and experimental animals. These variations may in part be due to variations in species studied and wide variations in methodology. Another potentially important source of variation is the fact that the calcitonin has been administered exogenously and originated in species other than the test animal. Often salmon calcitonin has been used, which is markedly different from the mammalian species that have been studied (Potts *et al.*, 1971a). For these reasons, the role of calcitonin in calcium absorption remains undefined.

The effects of calcitonin on the secretory activity of the GI tract seem better established. Calcitonin inhibits gastric secretion (Becker *et al.*, 1973; Fahrenkrug *et al.*, 1975) and bile flow (Dangoumau *et al.*, 1976), has a variable effect on secretin (Iwatsuki and Hashimoto, 1976; Tarnawski *et al.*, 1974), and promotes water and electrolyte secretion by the small intestine (Gray *et al.*, 1973). It stimulates salivary gland secretion (Koelz *et al.*, 1976), including amylase (Dreyfus *et al.*, 1976). Calcitonin decreases basal and gastrin- and histamine-stimulated gastric acid secretion and gastrin secretion (Becker *et al.*, 1973, 1974; Hesch *et al.*, 1971) and inhibits secretion of exocrine pancreatic enzymes (Schmidt *et al.*, 1971). Calcitonin only inhibits hormonally stimulated but not vagally stimulated pancreatic exocrine function (Hotz *et al.*, 1977). The effect of calcitonin may be more prominent on acinar than on ductular cells (Iwatsuki and Hashimoto, 1976).

4. Other Effects

A variety of other effects have been observed for calcitonin. It has been reported to be antiflammatory (Abdullahi *et al.*, 1977; Velo *et al.*, 1976), to promote fracture (Adachi *et al.*, 1974) and wound (Lupulescu, 1975) healing, to be uricosuric (Blahos *et al.*, 1975), to inhibit lipolysis (Werner and Low, 1974), to have pituitary (Leicht *et al.*, 1974) and CNS (Pecile *et al.*, 1975) effects, to be antihypertensive (Aldred *et al.*, 1976), to impair glucose tolerance (Blahos *et al.*, 1976), and to be analgesic (Braga *et al.*, 1978). The importance of these effects will be decided by future studies.

C. Secretion

1. Calcium and Related Minerals

Calcium is the best-studied secretagogue for calcitonin (Parthemore and Deftos, 1978). The secretion of calcitonin is directly related to blood calcium concentration. An acute increase in blood calcium results in a proportional increase in plasma calcitonin, and an acute decrease in blood calcium produces a corresponding decrease in plasma calcitonin in humans and experimental animals (Deftos, 1978a). Studies in humans suggest that females may have a decreased calcitonin reserve compared to males (Heath and Sizemore, 1977; Parthemore and Deftos, 1978). Although the effects of acute changes in blood calcium concentration on plasma calcitonin are well established, the effects of chronic hypercalcemia and hypocalcemia are not fully defined and contradictory results have been reported (Silva *et al.*, 1974c; Tashjian *et al.*, 1970). These variable responses of plasma calcitonin in patients with hypercalcemia may reflect a limited capacity of C cells to respond to chronic stimulation. Animal studies suggest that the C cells can become ''exhausted'' during prolonged exposure to elevated blood calcium (Ericson, 1968); however, these experiments have many limitations and their applicability to humans is not clear.

Elevated basal levels of calcitonin have been reported in some patients with hypercalcemia and malignancy, but it has been difficult in these studies to differentiate between hypercalcemia, ectopic calcitonin production by the tumor, impaired renal function, or other factors as the cause of increased plasma calcitonin (Coombes *et al.*, 1974a; Silva *et al.*, 1976). In hypercalcemia due to hyperparathyroidism, most studies have failed to demonstrate any consistent abnormalities in plasma calcitonin although normal, elevated, and decreased levels of the hormone have been reported (Adachi *et al.*, 1976; Goldsmith *et al.*, 1976; Heynen and Franchimont, 1974a; Lambert *et al.*, 1976; Morita *et al.*, 1975; Rojanasathit and Haddad, 1977; Silva *et al.*, 1974c; Tashjian *et al.*, 1970). Histological evidence of C-cell hyperplasia suggests increased calcitonin secretion in some hyperparathyroid patients (Kracht *et al.*, 1970; LiVolsi *et al.*, 1973; Ljungberg and Dymling, 1972; Tashjian and Voelkel, 1967). Recent studies have demonstrated increased plasma calcitonin secretion in patients, primarily males, with primary hyperparathyroidism (Parthemore, 1977; Parthemore *et al.*, 1977). As in normal subjects, females with primary hyperparathyroidism seem to have a decreased calcitonin reserve.

There are no definitive studies on the effect of chronic hypocalcemia on calcitonin secretion. It might be inferred from some studies that chronic hypocalcemia suppresses calcitonin secretion (Deftos *et al.*, 1973). Calcium and pentagastrin infusions in hypocalcemic patients produce a considerably greater increase in plasma calcitonin than seen in normal subjects. The chronic hypocalcemia in these subjects may result in increased storage of calcitonin in C cells, which is released by the secretagogues. Increased thyroidal calcitonin has been described in chronic hypocalcemic states (Aliapoulios *et al.*, 1966). Direct studies of secretion are necessary to establish this hypothesis.

Minerals related to calcium also seem to have an acute stimulatory effect on calcitonin secretion. In animal studies, the administration of magnesium and strontium stimulates the secretion of calcitonin but to a lesser degree than does calcium (Pento *et al.*, 1974). Magnesium also stimulates the secretion of calcitonin in normal human subjects (Deftos *et al.*, 1978c), but interestingly in some patients with medullary thyroid carcinoma, magnesium seems to suppress calcitonin secretion (Anast *et al.*, 1975).

2. *Gastrointestinal Factors*

Several gastrointestinal factors can also regulate the secretion of calcitonin. In both humans and experimental animals the intravenous administration of pentagastrin (or of the closely related cholecystokinin and caerulein) and glucagon produced a brisk increase in plasma calcitonin (Barlet and Garel, 1976; Deftos *et al.*, 1971; Parthemore and Deftos, 1978; Passeri *et al.*, 1975). In these studies, however, the dose of hormones was sufficiently great to increase their blood concentration to levels that are probably higher than even in the postprandial state. Thus, it is not clear if the relationship between GI hormones such as gastrin or glucagon is physiologically important. Furthermore, it has been possible to demonstrate an increase in plasma calcitonin related to eating and/or an oral calcium load in only a few clinical and experimental studies (Garel, 1978; Nozaka *et al.*, 1976). Although there is considerable clinical and experimental data to suggest a functional relationship between the gastrointestinal tract and C cells, the physiological significance of this relationship awaits further study.

3. *Neuroendocrine Factors*

Increasingly, there is evidence to indicate that neuroendocrine hormones can influence calcitonin secretion. Thus, adrenergic agents can stimulate and suppress the secretion of calcitonin (Care *et al.*, 1970). Similar effects have been observed in clinical studies in normal human subjects and in patients with primary and secondary abnormalities in calcitonin secretion. In humans, calcitonin was stimulated by the β-agonist isoproterenol and the α-antagonist phentolamine and decreased by the β-antagonist propranolol. The α-agonist methoxamine has also been reported to stimulate plasma calcitonin in humans (Metz *et al.*, 1978; Vora *et al.*, 1978). However, these studies have not excluded any possible secretory effect of changes in blood flow to the thyroid gland, small changes in ionized calcium, or alterations in hormone metabolism. An effect on calcitonin secretion of another neuroendocrine agent, somatostatin, has not been firmly established. High doses of somatostatin in animal studies suppress calcitonin (Hargis *et al.*, 1978), whereas this has not been apparent in lower doses in human studies (Metz *et al.*, 1978). The possibility of a somatostatin effect on calcitonin secretion is intriguing since somatostatin-containing cells have been demonstrated in the thyroid gland by immunohistological techniques (Hokfelt *et al.*, 1975). As with the gastrointestinal hormones, the physiological significance of the relationship between neuroendocrine factors and calcitonin secretion remains to be established.

4. *Age and Sex*

The effect of age and sex on plasma calcitonin appears to be species dependent. In the salmon, plasma calcitonin is higher in females than in males (Watts *et al.*, 1974). In the bovine species, the opposite is true, but age and dietary factors are also important in that calcitonin is decreased in older animals and increased in those on high-calcium diets (Deftos *et al.*, 1972). Female rats have higher plasma levels of calcitonin than male rats, and in both sexes hormone concentration increases as a function of age (Deftos *et al.*, 1975b; Roos *et al.*, 1978). Preliminary studies in humans indicate that age and sex also influence calcitonin secretion. Higher-than-normal plasma levels have been reported in pregnant females and newborn infants (Samaan *et al.*, 1973; Schedewiee *et al.*, 1978). Menstrual effects on plasma calcitonin have also been reported (Pitkin *et al.*, 1981; Whyte *et al.*, 1978). Preliminary studies suggested that plasma calcitonin decreases as a function of age in humans (Deftos *et al.*, 1980) and it seems reasonably well established that calcitonin secretion and calcitonin reserve are decreased in females (Heath and Sizemore, 1977; Parthemore and Deftos, 1978). Thus, although age and sex do influence calcitonin secretion, other factors, some of them species specific, also modulate these effects.

5. *Other Factors*

A surprising relationship has been observed between calcitonin secretion and iodine metabolism—surprising since C cells have not been classically regarded to participate in iodine metabolism (Hirsch and Munson, 1969). In rats made iodine deficient, C cells become hyperplastic and plasma calcitonin increased (Clark *et al.*, 1977; Peng *et al.*, 1975). This effect can be blocked or reversed by iodine replacement and perhaps by thyroxine (Deftos *et al.*, 1978c). In some instances the effect of iodine deficiency on calcitonin may be due to the development of hypercalcemia (Clark *et al.*, 1978). By contrast, athyreotic cretins may have a decreased calcitonin secretion (Carey *et al.*, 1978). Prostaglandins in high doses stimulate plasma calcitonin in the rat but this effect is difficult to reproduce consistently in humans (Metz et al., 1978; Roos and Deftos, 1976a). Some studies suggest that calcitonin may exert an autoregulatory effect on its own secretion (Bell, 1970).

D. Metabolism

The metabolism of calcitonin is a complex process that involves many organ systems. Evidence has been presented for degradation of the hormone by kidney, liver, bone, and even the thyroid gland. Unfortunately, most of the published data regarding calcitonin metabolism are of questionable physiologic significance, although of considerable pharmacologic interest. This is due to several reasons. Most of the studies have been done with either pharmacologic amounts or radioiodinated species of calcitonin (Ardaillou *et al.*, 1970; Clark *et al.*, 1974; Scarpace *et al.*, 1977; West *et al.*, 1969). More critical, however, is the fact that many studies have been performed with nonhomologous species of calcitonin—for example, salmon calcitonin studies in the dog, human calcitonin studies in the pig (Clark *et al.*, 1974; Ito *et al.*, 1976; Singer *et al.*, 1972b; West *et al.*, 1969). Additionally, many studies have assessed metabolism by measuring the immunological activity of calcitonin rather than biological activity (Ardaillou *et al.*, 1970; Singer *et al.*, 1972b; West *et al.*, 1969). These major reservations allow only the following tentative conclusions to be drawn regarding the metabolism of calcitonin. Similar to many other peptide hormones, calcitonin disappears from plasma in a multiexponential manner that includes an early half-life that can be measured in minutes and a later half-life of hours (Ardaillou *et al.*, 1970; Clark *et al.*, 1974; Scarpace *et al.*, 1977; West *et al.*, 1969). The rapid component(s) may represent mixing of calcitonin within its volume of distribution and the slower component(s) may represent the rate of true decay. In most studies, the kidney seems to be the most important organ of clearance for calcitonin (Ardaillou *et al.*, 1970; Clark *et al.*, 1974; West *et al.*, 1969). Peripheral inactivation of the hormone seems more important than renal excretion, since relatively little calcitonin can be detected in urine (Clark *et al.*, 1974; West *et al.*, 1969). Liver is also an important organ in calcitonin clearance and in some studies it is dominant (de Luise *et al.*, 1970; Singer *et al.*, 1972b). Bone, thyroid, and plasma degradation also contribute to the disappearance of calcitonin from the circulation (Clark *et al.*, 1974; Ito *et al.*, 1976; Pento, 1978; Scarpace *et al.*, 1977; Singer, *et al.*, 1972b; West *et al.*, 1969).

II. PHYSIOLOGY OF CALCITONIN

The physiological role of calcitonin in humans has not been established, either in terms of calcium homeostasis or skeletal metabolism. Athyreotic adults do not seem to have a clearly defined abnormality in skeletal metabolism that can be defined in short-term studies, but such studies should be interpreted with reservation. For example, it is difficult to determine if adults who have been thyroidectomized are, in fact, totally calcitonin deficient. Remnants of thyroid tissue may remain even after thyroidectomy or thyroid ablation with radioiodine. And, there may be extrathyroidal sources of calcitonin (Deftos *et al.*, 1978c). In fact, plasma and urinary calcitonin have been described in presumably athyreotic adults (Silva *et al.*, 1978). Furthermore, the role of potentially damaged parathyroid glands has not been carefully considered in such studies. No prospective long-term studies have been done to establish the presence or absence of mineral abnormalities in athyreotic adults. It is interesting to note that bone disease is common in athyreotic cretins. Although the bone disease is generally regarded to be due to deficiency of T_3 and T_4, some data suggest that calcitonin deficiency may play a role in the pathogenesis of thyroid-related bone disease (Carey *et al.*, 1978).

Studies in thyroidectomized patients have been interpreted to suggest that calcitonin may play a role in modulating perturbations in blood calcium, a view supported by the changes in plasma calcitonin seen in hypercalcemic states and perhaps renal disease. In some, but not all, studies, thyroidectomized patients have demonstrated a decreased tolerance to oral and parenteral calcium challenge, and patients with medullary thyroid carcinoma and high levels of calcitonin have demonstrated an increased calcium tolerance (Melvin *et al.*, 1970). It has been difficult to support this hypothesis by demonstrating in humans a postprandial increase in plasma calcitonin. However, in rats and cattle, plasma calcitonin is higher in the fed state than in the fasted state (Roos *et al.*, 1978).

Many early interpretations of the physiological role of calcitonin in humans were made before adequate methods were available to measure tissue, plasma, and urine calcitonin levels. It has taken the development of specific immunohistochemical techniques to identify consistently calcitonin in human thyroid glands (McMillan *et al.*, 1974); it has taken the development of highly sensitive and specific radioimmunoassay procedures to measure accurately the low plasma concentrations of hormone that are reported by most but not all laboratories (Parthemore and Deftos, 1978; Fig. 2).

A corollary to these problems was the difficulty that was initially encountered in demonstrating changes in plasma calcitonin during experimental protocols known to influence secretion of the hormone in experimental animals. However, with the development of sensitive assay procedures, it has now been established that agents such as calcium, EDTA, magnesium, pentagastrin, and glucagon, all can modify calcitonin secretion in humans (Deftos *et al.*, 1978c; Parthemore and Deftos, 1978).

In medullary thyroid carcinoma, characterized by increased plasma calcitonin, abnormalities in calcium or bone have not been consistently found. However, it is possible that the escape of bone from the biological effect of calcitonin has minimized such changes, perhaps in a homeostatistically appropriate manner (Raisz *et al.*, 1968). In addition, it still remains a plausible hypothesis that an increase in parathyroid hormone secretion in such patients, either in a compen-

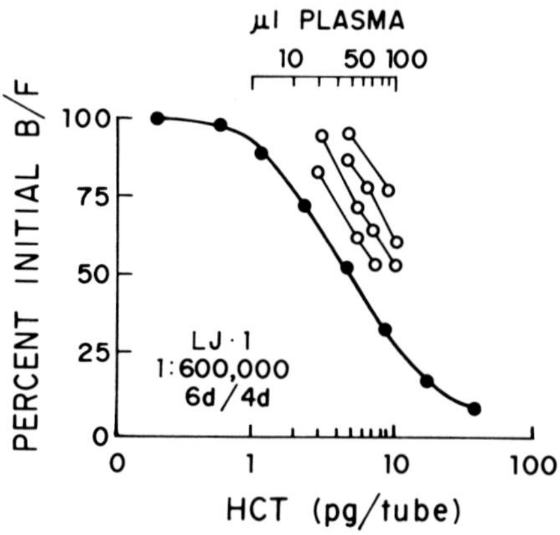

Fig. 2. Standard curve of the hCT RIA (●). Also shown is the displacement of tracer produced by increasing aliquots of several human plasma samples (○). (From Parthemore and Deftos, 1978.)

satory fashion or due to genetic factors, obviates the effects of calcitonin. Finally, in some careful studies, a presumed calcitonin effect on bone has been described in patients with medullary thyroid carcinoma (Melvin *et al.*, 1973).

On the basis of animal studies that demonstrated that the hypocalcemic effect of calcitonin decreases as a function of age and is most prominent in young animals, it has been suggested that calcitonin may play some role in the growth and development of bone (Deftos, 1978b). This view receives some support from clinical studies that have demonstrated elevated levels of plasma calcitonin in the neonate (Samaan *et al.*, 1974). However, an alternative explanation is that the response to exogenous calcitonin decreases with age because the endogenous plasma calcitonin levels increase with age, at least in rats (Deftos *et al.*, 1975b; Roos *et al.*, 1978).

The precise role of calcitonin in regulating calcium homeostasis and metabolism is as yet uncertain. It has always been puzzling why elimination of calcitonin has not led to a rise in the steady-state blood calcium level in normal animals or why it failed to affect the steady-state parameters of calcium metabolism (Bronner *et al.*, 1967; Sammon *et al.*, 1969). Studies utilizing an intraperitoneally injected calcium load (Bronner *et al.*, 1968; Sammon *et al.*, 1969; Talmadge *et al.*, 1965) revealed that in calcitonin-deficient (thyroidectomized with functioning parathyroid autografts) animals, it took longer than in controls for the plasma calcium level to return to the preinjection level. In other words, the ability to correct an acute positive error in plasma calcium regulation is diminished in animals without circulating calcitonin. This has been likened (Bronner, 1973; see also Chapter 2, this volume) to the absence of a derivative control. The physiological significance of this is not known, particularly as it is difficult to induce acute hypercalcemia by nutritional means, even in calcitonin-deficient animals. Moreover, one cannot distinguish parathyroidectomized from calcitonin-deficient animals in terms of their diminished ability to overcome an intraperitoneal calcium load. In other words, both groups have the same error–time curve (Bronner *et al.*, 1968). Consequently, a diminished ability to overcome acute hypercalcemia, while characteristic of the calcitonin-deficient animal, is not unique to that condition. However, clinical studies are beginning to uncover pathophysiological roles for calcitonin and to indicate new directions for research (Section III,A1,b–d and Section III,B–E). Recent studies have demonstrated that thyroidectomy in older rats, which have relatively high levels of plasma calcitonin, produces an increase in plasma calcium. However, this increase is slight and only transient (Kalu *et al.*, 1975).

Animal studies suggest another physiological role for calcitonin that finds some support in preliminary clinical studies. In rats, pregnancy and suckling and lactation results in an increase in plasma calcitonin (Cooper *et al.*, 1977; Toverud *et al.*, 1976). For the fetus and neonate, as discussed, this may protect against postprandial hypercalcemia and promote the assimilation of calcium into the developing skeleton. For the mother, the increased calcitonin may attenuate any increase bone resorption that occurs to provide calcium in milk (lactation).

Perhaps some of the more interesting information regarding the physiology of calcitonin comes from studies of sex-related changes in hormone secretion. In humans (as well as bovines), basal plasma calcitonin is lower in females than in males, and females have decreased calcitonin reserve during provocative testing (Deftos *et al.*, 1978c; Sizemore and Heath, 1975). It is interesting to note that in the bovine species a high-calcium diet can result in an increase to male levels of plasma calcitonin in females (Deftos *et al.*, 1972). It has been suggested that this relative calcitonin deficiency may play some role in the pathogenesis of certain bone diseases in females. Evidence for this view is provided by studies of plasma calcitonin in primary hyperparathyroidism. Females with primary hyperparathyroidism are unable to increase their plasma calcitonin concentrations in the face of this hypercalcemic (and bone hyperresorbtive) challenge, as are males (Parthemore *et al.*, 1977). This may account for the greater severity of bone disease reported for females with primary hyperparathyroidism (Pak *et al.*, 1975). This calcitonin deficiency in females may also play a role in the pathogenesis of postmenopausal osteoporosis. This view receives some support from the recent observation that calcitonin secretion in females decreases with increasing age (Davidson *et al.*, 1979).

Recent preliminary studies have led to a novel view regarding calcitonin physiology. Immunoreactive calcitonin, or a calcitonin-like substance, has been identified in the pituitary gland of several mammalian species (Deftos *et al.*, 1978a,b). When considered in connection with menstruation-related changes in plasma calcitonin in normal females (Pitkin *et al.*, 1981; Whyte *et al.*, 1978), it may be that calcitonin has a paracrine as well as an endocrine function. This possibility derives support from the wide variety of local, often inhibitory, effects attributed to calcitonin.

The physiologic significance of calcitonin thus still remains undefined. New, possible functions have emerged from recent studies but understanding of calcitonin function may come as we learn to ask new questions and test new approaches.

III. DISORDERS OF CALCITONIN SECRETION

A. Hypercalcitoninemia and Malignancy

1. *Eutopic Calcitonin Production*

Medullary Thyroid Carcinoma. Medullary thyroid carcinoma (MTC) is a tumor of the calcitonin-producing cells (C cells) of the thyroid gland. Whereas the follicular cells of the thyroid have been known for a long time, the presence of C cells within the human thyroid gland had attracted little attention until the discovery of (thyro)calcitonin in the early 1960s. Williams (1966) suggested in 1966 that C cells might be the origin of medullary carcinoma of the thyroid, a tumor that had been identified by Hazard and colleagues (Hazard *et al.*, 1959) as a pathologic entity different from other thyroid tumors. Williams's hypothesis was proved correct when several investigators demonstrated by bioassay the presence of abnormal calcitonin concentrations in medullary thyroid carcinoma (Cunliffe *et al.*, 1968; Melvin and Tashjian, 1968; Meyer and Abdel-Bari, 1968; Milhaud *et al.*, 1968). These findings were confirmed by specific radioimmunoassays of human calcitonin in tumor and blood (Clark *et al.*, 1969) and by histochemical studies (Kalina *et al.*, 1970). Subsequently, the tumor was shown to produce a wide variety of other bioactive substances (Deftos, 1978a). Of particular interest is the association of medullary thyroid carcinoma with other endocrine and nonendocrine neoplasms (Table I). This association may result from the fact that most of the tumor tissues have a common embryologic origin, namely the neural crest (LeDourain and LeLievre, 1970; Pearse and Takor, 1976).

(i). Embryology. Neural crest cells migrate to the ultimobranchial bodies. In submammals, these bodies form the ultimobranchial organ, where the C cells and their secretory product, calcitonin, are found. In mammals the C cells become incorporated in the thyroid gland and perhaps other sites.

(ii). Pathology. Medullary thyroid carcinoma usually presents as a firm, rounded tumor located in the middle or upper lobes of the thyroid gland (Williams, 1966). It is commonly bilateral and multifocal, especially in familial

TABLE I

Multiple Endocrine Neoplasia[a]

Type I	
Parathyroid	Adenoma or hyperplasia
Pancreas	Adenoma (islet cell)
Pituitary	Adenoma
Type II	
Thyroid	Medullary thyroid carcinoma
Adrenal	Pheochromocytoma
Parathyroid	Hyperplasia or adenoma
Type III	
Thyroid	Medullary thyroid carcinoma
Adrenal	Pheochromocytoma
Neural Tissue	Neurogangliomas
Somatic	Marfanoid habitus

[a] Adapted from Deftos (1978a).

cases. The histologic features of the tumor vary in appearance. The cells usually are polyhedral or polygonal in shape and are arranged in a variety of patterns (Ljungberg, 1972). The arrangement of the cells can be influenced by the distribution of stromal elements, which can be scanty or predominant. Sites of calcification are common in the tumor and tend to be denser and more irregular than the homogeneous psammoma bodies that occur in other thyroid cancers. Dense calcifications may be visible on X ray. A common feature of medullary thyroid carcinoma is the presence of amyloid with the histochemical characteristics of the immune amyloids, but immunochemical and immunohistological studies suggest that the material is also secreted by the C cells and is structurally related to calcitonin. Although in the past the present of amyloid was considered to be important for the diagnosis of medullary thyroid carcinoma, the diagnosis is now best established with specific immunohistochemical procecures for calcitonin that demonstrate the abnormal C cells (LiVolsi *et al.*, 1973; McMillan *et al.*, 1974).

(a). C-cell hyperplasia. Wolfe and colleagues (1973) defined C-cell hyperplasia as a distinct pathological entity. This had been preceded by the description of increased C-cell populations in animals (Williams, 1966) and humans (Ljungberg, 1972) with medullary thyroid carcinoma. Wolfe *et al.* (1973) were studying three patients at risk for medullary thyroid carcinoma because of their family history. These patients had small but progressive increases in plasma calcitonin during calcium infusion and consequently underwent thyroidectomy. The extirpated thyroid glands did not reveal the presence of medullary thyroid carcinoma. However, they did reveal clusters of hyperplastic parafollicular cells which were calcitonin positive by immunohistological studies. The presence of increased calcitonin in these cells was confirmed by bioassay and immunoassay. The distribution of these hyperplastic parafollicular cells was in the area where C cells are usually most prominent, the upper and middle portions of the lateral thyroid lobes. These cells exhibited no nuclear atypia or invasive tendencies. These observations suggested that, at least in familial cases of medullary thyroid carcinoma, the frank malignancy is preceded by a progressive hyperplasia of C cells.

This predecessor of medullary thyroid carcinoma can become manifest in early childhood or as late as the second decade (Carney *et al.*, 1976; Keiser *et al.*, 1973; Wolfe *et al.*, 1973). These early stages of medullary thyroid carcinoma are not only of fundamental importance for cancer pathogenesis, but also have considerable clinical significance. The early states of medullary thyroid carcinoma, when the neoplastic process is confined to the thyroid gland, are most amenable to surgery. While at present hyperplasia of the C cells and their subtle histological changes cannot be detected clinically, they may become identifiable with the calcitonin assay. Provocative testing is especially valuable in patients who have normal basal levels of plasma calcitonin (McKenna *et al.*, 1978).

(b). C-cell adenoma. Several instances of C-cell adenoma have been reported (Beskid, 1975; Milhaud *et al.*, 1972). These results must be considered as only preliminary evidence for the existence of such an adenoma. Definitive evidence will have to be provided by specific immunohistochemical studies that demonstrate the presence of calcitonin in the tumor and perhaps in peripheral blood.

(iii). Incidence. Medullary thyroid carcinoma has been reported to comprise 4–12% of all thyroid cancer, a relatively uncommon tumor (Hill *et al.*, 1973). The ratio of female to male involvement is closer to unity than in other thyroid tumors. Although the majority of cases reported in the earlier literature appeared to be sporadic, an appreciation of the familial incidence of the tumor is resulting in an increasing identification of inherited cases (Deftos, 1978a). Despite its rarity, the tumor has acquired clinical importance because it is distributed familially and in an autosomal dominant pattern. Its presence can be established by measuring calcitonin, its secretory product, and because it is associated with an intriguing array of clinical features (Table I). Moreover, the search for it in the family of an affected individual is often fruitful, as the tumor can be diagnosed biochemically even when there are no clinical signs. In turn, early diagnosis can lead to effective therapy and cure (Tashjian *et al.*, 1970).

(iv). Natural History. The natural history of a medullary thyroid carinoma can vary greatly, and this can make decisions regarding therapy difficult. The tumor is generally regarded to be intermediate to the aggressive behavior of anaplastic thyroid carcinoma and the more prolonged course of papillary and follicular thyroid carcinoma. However, it can be rapidly progressive, widely metastatic, and lead to death within weeks of diagnosis. By contrast, it can be indolent and compatible with decades of life (Hill *et al.*, 1973). Medullary thyroid carcinoma commonly spreads to regional lymphatics, a complication present in the majority of tumors reported. Distant metastases can involve any organ: lung, liver, bone, and adrenal gland are relatively common sites (Ibanez *et al.*, 1967).

(v). Calcitonin Secretion. Since medullary thyroid carcinoma is a neoplastic disorder of the C cells of the thyroid gland, the tumor produces abnormally high amounts of calcitonin, which can exceed normal thyroid content by orders of magnitude. As a result, patients with this tumor have elevated concentrations of calcitonin in peripheral blood and urine. In many patients, basal concentrations of the hormone are sufficiently elevated to be diagnostic of the tumor's presence. Therefore, the radioimmunoassay for calcitonin can be used to diagnose the presence of medullary thyroid carcinoma with an exceptional degree of accuracy and specificity when applied to measurements in random plasma samples. However, in a small but increasing percentage of patients, basal hormone levels are indistinguishable from normal (Deftos, 1974). Many of these cases represent early stages of C-cell neoplasia or perhaps even hyperplasia, and these early stages are, as stated above, most amenable to surgical cure. Provocative tests

have been developed for the diagnosis of medullary thyroid carcinoma and its histological antecedents (Melvin *et al.,* 1971a) and have led to the identification of the tumor in patients in whom the diagnosis could have been missed by only basal calcitonin determinations.

(a). Provocative testing.

1. Glucagon. Although glucagon can stimulate calcitonin secretion, it is not widely used as a diagnostic agent in the medullary thyroid carcinoma suspect. Glucagon is not a reliable calcitonin secretagogue, since its effect can be variable (Deftos *et al.,* 1971). Also, glucagon can release catecholamines and since patients with medullary thyroid carcinoma can have associated pheochromocytomas, an adrenergic crisis can be precipitated by its administration (Deftos, 1978a).

2. Calcium. Calcium by intravenous infusion has been the most widely used secretagogue for calcitonin in medullary thyroid carcinoma. In early studies calcium was infused at doses ranging from 3 to 5 mg per kg/hr for periods varying from 2 to 4 hr. The increase in calcium produced by such infusions, usually several mg/dl, consistently produced an abnormal increase in plasma calcitonin in patients with medullary thyroid carcinoma (Tashjian *et al.,* 1970). The abnormal increase in plasma calcitonin occurred even in tumor patients who had basal concentrations of the hormone that were indistinguishable from normal (Deftos, 1974). Thus, the measurement of calcitonin after calcium infusion served to identify patients with medullary thyroid carcinoma who had nondiagnostic concentrations of basal calcitonin (Deftos, 1974; McKenna *et al.,* 1978).

Prolonged calcium infusions have disadvantages. The procedure is fairly long and the dose of calcium often produces untoward effects such as hypertension, nausea, and vomiting. This has necessitated hospitalization in research wards. More recently, shorter infusions have been developed (Parthemore *et al.,* 1974, Rude and Singer, 1977). In these procedures, the increase in plasma calcium usually is less than 1 mg/dl, yet calcitonin release is reliably stimulated. The procedure can be completed in a few minutes and is relatively well tolerated (Deftos, 1974; Parthemore *et al.,* 1974).

3. Pentagastrin. Pentagastrin is another widely used provocative agent for calcitonin secretion in patients with medullary thyroid carcinoma (Hennessey *et al.,* 1974). When administered by rapid intravenous injection at a dose of 0.5 μg/kg, pentagastrin produces a prompt increase in plasma calcitonin. The response probably is a function of the dose and speed of injection, inasmuch as calcium, when given in similar fashion, produces a response similar to that seen with pentagastrin. Infusion of pentagastrin over several minutes produces a response similar to that produced by a calcium infusion (Deftos, 1978a; Rude and Singer, 1977). The rapidity of pentagastrin infusion also has drawbacks, as it leads to an unpleasant but poorly described sensation commonly called "burn-

ing'' or ''flushing.'' Moreover, the use of pentagastrin as a diagnostic test for suspected medullary thyroid carcinoma is not currently approved by the Food and Drug Administration; therefore, an institutionally approved protocol may be required for its administration.

Wells and colleagues (1975) have described an interesting modification of the pentagastrin test. They administered the peptide to patients while sampling plasma for calcitonin assay via an indwelling catheter in the inferior thyroid veins. This allows them to demonstrate a dramatic and diagnostic increase in thyroidal vein calcitonin whether or not peripheral calcitonin increased. However, such procedures cannot yet be considered routine, particularly as the concentration of thyroidal venous calcitonin is not well established and can be influenced by a small change in the position of the indwelling catheter. Moreover, more sensitive radioimmunoassays have better defined normal and abnormal ranges of basal as well as stimulated calcitonin concentrations in peripheral human plasma (Parthemore and Deftos, 1978). Accordingly, patients in whom provocative testing was previously required can now be identified by basal calcitonin measurements with assays of improved sensitivity.

A more practical use of selective venous catheterization is in the evaluation of the location and extent of medullary thyroid carcinoma (Wells *et al.*, 1975) or an ectopic calcitonin-producing tumor (Goltzman *et al.*, 1974; Wells *et al.*, 1975). The procedure can help localize a recurrent medullary thyroid carcinoma and thus lead to more effective treatment (Goltzman *et al.*, 1974). However, high circulating hormone levels may obscure the resulting calcitonin gradient, even when this difficult procedure is technically successful.

4. Pentagastrin versus calcium. The relative merits of pentagastrin and calcium infusions have been discussed (Hennessey *et al.*, 1974; Wells *et al.*, 1975). Most tumors respond to either agent and both procedures yield few false negative results, although some growths respond to calcium but not to gastrin and *vice versa* (Gagel *et al.*, 1975). Therefore, if one procedure gives negative results, the other should be considered before a medullary thyroid carcinoma is ruled out (Deftos, 1978a). So far, combined calcium-pentagastrin infusions have not yielded consistent results (McKenna *et al.*, 1978); Wells *et al.*, 1975). However, preliminary evidence suggests that calcium infusions may be more valuable for the diagnosis of early forms of the tumor (McKenna *et al.*, 1978). In general, the sensitivity and specificity of the calcitonin assay are probably as important as the choice of a particular test.

5. Whiskey. Another agent that has been used as a provocative test for calcitonin is scotch whiskey (Dymling *et al.*, 1976). When 50 ml are drunk by a patient with medullary thyroid carcinoma, there is an increase (usually within 15 min) of plasma calcitonin comparable to that produced by some calcium infusions. While the test is easy to administer, it can also lead to false negative results

and more experience is needed to establish its reliability. Since alcohol can produce diarrhea and flushing in patients with medullary thyroid carcinoma (Cohen *et al.*, 1973), the possibility of additional untoward effects exists.

6. Magnesium. While magnesium infusion increases plasma calcitonin levels in normal individuals and experimental animals (Deftos *et al.*, 1978c), Anast and colleagues (1975) have reported that it suppressed calcitonin secretion in three patients with medullary thyroid carcinoma. These results may reflect a difference between normal and malignant C cells.

(b). Venous catheterization procedures. The location as well as presence of medullary thyroid carcinoma can be established by calcitonin assay in conjunction with selective venous catheterization. A gradient of hormone concentration in a specific vein may localize the tumor to the site draining that vein. To do this requires accurate catheter placement and confirmation of location by appropriate venography studies. Several factors limit the usefulness of catheterization procedures. Since the high incidence of bilaterality in medullary thyroid carcinoma dictates bilateral neck surgery, the procedure has limited use in primary diagnosis. If recurrence or persistence after surgical treatment is being evaluated, this must be done in an area in which the venous pattern has been distorted by the surgery. Therefore, accurate correlation between venous sample and anatomical sites necessitates arteriography studies to establish blood flow patterns. Such studies add considerable risk, time, and expense to venous catheterization. Therefore, the greatest potential value of catheterization studies is probably in the location of tumor metastases (or ectopic calcitonin production). Prior knowledge of the presence of metastatic (or ectopic) disease could greatly influence therapy (Goltzman *et al.*, 1974).

(c). Calcitonin measurements in the evaluation of therapy. The effectiveness of therapy in patients with calcitonin-producing tumors can be monitored by serial measurements of plasma calcitonin (Deftos *et al.*, 1976b). This application of the calcitonin assay pertains to surgical as well as chemotherapeutic treatment (Fig. 3). In addition to determining the relatively acute effects of a given treatment regimen, a periodic surveillance with appropriate provocative testing can be conducted for recurrence of tumor (Deftos *et al.*, 1976b; Gagel *et al.*, 1975; Silva *et al.*, 1975).

(d). Immunochemical heterogeneity. There are multiple immunochemical forms of calcitonin in tumors and in plasma (Deftos *et al.*, 1975a; Singer and Habener, 1974; Sizemore and Heath, 1975; Snider *et al.*, 1977). When the plasma or tumor of a patient with medullary thyroid carcinoma is immunoassayed after gel filtration chromatography, several peaks of immunoreactive calcitonin are seen. Their number is a function of the size of the column, the nature of the matrix gel, and the elution conditions. Calcitonin auto- or homoaggregation (e.g., dimerization or polymerization) or heteroaggregation (e.g., with other proteins) also affect the elution profile. Thus, only some of the peaks actually

reflect the biosynthesis, secretion, and metabolism of calcitonin. Since a metabolic precursor for calcitonin has been described (Roos *et al.*, 1974) and a preprocalcitonin is likely to exist, these species may also be represented in plasma. Moreover, since calcitonin is metabolized at least after secretion and perhaps intracellularly, such metabolic derivatives may also be represented in plasma. Therefore, the multiple forms of immunoassayable plasma calcitonin represent a complex mixture of calcitonin forms, its precursors, and metabolites.

The immunochemical profile of calcitonin may vary among certain disease states. This variation has been demonstrated for calcitonin-producing tumors and for renal disease (Lee *et al.*, 1977b; Deftos, 1978a; Snider *et al.*, 1977). The various species of plasma calcitonin seen in renal disease and malignancy are produced in part by abnormalities in hormone metabolism and secretion. Thus the calcitonin peak representing the monomer seen in medullary thyroid carcinoma plasma is nearly absent in renal disease where most of the calcitonin elutes at or near the void volume (Lee *et al.*, 1977b). This also appears to be true in some instances of ectopic calcitonin production where the hormone may also elute at or near the position of the biosynthetic precursor(s) of calcitonin (Roos *et al.*, 1974). In other malignancies, the calcitonin monomer may predominate (Snider *et al.*, 1977). Therefore, it may become possible to use the immunochemical elution pattern of plasma calcitonin for the differential diagnosis of hypercalcitoninemic states. Therefore, both specificity and sensitivity must be considered in assessing the diagnostic value of a calcitonin assay system.

Antibodies of a given specificity for the calcitonin molecule will react preferentially with hormone species which have that specificity. For example, if calcitonin is metabolized to a fragment that contains a carboxy-terminal peptide, an antiserum with specificity for the carboxy-terminal region of calcitonin will detect that fragment, whereas an antiserum with specificity for another region of the molecule may not. Therefore, immunochemical heterogeneity is a function of the hormone species being measured as well as of the analytical procedure in use.

Assessment of the immunochemical heterogeneity of plasma calcitonin can also provide information about C-cell function because it will indicate whether excess production occurs at the prehormone, hormone, or metabolic product level. However, the most important use of calcitonin heterogeneity is to screen patients in the early diagnosis of medullary thyroid carcinoma or other calcitonin-producing tumors. Some assay procedures, because of their immunochemical specificity or sensitivity, may more effectively identify slightly increased basal concentrations of calcitonin that occur in early medullary thyroid carcinoma. Furthermore, different provocative agents may stimulate the secretion (or release) of different species of calcitonin (Heath and Sizemore, 1975; Silva *et al.*, 1977). Thus, the optimal diagnostic procedure is that which best recognizes the species produced in response to a provocative test.

(vi). Treatment. The treatment of choice for medullary thyroid carcinoma is

surgery, adapted to each patient (Hill *et al.*, 1973) by a surgeon prepared to make many procedural decisions in the course of the operation. Thus, in tumors confined to the thyroid gland, a total thyroidectomy should be performed, even if only one lobe appears to be involved, since the other lobe is quite likely to be involved as well, especially in familial medullary thyroid carcinoma. However, tumor bilaterality occurs often enough in what appear to be sporadic cases to warrant total thyroidectomy. When even a rim of apparently normal thyroid tissue is left behind, the malignancy is likely to recur locally or metastatically (Keiser *et al.*, 1973).

If there is regional lymph node involvement, surgical intervention should be aggressive. Since the tumor sometimes behaves indolently, removal of regional lymphatics may retard the complications of a locally invasive tumor. Therefore, the surgeon should be prepared to remove as many lymph nodes as possible. To do so, a central dissection of lymph nodes may be indicated (Hill *et al.*, 1973); neck dissection may be performed if the lateral cervical nodes are involved. The neck dissection may be radical or a modified radical procedure (Kaplan, 1973; Nathaniels *et al.*, 1970). The sternum may be split for more extensive node removal if that is indicated by the findings at surgery (Block *et al.*, 1967, 1975).

Although ^{131}I and suppressive doses of T_4 have been reported to be useful in some patients, this form of treatment generally cannot be recommended but may be useful in some patients (Didolker and Moore, 1974). The C cells do not concentrate iodine, as do the follicular cells of the thyroid, and the secretory activity of the tumor does not respond to either T_4 or TSH (Melvin *et al.*, 1971a). Chemotherapy has not been evaluated extensively in the treatment of medullary thyroid carcinoma since surgery is beneficial in a majority of treatable patients. However, chemotherapy with adriamycin or in combination with other agents (Gottlieb and Hill, 1975) must be considered in patients with metastatic and recurrent disease who have already been treated surgically.

(vii). Multiple Endocrine Neoplasia (MEN). There is a striking association between medullary thyroid carcinoma and pheochromocytomas, mucosal neuromas, and hyperparathyroidism (Table I). This thyroid tumor is thus part of a MEN syndrome that can be distinguished from MEN, Type I (Steiner *et al.*, 1968). When medullary thyroid carcinoma occurs with these other endocrine tumors, two distinct patterns can be defined. One of them includes medullary thyroid carcinoma, pheochromocytomas, and hyperparathyroidism and is referred to as MEN, Type II or IIa, or Sipple's syndrome. The other, MEN Type III (or IIb), includes medullary thyroid carcinoma, pheochromocytomas, and mucosal neuromas. (These tumors are also called ganglioneurom as to indicate the presence of ganglion cells, but they probably are most accurately referred to as neurognagliomas, since neural tissue predominates.). Also, these patients can have a Marfanoid habitus.

There is an embryologic as well as a genetic basis for the association of medullary thyroid carcinoma with these other tumors. The cells of medullary thyroid carcinoma, pheochromocytomas, and the neurogangliomas are all of neural crest origin (Pearse, 1968). The associated hyperparathyroidism does not fit into this unitary concept of embryogenesis, since parathyroid cells are not classically considered to be of neural crest origin. However, some authorities have suggested a neural crest origin for the parathyroid gland (Pearse and Takor, 1976). An alternative explanation is a functional relationship between hyperparathyroidism and medullary thyroid carcinoma. According to this hypothesis, the abnormal concentrations of calcitonin produce a hyperparathyroidism that is secondary to the hypocalcemic actions of the calcitonin (Deftos and Parthemore, 1974). Although this type of functional relationship between the neoplasias may exist, the most convincing evidence supports a genetic relationship between medullary thyroid carcinoma and hyperparathyroidism (Melvin *et al.*, 1971a).

The association of medullary thyroid carcinoma with other tumors leads to mucosal neurogangliomas that may be the first manifestation of the MEN syndrome. These lesions thus may provide an early warning of the presence of two potentially lethal tumors—medullary thyroid carcinoma and pheochromocytoma. Additionally, the existence of pheochromocytoma or medullary thyroid carcinoma should suggest a possible coexistence with other tumors. Hyperparathyroidism can be similarly regarded. The diagnosis of medullary thyroid carcinoma should therefore stimulate a search for other tumors in the patients' family. If diagnosed early, all of the serious features of MEN are treatable and even curable.

(a). Pheochromocytoma. There are several distinct features of pheochromocytomas occurring in association with medullary thyroid carcinoma. In this circumstance, bilateral and multifocal pheochromocytomas are very common and have an incidence of greater than 70%. This contrasts with a bilateral incidence of usually less than 10% for sporadic pheochromocytomas. Pheochromocytomas are much more likely to occur in patients with familial rather than sporadic medullary thyroid carcinoma (Khairi *et al.*, 1975; Steiner *et al.*, 1968). When pheochromocytomas and medullary thyroid carcinoma occur together in the same patient, the medullary thyroid carcinoma is likely to be diagnosed first (Hill *et al.*, 1973; Khairi *et al.*, 1975; Steiner *et al.*, 1968). The thyroid tumor may antedate the pheochromocytomas by as much as 21 years (Nathaniels *et al.*, 1970). Furthermore, a second pheochromocytoma may become manifest after removal of the first (Hill *et al.*, 1973). This sequence of events results in a greater incidence of pheochromocytomas in older patients with medullary thyroid carcinoma. Less often, the thyroid and adrenal tumor may be discovered contemporaneously and, in some cases, pheochromocytomas may be diagnosed before medullary thyroid carcinoma. If hyperparathyroidism also exists, it, too, is likely to antedate pheochromocytoma (Hill *et al.*, 1973; Khairi *et al.*, 1975; Steiner *et al.*, 1968).

Since different reports have emphasized different aspects of the MEN syndrome, it is difficult to determine how commonly pheochromocytomas occur in association with medullary thyroid carcinoma. It has become apparent that the incidence of pheochromocytomas is much higher than previously appreciated. In MEN III, the incidence of pheochromocytomas usually approaches 50% (Khairi *et al.*, 1975), whereas in the MEN II syndrome it usually is less than 20% (Hill *et al.*, 1973). However, it is likely that these represent underestimations, especially in MEN type III, since most recent studies suggest a much higher incidence (Deftos, 1978a).

Adrenal medullary hyperplasia may be a predecessor of the pheochromocytomas seen with medullary thyroid carcinoma, just as C-cell hyperplasia may be a predecessor of medullary thyroid carcinoma (Carney *et al.*, 1975; Ljungberg, 1972). Although cases of adrenal medullary hyperplasia had been reported in the literature, none of them occurred in patients with medullary thyroid carcinoma (Bialestock, 1961; Drukker *et al.*, 1957; Montalbano *et al.*, 1962; Sherwin, 1964; Visser and Axt, 1975). DeLellis and colleagues (1976) described the adrenal glands of ten patients from a large kindred with familial medullary thyroid carcinoma. There is hypertrophy as well as hyperplasia of the cells and they show increased mitotic activity and increased total catecholamine content (Carney *et al.*, 1975). In addition, the ratio of epinephrine to norepinephrine was increased in the tumor and in the urine (DeLellis *et al.*, 1976). These findings suggest that a sequence of events similar to those postulated for medullary thyroid carcinoma and hyperparathyroidism takes place in the development of pheochromocytomas: Hypertrophy develops into hyperplasia, multifocal hyperplasia develops into nodularity, and neoplastic transformation to pheochromocytomas is the final stage of the sequence in most cancers, but malignancy can also be seen.

(b). Hyperparathyroidism. It is difficult to establish the exact incidence of hyperparathyroidism in patients with medullary thyroid carcinoma. Melvin and colleagues (1971a) made the diagnosis of hyperparathyroidism in ten of 12 patients of a kindred with medullary thyroid carcinoma, whereas Hill and colleagues (1973) could establish the diagnosis of hyperparathyroidism in only two of 73 patients with medullary thyroid carcinoma. The most recent literature suggest that hyperplasia is more common than adenoma (Deftos, 1978a). There are several possible explanations for this disparity. There is disagreement regarding the criteria necessary to distinguish between a normal and abnormal parathyroid gland and the criteria to classify parathyroid abnormalities (Block *et al.*, 1975). Another explanation for the reported incidence of hyperparathyroidism in medullary thyroid carcinoma is the developing appreciation of the differing incidence of hyperparathyroidism in MEN II and MEN III. Despite these differences, the concurrence of hyperparathyroidism and medullary thyroid carcinoma is well established and, although it cannot be quantitated, the presence of one tumor should always make the presence of the other suspect.

Two hypotheses prevail regarding the link between hyperparathyroidism and medullary thyroid carcinoma. One possibility is that the hyperparathyroidism is a functional disorder representing a compensatory response of the parathyroid glands to a hypocalcemic effect of the calcitonin. This view does have some clinical and experimental support (Deftos and Parthemore, 1974). There are also, however, equally convincing data that the hyperparathyroidism is an inherited rather than functional component of medullary thyroid carcinoma (Deftos, 1978a). The genetic view would be more attractive if the embryologic origin of the parathyroid gland were neural crest, as is the embryologic origin of the other prominent features of the syndrome—pheochromocytoma, medullary thyroid carcinoma, and mucosal neuromas. Most evidence suggest that the parathyroid glands are of endodermal origin, arising from the third and fourth branchial pouches. However, there are data to suggest that the parathyroid glands may, indeed, be of neural crest origin (Pearse and Takor, 1976). If this is confirmed, it would provide a more unifying genetic basis for MEN II and III.

(c). Multiple mucosal neuromas (MMN). The presence of neuromas with a centrofacial distribution is the most consistent component of this syndrome. The most common location of neuromas is in the oral cavity. The most prominent microscopic feature of the neuromas is an increase in the size and number of nerves. The lips, tongue, and buccal mucosa are the most common sites for the oral mucosal neuromas. The oral lesions usually are the first components of the syndrome to appear. They are almost invariably present by the first decade and can even be present at birth (Khairi *et al.*, 1975). The mucosal neuromas along with the subsequently described ocular findings give the involved patients a very characteristic facial appearance. Mucosal neuromas can be present in the eyelids, conjunctiva, and cornea.

A Marfanoid habitus is seen commonly in the MMN syndrome (Khairi *et al.*, 1975). The Marfanoid habitus refers to a tall, slender body with an abnormal upper to lower body segment ratio and poor muscle development. The extremities are thin and long and there may be lax joints and hypotonic muscles. Associated with the Marfanoid habitus may be dorsal kyphosis, pectus excavatum, pectus carinatum, pes cavus, and a high-arched palate. In contrast to true Marfan's syndrome, no patients with MMN have been reported who have aortic abnormalities, ectopic lentis, homocystinuria, or mucopolysaccharide abnormalities.

b. Tumor-Associated Hypercalcemia. An acute increase in blood calcium has long been known to be a potent calcitonin secretagogue (Potts and Deftos, 1969). Recent studies indicate that chronic hypercalcemia can also stimulate thyroidal calcitonin secretion in humans (Lee *et al.*, 1977d; Parthemore *et al.*, 1977) and may account for some instances of the hypercalcitoninemia of malignancy (Deftos, 1978a).

c. Tumor-Associated Calcitonin Secretagogue. This intriguing hypothesis is supported by the observation that in patients with some tumors (not associated with hypercalcemia), the thyroid gland seems to be the source of the elevated plasma calcitonin (Silva *et al.*, 1975). Several candidates for such a secretagogue exist. They include prostaglandins, which are produced by a variety of tumors and which can stimulate the secretion of calcitonin and gastrin. The latter can also be an ectopic product of tumors and stimulate calcitonin secretion (Hennessey *et al.*, 1973a; Seyberth *et al.*, 1975; Roos and Deftos, 1976b).

d. Tumor Metastases to Bone. This could result from hypercalcemia due to the metastases to the skeleton and/or the production by the tumor of a bone-resorbing agent such as parathyroid hormone, prostaglandin, a vitamin D-like sterol, or an osteocyte-activating factor (OAF) (Deftos and Neer, 1974; Gordan *et al.*, 1966; Mundy *et al.*, 1974; Powell *et al.*, 1973; Seyberth *et al.*, 1975). An equally interesting possibility is the release of a calcitonin secretagogue from bone cells perturbed by either the tumor or a bone resorptive product of the

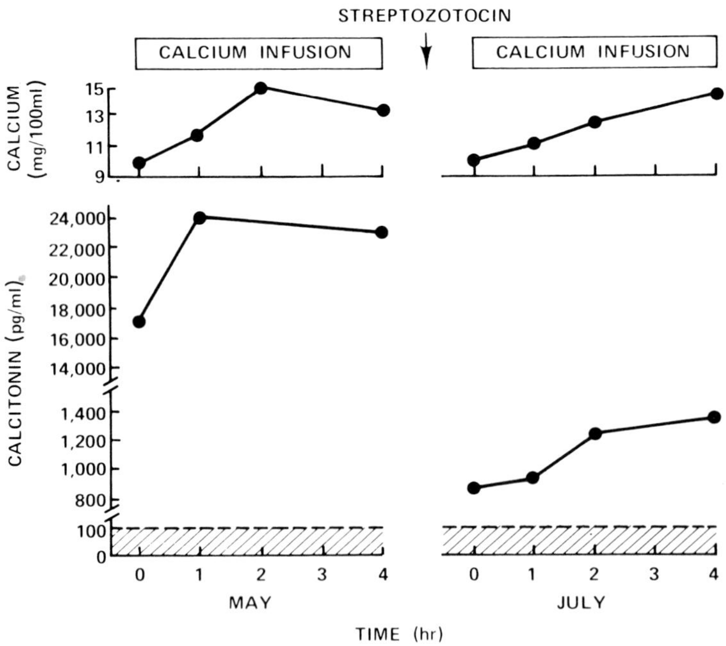

Fig. 3. Changes in calcitonin following 18.4 mg total dose of streptozotocin in a patient with pancreatic isletcell carcinoma. Illustrated is the effect of calcium infusion (time in hours) on plasma calcitonin before (left) and after (right) treatment. Although calcitonin concentration changes appropriately upon calcium challenge before and after treatment, there was a marked drop in the absolute plasma level of hormone. Standard errors for the calcitonin determinations were <10%. Shaded area represents normal calcitonin assay ranges. (From Deftos *et al.*, 1976a.)

tumor (Deftos, 1978b; Deftos *et al.*, 1975b). This would imply that bone cells "protect" themselves against increased bone resorption by stimulating calcitonin secretion (Deftos, 1978b).

2. *Ectopic Calcitonin Production*

On the basis of concurrent hypercalcitoninemia and malignancy, a variety of nonthyroidal tumors has been reported to produce calcitonin (Coombes *et al.*, 1974b; Hillyard *et al.*, 1975, 1976; Milhaud *et al.*, 1974; Silva *et al.*, 1974a; Fig. 3). However, such an association does not establish causality, even though some tumors have been shown to produce calcitonin (Coombes *et al.*, 1974b; David *et al.*, 1975; Ellison *et al.*, 1975; Hillyard *et al.*, 1975, 1976; Milhaud *et al.*, 1974; Silva and Becker, 1976; Silva *et al.*, 1974a, 1976).

It is also possible that calcitonin-producing tumors may produce abnormal amounts of calcitonin precursors, such as pro(or pre-)calcitonin or calcitonin peptides. Many of the tumors that ectopically secrete calcitonin are of neural crest origin and therefore embryologically related to each other (Weichert, 1970). (This, of course, raises questions about the distinction between eutopic and ectopic calcitonin production.) Calcitonin and its precursor molecules may be part of a large "neural crest" molecule (Lips *et al.*, 1978). This possibility is suggested by several observations: (1) Calcitonin is of neural crest origin; (2) oat-cell carcinoma of the lung, thought to derive from cells of neural crest origin, concurrently secretes calcitonin, ACTH, and β-endorphin (Deftos *et al.*, 1979); (3) there is structural homology between calcitonin and the ACTH-LPH precursor (Nakanishi *et al.*, 1979); and, (4) immunoreactive calcitonin has been demonstrated in the pituitary gland of several species (Deftos *et al.*, 1978b).

3. *Artifactual Elevations in Plasma Calcitonin*

Although it is now established that true hypercalcitoninemia occurs in a variety of cancers, the immunological measurement may indicate hypercalcitoninemia that is the result of a nonspecific effect of the malignant state on calcitonin measurement (David *et al.*, 1975; Deftos, 1971; Deftos *et al.*, 1971). Possible examples of this would include the presence of (1) abnormal immunoglobulins or other proteins (especially in myelomas and lymphomas) that would interfere with the immunology of the radioimmunoassay or (2) the presence of enzymes that might affect in a nonspecific manner either plasma calcitonin or the calcitonin tracer or antibody used in the radioimmunoassay (David *et al.*, 1975; Deftos and O'Riordan, 1978; Strauss and Yalow, 1976).

A number of studies have demonstrated that many of these hypotheses are plausible in at least some instances of the hypercalcitoninemia of malignancy. The studies have shown that (1) nonthyroidal malignancies produce calcitonin (Baylin, 1975; Coombes *et al.*, 1974a; Deftos *et al.*, 1976a; Hillyard *et al.*, 1976; Silva *et al.*, 1976), (2) that tumor-associated hypercalcemia increases plasma calcitonin (Parthemore *et al.*, 1977), (3) that tumor-associated factors can act as calcitonin secretagogues (Roos and Deftos, 1976b; Seyberth *et al.*, 1975), (4) that calcitonin associated with malignancy exists in "abnormal" forms (Deftos *et al.*, 1975b, 1976; Snider *et al.*, 1977), and (5) that nonspecific factors in malignant disease can influence calcitonin assays (Deftos and O'Riordan, 1978).

B. Hypercalcemia and Primary Hyperparathyroidism

Acutely induced hypercalcemia is a well-documented stimulus for calcitonin secretion (Deftos, 1978b). It is now becoming evident that chronic hypercalcemic and hypercalciuric states may also be associated with increased calcitonin secretion (Lee *et al.*, 1977d; Parthemore *et al.*, 1977). This presumably represents a homeostatic response of the C cells to defend against the challenge to calcium homeostasis (Fig. 4). Provocative testing of calcitonin secretion may be necessary to demonstrate fully the hypersecretory state of calcitonin that exists in chronic hypercalcemic states such as primary hyperparathyroidism (Deftos *et*

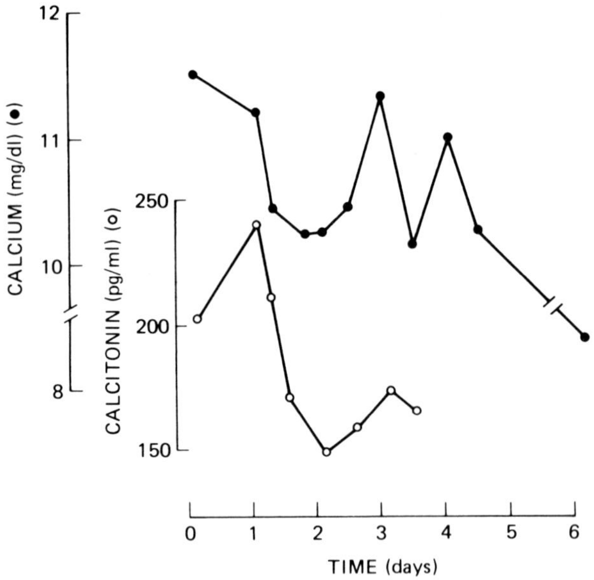

Fig. 4. Changes in calcium (●) and calcitonin (○) in a patient with coccidioidomycosis during treatment with salmon calcitonin. The drug, 4 MRC units per kilogram of body weight, was given subcutaneously every 12 hr. Basal calcitonin was increased above the upper limit of normal of 100 pg/ml and decreased with treatment (Lee *et al.*, 1977a). Calcitonin was determined by a radioimmunoassay specific for human calcitonin. The assay does not cross-react with salmon calcitonin.

al., 1978c). It is of note that females with primary hyperparathyroidism, like normal females, have less calcitonin reserve than males (Parthemore *et al.*, 1977).

C. Renal Disease

The importance of abnormalities of parathyroid hormone and vitamin D in renal failure is well known. Recently there has been renewed interest in the hypothesis that there may also be a role of calcitonin in the pathogenesis of renal osteodystrophy. However, even these preliminary studies have generated controversy. There is general agreement that the immunoassayable levels of calcitonin are increased in patients with both acute and chronic renal failure (Ardaillou *et al.*, 1975; Cochran *et al.*, 1976; Deftos *et al.*, 1976a; Heynen and Franchimont, 1974a,b; Heynen *et al.*, 1977; Isaac *et al.*, 1975; Lee *et al.*, 1977c; Parthemore, 1977; Parthemore and Roos, 1976; Parthemore *et al.*, 1976; Roos *et al.*, 1977; Silva *et al.*, 1974b), but there is considerable disagreement regarding the degree of increase. Some investigators have reported that when patients with renal disease are dialyzed or receive a calcium infusion, their already-high plasma calcitonin increases further (Deftos, *et al.*, 1976a; Heynen and Franchimont, 1974a; Heynen *et al.*, 1977; Lee *et al.*, 1977a; Parthemore, 1977; Parthemore and Roos, 1976; Parthemore *et al.*, 1975a, 1976; Roos *et al.*, 1977). By contrast, other investigators report that dialysis or calcium infusion does not lead to a further increase in plasma calcitonin in patients with renal failure (Isaac *et al.*, 1975; Silva *et al.*, 1974c). Additionally, it is unclear whether these high plasma levels represent an abnormality of hormone secretion, metabolism, or both. It is likely that abnormalities of calcitonin metabolism are associated with renal failure, since the kidney is important in the metabolism of the hormone (Ardaillou *et al.*, 1971; Foster *et al.*, 1972) and since the metabolic clearance rate of calcitonin is decreased in renal failure (Ardaillou *et al.*, 1970). Moreover, calcitonin levels return toward normal if renal failure resolves (Deftos *et al.*, 1976a; Lee *et al.*, 1977a; Parthemore, 1977; Parthemore *et al.*, 1976; Parthemore and Roos, 1976; Roos *et al.*, 1977) or if renal transplantation has taken place (Heynen *et al.*, 1977). Since the secretion and/or metabolism of calcitonin is abnormal in renal disease and since renal osteodystrophy is characterized by, among other parameters, increased bone resorption, it is possible that calcitonin, which acts to inhibit bone resorption, could be implicated in the pathogenesis of uremic osteodystrophy (Cochran *et al.*, 1976; Feletti and Bonomini, 1981; Lee *et al.*, 1977a; Parthemore, 1977; Roos *et al.*, 1977). The greatest elevations, perhaps compensatory to the increased bone resorption, are reported to occur in patients with lesser bone disease (Kanis *et al.*, 1977).

Several possible mechanisms might contribute to the hypercalcitoninemia of renal failure. Hormone secretion could be increased, hormone catabolism could be decreased, or both. There is no obvious explanation for increased calcitonin secretion in these patients, since plasma calcium levels are usually low in renal disease. Gastrin levels are increased in renal failure (Korman *et al.*, 1972) and pentagastrin is a potent calcitonin secretagogue when administered acutely. In addition, chronic hypergastrinemic states, as in pernicious anemia, have been reported to be associated with elevated levels of plasma calcitonin (Heynen and Franchimont, 1974a). However, in renal disease, there is no correlation between plasma gastrin and calcitonin.

The data of Lee *et al.* (1977a) indicate that the species of calcitonin found in the plasma from patients with renal disease differs markedly from that seen in patients with other hypercalcitoninemic states such as medullary thyroid carcinoma. In the latter, multiple forms of calcitonin occur and a predominant component of these multiple forms is calcitonin monomer. By contrast, patients with chronic renal failure who are on dialysis have relatively small amounts of the calcitonin monomer in their plasma, with the predominant form being of much higher molecular weight and unknown biological significance. The species of plasma calcitonin seen in patients with acute renal failure also appears to differ from that seen in dialysis patients (Lee *et al.*, 1977a).

These observations may explain some of the discrepancies. In the patient undergoing dialysis, the smaller species of calcitonin, like the monomer, are more likely to be lost through dialysis. This will tend to decrease the plasma calcitonin concentration. On the other hand, the calcium load of the dialysis may stimulate calcitonin secretion involving both smaller and larger species, with the latter least likely to be removed by dialysis. Little is known about the biological activity of the circulating hormone in renal disease and it is possible that the abnormal immunochemical forms of calcitonin found in renal disease are less active biologically or even are inactive. In the rat, acute renal failure results in a decrease in immunoassayable calcitonin and the response of calcitonin to stimulation by calcium infusion is blunted (Lee *et al.*, 1977b). The abnormality of calcitonin secretion in renal disease could vary with the course (and severity) of the illness. Early renal failure would then be characterized by calcitonin deficiency, while established renal failure would be characterized by low levels of biologically active calcitonin with high levels of inactive hormone.

D. Bone Disease

The secretion of calcitonin is abnormal in pycnodysostosis, and may also be abnormal in other hyperostotic states (Baker *et al.*, 1973; Table II). The decreased calcitonin reserve in females may play a role in the greater severity of osteitis fibrosa cystica in women with primary hyperparathyroidism and in the pathogenesis of osteoporosis (Davidson *et al.*, 1979; Heath and Sizemore, 1977; Milhaud *et al.*, 1974; Parthemore, 1977; Parthemore *et al.*, 1977). Calcitonin deficiency may also play a role in some cases of osteoporosis if the disease is

TABLE II

Conditions Reported or Postulated to Be Associated with Abnormalities of Calcitonin Secretion and/or Metabolism[a]

Condition	Possible mechanism
1. Medullary thyroid carcinoma	Genetic/functional
a. C-cell hyperplasia	
b. Prehyperplasia	
2. Ectopic calcitonin production	Malignancy
3. Hypocalcemia	Calcium
4. Hypercalcemia/hypercalciuria	Calcium/gastrin
5. Hyperparathyroidism	Calcium/PTH/GI hormones
6. Malignancy	Possible factors
	Calcium
	Bone resorption
	Prostaglandins
	CT secretagogues
7. Pancreatitis	Glucagon/nonthyroidal calcitonin
8. Pregnancy	Calcium/bone resorption
9. Neonatal hypocalcemia	Calcium/bone resorption
10. Renal disease	Metabolism/bone resorption/vitamin D
11. Bone disease	Bone resorption/CT secretagogues
a. Hyperostotic states	
Pycnodysostosis	
Engelman's disease	
Osteopetrosis	
b. Hyperresorptive states	
Osteitis fibrosa cystica	
Osteoporosis	
Renal osteodystrophy	

[a] Adapted from Deftos (1978a).

due to higher than normal bone resorption (Baud *et al.*, 1969; Bloch-Michel *et al.*, 1970; Caniggia *et al.*, 1970; Cohn *et al.*, 1971; Milhaud *et al.*, 1975; Tamburino *et al.*, 1976). In some studies calcitonin has had a beneficial therapeutic effect (Baud *et al.*, 1969; Bloch-Michel *et al.*, 1970; Caniggia *et al.*, 1970; Cohn *et al.*, 1971; Milhaud *et al.*, 1975). However, in most instances of osteoporosis, calcitonin treatment has not been of therapeutic value (Riggs *et al.*, 1976). Thus, a possible role for relative calcitonin deficiency in the pathogenesis of osteoporosis remains hypothetical.

E. Pancreatitis

Increased calcitonin secretion has been implicated in the pathogenesis of the hypocalcemia of pancreatitis. Although this view is supported by some radioimmunoassay studies, others cannot demonstrate any calcitonin abnormalities in pancreatitis (Canale and Donabedian, 1975; Robertson *et al.*, 1976) and there is much disagreement in the published literature (Avioli, 1972; Avioli *et al.*, 1969; Canale and Donabedian, 1975; Condon *et al.*, 1975; Lawrence, 1972; Marshall *et al.*, 1975; Norberg *et al.*, 1975; Paloyan *et al.*, 1967; Robertson *et al.*, 1976; Weir *et al.*, 1975). Studies in which elevated levels of calcitonin have been reported (Canale and Donabedian, 1975; Robertson *et al.*, 1976) have been regarded as support for the hypothesis that pancreatitis is characterized by the release of glucagon and that glucagon stimulates calcitonin secretion (Avioli, 1972; Avioli *et al.*, 1969; Lawrence, 1972; Norberg *et al.*, 1975; Paloyan *et al.*, 1967). It is intriguing to speculate that the pancreas or adjacent gastrointestinal cells may be a source of calcitonin-like activity (Sowa *et al.*, 1977; Takaoka *et al.*, 1969). Plasma artifacts affecting radioimmunoassay performance may be exaggerated in pancreatitis, and this problem must be overcome before an accurate assessment can be made of calcitonin secretion in pancreatitis (Deftos, 1978b; Deftos and O'Riordan, 1978; Strauss and Yalow, 1976).

IV. THERAPEUTIC APPLICATIONS OF CALCITONIN

The therapeutic applications of calcitonin utilize its major biologic actions (1) to inhibit bone resorption and (2) to lower blood calcium. Three forms of calcitonin have been used—porcine, salmon, and human. Porcine calcitonin has been most widely used in continental Europe, human calcitonin in England, and salmon calcitonin in the United States. Salmon calcitonin has the advantage of being the most potent form of the hormone. Unlike human calcitonin, it is a foreign protein, and since it must be given parenterally, it can produce antibodies. These antibodies may neutralize the biologic effect of the hormone (Bijvoet *et al.*, 1968; DeRose *et al.*, 1974; Greenberg *et al.*, 1974; Singer, 1975; Woodhouse *et al.*, 1971).

A. Bone Diseases

1. Paget's Disease

Calcitonin, which acts to inhibit bone resorption, has been an effective agent in treating patients with Paget's disease (Bijvoet *et al.*, 1968). The recommended parenteral dose of calcitonin is 100 MRC units per day. Smaller doses may be effective also (Avramides *et al.*, 1975). The drug results in improvement of the clinical and biochemical parameters of the disease. Bone pain usually is improved or relieved within several weeks of starting therapy, but this effect has not been evaluated in a double-blind study. Skin temperature may decrease toward normal and there can be a dramatic improvement in the neurologic complications of the illness. If cardiac output is elevated as a complication of Paget's disease, it can be returned toward normal by calcitonin (Singer, 1975). The biochemical abnormalities of Paget's disease are also improved by the administration of calcitonin. Elevated levels of plasma and urine hydroxyproline and of plasma alkaline phosphatase fall soon after the initiation of calcitonin therapy. This reflects the hormone's inhibition of osteoclast activity (Avramides *et al.*, 1974; Singer, 1975). In patients with mild Paget's disease, alkaline phosphatase and hydroxyproline may return to normal but in cases of severe disease they may decline only to a plateau above normal levels. Nevertheless, calcitonin treatment leads to continued radiological and histological improvement of bone. Therefore, in some patients, the persistence of elevated alkaline phosphatase and hydroxyproline actually may be associated with bone healing (DeRose *et al.*, 1974; Greenberg *et al.*, 1974). However, it is clear that some patients with Paget's disease become resistant to the therapeutic effects of the hormone. This refractoriness may or may not be associated with the development of antibodies to the calcitonin (Haddad and Caldwell, 1972; Singer *et al.*, 1972a). An advantage of calcitonin over other forms of treatment for Paget's disease is relative freedom from side effects. In addition to its effectiveness, calcitonin is the least toxic agent for the treatment of Paget's disease (Singer and Habener, 1974). Nausea may occur after administration of the drug but it is usually mild and transient (Singer and Habener, 1974).

Mithramycin and the diphosphonates, the former on an investigational basis, are available for the treatment of Paget's disease. Their use has been discussed in several reviews (Ryan *et al.*, 1969; Singer and Habener, 1974; Smith *et al.*, 1971).

2. *Osteopenic States*

Calcitonin has been used in the treatment of patients with a variety of osteopenic states, including generalized and localized osteoporosis and osteogenesis imperfecta. Results have been variable and further evaluation is necessary.

B. Hypercalcemic States

Treatment of the patient with hypercalcemia utilizes another of the biologic actions of calcitonin, the lowering of blood calcium. Calcitonin manifests its hypocalcemic effect primarily by inhibiting bone resorption; it is also weakly calciuretic (Bijvoet *et al.*, 1968; Deftos and Neer, 1974). Thus, at least acutely, calcitonin commonly is effective in producing a rapid decrease of 1–2 mg in blood calcium in the hypercalcemic patient. In some patients, the results can be more dramatic but in others there may be little effect. A primary advantage of calcitonin in treating hypercalcemia is its ease of administration and its freedom from toxicity. Calcitonin is especially useful in the treatment of the hypercalcemic patient who is also hyperphosphatemic, since the hormone can lower the concentration of both minerals (Deftos and Neer, 1974).

ACKNOWLEDGMENTS

This work was supported by the American Cancer Society, the Veterans Administration, the National Institutes of Health, and CIBA-GEIGY. Susan Murphy and Elaine Kimbler provided secretarial assistance.

REFERENCES

Abdullahi, S. E., Arrigoni-Martelli, E., Gramm, E., Franco, L., and Velo, G. P. (1977). Effect of calcitonin in different inflammatory models. *Agents Actions* **7,** 533-538.

Adachi, I., Abe, K., Tanaka, M., Miyakawa, S., and Kumaoaka, S. (1974). Phosphaturic effect of I.V. administered calcitonin in man. *Endocrinol. Jpn.* **21,** 317-322.

Adachi, I., Abe, K., Tanaka, M., Yamaguchi, K., Miyakawa, S., Hiradawa, H., and Tanaka, N. (1976). Plasma human calcitonin (hCT) levels in normal and pathologic conditions, and their responses to short calcium or tetragastrin infusion. *Endocrinol. Jpn.* **23,** 517-526.

Aldred, J. P., Luna, P. D., Zeedyk, R. A., and Bastian, J. W. (1976). Inhibition by salmon calcitonin (sCT) of desoxycorticosterone acetate (DOCA) induced hypertension in the rat. *Proc. Soc. Exp. Biol. Med.* **152,** 557-559.

Aliapoulios, M. A., Voelkel, E. F., and Munson, P. L. (1966). Assay of human thyroid glands for thyrocalcitonin activity. *J. Clin. Endocrinol. Metab.* **26,** 897-901.

Anast, C., David, L., Winnacker, J., Glass, R., Baskin, W., Brubaker, L., and Burns, T. (1975). Serum calcitonin-lowering effect of magnesium in patients with medullary thyroid carcinoma. *J. Clin. Invest.* **56,** 1615-1621.

Ardaillou, R. (1975). Kidney and calcitonin. *Nephron* **15,** 250-260.

Ardaillou, R., Vuagnat, P., Milhaud, G., and Richet, G. (1967). Effets de la thyrocalcitonine sur l'excrétion rénale des phosphates, du calcium et des ions H+ chez l'homme. *Nephron* **4,** 298-314.

Ardaillou, R., Sizonenko, P., Meyrier, A., Vallee, G., and Beaugas, C. (1970). Metabolic clearance rate of radioiodinated human calcitonin in man. *J. Clin. Invest.* **49,** 2345-2352.

Ardaillou, R., Paillard, F., Savier, C., and Bernier, A. (1971). Renal uptake of radioiodinated human calcitonin in man. *Rev. Eur. Etud. Clin. Biol.* **16,** 1031-1036.

Ardaillou, R., Beaufils, M., Nivez, M. P., Mayaud, C., and Sraer, J. D. (1975). Increased plasma calcitonin in early acute renal failure. *Clin. Sci. Mol. Med.* **49,** 301-304.

Avioli, L. V. (1972). The effect of glucagon on mineral and electrolyte metabolism. *In* "Glucagon" (P. J. Lefebvre and R. H. Unger, eds.), pp. 181-186. Pergamon, Oxford.

Avioli, L. V., Birge, S., Scott, S., and Shuber, W. (1969). Role of the thyroid gland during glucagon-induced hypocalcemia in the dog. *Am. J. Physiol.* **216,** 936-945.

Avramides, A., Baker, R. K., and Wallach, S. (1974). Metabolic effects of synthetic salmon calcitonin in Paget's disease of bone. *Metab., Clin. Exp.* **23,** 1037-1046.

Avramides, A., Flores, A., DeRose, J., and Wallach, S. (1975). Treatment of Paget's disease of bone with once-a-week injections of salmon calcitonin. *Br. Med. J.* **3,** 632.

Baber, E. C. (1876). Contributions to the minute anatomy of the thyroid gland of the dog. *Philos. Trans. R. Soc. London* **166,** 557-568.

Baker, R. K., Wallach, S., and Tashjian, A. H., Jr. (1973). Plasma calcitonin in pycnodysostosis: Intermittently high basal levels and exaggerated responses to calcium and glucagon infusions. *J. Clin. Endocrinol. Metab.* **37,** 46–55.

Barlet, J. P., and Garel, J. M. (1976). Effect of an intravenous injection of cholecystokinin-pancreozymin on plasma calcium and calcitonin levels in newborn lambs. *J. Endocrinol.* **70,** 151–152.

Baud, C. A., deSiebenthal, J., Langer, B., Tupling, M. R., and Mach, R. S. (1969). Effets de l'ademinstration prolonge de thyrocalcitonine dans l'ostéoporose senile humaine. Etude clinique histologique et microradiographique. *Schweiz. Med. Wochenschr.* **99,** 657–661.

Baylin, S. B. (1975). Ectopic production of hormones and other proteins by tumors. *Hosp. Pract.* **10,** 117–126.

Becker, H. D., Konturek, S. J., Reeder, D. D., and Thompson, J. C. (1973). Effect of calcium and calcitonin on gastrin and gastric secretion in cats. *Am. J. Physiol.* **225,** 277–280.

Becker, H. D., Reeder, D. D., Scurry, M. T., and Thompson, J. C. (1974). Inhibition of gastrin release and gastric secretion by calcitonin in patients with peptic ulcer. *Am. J. Surg.* **127,** 71–75.

Bell, N. H. (1970). The effects of glucagon, dibutyryl cAMP and theophylline on calcitonin secretion in vitro. *J. Clin. Invest.* **49,** 1368–1373.

Beskid, M. (1975). Thyroid C-cells in normal and goitrous gland: A histochemical study. *Acta Histochem.* **54,** 313–321.

Bialestock, D. (1961). Hyperplasia of the adrenal medulla in hypertension in children. *Arch. Dis. Child.* **36,** 465–473.

Bijvoet, O. L. M., van der Sluys Veer, J., and Jansen, A. P. (1968). Effect of calcitonin on patients with Paget's disease, thyrotoxicosis, or hypercalcemia. *Lancet* **1,** 876–881.

Bijvoet, O. L. M., van der Sluys Veer, J., de Vries, H. R., and van Koppen, A. T. J. (1971). Natriuretic effect of calcitonin in man. *N. Engl. J. Med.* **284,** 681–688.

Blahos, J., Osten, J., Mertl, L., Kotas, J., Gregor, O., and Reisenauer, R. (1975). Uricosuric effect of calcitonin. *Horm. Metab. Res.* **7,** 445–446.

Blahos, J., Svoboda, Z., and Hoschl, C. (1976). The effect of calcitonin on glucose metabolism. *Endocrinologie* **68,** 226–230.

Bloch-Michel, H., Milhaud, G., Coutris, G., Waltzing, P., Charret, A., Morin, Y., Verger, D., and Dussart, N. (1970). Traitement au long cours de l'ostéoporose par la thyrocalcitonine. A propos de 7 observations. *Rev. Rhum. Mal. Osteo-Articulaires* **37,** 629–638.

Block, M. A., Horn, R. C., Jr., Miller, J. M., Barrett, J. L., and Brush, B. E. (1967). Familial medullary carcinoma of the thyroid. *Ann. Surg.* **166,** 403–412.

Block, M. A., Xavier, A., and Brush, B. E. (1975). Management of primary hyperparathyroidism in the elderly. *J. Am. Geriatr. Soc.* **23,** 385–389.

Braga, P., Ferri, S., Santagostino, A., Olgiati, V. R., and Pecile, A. (1978). Lack of opiate receptor involvement in centrally induced calcitonin analgesia. *Life Sci.* **22,** 971–978.

Brewer, H. B., Jr., and Ronan, R. (1969). Amino acid sequence of bovine thyrocalcitonin. *Proc. Natl. Acad. Sci. U.S.A.* **63,** 940–947.

Bronner, F. (1973). Kinetic and cybernetic analysis of calcium metabolism. *In* "Calcium and Phosphorus Metabolism" (J. T. Irving, ed.), pp. 149–185. Academic Press; New York.

Bronner, F., Sammon, P. J., Stacey, R. E., and Shah, B. G. (1967). Role of thyrocalcitonin in the regulation of the blood calcium level. *Biochem. Med.* **1,** 261–279.

Bronner, F., Sammon, P. J., Nicholas, C., Stacey, R. E., and Shah, B. G. (1968). Thyrocalcitonin and plasma calcium homeostasis in the rat. *In* "Parathyroid Hormone and Thyrocalcitonin (Calcitonin)" (R. V. Talmage and L. F. Bélanger, eds.), pp. 353–369. Excerpta Medica, Amsterdam.

Bussolati, G., and Pearse, A. G. E. (1967). Immunofluorescent localization of calcitonin in the C-cells of pig and dog thyroid. *J. Endocrinol.* **37,** 205–209.

Byfield, P. G. H., McLoughlin, J. L., Matthews, E. W., and MacIntyre, I. (1976). A proposed structure for rat calcitonin. *FEBS Lett.* **65,** 242–245.

Canale, D. D., and Donabedian, R. K. (1975). Hypercalcitoninemia in acute pancreatitis. *J. Clin. Endocrinol. Metab.* **40,** 738–741.

Caniggia, A., Gennari, C., Bencini, M., Cesari, L., and Borrello, G. (1970). Calcium metabolism and 47-calcium kinetics before and after long-term thyrocalcitonin treatment in senile osteoporosis. *Clin. Sci.* **38,** 397–407.

Care, A. D., Bates, R. F. L., and Gitelman, H. J. (1970). A possible role for the adenyl cyclase system in calcitonin release. *J. Endocrinol.* **48,** 1–15.

Carey, D., Jones, K. L., Parthemore, J. G., and Deftos, L. J. (1978). Studies of plasma calcitonin in agoitrous cretins. *Clin. Res.* **26,** 72A.

Carney, A. J., Sizemore, G. W., and Tyce, G. M. (1975). Bilateral adrenal medullary hyperplasia in MEN, Type 2. *Mayo Clin. Proc.* **50,** 3–10.

Carney, A. J., Sizemore, G. W., and Lovestedt, S. A. (1976). Mucosal ganglioneuromatosis, medullary thyroid carcinoma, and pheochromocytoma: MEN, Type 2B. *Oral Surg., Oral Med. Oral Pathol.* **41,** 739–752.

Clark, M. B., Byfield, P. G. H., Boyd, G. W., and Foster, G. V. (1969). A radioimmunoassay for human calcitonin M. *Lancet* **2,** 74–77.

Clark, M. B., Williams, C. C., Nathanson, B. M., Horton, R. E., Glass, H. I., and Foster, G. V. (1974). Metabolic fate of human calcitonin in the dog. *J. Endocrinol.* **61,** 199–210.

Clark, O. H., Rollo, D., Stroop, J., Castner, B., Rehfeld, S. J., Loken, H. F., and Deftos, L. J. (1977). Thyroid stimulation and sensitivity of thyroid and parathyroid glands to radiation exposure. *Assoc. Acad. Surg.*

Clark, O. H., Rehfeld, S. J., Castner, B., Stroop, J., Loken, H. F., and Deftos, L. J. (1978). Iodine deficiency produces hypercalcemia and hypercalcitoninemia in rats. *Surgery* **83,** 626–632.

Cochran, M., Hillyard, C. J., Dew, G. J., and Martin, T. J. (1976). Acute responsiveness to calcitonin in chronic renal failure. *Br. Med. J.* **2,** 396–398.

Cohen, S. L., MacIntyre, I., Grahame-Smith, D., and Walker, J. G. (1973). Alcohol-stimulated calcitonin release in medullary carcinoma of the thyroid. *Lancet* **2,** 1172–1174.

Cohn, S. H., Dombrowski, C. S., Hauser, W., Klopper, J., and Atkins, H. L. (1971). Effects of porcine calcitonin on calcium metabolism in osteoporosis. *J. Clin. Endocrinol. Metab.* **33,** 719–728.

Condon, J. R., Ives, D., Knight, M. J., and Day, J. (1975). The aetiology of hypocalcemia in acute pancreatitis. *Br. J. Surg.* **62,** 115–118.

Coombes, R. C., Hillyard, C. J., Greenberg, P. B., and MacIntyre, I. (1974a). Plasma-immunoreactive-calcitonin in patients with non-thyroid tumors. *Lancet* **1,** 1080–1083.

Coombes, R. C., Hillyard, C., Greenberg, P. B., and MacIntyre, I. (1974b). Reply to a letter by Greenfield entitled Plasma-calcitonin and non-thyroid tumors. *Lancet* **2,** 164.

Cooper, C. W., Obie, J. F., Toverud, S. U., and Munson, P. L. (1977). Elevated serum calcitonin and serum calcium during suckling in the baby rat. *Endocrinology (Baltimore)* **101,** 1657–1664.

Copp, D. H., Cameron, E. C., Cheney, B. A., Davidson, A. G. F., and Henze, K. G. (1962). Evidence for calcitonin—a new hormone from the parathyroid that lowers blood calcium. *Endocrinology (Baltimore)* **70,** 638–649.

Copp, D. H., Cockroft, D. W., and Kueh, Y. (1967). Calcitonin from ultimobranchial glands of dogfish and chickens. *Science* **158,** 924–925.

Cramer, C. F. (1973). Effect of salmon calcitonin on in vivo calcium absorption in rats. *Calcif. Tissue Res.* **13,** 169–172.

Cramer, C. F., Parkes, C. O., and Copp, D. H. (1969). The effect of chicken and hog calcitonin on some parameters of Ca, P, and Mg metabolism in dogs. *Can. J. Physiol. Pharmacol.* **47,** 181–184.

Cunliffe, W. J., Black, M. M., Hall, R., Johnston, I. D. A., Hudgson, P., Shuster, S., Gudmundsson, T. V., Joplin, G. F., Williams, E. D., Woodhouse, N. J. Y., Galante, L., and MacIntyre, I. (1968). A calcitonin-secreting thyroid carcinoma. *Lancet* **2,** 63–66.

Cutler, G. B., Jr., Habener, J. F., Dee, P. C., and Potts, J. T., Jr. (1974a). Radioimmunoassay for chicken calcitonin. *FEBS Lett.* **38,** 209–212.

Cutler, G. B., Jr., Habener, J. F., and Potts, J. T., Jr. (1974b). Comparative immunochemical studies of chicken ultimobranchial calcitonin. *Gen. Comp. Endocrinol.* **24,** 183–190.

Dangoumau, J., Bussiere, C., Noel, M., and Balahaud, C. (1976). Influence of calcitonin on bile production in the rat. *J. Pharmacol.* **7,** 69–76.

David, L., Cohn, D. V., and Anast, C. S. (1975). Identification of artifacts introduced to radioimmunoassays by the treatment of sera with charcoal in order to obtain 'dehormonized' sera. Applications to the radioimmunoassay of parathormone and calcitonin. *Pathol. Biol.* **23,** 833–834.

Deftos, L. J. (1971). An immunoassay for human calcitonin. I. The method. *Metab., Clin. Exp.* **20,** 1122–1128.

Deftos, L. J. (1974). Radioimmunoassay for calcitonin in medullary thyroid carcinoma. *JAMA, J. Am. Med. Assoc.* **227,** 403–406.

Deftos, L. J. (1978a). Calcitonin in clinical medicine. *Adv. Intern. Med.* **23,** 159–193.

Deftos, L. J. (1978b). Regulation of skeletal homeostasis. *Clin. Res.* **26,** 528A.

Deftos, L. J., and Neer, R. (1974). Medical management of the hypercalcemia of malignancy. *Annu. Rev. Med.* **25,** 323–331.

Deftos, L. J., and O'Riordan, J. L. H. (1978). Problems in radioassays of the calcitropic hormones. *In* "Endocrinology of Calcium Metabolism" (D. H. Copp and R. V. Talmage, eds.), pp. 345–348. Excerpta Medica, Amsterdam.

Deftos, L. J., and Parthemore, J. G. (1974). Secretion of parathyroid hormone in patients with medullary thyroid carcinoma. *J. Clin. Invest.* **54,** 416–420.

Deftos, L. J., Bury, A. W., Habener, J. F., Singer, F. R., and Potts, J. T., Jr. (1971). Immunoassay for human calcitonin. II. Clinical studies. *Metab., Clin. Exp.* **20,** 1129–1137.

Deftos, L. J., Habener, J. F., Krook, L., and Mayer, G. P. (1972). Multiple endocrine adenomatosis and calcitonin secretion in the bovine species. *Clin. Res.* **20,** 544.

Deftos, L. J., Powell, D., Parthemore, J. G., and Potts, J. T., Jr. (1973). Secretion of calcitonin in hypocalcemic states in man. *J. Clin. Invest.* **52,** 3109–3114.

Deftos, L. F., Roos, B. A., Bronzert, D., and Parthemore, J. G. (1975a). Immunochemical heterogeneity of calcitonin in plasma. *J. Clin. Endocrinol. Metab.* **40,** 407–410.

Deftos, L. J., Roos, B. A., and Parthemore, J. G. (1975b). Calcium and skeletal metabolism. *West. J. Med.* **123,** 447–458.

Deftos, L. J., Gogo, A., Lee, J. C., and Parthemore, J. G. (1976a). Hypercalcitoninism and hyperparathyroidism in chronic renal disease: Immunochemical heterogeneity. *Proc. 58th Annu. Meet. Endocr. Soc.* p. 254.

Deftos, L. J., McMillan, P. J., Sartiano, G. P., Abuid, J., and Robinson, A. G. (1976b). Simultaneous ectopic production of parathyroid hormone and calcitonin. *Metab., Clin. Exp.* **25,** 543–550.

Deftos, L. J., Burton, D., Bone, H. G., Catherwood, B. D., Parthemore, J. G., Moore, R. Y., Minick, S., and Guillemin, R. (1978a) Immunoreactive calcitonin is present in the intermediate lobe of the pituitary gland. *Life. Sci.* **23,** 743–748.

Deftos, L. J., Burton, D., Catherwood, B. D., Bone, H. G., Parthemore, J. G., Guillemin, R., Watkins, W., and Moore, R. Y. (1978b) Demonstration by immunoperoxidase histochemistry of calcitonin in the anterior lobe of the rat pituitary. *J. Clin. Endocrinol. Metab.* **47,** 457–460.

Deftos, L. J., Roos, B. A., Knecht, G. L., Lee, J., Pavlinac, D., Bone, H. G., and Parthemore, J. G. (1978c). Calcitonin secretion. *In* "Endocrinology of Calcium Metabolism" (D. H. Copp and R. V. Talmage, eds.), pp. 134–142. Excerpta Medica, Amsterdam.

DeLellis, R. A., Wolfe, H. J., Gagel, R. F., Feldman, Z. T., Miller, H. H., Gang, D. L., and Reichlin, S. (1976). Adrenal medullary hyperplasia. *Am. J. Pathol.* **83,** 177–196.

deLuise, M., Martin, T. J., and Melick, R. A. (1970). Inactivation and degradation of porcine calcitonin by rat liver and relative stability of salmon calcitonin. *J. Endocrinol.* **48,** 181–188.

DeRose, J., Singer, F. R., Avramides, A., Flores, A., Dziadiw, R., Baker, R. K., and Wallach, S. (1974). Response of Paget's disease to porcine and salmon calcitonin: Effects of long-term treatment. *Am. J. Med.* **56,** 858–866.

Didolker, M. S., and Moore, G. E. (1974). Hormone-dependent medullary carcinoma of the thyroid. *Am. J. Surg.* **128,** 100–102.

Dreyfus, C. F., Gershon, M. D., Haymovits, A., and Nunez, E. (1976). Calcitonin: Antagonism at intestinal muscarinic receptors. *Br. J. Pharmacol.* **57,** 155–157.

Drukker, W., Formijne, P., and Schoot, J. B. (1957). Hyperplasia of the adrenal medulla. *Br. Med. J.* **1,** 186–189.

Dymling, J. F., Ljungberg, O., Hillyard, C. J., Greenberg, P. B., Evans, I. M. A., and MacIntyre, I. (1976). Whiskey: A new provocative test for calcitonin secretion. *Acta Endocrinol. (Copenhagen)* **82,** 500–509.

Ellison, M., Woodhouse, D., Hillyard, C., Dowsett, M., Coombes, R. C., Gilby, E. D., Greenberg, P. B., and Neville, A. M. (1975). Immunoreactive calcitonin production by human lung carcinoma cells in culture. *Br. J. Cancer* **32,** 373–379.

Ericson, L. E. (1968). Degranulation of the parafollicular cells of the rat thyroid by vitamin D_2-induced hypercalcemia. *J. Ultrastruct. Res.* **24,** 145–149.

Fahrenkrug, J., Hornum, I., and Rehfeld, J. F. (1975). Effect of calcitonin on serum gastrin concentration and component pattern in man. *J. Clin. Endocrinol. Metab.* **41,** 149–152.

Feletti, C., and Bonomini, V. (1980). Effect of calcitonin on bone lesions in chronic dialysis patients. *Nephron* (in press).

Foster, G. V., Baghdiantz, A., Kumar, M. A., Slack, E., Soliman, H. A., and MacIntyre, I. (1964a). Thyroid origin of calcitonin. *Nature (London)* **202,** 1303–1305.

Foster, G. V., MacIntyre, I., and Pearse, A. G. E. (1964b). Calcitonin production and the mitochondrion-rich cells of the dog thyroid. *Nature (London)* **203,** 1029–1030.

Foster, G. V., Clark, M. B., Williams, C., Nathanson, B. M., Horton, R., Buranapong, P., and Glass, H. I. (1972). Metabolic fate of human calcitonin in the dog. *In* "Endocrinology 1971," pp. 71–78. Heinemann, London.

Gagel, F. R., Melvin, K. E. W., Tashjian, A. H., Jr., Miller, H. H., Feldman, Z. T., Wolfe, H. J., DeLellis, R. A., Cervi-Skinner, S., and Reichlin, S. (1975). Natural history of the familial medullary thyroid carcinoma-pheochromocytoma syndrome and the identification of preneoplastic stages by screening studies: A five-year report. *Trans. Assoc. Am. Physicians* **88,** 177–191.

Garel, J. M. (1978). Stimulation of calcitonin secretion in the fasting newborn rat by ingestion of triglycerides. *C. R. Hebd. Seances Acad. Sci.* **286,** 643–646.

Goldsmith, R. E., Sizemore, G. W., Chen, I. W., Zalme, E., and Altemeier, W. A. (1976). Familial hyperparathyroidism. *Ann. Intern. Med.* **84,** 36–43.

Goltzman, D., Potts, J. T., Jr., Ridgeway, E. C., and Maloof, F. (1974). Calcitonin as a tumor marker: Use of a radioimmunoassay for calcitonin in the post-operative evaluation of patients with medullary thyroid carcinoma. *N. Engl. J. Med.* **290,** 1035–1039.

Gordan, G. S., Cantino, T. J., Erhardt, L., Hansen, J., and Lubich, W. (1966). Osteolytic sterol in human breast cancer. *Science* **151,** 1226–1228.

Gottlieb, J. A., and Hill, C. S., Jr. (1975). Adriamycin (NSC-123127) therapy in thyroid carcinoma. *Cancer Chemother. Rep.* **6,** 283–296.

Gray, T. K., Bieberdorf, F. A., and Fordtran, J. S. (1973). Thyrocalcitonin and the jejunal absorption of calcium, water, and electrolytes in normal subjects. *J. Clin. Invest.* **52,** 3084–3088.

Greenberg, P. B., Doyle, E. H., Fisher, M. T., Hillyard, C. J., Joplin, G. F., Pennock, J., and MacIntyre, I. (1974). Treatment of Paget's disease of bone with synthetic human calcitonin: Biochemical and roentgenologic changes. *Am. J. Med.* **56,** 867–870.

Guttmann, St., Pless, J., Sandrin, E., Jaquenoud, P. A., Bossert, H., and Willems, H. (1968). Synthèse des thyrocalcitonins. *Helv. Chim. Acta* **51,** 1155–1161.

Habener, J. F., Singer, F. R., Neer, R. M., Deftos, L. J., and Potts, J. T., Jr. (1971). An explanation for the unusual potency of salmon calcitonin. *Nature (London)* **232,** 91–92.

Haddad, J. G., Jr., and Caldwell, J. G. (1972). Calcitonin resistance: Clinical and immunological studies in subjects with Paget's disease of bone treated with porcine and salmon calcitonins. *J. Clin. Invest.* **51,** 3133–3141.

Hargis, G. K., Williams, G. A., Reynolds, W. A., Chertow, B. S., Kukreja, S. C., Bowser, E. N., and Henderson, W. J. (1978). Effect of somatostatin on parathyroid hormone and calcitonin secretion. *Endocrinology (Baltimore)* **102,** 745–750.

Hazard, J. B., Hawk, W. A., and Crile, G. (1959). Medullary (solid) carcinoma of the thyroid—a clinicopathologic entity. *J. Clin. Endocrinol. Metab.* **19,** 152–161.

Heath, H., and Sizemore, G. W. (1977). Plasma calcitonin in normal man. Differences between men and women. *J. Clin. Invest.* **60,** 1135–1140.

Heersche, J. N. M., Marcus, R., and Aurbach, G. D. (1974). Calcitonin and the formation of 3′,5′-AMP in bone and kidney. *Endocrinology (Baltimore)* **94,** 241–247.

Hennessey, J. F., Gray, T. K., Cooper, C. W., and Ontjes, D. A. (1973a). Stimulation of thyrocalcitonin secretion by pentagastrin and calcium in two patients with medullary thyroid carcinoma of the thyroid. *J. Clin. Endocrinol. Metab.* **36,** 200–203.

Hennessey, J. F., Wells, S. A., Cooper, C. W., and Ontjes, D. A. (1973b). Calcium infusion and pentagastrin injection as provocative tests for medullary carcinoma of the thyroid. *Proc. 56th Annu. Meet. Endocr. Soc.* A205.

Hennessey, J. F., Wells, S. A., Ontjes, D. A., and Cooper, C. W. (1974). A comparison of pentagastrin injection and calcium infusion as provocative agents for the detection of medullary thyroid carcinoma. *J. Clin. Endocrinol. Metab.* **39,** 487–495.

Hesch, R. D., Hufner, M., Hasenjager, M., and Creutzfeldt, W. (1971). Inhibition of gastric secretion by calcitonin in man. *Horm. Metab. Res.* **3,** 140.

Heynen, G., and Franchimont, P. (1974a). Human calcitonin radioimmunoassay in normal and pathological conditions. *Eur. J. Clin. Invest.* **4,** 213–222.

Heynen, G., and Franchimont, P. (1974b). Human calcitonin and serum phosphate. *Lancet* **1,** 627.

Heynen, G., Kanis, J., Earnshaw, M., Ledingham, J., Oliver, D., Russell, R., Walton, R., and Woods, C. (1977). A possible role for endogenous calcitonin (CT) in renal osteodystrophy. *Proc. Int. Cong. Endocrinol. 5th, 1976* p. 159.

Hill, C. S., Jr., Ibanez, M. L., Samaan, N. A., Ahearn, M. J., and Clark, R. L. (1973). Medullary (solid) carcinoma of the thyroid gland: An analysis of the M. D. Anderson Hospital experience with patients with the tumor, its special features and its histogenesis. *Medicine (Baltimore)* **52,** 141–171.

Hillyard, C. J., Coombes, R. C., Greenberg, P. B., and MacIntyre, I. (1975). Immunoreactive calcitonin in patients with carcinomata. *J. Endocrinol.* **66,** 2p–3p.

Hillyard, C. J., Coombes, R. C., Greenberg, P. B., Galante, L. S., and MacIntyre, I. (1976). Calcitonin in breast and lung cancer. *Clin. Endocrinol. (Oxford)* **5,** 1–8.

Hioco, D., Bordier, P., Miravet, L., Denys, H., and Tun-Chot, S. (1970). Prolonged administration of calcitonin in man: Biological, isotopic and morphological effects. *Calcitonin, Proc. Int. Symp., 2nd,* pp. 514–522.

Hirsch, P. F., and Munson, P. L. (1969). Thyrocalcitonin. *Physiol. Rev.* **49,** 548–622.

Hirsch, P. F., Gauthier, G. F., and Munson, P. L. (1963). Thyroid hypocalcemic principle and recurrent laryngeal nerve injury as factors affecting the response to parathyroidectomy in rats. *Endocrinology (Baltimore)* **73,** 244–252.

Hirsch, P. F., Voelkel, E. F., and Munson, P. L. (1964). Thyrocalcitonin: Hypocalcemic hypophosphatemic principle of the thyroid gland. *Science* **146,** 412–413.

Hirsch, P. F., Cooper, C. W., Peng, T. C., Burford, H. J., Toverud, S. U., Gray, T. K., Juan, D., Ontjes, D. A., Hennessey, J. F., and Munson, P. L. (1974). Effects, functions and endocrine interrelations of thyrocalcitonin. *In* "Calcium-Regulating Hormones" (R. V. Talmage, M. Owen, and J. A. Parsons, eds.), pp. 89–99. Excerpta Medica, Amsterdam.

Hokfelt, T., Efendic, S., Hellerström, C., Johansson, O., Luft, R., and Arimura, A. (1975). Cellular localization of somatostatin in endocrine-like cells and neurons of the rat with special references to the A_1-cells of the pancreatic islets and to the hypothalamus. *Acta Endocrinol. (Copenhagen)* **80,** 5–41.

Hotz, J., Goebell, H., and Ziegler, R. (1977). Calcitonin and exocrine pancreatic secretion in man: Inhibition of enzymes stimulated by CCK-pancreozymin, caerulein, or calcium—no response to vagal stimulation. *GT* **18,** 615–622.

Ibanez, M. L., Cole, V. W., Russell, W. O., and Clark, R. I. (1967). Solid carcinoma of the thyroid gland. *Cancer* **20,** 706–723.

Isaac, R., Nivez, M. P., Piamba, G., Fillastre, J. P., and Ardaillou, R. (1975). Influence of calcium infusion on calcitonin and parathyroid hormone concentrations in normal and hemodialyzed subjects. *Clin. Nephrol.* **3,** 14–17.

Ito, H., Ooyama, T., and Orimo, H. (1976). Inactivation of porcine calcitonin by rat kidney microsome. *Endocrinol. Jpn.* **23,** 109–114.

Iwatsuki, K., and Hashimoto, K. (1976). Effects of calcitonin on the secretion of pancreatic juice induced by dopamine, secretin, and pancreozymin. *Clin. Exp. Pharmacol. Physiol.* **3,** 159–165.

Kalina, M., Foster, G. V., Clark, M. B., and Pearse, A. G. E. (1970). C-cells in man. *Calcitonin, Proc. Int. Symp., 2nd, 1969* pp. 268–273.

Kalu, D. N., Hadji-Georgopoulos, A., and Foster, G. V. (1975). Evidence for physiological importance of calcitonin in the regulation of plasma calcium in rats. *J. Clin. Invest.* **55,** 722–727.

Kanis, J. A., Earnshaw, M., Heynen, G., Russell, R. G. G., and Woods, C. G. (1977). The possible role of calcitonin deficiency in the development of bone disease due to chronic renal failure. *Calcif. Tissue Res.* **22,** 147–153.

Kaplan, E. L. (1973). Recent advances in calcium metabolism. Application to medullary carcinoma of the thyroid and hyperparathyroidism. *Surg. Annu.* **5,** 97–119.

Keiser, J. R., Beaven, M. A., Doppman, J., Wells, S., and Buja, L. M. (1973). Medullary thyroid carcinoma, pheochromocytoma, and parathyroid disease. *Ann. Intern. Med.* **78,** 561–579.

Keutmann, H. T., Parsons, J. A., Potts, J. T., Jr., and Schlueter, R. J. (1970). Isolation and chemical properties of two calcitonins from salmon ultimobranchial glands. *J. Biol. Chem.* **245,** 1491–1496.

Keutmann, H. T., Lequin, R. M., Habener, J. F., Singer, F. R., Niall, H. D., and Potts, J. T., Jr. (1972). Chemistry and physiology of the calcitonins: Some recent advances. *In* "Endocrinology 1971," pp. 316–323. Heinemann, London.

Khairi, M. R. A., Dexter, R. N., Burzynski, N. J., and Johnston, C. C., Jr. (1975). Mucosal neuroma, pheochromocytoma, and medullary thyroid carcinoma: MEN, Type III. *Medicine (Baltimore)* **54,** 89–112.

Koelz, H. R., Drack, G. T., and Blum, A. L. (1976). Effect of calcitonin on salivary amylase secretion in vivo and in vitro. *Schweiz. Med. Wochenschr.* **106,** 298–299.

Korman, M. G., Lauer, M. C., and Hansky, J. (1972). Hypergastrinemia in chronic renal failure. *Br. Med. J.* **1,** 209–210.

Kracht, J., Hachmeister, U., and Christ, U. (1970). C-cells in the human thyroid. *Calcitonin, Proc.* investigation on C-cells. *Calcitonin, Proc. Symp. Thyrocalcitonin C Cells, 1967* pp. 143–151.

Kracht, J., Hachmeister, U., an :Christ, U. (1970). C-cells in the human thyroid. *Calcitonin, Proc. Int. Symp., 2nd, 1969* pp. 274–280.

Lambert, P. W., Heath, H., and Sizemore, G. W. (1976). Basal and stimulated plasma immunoreactive calcitonin (iCT) values are not high in primary hyperparathyroidism (1°HPT). *Clin. Res.* **24,** 581A.

Lawrence, A. M. (1972). Pancreatic alpha-cell function in miscellaneous clinical disorders. *In* "Glucagon" (P. J. Lefebvre and R. H. Unger, eds.), pp. 259–274. Pergamon, Oxford.

LeDourain, N., and LeLievre, C. (1970). Demonstration de l'origine neural des cellules a calcitonine du corps ultimobranchial chez l'embryon de poulet. *C. R. Hebd. Seances Acad. Sci.* **270,** 2857–2860.

Lee, J. C., Catanzaro, A., Parthemore, J. G., Roach, B., and Deftos, L. J. (1977a). Hypercalcemia in disseminated coccidioidomycosis. *N. Engl. J. Med.* **297,** 431–433.

Lee, J. C., Larsen, M. A., Roos, B. A., and Deftos, L. F. (1977b). Decreased calcitonin (CT) responsiveness and calcium intolerance in renal failure. *Clin. Res.* **25,** 394A.

Lee, J. C., Parthemore, J. G., and Deftos, L. J. (1977c). Calcitonin secretion in renal disease. *Calcif. Tissue Res.* **22S,** 154–157.

Lee, J. C., Parthemore, J. G., and Deftos, L. J. (1977d). Immunochemical heterogeneity of calcitonin in renal failure. *J. Clin. Endocrinol. Metab.* **45,** 528–533.

Leicht, E., Biro, G., and Weinges, K. F. (1974). Inhibition of releasing hormone induced secretion of TSH and LH by calcitonin. *Horm. Metab. Res.* **6,** 410–414.

Lips, C. J. M., van der Sluys Veer, J., van der Donk, J. A., van Dam, R. H., and Hackeng, W. H. L. (1978). Common precursor molecule as origin for the ectopic hormone producing tumor syndrome. *Lancet* **1,** 16–18.

LiVolsi, V. A., Feind, C. R., LoGerfo, P., and Tashjian, A. H., Jr. (1973). Demonstration by immunoperoxidase staining of hyperplasia of parafollicular cells in the thyroid gland in hyperparathyroidism. *J. Clin. Endocrinol. Metab.* **37,** 550–559.

Ljungberg, O. (1972). On medullary carcinoma of the thyroid: A clinicopathologic entity. *Acta Pathol. Microbiol. Scand.* **231,** 1–57.

Ljungberg, O., and Dymling, J. F. (1972). Pathogenesis of C-cell neoplasia in thyroid gland. C-cell preliferation in a case of chronic hypercalcemia. *Acta Pathol. Microbiol. Scand.* **80,** 577–588.

Lupulescu, A. (1975). Effect of calcitonin on DNA synthesis in experimental wounds. *Proc. Soc. Exp. Biol. Med.* **150,** 703–706.

McKenna, T. J., McLean, D., Lorber, D. L., Bone, H. G., Parthemore, J. G., and Deftos, L. J. (1978). Comparison of calcitonin stimulation gests used in screening for medullary carcinoma of the thyroid. *Proc. 60th Annu. Meet. Endocr. Soc.* p. 370.

McMillan, P. J., Hooker, W. M., and Deftos, L. J. (1974). Distribution of calcitonin-containing cells in human thyroid. *Am. J. Anat.* **140,** 73–80.

Maier, R., Kamber, B., Riniker, B., and Rittel, W. (1975). Analogues of human calcitonin. II. Influence of modifications in amino acid positions 1, 8, and 22 on hypocalcemic activity in rat. *Horm. Metab. Res.* **7,** 511–514.

Marshall, J. P., Winnacker, J. L., and Anast, C. (1975). Hypercalcitoninemia (HCT) in acute pancreatitis (AP). *Clin. Res.* **23,** 325A.

Marx, S. J., and Aurbach, G. D. (1975). Renal receptors for calcitonin: Coordinate occurrence with calcitonin-activated adenylate cyclase. *Endocrinology (Baltimore)* **97,** 448–453.

Melvin, K. E. W., and Tashjian, A. H., Jr. (1968). The syndrome of excessive thyrocalcitonin produced by medullary carcinoma of the thyroid. *Proc. Natl. Acad. Sci. U.S.A.* **59,** 1216-1222.

Melvin, K. E. W., Voelkel, E. F., and Tashjian, A. H., Jr. (1970). Medullary carcinoma of the thyroid: Stimulation by calcium and glucagon of calcitonin secretion. *Calcitonin, Proc. Int. Symp., 2nd, 1969* pp. 487-496.

Melvin, K. E. W., Tashjian, A. H., Jr., and Miller, H. H. (1971a). Studies in familial thyroid cancer. *Trans. Assoc. Am. Physicians* **84,** 144-151.

Melvin, K. E. W., Miller, H. H., and Tashjian, A. H., Jr. (1971b). Early diagnosis of medullary carcinoma of the thyroid gland by means of calcitonin assay. *N. Engl. J. Med.* **285,** 1115-1120.

Melvin, K. E. W., Tashjian, A. H., Jr., and Bordier, P. (1973). The metabolic significance of calcitonin-secreting thyroid carcinoma. *In* "Clinical Aspects of Metabolic Bone Disease" (W. Frame, A. M. Parfitt, and H. Duncan, eds.), pp. 193-201. Excerpta Medica; Amsterdam.

Metz, S. A., Deftos, L. J., Baylink, D., and Robertson, R. P. (1978). Neuroendocrine modulation of calcitonin and parathyroid hormone in man. *J. Clin. Endocrinol. Metab.* **47,** 151-159.

Meyer, J. S., and Abdel-Bari, W. (1968). Granules and thyrocalcitonin-like activity in medullary carcinoma of the thyroid. *N. Engl. J. Med.* **278,** 523-529.

Milhaud, G., and Moukhtar, M. S. (1966). Thyrocalcitonin: Effects on calcium kinetics in the rat. *Proc. Soc. Exp. Biol. Med.* **123,** 207-209.

Milhaud, G., Tubiana, M., Parmentier, C., and Coutris, G. (1968). Epithelioma de la thyroide secretant de la thyrocalcitonine. *C. R. Hebd. Seances Acad. Sci.* **266,** 608-610.

Milhaud, G., Calmettes, C., Jullienne, A., Tharaud, D., Bloch-Michel, H., Cavaillon, J. P., Colin, R., and Moukhtar, M. S. (1972). A new chapter in human pathology: Calcitonin disorders and therapeutic use. *In* "Calcium, Parathyroid Hormone and the Calcitonins" (R. V. Talmage and P. L. Munson, eds.), pp. 56-70. Excerpta Medica, Amsterdam.

Milhaud, G., Calmettes, C., Taboulet, J., Jullienne, A., and Moukhtar, M. S. (1974). Hypersecretion of calcitonin in neoplastic conditions. *Lancet* **1,** 462-463.

Milhaud, G., Talbot, J. N., and Coutris, G. (1975). Calcitonin treatment of post-menopausal osteoporosis. Evaluation of efficacy by principal components analysis. *Biomedicine* **22,** 223-232.

Montalbano, F. P., Baronofsky, I. D., and Ball, H. (1962). Hyperplasia of the adrenal medulla. *JAMA, J. Am. Med. Assoc.* **182,** 264-267.

Morita, R., Fukunaga, I., Yamamoto, I., Mori, T., and Torizuka, K. (1975). Radioimmunoassay for human calcitonin employing synthetic calcitonin M: Its clinical application. *Endocrinol. Jpn.* **22,** 419-426.

Mundy, G. R., Raisz, L. G., Cooper, R. A., Schechter, G. P., and Salmon, S. E. (1974). Evidence for the secretion of an osteoclast stimulating factor in myeloma. *N. Engl. J. Med.* **291,** 1041-1046.

Nathaniels, E. K., Nathaniels, A. M., and Wang, C. A. (1970). Mediastinal parathyroid tumors: A clinical and pathological study of 84 cases. *Ann. Surg.* **171,** 165-170.

Neher, R., Riniker, B., Zuber, H., Rittel, W., and Kahnt, F. W. (1968a). Thyrocalcitonin. II. Strukture von alpha-thyrocalcitonin. *Helv. Chim. Acta* **51,** 917-924.

Neher, R., Riniker, B., Rittel, W., and Zuber, H. (1968b). Menschliches calcitonin. III. Strukture von calcitonin M und D. *Helv. Chim. Acta* **51,** 1900-1905.

Niall, H. D., Keutmann, H. T., Copp, D. H., and Potts, J. T., Jr. (1969). Amino acid sequence of salmon ultimobranchial calcitonin. *Proc. Natl. Acad. Sci. U.S.A.* **64,** 771-778.

Noda, T., and Narita, K. (1976). Amino acid sequence of eel calcitonin. *J. Biochem. (Tokyo)* **79,** 353-359.

Nonidez, J. F. (1932). The origin of the 'parafollicular' cell, a second epithelial component of the thyroid gland in the dog. *Am. J. Anat.* **49,** 479–505.

Norberg, H. P., DeRoos, J., and Kaplan, E. L. (1975). Increased parathyroid hormone secretion and hypocalcemia in experimental pancreatitis: Necessity for an intact thyroid gland. *Surgery* **77,** 773–779.

Nozaki, K., Noda, S., Obi, S., Nishizawa, Y., Morii, H., and Wada, M. (1976). Secretion of gastrin and calcitonin after ingestion of meat extract in patients with peptic ulcer. *Endocrinol. Jpn.* **23,** 83–86.

Olson, E. B., DeLuca, H. F., and Potts, J. T., Jr. (1972). The effect of calcitonin and parathyroid hormone on calcium transport of isolated intestine. *In* "Calcium, Parathyroid Hormone and the Calcitonins" (R. V. Talmage and P. L. Munson, eds.), pp. 240–246. Excerpta Medica, Amsterdam.

Otani, M., Yamauchi, H., Meguro, T., Kitazawa, S., Tatanabe, S., and Orimo, H. (1976). Isolation and characterization of calcitonin from pericardium and esophagus of eel. *J. Biochem. (Tokyo)* **79,** 345–352.

Pak, C. Y. C., Steward, A., Kaplan, R., Bone, H., Notz, C., and Browne, R. (1975). Photon absorptiometric analysis of bone density in primary hyperparathyroidism. *Lancet* **2,** 7–8.

Paloyan, E., Paloyan, D., and Harper, P. V. (1967). The role of glucagon hypersecretion in the relationship of pancreatitis and hyperparathyroidism. *Surgery* **62,** 167–173.

Parthemore, J. G. (1977). Compensatory hypercalcitoninism in primary hyperparathyroidism. *Proc. 59th Annu. Meet. Endocr. Soc.* p. 235.

Parthemore, J. G., and Roos, B. A. (1976). Calcitonin heterogeneity: In vivo and in vitro studies. *Proc. 58th Annu. Meet. Endocr. Soc.* p. 65.

Parthemore, J. G., and Deftos, L. J. (1978). Calcitonin secretion in normal human subjects. *J. Clin. Endocrinol Metab.* **47,** 184–188.

Parthemore, J. G., Bronzert, D., Roberts, G., and Deftos, L. F. (1974). A short calcium infusion in the diagnosis of medullary thyroid carcinoma. *J. Clin. Endocrinol. Metab.* **39,** 108–111.

Parthemore, J. G., Deftos, L. J., and Bronzert, D. (1975a). The regulation of calcitonin in normal human plasma as assessed by immunoprecipitation and immunoextraction. *J. Clin. Invest.* **56,** 835–841.

Parthemore, J. G., Roos, B. A., and Deftos, L. J. (1975b). Immunochemical heterogeneity of calcitonin in plasma. *Clin. Res.* **23,** 113.

Parthemore, J. G., Roos, B. A., and Deftos, L. J. (1976). Calcitonin heterogeneity: In vivo and in vitro studies. *Proc. Eur. Symp. Calcif. Tissues, 12th, 1976* p. 68.

Parthemore, J. G., Moriguchi, M., and Deftos, L. J. (1977). Secondary hypercalcitoninism in primary hyperparathyroidism. *Clin. Res.* **25,** 498A.

Passeri, M., Carapezzi, C., Seccato, S., Monica, C., Storzzi, D., and Palummeri, E. (1975). Possible effect of caerulein on calcitonin secretion in man. *Experientia* **31,** 1234–1235.

Pearse, A. G. E. (1966). The cytochemistry of the thyroid cells and their relationship to calcitonin. *Proc. R. Soc. London* **164,** 478–487.

Pearse, A. G. E. (1968). Common cytochemical and ultrastructural characteristics of cells producing polypeptide hormones (the APUD series) and their relevance to thyroid and ultimobranchial C-cells and calcitonin. *Proc. R. Soc. London* **170,** 71–80.

Pearse, A. G. E., and Takor, T. T. (1976). Neuroendocrine embryology and the APUD concept. *Clin. Endocrinol. (Oxford)* **5,** 299–244.

Pecile, A., Ferri, S., Braga, P. C., and Oligiati, V. R. (1975). Effects of intracerebroventricular calcitonin in the conscious rabbit. *Experientia* **31,** 332–333.

Peng, T. C., Cooper, C. W., Pterusz, P., and Volpert, E. M. (1975). Identification of C-cells in normal and goitrous rat thyroid tissues using antiserum to rat thyrocalcitonin and the immunoperoxidase bridge technique. *Endocrinology* **97,** 1537–1544.

Pento, J. T. (1978). Characteristics of calcitonin degradation in vitro produced by incubation with porcine thyroid tissue. *Mol. Cell. Endocrinol.* **12,** 31–40.

Pento, J. T., Glick, S. M., Kagen, A., and Gorfein, P. C. (1974). The relative influence of calcium, strontium, and magnesium on calcitonin secretion in the pig. *Endocrinology (Baltimore)* **94,** 1176–1180.

Pitkin, M., Reynolds, W. A., Williams, G. A., and Hargis, G. K. (1981). Calcium-regulating hormones during the menstrual cycle. *J. Clin. Endocrinol. Metab.* (in press).

Potts, J. T., Jr., and Deftos, L. J. (1969). Parathyroid hormone, thyrocalcitonin, vitamin D and diseases of bone and bone mineral metabolism. *In* ''Duncan's Diseases of Metabolism, Endocrinology and Nutrition'' (P. K. Bondy, ed.), 6th ed., Vol. 2, pp. 904–1082. Saunders, Philadelphia, Pennsylvania.

Potts, J. T., Jr., Niall, H. D., Keutmann, H. T., Brewer, H. T., and Deftos, L. J. (1968). The amino acid sequence of porcine thyrocalcitonin. *Proc. Natl. Acad. Sci. U.S.A.* **59,** 1321–1328.

Potts, J. T., Jr., Keutmann, H. T., Niall, H. D., and Tregear, G. W. (1971a). The chemistry of parathyroid hormone and the calcitonins. *Vitam. Horm. (N.Y.)* **29,** 41–93.

Potts, J. T., Jr., Niall, H. D., and Deftos, L. J. (1971b). Calcitonin. *Curr. Top. Exp. Endocrinol.* **1,** 151–173.

Powell, D., Singer, F. R., Murray, T. M., Minkin, C., and Potts, J. T., Jr. (1973). Non-parathyroid humoral hypercalcemia in patients with neoplastic diseases. *N. Engl. J. Med.* **289,** 176–181.

Putter, I., Kacka, E. A., Harman, R. E., Rickes, E., Kempf, A. J., Chaiet, L., Rothrock, J. W., Wase, A., and Wolf, F. J. (1968). Thyrocalcitonin: Isolation and chemial properties. *Calcitonin, Proc. Symp. Thyrocalcitonin C Cells, 1967* pp. 74–76.

Raisz, L. G., Au, W. Y. W., Friedman, J., and Niemann, I. (1968). Inhibition of bone resorption in tissue culture by thyrocalcitonin. *Calcitonin, Proc. Symp. Thyrocalcitonin C Cells, 1967,* pp. 215–222.

Raulais, D., Merle, M., and Milhaud, G. (1974). Horse calcitonin: Isolation and biological properties. *In* ''Endocrinology 1973,'' pp. 117–184. Heinemann, London.

Riggs, B. L., Jowsey, J., Kelly, P. J., and Arnaud, C. D. (1976). Role of hormonal factors in the pathogenesis of postmenopausal osteoporosis. *Isr. J. Med. Sci.* **12,** 615–619.

Riniker, B., Neher, R., Maier, R., Kahnt, F. W., Byfield, P. G. H., Gudmundsson, T. V., Galante, L., and MacIntyre, I. (1968). Menschliches calcitonin. I. Isolierung und charakterisierung. *Helv. Chim. Acta* **51,** 1738–1742.

Rittel, W., Brugger, M., Kamber, B., Riniker, B., and Sieber, P. (1968). Thyrocalcitonin. III. Die synthese des alpha-thyrocalcitonins. *Helv. Chim. Acta* **51,** 924–928.

Rittel, W., Maier, R., Brugger, M., Kamber, B., Riniker, B., and Sieber, P. (1976). Structure-activity relationship of human calcitonin. III. Biological activity of synthetic analogues with shortened or terminally modified peptide chaims. *Experientia* **32,** 246–248.

Robertson, G. M., Jr., Moore, E. W., Switz, D. M., Sizemore, G. W., and Estep, H. L. (1976). Inadequate parathyroid response in acute pancreatitis. *N. Engl. J. Med.* **294,** 512–516.

Rojanasathit, S., and Haddad, J. G., Jr. (1977). Human calcitonin radioimmunoassay: Characterization and application. *Clin. Chim. Acta* **78,** 425–437.

Roos, B. A., and Deftos, L. J. (1976a). Radioimmunoassay of calcitonin in plasma, normal thyroid, and medullary thyroid carcinoma of the rat. *J. Lab. Clin. Med.* **88,** 173–182.

Roos, B. A., and Deftos, L. J. (1976b). Regulation of calcitonin secretion in vitro. *Clin. Endocrinol. (Oxford)* **5,** 217s–222s.

Roos, B. A., Okano, K., and Deftos, L. J. (1974). Evidence for a pro-calcitonin. *Biochem. Biophys. Res. Commun.* **60,** 1134–1140.

Roos, B. A., Parthemore, J. G., Lee, J., and Deftos, L. J. (1977). Calcitonin heterogeneity: In vivo and in vitro studies. *Calcif. Tissue Res.* **22S,** 298–302.

Roos, B. A., Cooper, C. W., Frelinger, A. L., and Deftos, L. J. (1978). Calcitonin in murine physiology. Acute and chronic fluctuations in biologically active calcitonin. *Endocrinology (Baltimore)* **103,** 2180–2186.

Rude, R. K., and Singer, F. R. (1977). Comparison of serum levels after a one-minute calcium injection and after pentagastrin injection in diagnosis of medullary thyroid carcinoma. *J. Clin. Endocrinol. Metab.* **44,** 980–983.

Ryan, W. G., Schwartz, T. B., and Perlia, C. P. (1969). Effects of mithramycin on Paget's disease of bone. *Ann. Intern. Med.* **70,** 549–557.

Samaan, N. A., Hill, C. S., Jr., Beceiro, J. R., and Schultz, P. N. (1973). Immunoreactive calcitonin in medullary carcinoma of the thyroid and in maternal and cord serum. *J. Lab. Clin. Med.* **81,** 671–681.

Samaan, N. A., Wigoda, C., and Castillo, S. G. (1974). Human serum calcitonin and parathyroid hormone levels in the maternal, umbilical cord blood and postpartum. *In* "Endocrinology 1973," pp. 364–372. Heinemann, London.

Sammon, P. J., Stacey, R. E., and Bronner, F. (1969). Further studies on the role of thyrocalcitonin in calcium homeostasis and metabolism. *Biochem. Med.* **3,** 252–270.

Sauer, R., Niall, H. D., and Potts, J. T., Jr. (1970). Accelerated procedures for automated peptide degradation. *Fed. Proc., Fed. Am. Soc. Exp. Biol.* **29,** 728/2723.

Scarpace, P. J., Neuman, W. F., and Raisz, L. G. (1977). Metabolism of radioiodinated salmon calcitonin in rats. *Endocrinology (Baltimore)* **100,** 1260–1267.

Schedewid, H., Odell, W., Fisher, D., Kurtzik, S., Deftos, L. J., Cousins, L., Cantor, T., and Fiser, W. (1978). Calcitonin and PTH in the control of perinatal calcium homeostasis. *Clin. Res.* **26,** 72A.

Schimke, R. N., Hartmann, W. H., Prout, T. E., and Rimoin, D. L. (1968). Syndrome of bilateral pheochromocytoma, medullary thyroid carcinoma, and multiple neuromas. *N. Engl. J. Med.* **279,** 1–7.

Schmidt, H., Hesch, R. D., Hufner, M., Paschen, K., and Creutzfeldt, W. (1971). Hemmung der exokrinen pankreassekretion des menschen durch calcitonin. *Dtsch. Med. Wochenschr.* **96,** 1773–1775.

Seyberth, H. W., Segre, G. V., Morgan, J. L., Sweetman, B. J., Potts, J. T., Jr., and Oates, J. A. (1975). Prostaglandins as mediators of hypercalcemia associated with cancer. *N. Engl. J. Med.* **293,** 1278–1283.

Sherwin, R. P. (1964). Present status of the pathology of the adrenal gland in hypertension. *Am. J. Surg.* **107,** 136–143.

Sieber, P., Brugger, M., Kamber, B., Riniker, B., and Rittel, W. (1968). Menschliches calcitonin. IV. 1) Diesynthese von calcitonin M. *Helv. Chim. Acta* **51,** 2057–2061.

Sieber, P., Brugger, M., Kamber, B., Riniker, B., Rittel, W., Maier, R., and Staehelin, M. (1970). Synthesis and biological activity of peptide sequences related to porcine a-thyrocalcitonin. *Calcitonin, Proc. Int. Symp., 2nd, 1969,* pp. 28–33.

Silva, O. L., and Becker, K. L. (1976). High plasma calcitonin levels in breast cancer. *Br. Med. J.* **1,** 460.

Silva, O. L., Becker, K. L., Primack, A., Doppman, J., and Snider, R. H. (1974a). Ectopic secretion of calcitonin by oat-cell carcinoma. *N. Engl. J. Med.* **290,** 1122–1124.

Silva, O. L., Becker, K. L., Selawry, H. F., Snider, R. H., Moore, C. F., Bivins, L. E., and Shalhoub, R. J. (1974b). Human calcitonin and serum-phosphate. *Lancet* **1,** 1055.

Silva, O. L., Snider, R. H., and Becker, K. L. (1974c). Radioimmunoassay of calcitonin in human plasma. *Clin. Chem.* **20,** 337–339.

Silva, O. L., Becker, K. L., Primack, A., Doppman, J. L., and Snider, R. H. (1975). Hypercalcitoninemia in bronchogenic cancer. *JAMA, J. Am. Med. Assoc.* **234,** 183–185.

Silva, O. L., Becker, K. L., Primack, A., Doppman, J. L., and Snider, R. H. (1976). Increased serum calcitonin levels in bronchogenic cancer. *Chest* **69,** 495–499.

Silva, O. L., Snider, R. H., Becker, K. L., and Moore, C. F. (1977). Altered immunochemical heterogeneity of calcitonin induced by calcium infusion. *J. Endocrinol.* **73,** 183–184.

Silva, O. L., Wisneski, L. A., Cyrus, J., Snider, R. H., Moore, C. F., and Becker, K. L. (1978). Calcitonin in thyroidectomized patients. *Am. J. Med. Sci.* **275,** 159–164.

Singer, F. R. (1975). Treatment of Paget's disease of bone. *Postgrad. Med.* **57,** 117–120.

Singer, F. R., and Habener, J. F. (1974). Multiple immunoreactive forms of calcitonin in human plasma. *Biochem. Biophys. Res. Commun.* **61,** 660–666.

Singer, F. R., Aldred, J. P., Neer, R. M., Krane, S. M., Potts, J. T., Jr., and Bloch, K. J. (1972a). An evaluation of antibodies and clinical resistance to salmon calcitonin. *J. Clin. Invest.* **51,** 2331–2338.

Singer, F. R., Habener, J. F., Greene, E., Godin, P., and Potts, J. T., Jr. (1972b). Inactivation of calcitonin by specific organs. *Nature (London), New Biol.* **237,** 269–270.

Sizemore, G. W., and Heath, H. (1975). Immunochemical heterogeneity of calcitonin in plasma of patients with medullary thyroid carcinoma. *J. Clin. Invest.* **55,** 111–118.

Sizemore, G. W., and Heath, H. (1976). Pentagastrin injection is superior to calcium infusion for the diagnosis of familial medullary thyroid carcinoma. *Clin. Res.* **24,** 584A.

Smith, R., Russell, R. G., and Bishop, M. (1971). Diphosphonates and Paget's disease of bone. *Lancet* **1,** 945–946.

Snider, R. H., Silva, O. L., Moore, C. F., and Becker, K. L. (1977). Immunochemical heterogeneity of calcitonin in man. Effect on radioimmunoassay. *Clin. Chim. Acta.* **76,** 1–14.

Solcia, E., and Sampietro, R. (1968). New methods for staining secretory granules and 5-hydroxytryptamine in the thyroid C-cells. *Calcitonin, Proc. Symp. Thyrocalcitonin C Cells, 1967* pp. 127–132.

Sowa, M., Appert, H. E., and Howard, J. M. (1977). Hypocalcemic activity of pancreatic tissue homgenate in dog. *Surg., Gynecol. Obstet.* **144,** 365–370.

Steiner, A. L., Goodman, A. D., and Powers, S. R. (1968). Study of kindred with pheochromocytoma, medullary thyroid carcinoma hyperparathyroidism, and Cushing's disease: MEN, Type II. *Medicine (Baltimore)* **47,** 371–409.

Strauss, E., and Yalow, R. S. (1976). Artifacts in the radioimmunoassay of peptide hormones in gastric and duodenal secretions. *J. Lab. Clin. Med.* **87,** 292–298.

Swaminathan, R., Ker, J., and Care, A. D. (1974). Calcitonin and intestinal calcium absorption. *J. Endocrinol.* **61,** 83–94.

Takaoka, Y., Takamori, M., Ichinose, M., Shikaya, T., Igawa, N., Kikutani, M., and Yamamoto, Y. (1969). Hypocalcemic action of a pancreatic factor and its clinical significance on the myasthenic patients. *Acta Med. Nagasak.* **13,** 28–35.

Talmage, R. V., Neuenschwander, J., and Kraintz, L. (1965). Evidence for the existence of thyrocalcitonin in the rat. *Endocrinology (Baltimore)* **76,** 103–107.

Tamburino, G., Fiore, C. E., Cottini, E., and Petralito, A. (1976). Plasma calcitonin after calcium infusion in normal adults and in senile osteoporosis. *IRCS Med. Sci.* **4,** 41.

Tarnawski, A., Bogdal, J., Dura, K., Marsnalek, Z., and Jedrychowski, A. (1974). Effect of calcitonin on the formation, composition, and enzymatic activity of the hepatic bile in guinea pigs. *GT* **15,** 703–705.

Tashjian, A. H., Jr., and Voelkel, E. F. (1967). Decreased thyrocalcitonin in thyroid glands from patients with hyperparathyroidism. *J. Clin. Endocrinol. Metab.* **27,** 1353–1357.

Tashjian, A. H., Jr., Howland, B. G., Kenneth, B. A., Melvin, K. E. W., and Hill, C. S., Jr. (1970). Immunoassay of human calcitonin. (Clinical measurement, relation to serum calcium and studies in patients with medullary thyroid carcinoma.) *N. Engl. J. Med.* **283,** 890–895.

Tauber, S. D. (1967). The ultimobranchial origin of thyrocalcitonin. *Proc. Natl. Acad. Sci. U.S.A.* **58,** 1684–1687.

Toverud, S. U., Harper, C., and Munson, P. L. (1976). Calcium metabolism during lactation: Enhanced effects of thyrocalcitonin. *Endocrinology (Baltimore)* **99,** 371–378.

Velo, G. P. DeBastiani, G., Nogarin, L., and Abdullahi, S. E. (1976). Anti-inflammatory effect of calcitonin. *Agents Actions* **6,** 284.

Visser, J. W., and Axt, R. (1975). Bilateral adrenal medullary hyperplasia: A clinicopathological entity. *J. Clin. Pathol.* **28,** 298–304.

Vora, N. M., Williams, G. A., Hargis, G. K., Bowser, E. N., Kawahara, W., Jackson, B. L., Henderson, W. J., and Kukreja, S. C. (1978). Comparative effect of calcium and of the adrenergic system on calcitonin secretion in man. *J. Clin. Endocrinol. Metab.* **46,** 567–571.

Watts, E. G., Copp, D. H., and Deftos, L. F. (1974). Changes in plasma calcitonin and calcium during the migration of salmon. *Endocrinology (Baltimore)* **96,** 214–218.

Weichert, R. F., III (1970). The neural ectodermal origin of the peptide-secreting endocrine glands. A unifying concept for the etiology of multiple endocrine adenomatosis and the inappropriate secretion of peptide hormones by nonendocrine tumors. *Am. J. Med.* **49,** 232–241.

Weir, G. C., Lesser, P. G., Drop, L. J., Fischer, J. E., and Warshaw, A. L. (1975). The hypocalcemia of acute pancreatitis. *Ann. Intern. Med.* **83,** 185–189.

Wells, S. A., Jr., Ontjes, D. A., Cooper, C. W., Hennessey, J. F., Ellis, G. J., MacPherson, H. T., and Sabiston, D. C., Jr. (1975). The early diagnosis of medullary carcinoma of the thyroid gland in patients with multiple endocrine neoplasia, Type II. *Ann. Surg.* **182,** 362–370.

Werner, S., and Low, H. (1974). Inhibitory effects of calcitonin on lipolysis and 47-calcium accumulation in rat adipose tissue in vivo. *Horm. Metab. Res.* **6,** 30–36.

West, T. E. T., O'Riordan, J. L. H., and Care, A. D. (1969). The clearance of homologous calcitonin. *J. Endocrinol.* **45,** 495–504.

Wetzel, B. K., and Gittes, R. F. (1966). Changes in the light (parafollicular) cells of the rat thyroid gland following parathyroidectomy. *Proc. 48th Annu. Meet. Endocr. Soc.* p. 71.

Whyte, M. P., Aran, D. T., Deftos, L. J., Slatopolsky, E., and Avioli, L. V. (1978). Menstrual cycle effect on calcitonin secretion in normal young women. *Proc. 60th Annu. Meet. Endocr. Soc.* p. 475.

Williams, E. D. (1966). Histogenesis of medullary carcinoma of the thyroid. *J. Clin. Pathol.* **19,** 114–118.

Wolfe, H. J., Melvin, K. E. W., Cervi-Skinner, S. J., Al Saadi, A. A., Juliar, J. F., Jackson, C. E., and Tashjian, A. H., Jr. (1973). C-cell hyperplasia preceding medullary thyroid carcinoma. *N. Engl. J. Med.* **289,** 437–441.

Wolfe, H. J., Voelkel, E. F., and Tashjian, A. H., Jr. (1974). Distribution of calcitonin-containing cells in the normal adult human thyroid gland: A correlation of morphology with peptide content. *J. Clin. Endocrinol. Metab.* **38,** 688–694.

Woodhouse, N. J. Y., Bordier, P., Fisher, M., Joplin, G. F., Reiner, M., Kalu, D. N., Foster, G. V., and MacIntyre, I. (1971) Human calcitonin in the treatment of Paget's bone disease. *Lancet* **1,** 1139–1143.

9

Hormonal Modifiers of Mineral Metabolism Other Than Parathyroid Hormone, Vitamin D, and Calcitonin

Robert K. Rude and Frederick R. Singer

Disorders of Mineral Metabolism, Vol. II

ISBN 0-12-135302-8

I. ADRENAL GLUCOCORTICOIDS

A. Mode of Action of Steroid Hormones

Steroid hormones are ubiquitous, affecting all tissues either directly or indirectly. Even though different classes of steroid hormones may differ in their target cells and bring about different physiologic responses, their mode of action seems similar (Baxter, 1976).

Steroid hormones in the plasma generally are bound to specific transport proteins. For example, cortisol is bound to a specific α-globulin termed the corticosteroid-binding globulin. Protein bound steroids probably serve as a reservoir while the circulating free hormones, which usually account for less than 10% of the total plasma concentration (Thompson and Lippman, 1974), represent the biologically active forms.

Steroid hormones can readily penetrate the cell membrane that appears devoid of specific receptors. Nevertheless, some hormones such as the glucocorticoids interact with plasma membranes and modify their properties. Inside the cell steroid hormones bind to specific cytoplasmic protein receptors. The formation of the steroid-cytosol receptor complex leads to a conformational change in the receptor. As a result, the complex migrates to the nucleus where it becomes bound to binding sites that are specific for the type and tissue of origin. This binding initiates transcriptional and translational events that result in the synthesis of proteins responsible for the steroid action (Gorski and Gannon, 1976).

The effects of these hormones may be either anabolic or catabolic, and target tissues are profoundly influenced by either an excess or lack of the effectors. For example, biochemical differentiation of several systems in fetal life may require glucocorticoids whereas the same steroids inhibit growth in the same tissue later in life. In addition to a role in biochemical differentiation and cell growth, induction of specific proteins in differentiated cells is a prominent physiologic and pharmacologic effect of steroid hormones (O'Malley, 1971). Another aspect of steroid function, particularly of the glucocorticoids, is their "permissive" action in allowing other nonsteroidal hormones to express their metabolic function fully (Thompson and Lippman, 1974).

B. Interaction with Bone

Glucocorticoids have a pronounced effect on bone metabolism (Storey, 1963; Gallagher *et al.*, 1973a). Cushing's syndrome and the exogenous administration of glucocorticoids are both associated with decreased bone growth in children (Follis, 1951; Blodgett *et al.*, 1956; Iannaccone *et al.*, 1960) and growing animals (Yasumura *et al.*, 1976; Sheagren *et al.*, 1977), and marked loss of bone volume in the adult (Follis, 1951; Iannaccone *et al.*, 1960; Isaksson and Lindholm, 1965). Fracture healing is also impaired during cortisone therapy (Blunt *et al.*, 1950).

The glucocorticoids inhibit cartilage growth and development *in vitro* as demonstrated by the inhibition of sulfation of cartilage and decreased accumulation of acid mucopolysaccharides (Schryver, 1965; Barrett *et al.*, 1966). In addition, an inhibition of the incorporation of radioactive amino acids into cartilage collagen has been demonstrated (Daughaday and Mariz, 1962). Studies also suggest that there is impaired synthesis of the organic matrix of bone and decreased new bone formation (Reynolds, 1966; Peck *et al.*, 1967; Oikarinen, 1977). Cortisol was found to decrease the incorporation of radioactive amino acids into collagen in bone culture (Peck *et al.*, 1967). Cortisol also decreased the incorporation of radioactive labeled nucleosides into RNA (Peck *et al.*, 1969). Evidence that the latter antianabolic effect of cortisol is dependent on protein synthesis is provided by the fact that the simultaneous administration of protein synthesis inhibitors abolished this action of cortisol (Peck *et al.*, 1969).

In addition to this antianabolic effect of glucocorticoids, a direct effect on bone cell development has been demonstrated. High-affinity glucocorticoid-binding proteins have been found in bone cells from fetal rat calvaria (Feldman *et al.*, 1975; Manolagas *et al.*, 1979). After steroid binding, the steroid-receptor complex is transferred from the cytosol and bound to the nucleus (Chen *et al.*, 1977). Glucocorticoid administration results in impaired bone cell growth, development, and maturation (Epker, 1970; Jee *et al.*, 1970; Jett *et al.*, 1970; Liskova-Kiar, 1979). Progesterone, an antagonist of glucocorticoids, partially blocked the glucocorticoid inhibition of bone cell growth (Chen *et al.*, 1977). There appears to be decreased mesenchymal cell differentiation into osteoclasts and osteoblasts. The result is a diminished number of bone cellular elements. This effect may be dose- and time-dependent. In short-term studies, high doses of cortisol (25–50 mg/kg/day) suppressed osteoprogenitor cell proliferation and bone formation. Lower doses (0.5–5.0 mg/kg/day) initially resulted in increased osteoprogenitor cell proliferation and increased numbers of osteoclasts (Jee *et al.*, 1970). With chronic glucocorticoid excess, regardless of dose, the number of bone cells was decreased (Jett *et al.*, 1970).

Measurements of skeletal dynamics in man, dog, and rabbit with Cushing's syndrome, either endogenous or exogenous, complement these findings. Bone formation is markedly suppressed as measured histologically (Jett *et al.*, 1970; Bressot *et al.*, 1976), autoradiographically (Rigg *et al.*, 1966), by tetracycline labeling (Jowsey and Riggs, 1970), or in radiocalcium kinetic studies (Bohr and Dawids, 1964). The suppression of bone formation is most apparent when bone is examined after prolonged glucocorticoid excess, thereby allowing for a new steady-state remodeling system of the basic metabolic unit of bone cells (osteon) to occur (Jett *et al.*, 1970). The degree of this suppressive effect on bone formation appears to be more severe with higher doses of glucocorticoids.

In addition to decreasing bone formation, the glucocorticoids also affect bone resorption (Storey, 1961; Riggs *et al.*, 1966; Jee *et al.*, 1970; Jett *et al.*, 1970; Bressot *et al.*, 1976). Cortisol in doses of from 0.5 to 5.0 mg/kg/day causes increased mesenchymal cell proliferation and an increased number of osteoclasts (Jee *et al.*, 1970). Bone resorption is stimulated as evidenced by accelerated removal of previously incorporated strontium 85 in the rat (Jee *et al.*, 1970), and the presence of increased resorption surfaces in bone from patients with endogenous or exogenous Cushing's syndrome (Riggs *et al.*, 1966; Jett *et al.*, 1970; Bressot *et al.*, 1976). As this effect appears to be abolished by parathyroidectomy, the elevated levels of parathyroid hormone seen following glucocorticoid administration may mediate the increase in bone resorption (Jee *et al.*, 1970). A direct stimulatory effect is also possible since glucocorticoids have been reported to enhance bone resorption by peritoneal macrophages in vitro in the rat (Teitelbaum *et al.*, 1981). Glucocorticoids have also been observed to maintain the content of cytosol receptors for $1,25(OH)_2D_3$ in bone that might enhance bone resorption (Manolagas *et al.*, 1979). Jett *et al.*, (1970) concluded after studying the effects of cortisol on Haversian bone that, although an initial "burst" of osteoclasts may occur, both resorption and accretion are decreased. These investigators felt that the increase in resorption surfaces was due to an early rise in osteoclastic activity and to subsequent failure of new bone formation in areas where previous bone resorption had occurred. They also concluded that there was an uncoupling of bone resorption and formation and that, although both parameters were impaired, bone formation was slowed more than bone resorption, thus leading to a net increase in the rate of bone loss. At higher levels of cortisol administration (25–50 mg/kg/day), bone resorption is inhibited (Yasumura, 1976). Histologically, there initially occurs a decrease in osteoprogenitor cell proliferation (Jee *et al.*, 1970). *In vitro* studies also demonstrate that glucocorticoids inhibit bone resorption induced by parathyroid hormone (Stern, 1969; Liskova-Kiar, 1979).

C. Interaction with Kidney

Glucocorticoids are required for some renal functions, such as free water clearance to proceed optimally (Kleeman *et al.*, 1975). Cortisol does not affect the acute renal handling of calcium or magnesium (Massry and Coburn, 1973). However, during prolonged glucocorticoid excess hypercalciuria and hypermagnesuria are seen whether or not plasma concentrations are normal or decreased (Clark *et al.*, 1959; Pechet *et al.*, 1959; Laake, 1960; Molinatti *et al.*, 1960; Collins *et al.*, 1962; Wajchenberg *et al.*, 1969). The chronic administration of cortisol or mineralocorticoids results in plasma volume expansion, increased renal blood flow and glomerular filtration rate, with a consequent increase in the renal excretion of sodium, calcium, and magnesium (Massry and Coburn, 1973; Kleeman *et al.*, 1975). Dietary sodium restriction in the experimental animal reverses this trend and leads to reduction in urinary calcium excretion (Suki *et al.*, 1968). In addition to chronic volume expansion, the soft tissue and skeletal breakdown seen in chronic glucocorticoid excess is also thought to contribute to the hypercalciuria (Kleeman *et al.*, 1975).

Glucocorticoids have been observed acutely to decrease urinary phosphate excretion (Persky *et al.*, 1955; Goldsmith *et al.*, 1965). During chronic glucocorticoid administration, however, urinary phosphate excretion has been found to be high (Ingbar *et al.*, 1951; Roberts and Pitts, 1953; Anderson and Foster, 1959). Both the increase in urinary phosphate excretion and an increase in urinary cyclic AMP excretion in prednisone-treated patients can be suppressed with calcium infusion (Lukert and Adams, 1976). An increase in the plasma concentration of parathyroid hormone, as described below, may therefore be responsible for the increase in renal phosphate excretion. Plasma phosphate concentration in prednisone-treated patients is not significantly different than normal (Lukert and Adams, 1976) suggesting an increased flow of skeletal phosphate into the extracellular pool.

Glucocorticoid deficiency is associated with a decrease in urinary calcium excretion in man and animals (Lamberg and Torst, 1964; Kenny, 1966). This may be related to a reduction in the renal blood flow or glomerular filtration rate (Kleeman *et al.*, 1975).

D. Interaction with Vitamin D and Intestine

The antagonistic effect glucocorticoids have on the intestinal action of vitamin D was recognized in 1960 (Harrison and Harrison, 1960). Glucocorticoids have been shown to decrease the intestinal absorption of calcium *in vivo* (Fischer and Hastrup, 1954; Fox *et al.*, 1978; Hahn *et al.*, 1979a) and the active transport of calcium *in vitro* (Kimberg *et al.*, 1971). The mechanism by which this occurs remains unclear. Studies of vitamin D metabolism in the cortisol-treated rat have led to conflicting results. The original studies concerning the effect of glucocorticoids on vitamin D metabolism demonstrated normal 25-hydroxylation of vitamin D_3 in the liver and normal renal 1α-hydroxylation of 25-hydroxyvitamin D_3 [25(OH)D_3] in the rat (Kimberg *et al.*, 1971). In subsequent studies both a decrease in renal 1,25-dihydroxyvitamin D_3 [1,25$(OH)_2D_3$] production in the rat (Edelstein and Noff, 1977) and an increase in renal 1α-hydroxylase activity in the chick (Spanos *et al.*, 1977) have been reported. Studies in man suggest that chronic glucocorticoid excess does not affect production or degradation of 1,25$(OH)_2D_3$ (Seeman *et al.*, 1980). Conversion of 1,25$(OH)_2D_3$ in the intestine of cortisol-treated rats into a more polar, biologically inactive metabolite than 1,25$(OH)_2D_3$ has also been postulated as causing the alteration in intestinal calcium transport (Miravet *et al.*, 1975).

The possibility that glucocorticoids interfere with vitamin D action at its target organ has also been investigated. Intestinal localization and nuclear binding of the vitamin D metabolites occur in cortisone-treated rats (Favus *et al.*, 1973a). The levels of intestinal 1,25$(OH)_2D_3$ were observed to be normal or reduced (Lukert *et al.*, 1973; Miravet *et al.*, 1975; Edelstein and Noff, 1977) following cortisol administration. One of the direct physiologic effects of vitamin D, the production of an intestinal calcium-binding protein, was found to be either normal (Kimberg *et al.*, 1971; Krawitt, 1972) or decreased (Edelstein and Noff, 1977) following cortisol administration in the rat. Cortisol decreased both intestinal calcium absorption and calcium-binding protein in the vitamin D-treated rachitic chick (Feher and Wasserman, 1978). It was initially observed that the administration of vitamin D or its metabolites, $25(OH)D_3$ (Favus *et al.*, 1973a) and $1,25(OH)_2D_3$ (Favus *et al.*, 1973b) to cortisol-treated rats did not return intestinal calcium absorption to normal. Similar observations were made in the rachitic chick (Feher and Wasserman, 1978). Miravet *et al.* (1975), however, found $1,25(OH)_2D_3$ returned calcium absorption to normal in cortisol-treated vitamin D-deficient rats. Glucocorticoid-mediated decrease in intestinal calcium absorption in the pig was also reversed by 1α-hydroxyvitamin D (Fox *et al.*, 1978).

Studies in man demonstrated that $25(OH)D_3$ was effective in improving calcium absorption in iatrogenic Cushing's syndrome (Caniggia and Gennari, 1973; Hahn *et al.*, 1979a). Similarly, physiologic doses of $1,25(OH)_2D_3$ and 1α-hydroxyvitamin D_3 in prednisone-treated patients resulted in enhanced intestinal calcium absorption (Klein *et al.*, 1977, Lindgren *et al.*, 1978). Evidence that cortisol may cause an end-organ resistance to vitamin D in man is the finding that the plasma concentration of $1,25(OH)_2D_3$ is normal or elevated in corticosteroid-treated patients (Hahn *et al.*, 1979b; Seeman *et al.*, 1980) and rats (Lukert *et al.*, 1973). Plasma $25(OH)D_3$ has been found to either be normal (Aloia *et al.*, 1974, Hahn *et al.*, 1977) or low (Klein *et al.*, 1977; Seeman *et al.*, 1980).

Glucocorticoids alter the absorption of other substances such as iron and galactose (Kimberg *et al.*, 1971) and phosphate (Fox *et al.*, 1981). A generalized defect in the intestinal mucosal cell may then result in nonspecific malabsorption of a number of substances including calcium.

Little work has been carried out on the effect of glucocorticoids on the metabolic action of vitamin D on bone. Cortisol was found to decrease the resorptive capacity of $25(OH)D_3$ in tissue culture (Raisz *et al.*, 1972) and vitamin D-induced ultrastructural changes in bone cells have been observed to be unaffected by cortisol (Weisbrode and Capen, 1976). Recently glucocorticoids were observed to maintain the stability of cytosol $1,25(OH)_2D_3$ receptors in bone (Manolagas *et al.*, 1979).

E. Interaction with Parathyroid Hormone

Early investigation into the effect of corticosteroids on parathyroid gland function suggested that corticosteroids decreased parathyroid hormone secretion (Eliel *et al.*, 1965). This inference found further support in studies that showed pharmacologic doses of glucocorticoids decreased parathyroid gland volume and mitotic rate in rats (Hansson, 1967). The excretion of parathyroid extract as determined by a rat bioassay system was unaltered by large doses of prednisone, indicating that glucocorticoids do not increase the degradation of parathyroid hormone (Eliel *et al.*, 1965). Glucocorticoids do have an antagonistic effect on the peripheral action of parathyroid hormone (Stoerk *et al.*, 1963; Eliel *et al.*, 1965; Raisz, 1965; Wajchenberg *et al.*, 1965; Margargal *et al.*, 1969; Gozariu *et al.*, 1971; Raisz *et al.*, 1972; Williams *et al.*, 1974). Cortisol will worsen hypocalcemia and tetany in hypoparathyroidism and lower the serum calcium concentration in hypoparathyroid patients on vitamin D or parathyroid extract (Stoerk *et al.*, 1963; Eliel *et al.*, 1965; Canas *et al.*, 1967). This effect should lead to a compensatory increase in parathyroid hormone secretion in the parathyroid-intact subject (Williams *et al.*, 1974). Glucocorticoid administration has been shown to result in elevated plasma concentrations of immunoreactive parathyroid hormone in rat and man without a simultaneous change in serum calcium concentration (Williams *et al.*, 1974; Fucik *et al.*, 1975; Kukreja *et al.*, 1976; Lukert and Adams, 1976; Hahn *et al.*, 1979a). This has been observed during both acute and chronic glucocorticoid therapy (Fucik *et al.*, 1975). The reason for the increase in plasma parathyroid hormone concentration remains unclear. Although it may be secondary to the peripheral antagonism of parathyroid hormone or vitamin D, a direct stimulation of parathyroid hormone secretion by cortisol in parathyroid gland culture has also been observed (Au, 1976).

Parathyroid hormone is capable of eliciting its physiologic effect in the adrenalectomized or cortisol-excess animal (Stoerk *et al.*, 1963; Williams *et al.*, 1974). Greater amounts of parathyroid hormone are needed to exert the same hypercalcemic effect in cortisol excess animals as compared to normal controls (Stoerk *et al.*, 1963; Margargal *et al.*, 1969). Conversely, a greater rise in the serum calcium concentration in response to parathyroid hormone is seen in adrenalectomized than in intact rats (Williams *et al.*, 1974).

F. Interaction with Calcitonin

Determinations of serum calcitonin concentration in glucocorticoid excess or deficiency states have not yet been reported. Exogenous cortisol administration appears to increase the calcitonin content of the thyroid gland in the rat (deGuiseppe and Rindi, 1969; Yasumura *et al.*, 1976). Since cortisone decreases the protein content of the thyroid gland (Yatvin *et al.*, 1966), this increase in calcitonin may be due to decreased secretion rather than increased synthesis. Decreased calcitonin secretion could result from the lowered serum calcium induced by pharmacologic doses of glucocorticoids as discussed above.

The hypocalcemic effects of exogenous porcine calcitonin in the rat is decreased by the prior administration of pharmacologic doses (50–100 mg/kg/day) of cortisol (Thompson *et al.*, 1968; Eliel *et al.*, 1971). No change was noted in its hypophosphatemic effect (Thompson *et al.*, 1974). In contrast, adrenalectomy does not alter the hypocalcemic action of calcitonin (Thompson *et al.*, 1968; Meyer and Brinkley 1972), although recovery from hypocalcemia is delayed (Lineberry and Waite, 1978). Studies in the rat indicate normal physiologic function of endogenous calcitonin in states of either cortisol excess or deficiency (Talmage *et al.*, 1970; Talmage and Kennedy, 1970). The apparent contradictory effect of cortisol on the hypocalcemic action of exogenous calcitonin cited above with endogenous calcitonin may be explained by the lower dose of cortisol given (5 mg/kg/day) in the study by Talmage *et al.* (1970).

Calcitonin has been demonstrated to prevent bone loss partially during corticosteroid therapy in the rabbit (Thompson and Urist, 1973; Eliel *et al.*, 1971; J. S. Thompson *et al.*, 1972). This suggests that calcitonin may serve to protect against the catabolic effect pharmacologic amounts of glucocorticoids have on the skeleton.

G. Glucocorticoid Excess

Pharmacologic amounts of glucocorticoids are commonly used in a variety of clinical disorders and, as described above, can result in significant clinical complications.

The inhibition of growth in children with Cushing's syndrome and those receiving glucocorticoids for disorders such as severe allergic disease, rheumatoid arthritis, and the nephrotic syndrome has been well documented (Follis, 1951; Blodgett *et al.*, 1956; Iannaccone *et al.*, 1960; Strickland *et al.*, 1972). Cortisol will diminish the rate of longitudinal growth and skeletal maturation within a few weeks of onset of therapy (Blodgett *et al.*, 1956). While pharmacologic amounts of glucocorticoids are needed to suppress growth in endocrine intact children, physiologic amounts have a growth-suppressing effect in hypopituitary patients (Blodgett *et al.*, 1956); this may indicate an antagonism of glucocorticoids to the action of growth hormone. Studies in rats have demonstrated that the suppression of linear growth by corticosteroids or adrenocorticotropic hormone (ACTH) can be overcome by administration of growth hormone (Becks *et al.*, 1944; Selye, 1952; Soyka and Crawford, 1965). Greater amounts of growth hormone were needed to offset the growth-suppressing effect of higher doses of glucocorticoids; this suggests a dose-related effect. Similarly, the optimum growth hormone effect in hypopituitary patients can be blunted with physiologic doses of cortisol (Soyka and Crawford, 1965). Prolonged administration of human growth hormone did not result in any improvement in growth rate, or retention of nitrogen, potassium, or phosphate in eight corticosteroid-treated children studied by Morris *et al.* (1968b). Others (Matiasevic and Gershberg, 1966) have reported some improvement in growth in similar patients while a positive nitrogen balance was obtained in a child with Cushing's syndrome after the administration of human growth hormone (Bergenstal and Lipsett, 1960).

Abnormal growth hormone secretion has also been proposed as a factor in the diminished growth rate in Cushing's syndrome. A diminished or absent response of growth hormone secretion to insulin-induced hypoglycemia has been reported in Cushing's syndrome secondary to a hypothalamic–pituitary disorder or adrenal tumors (Frantz and Rabkin, 1964; Hartog *et al.*, 1964; Krieger and Glick, 1972). Patients and normal volunteers receiving long-term corticosteroid administration for nonendocrine diseases also show similar abnormalities in growth hormone dynamics (Frantz and Rubkin, 1964; von Werder *et al.*, 1971; R. G. Thompson *et al.*, 1972). When glucocorticoid status was restored to normal in volunteers in patients with high dose exogenous glucocorticoids and in those whose Cushing's syndrome was secondary to adrenal tumors, growth hormone response to insulin-induced hypoglycemia returned to normal. Those patients with bilateral adreno-cortical hyperplasia continued to lack normal growth hormone responsiveness following therapy (Krieger and Blick, 1972). This suggests a central abnormality is present in these patients. In contrast, studies of steroid-treated children have shown growth hormone dynamics to be normal (Root *et al.*, 1967; Morris *et al.*, 1968a; Strickland *et al.*, 1972).

In the adult, the disturbance in mineral metabolism most frequently manifests itself as osteoporosis. Cushing's syndrome is not infrequently associated with an increased incidence of fractures, particularly of the vertebrae (Demartini *et al.*, 1952; Curtiss *et al.*, 1954; McAllen, 1970). Findings of decreased total body calcium and phosphorus in Cushing's syndrome (Aloia *et al.*, 1974) complement the histologic picture described above and explain the propensity toward fractures encountered in these patients.

Patients with disorders such as rheumatoid arthritis, asthma, nephrosis, and systemic lupus erythematosis frequently are treated with pharmacologic amounts of glucocorticoids for prolonged periods of time (Demartini *et al.*, 1952; Soffer and Bader, 1952; Curtiss *et al.*, 1954; Klein *et al.*, 1965; McAllen, 1970). Although these patients appear to exhibit a greater than normal incidence of osteoporosis and fractures, the incidence of osteoporosis in patients treated with glucocorticoids does not seem to differ from that in patients who did not receive steroid therapy (McConkey *et al.*, 1962; Saville and Kharmosh, 1967). One study (Saville and Kharmosh, 1967) did report increased osteoporosis in female patients over the age of 50 who received glucocorticoids, but not in younger females or males. Thus it appears that age, sex, and underlying disease contribute to the development of osteoporosis. Although photon absorptiometry demonstrated bone loss during prednisone therapy over a 12-week period (Deding *et al.*, 1977), in another study in which five patients were treated with glucocorticoids *in vivo,* neutron activation analysis revealed no evidence of bone loss over a 20- to 33-month treatment period (Hosking and Chamberlain, 1973). It was suggested that when immobilization is not prominent in the disease, osteoporosis is a less common feature.

H. Glucocorticoid Insufficiency

Glucocorticoid insufficiency is quite uncommon and if untreated will rapidly lead to the demise of the patient. Little information is therefore available concerning the effects of chronic glucocorticoid deficiency on mineral metabolism. In 1911 adrenalectomy was first shown to ameliorate tetany in parathyroidectomized animals (Guleke, 1911). Hypercalcemia following adrenalectomy has been demonstrated in rabbits (Kisch, 1924), cats (Taylor and Caven, 1927), dogs (Rogoff and Stewart, 1928; Myers and Lawrence, 1958), and rats (Raman, 1970a). Hypercalcemia has also been observed in patients with Cushing's syndrome and in Addison's disease after adrenalectomy (Loeb, 1932; Leeksma *et al.*, 1957; Walser *et al.*, 1963; Jorgenson, 1973).

The cause of the hypercalcemia in adrenal insufficiency is unclear. Actual elevation of serum ionized calcium has not been documented in man. Walser *et al.* (1963) were also unable to show an elevation in the plasma free calcium ion concentration in adrenalectomized dogs. Raman (1970a) did find elevated plasma ionized calcium levels in adrenalectomized rats, although others (Walser *et al.*, 1963) were unable to demonstrate any change in plasma ionized calcium concentration in this animal. Several mechanisms probably contribute to the development of hypercalcemia. Sodium and water loss lead to hemoconcentration with subsequent elevated plasma proteins and elevated total serum calcium concentration (Walser *et al.*, 1963; Raman, 1970a). When the ionic strength of plasma is decreased, there is a greater affinity of plasma proteins for calcium (Walser *et al.*, 1963). Hyponatremia may therefore result in an increase in the total plasma calcium concentration. Increased amounts of filterable and nonfilterable complexes of calcium with phosphate and citrate have also been found (Walser *et al.*, 1963). It seems unlikely that the parathyroid gland plays a role because of the occurrence of hypercalcemia in parathyroidectomized, adrenalectomized dogs (Myers and Lawrence, 1961). Increased intestinal absorption of calcium has not been shown to be a significant factor in the hypercalcemia of adrenal insufficiency (Rubin and Krick, 1936; Tibbets and Aub, 1937; Walser *et al.*, 1963). The possibility of an increased flux of calcium out of bone into the extracellular fluid remains (Myers and Lawrence, 1961; Schartum and Nichols, 1961; Canas *et al.*, 1967). *In vitro* studies have demonstrated that physiological concentrations of glucocorticoids decrease osteoclast activity without altering function and suggest that during adrenal insufficiency an increase in osteoclast activity may be responsible for the hypercalcemia seen in this disorder (Wong, 1979).

I. Summary

The effect of glucocorticoid excess on mineral metabolism is manifest primarily by its influence on the skeleton. These steroid hormones inhibit both cartilage and bone growth and development. In addition, loss of bone volume in the adult is seen. Bone formation is decreased by impaired organic matrix synthesis and also a decrease in mesenchymal cell differentiation into mature bone cells. Increased bone resorption and/or uncoupling of bone turnover with resorption exceeding formation may also be observed during glucocorticoid therapy.

The enhanced skeletal resorption appears to be secondary to an increase in parathyroid hormone secretion. During glucocorticoid therapy or in Cushing's syndrome a negative calcium balance is incurred. A decrease in intestinal calcium absorption may be secondary to alteration in vitamin D metabolism, impairment of the effect of vitamin D or its metabolites on the gut, or a nonspecific effect of glucocorticoid excess on intestinal absorption. In addition, hypercalciuria is seen and together with the increased fecal calcium excretion, is associated with an increased parathyroid hormone secretion.

Glucocorticoid insufficiency can result in hypercalcemia. This may be secondary to increased affinity of plasma protein for calcium, increased complexes of calcium with phosphate and citrate, plasma volume contraction, and an actual increase in ionized calcium.

II. GONADAL STEROIDS

A. Mode of Action

The mode of action of the gonadal steroids is similar to that of the glucocorticoids. They provide an example of a steroid hormone-mediated growth response. The first physiologic effects of these hormones are on the development of secondary sex tissues during embryogenesis. The effect of such hormones on secondary sex tissue in the adult is also well appreciated.

Although the skeleton, intestine, and kidney are not primary sites of action for the gonadal steroids, the interaction of sex hormones with these tissues has been under investigation because of the profound alterations in mineral metabolism in states of sex steroid deficiency. The mechanisms by which the gonadal steroids influence mineral metabolism is yet unclear. These effects will be discussed in the subsequent sections.

B. Interaction with Bone

The effect of the sex steroids on bone metabolism has been under intense investigation ever since the hypothesis was put forth that senile osteoporosis was related to the menopause (Albright *et al.*, 1941). Following natural or artificial menopause, radiographic morphometry (Nordin *et al.*, 1966; Meema and Meema, 1968; Nordin, 1971; Horsman *et al.*, 1977; Recker *et al.*, 1977), photodensitometry (Meema *et al.*, 1965; Aitken *et al.*, 1973a; Recker *et al.*, 1977), photon absorption (Davis *et al.*, 1966; Aitken *et al.*, 1972; Riggs *et al.*, 1981; Recker *et al.*, 1977; Lindsay *et al.*, 1978a), and total body neutron activation analysis (Aloia *et al.*, 1977; Chestnut *et al.*, 1977) techniques have demonstrated an accelerated loss of bone and/or a decrease in bone mass. Estrogen and/or androgen therapy in these patients results in a slowing or cessation of this loss of bone (Davis *et al.*, 1966; Aitken *et al.*, 1973b; Meema *et al.*, 1975; Chestnut *et al.*, 1977; Recker *et al.*, 1977; Lindsay *et al.*, 1978a, 1980; Christiansen *et al.*, 1980). Similar changes were also seen following progestogen therapy alone (Lindsay *et al.*, 1978a). An actual increase in bone mass was seen following estrogen therapy when the treatment was started within 3 years of the onset of the menopause (Aitken *et al.*, 1973b). It is during this period that the greatest loss of skeletal mass is seen (Davis *et al.*, 1966; Aitken *et al.*, 1973a; Horsman *et al.*, 1977). Withdrawal of estrogen therapy in ovariectomized (Lindsay *et al.*, 1978b) or postmenopausal (Horsman *et al.*, 1979) patients resulted in an accelerated loss of bone mineral comparable to that seen in patients who did not receive estrogen therapy. Christiansen *et al.* (1981), however, found that the rate of bone loss in postmenopausal women after discontinuation of estrogen/gestagen treatment was similar to an untreated control group.

Albright *et al.* (1941) originally noted that following the menopause there occurred a decrease in bone mass with a subsequent increase in fracture rate. He hypothesized that sex hormones were needed for optimal osteoblastic function and bone matrix synthesis. An estrogen-induced increase in the organic and mineral component of medullary bone in birds supports the concept that estrogens have an anabolic effect on bone (Turner and Schraer, 1977). Sex steroids also have been shown to have an effect on collagen metabolism. Estrogen has been demonstrated to inhibit collagen breakdown in rat uterus (Woessner, 1969), while both estrogen and testosterone were shown to have anabolic actions on bone collagen in the rat (Kowalewski *et al.*, 1971). A change in the lysine and hydroxylysine content of the insoluble bone collagen from rats treated with estrogens has been reported (Igarashi *et al.*, 1976). Studies demonstrating an improved calcium balance along with a decreased incidence of fractures and loss of height in postmenopausal women treated with estrogen convincingly demonstrated a role of estrogens in the maintenance of a normal skeleton (Wallach and Henneman, 1959; Hernberg, 1960; Gordan *et al.*, 1973; Lindsay *et al.*, 1980; Weiss *et al.*, 1980). However, the hypothesis of a decreased synthesis of bone matrix as the primary abnormality in postmenopausal osteoporosis is controversial. In 1958, radiocalcium kinetic studies demonstrated normal bone formation in patients with osteoporosis (Heaney and Whedon, 1958). This has been confirmed by others (Nordin, 1959; Lafferty *et al.*, 1964; Melick, 1966). Bronner *et al.* (1963), using similar techniques, however, demonstrated lower bone turnover in women with postmenopausal osteoporosis as compared to patients without osteoporosis. Skeletal accretion rates utilizing stable strontium have shown either normal (Fraser *et al.*, 1960; Lafferty *et al.* 1964) or low values (Eisenberg and Gordan, 1961). Estrogen or androgen therapy in these patients resulted in a further lowering of bone accretion rates after prolonged treatment (Gordan and Eisenberg, 1963; Lafferty *et al.*, 1964). Tetracycline-labeling studies have usually shown low bone formation rates in postmenopausal and senile osteoporosis (Villanueva *et al.*, 1966; Wu and Frost, 1969). Increased bone resorption was demonstrated by the kinetic studies of Gordan and Eisenberg (1963), Lafferty *et al.* (1964), and Joly *et al.* (1980) in postmenopausal women with osteoporosis which was decreased with androgen or estrogen therapy. Subsequent calcium-kinetic studies have confirmed an increase in skeletal resorption in postmenopausal women as compared to perimenopausal or estrogen-treated postmenopausal women (Heaney *et al.*, 1978b). Quantitative morphologic analyses of bone have also demonstrated an increase in bone resorption in sex steroid deficiency states (Bordier *et al.*, 1965; Jowsey *et al.*, 1965; Wu *et al.*, 1967; Brown *et al.*, 1974; Bressot *et al.*, 1976; Joly *et al.*, 1980); however, no difference was noted in age-matched patients with and without osteoporosis (Meunier *et al.*, 1973). Estrogen has been shown to retard this process (Riggs *et al.*, 1969).

The mechanism by which the sex steroids slow bone loss during estrogen deficiency is uncertain. While estrogens appear to have no local effect on bone cells (Nutik and Cruess, 1974; Atkins and Peacock, 1975), concentrations of these steroids two- to tenfold greater than the concentrations that inhibit parathyroid hormone-stimulated calcium release, from bone, cause a net accretion of calcium *in vitro* (Stern, 1969; Atkins and Peacock, 1975). The most probable mechanism is the antagonistic effect of estrogens on the action of parathyroid hormone on bone as discussed below. The decrease in urinary excretion of hydroxyproline with sex steroid therapy would support this contention (Young *et al.*, 1968; Riggs *et al.*, 1969; Gallagher and Nordin, 1972; Lindsay *et al.*, 1976, 1978a). Estrogens also antagonize the peripheral effects of growth hormone as determined by the fall in urinary calcium and hydroxyproline when administered to patients with acromegaly (Schwartz *et al.*, 1969a) or to patients receiving growth hormone therapy (Schwartz *et al.*, 1969b).

There may be other, as yet unidentified, direct effects of estrogen on bone, as suggested by the observation that estrogens may induce tetany in idiopathic hypoparathyroidism (Burckhardt *et al.*, 1975). Hypercalcemia has also been reported to occur following estrogen withdrawal in vitamin D-treated hypoparathyroidism (Verbeelen and Fuss, 1979).

C. Interaction with Kidney

Patients with postmenopausal or senile osteoporosis excrete normal amounts of calcium in the urine, but the fact that they are in negative calcium balance

(Henneman and Wallach, 1957) suggests that there may be an inappropriate urinary loss of calcium. As discussed below there is an improved calcium balance following estrogen or androgen therapy, brought about largely by a decrease in urinary calcium output.

The effect of testosterone and estrogen in decreasing urinary calcium excretion in postmenopausal osteoporosis was noted originally by Reifenstein and Albright (1947). A number of subsequent studies have confirmed their observations (Shorr, 1945; Bogdonoff *et al.*, 1954; Henneman and Wallach, 1957; Young *et al.*, 1968; Gallagher *et al.*, 1973b; Heaney *et al.*, 1978a). Young and Nordin (1967) observed a rise in urinary calcium following natural or artificial menopause. They showed that estrogen administration caused a lowering of urinary calcium excretion to levels similar to those of the premenopausal state (Young *et al.*, 1968). A recent study demonstrated a significant inverse relationship of urinary calcium to endogenous estradiol production in oophorectomized women (Lindsay *et al.*, 1977).

The principal mechanism by which the sex steroids decrease urinary calcium excretion is thought to be secondary to decreased bone resorption. This results in a lowered serum calcium concentration and a reduced filtered load of calcium (Young *et al.*, 1968; Riggs *et al.*, 1969; Aitken *et al.*, 1971; Gallagher *et al.*, 1973b). This does not exclude a concomitant effect of these hormones on the kidney. Evidence for estrogen receptors in the kidney has been reported (Christy and Shaver, 1974). The administration of estrogens does not result in any significant change in renal blood flow or glomerular filtration rate (Christy and Shaver, 1974; Katz and Lindheimer, 1977), despite a significant decrease in urinary calcium excretion. It does appear that estrogens play a direct role in increasing sodium and water reabsorption (Christy and Shaver, 1974). Since there is a close relationship between sodium and calcium clearance (Massry *et al.*, 1973), estrogens may have a direct effect on renal tubular calcium transport via their action on sodium reabsorption in the proximal tubule.

Estrogen also affects phosphate metabolism. Elevated serum phosphate levels are frequently seen in estrogen-deficient states (Young and Nordin, 1967; Lindsay *et al.*, 1977) and can be lowered with estrogen therapy (Young *et al.*, 1968; Aitken *et al.*, 1971). Increased urinary phosphate excretion in patients with postmenopausal osteoporosis (Young and Nordin, 1967) is found to decrease with estrogen therapy (Bogdonoff *et al.*, 1954; Young *et al.*, 1968). In one of these studies no change in the phosphate excretion index was noted (Young *et al.*, 1968), whereas in another study urinary phosphate excretion increased following estrogen therapy and was accompanied by an elevated index of phosphate excretion (Aitken *et al.*, 1971). The divergent results can be explained by an influence of calcium on the renal handling of phosphate (Lavender and Pullman, 1963), since dietary calcium in these studies was either not monitored (Aitken *et al.*, 1971) or varied widely (Young *et al.*, 1968). The maximal renal tubular reabsorption of phosphate was found to be elevated in estrogen deficiency (Lindsay *et al.*, 1977) and in another study in postmenopausal patients, stilbesterol lowered the renal tubular maximum for phosphate (Nassim *et al.*, 1956). Increased levels of urinary cyclic AMP have been found in oophorectomized women receiving mestronal (Lindsay *et al.*, 1976). These observations support the concept that changes in urinary phosphate excretion are secondary to changes in parathyroid hormone secretion.

D. Interaction with Intestine

Intestinal calcium absorption has usually been found to be low in patients with postmenopausal or senile osteoporosis (Bronner *et al.*, 1963; Caniggia *et al.*, 1963; Jaworski *et al.*, 1963; Munck, 1964; Spencer *et al.*, 1964; Avioli *et al.*, 1965; Parsons *et al.*, 1968; Gallagher *et al.*, 1973b, 1979) but not significantly different than in age- and sex-matched normal individuals (Avioli *et al.*, 1965; Bullamore *et al.*, 1970; Gallagher *et al.*, 1973b; Ireland and Fordtran, 1973). This abnormality may represent merely an effect of aging. Additional evidence that malabsorption of calcium may be present in many elderly individuals is the observation that a calcium intake as high as 1.5 gm may be required to produce a positive calcium balance (Heaney *et al.*, 1974, 1978a). This is approximately twice the usual dietary calcium intake in this population.

Although there has been no evidence to indicate that estrogens or androgens have a direct effect on intestinal calcium transport, these steroids do appear to affect calcium balance. Estrogens and androgens have been observed to improve calcium balance in patients with postmenopausal or senile osteoporosis (Reifenstein and Albright, 1947; Anderson, 1950; Bogdonoff *et al.*, 1954; Henneman and Wallach, 1957; Young *et al.*, 1968; Caniggia and Gennari, 1972; Gallagher *et al.*, 1973a; Heaney *et al.*, 1978b). It has been demonstrated in sheep that estrogens increase the efficiency of absorption of dietary calcium (Braithwaite *et al.*, 1972). Similarly, the intestinal absorption of radioactive calcium and stable calcium has been shown to improve following the administration of sex steroids to patients with postmenopausal osteoporosis (Jaworski *et al.*, 1963; Caniggia and Gennari, 1972; Gallagher *et al.*, 1980). In other studies, however, little effect on these parameters were noted despite achievement of a positive calcium balance (Gallagher *et al.*, 1973b; Spencer *et al.*, 1976; Recker *et al.*, 1977). Finally, twice-elevated values for intestinal calcium absorption have been found in pregnancy (Heaney and Skillman, 1971). Although estrogens may be responsible, in part, for this observation, placental lactogen has also been implicated (Heaney and Skillman, 1971). As discussed in a later section, prolactin is also capable of increasing intestinal calcium absorption.

Impaired intestinal absorption of phosphate has also been reported in postmenopausal women (Caniggia and Gennari, 1972). Estrogen therapy was observed to improve intestinal phosphate absorption (Young *et al.*, 1968; Caniggia and Gennari, 1972), and phosphate balance (Bogdonoff *et al.*, 1954). If, as discussed below, estrogens can increase the synthesis of $1,25(OH)_2D_3$, the expected end result would be enhanced absorption of both calcium and phosphate.

E. Interaction with Parathyroid Hormone

Parathyroid hormone has been shown to be required for the development of immobilization osteoporosis (Burkhart and Jowsey, 1967) and calcium-deficient osteoporosis (Jowsey and Raisz, 1968). Because of the striking preponderance of osteoporosis in the postmenopausal or estrogen-deficient female (Meema *et al.*, 1965; Davis *et al.*, 1966; Nordin *et al.*, 1966), the interaction of sex steroids with parathyroid hormone has received considerable attention. The concentration of serum immunoreactive parathyroid hormone in estrogen-deficient patients has usually been found to be normal or low (Gallagher *et al.*, 1973b; Riggs *et al.*, 1973; Brown *et al.*, 1974; Teitelbaum *et al.*, 1976; Aloia *et al.*, 1977; Davies *et al.*, 1977; Joly *et al.*, 1980) although a number of patients with postmenopausal osteoporosis have been found to have elevated levels of serum parathyroid hormone (Riggs *et al.*, 1973; Berlyne *et al.*, 1974; Teitelbaum *et al.*, 1976; Joly *et al.*, 1980). These divergent results may reflect assay specificity, variable renal function, early primary hyperparathyroidism, or a subpopulation of these patients. The finding of increased resorption lacunae in postmenopausal and hypogonadal patients with osteoporosis (Bordier *et al.*, 1965; Jowsey, 1966; Brown *et al.*, 1974; Bressot *et al.*, 1976; Joly *et al.*, 1980) does suggest increased parathyroid hormone activity.

There is experimental evidence that the sex steroids may modulate the peripheral effects of parathyroid hormone. *In vivo* studies have shown an increased sensitivity of bone to parathyroid hormone in ovariectomized rats (Orimo *et al.*, 1972). In two *in vitro* bone culture systems, estrogens were found to decrease the bone resorptive response to parathyroid hormone (Stern, 1969; Atkins *et al.*, 1972). However, in a third study no effect of 17β-estradiol on parathyroid hormone resorption was demonstrated (Caputo *et al.*, 1976). Estrogens have been shown to interfere with the metabolic effects of parathyroid hormone on bone cells as manifested by both reduced glycolysis and accumulation of citric acid (Atkins *et al.*, 1972); this may explain the antagonism to the skeletal effect of parathyroid hormone. Liskova (1976) observed that ethinyl estradiol decreased calcium release from parathyroid hormone-treated bone as well as control bone and concluded the inhibitory action was caused by a toxic effect on bone cells. Progesterone, testosterone, and androstenedione have also been observed to inhibit the resorptive action of parathyroid hormone in bone culture (Atkins and Peacock, 1975; Peacock *et al.*, 1977).

Further evidence that estrogens might antagonize the peripheral effects of parathyroid hormone is derived from clinical studies. Greater bone loss has been found in postmenopausal women with primary hyperparathyroidism as compared to premenopausal primary hyperparathyroid patients (Hossain *et al.*, 1970). Ethinyl estradiol was found to decrease bone resorption and urinary hydroxyproline excretion in postmenopausal women with primary hyperparathyroidism (Gallagher and Wilkinson, 1973). Estrogen therapy in ovariectomized patients resulted in a fall in the serum calcium and a rise in the serum parathyroid hormone concentration (Riggs *et al.*, 1972a; Gallagher *et al.*, 1980). This effect of estrogens on the serum calcium concentration has been applied successfully in the treatment of postmenopausal women with primary hyperparathyroidism (Gallagher and Wilkinson, 1973) and patients with parathyroid carcinoma (Goepfert *et al.*, 1966; Sigurdsson *et al.*, 1973b). Testosterone also has been found to be effective in lowering the serum calcium concentration in primary hyperparathyroidism due to parathyroid carcinoma or adenoma (Landau and Kappas, 1965).

F. Interaction with Calcitonin

The observation that the rise in the serum calcium concentration following an oral calcium load was greater in female than in male rats suggests that either there is a sex difference in calcitonin secretion or in its peripheral action (Sorenson and Hindberg, 1971; Peng and Garner, 1980). Thyroidectomy has been shown to result in a rise in the serum calcium concentration in the female rat, which was prevented by prior oophorectomy (Foster *et al.*, 1977). These results suggest that estrogens antagonize the effect of calcitonin. Estrogens have been shown to antagonize the hypocalcemic effects of exogenously administered calcitonin in the rabbit (Currie and Black, 1972) and rat (Shai and Wallach, 1972). Androgens have been observed to enhance the hypocalcemic response to calcitonin in the rat (Hinde and Phillippo, 1968; Ogata *et al.*, 1970; Sorenson and Hindberg, 1971); however, in one study this was only true in castrated rats (Sorenson and Hindberg, 1971). In addition, a lack of endogenous androgen decreased calcitonin's hypocalcemic action (Ogata *et al.*, 1970; Hollo *et al.*, 1971). The effects of both androgens and estrogens on the hypocalcemic effects of calcitonin are thought to reflect an effect on bone.

Comparison of basal serum calcitonin concentrations in men and women has yielded conflicting results. Delorme *et al.* (1976) reported higher values in women than in men whereas others found opposite results (Heath and Sizemore, 1977; Hillyard *et al.*, 1978). Other studies found no sex differences in basal serum calcitonin concentration (Parthemore and Deftos, 1978; Deftos *et al.*, 1980). In the study of DeLorme *et al.* (1976), estrogen-deficient women had serum calcitonin levels that were similar to males, and estrogen therapy in these women returned the serum calcitonin concentration to the normal range for estrogen-sufficient women. In addition, there was a significantly greater rise in the serum calcitonin concentration to calcium stimulus in the estrogen-replete women than in estrogen-deficient women. The ability of estrogen to increase the basal and calcium-stimulated serum calcitonin concentration has been confirmed by others (Hillyard *et al.*, 1978; Morimoto *et al.*, 1980; Stevenson *et al.*, 1980). Heath and Sizemore (1977) and Deftos *et al.* (1980) noted a greater rise in plasma calcitonin in response to both calcium and/or pentagastrin infusion in men as compared to premenopausal women, while Parthemore and Deftos (1978) found this sex difference only with pentagastrin. The reason for the differences between these studies is unclear.

G. Interaction with Vitamin D

Patients with postmenopausal osteoporosis have decreased intestinal calcium absorption and frequently a negative calcium balance. Since vitamin D plays an important role in intestinal calcium transport, an interaction of sex steroids with vitamin D has been sought. Low serum concentrations of $1{,}25(OH)_2D$ in osteoporotic patients and elderly subjects (Gallagher *et al.*, 1979) along with a decreased conversion of $25(OH)D_3$ to $1{,}25(OH)D_3$ in aging rats (Armbrecht *et al.*, 1980) suggest impaired metabolism of vitamin D may contribute to the decrease in intestinal calcium absorption. One study however reported appropriate formation of $25(OH)D_3$ and $1{,}25(OH)D_3$ from isotopically labeled cholecalciferol in osteoporotic women (Davies *et al.*, 1977). Vitamin D_3 has been found to increase calcium absorption in postmenopausal women, but only with doses over 20,000 units per day (Hall *et al.*, 1969; Gallagher *et al.*, 1973b). The effects of physiologic doses of $1{,}25(OH)D_3$ have been found to be normal in patients with postmenopausal osteoporosis (Davies *et al.*, 1977; Gallagher *et al.*, 1979). The concentration of plasma $25(OH)D_3$ in estrogen-deficient postmenopausal patients with osteoporosis is not different from that in age-matched normal individuals (Lund *et al.*, 1975; Gallagher *et al.*, 1979; Davies *et al.*, 1977). In one study the level of $1{,}25(OH)_2D_3$ was found to be significantly below normal in such patients (Gallagher *et al.*, 1976); however, in a similar study this finding was not confirmed (Haussler and McCain, 1978). Estrogen administration to postmenopausal women has been found to cause a rise in the plasma concentration of $1{,}25(OH)_2D_3$ with a simultaneous increase in intestinal calcium absorption (Gallagher *et al.*, 1980). The increased $1{,}25(OH)_2D_3$ levels could be secondary to the simultaneous increase in serum parathyroid hormone concentration (Gallagher *et al.*, 1980), or to a direct effect of estrogen itself on vitamin D metabolism. Kenny (1976) observed an increased synthesis of $1{,}25(OH)_2D_3$ in the Japanese quail during ovulation and later demonstrated that the *in vivo* administration of estrogen enhanced the *in vitro* synthesis of $1{,}25(OH)_2D_3$ by kidney homogenates (Baksi and Kenny, 1977). This finding confirmed similar observations by Tanaka *et al.* (1976) in the Japanese quail and in the chick.

Estrogen in these studies was found to increase $1,25(OH)_2D_3$ formation while decreasing the synthesis of 24,25-dihydroxyvitamin D_3 [$24,25(OH)_2D_3$]. Estradiol has also been observed to stimulate *in vivo* production of $1,25(OH)_2D_3$ in the rat (Baksi and Kenny, 1978). Recent preliminary studies have shown that estradiol added to a chick kidney cell culture (Henry, 1978) decreases $1,25(OH)_2D_3$ production. This suggests that the *in vivo* effects of estrogens on $1,25(OH)_2D_3$ production are indirect. Progesterone has also been found to increase $1,25(OH)_2D_3$ production in the Japanese quail, but was less effective than estrogen (Baksi and Kenny, 1977). Testosterone itself does not cause a similar increase in $1,25(OH)_2D_3$ formation, but may be required to show the estrogen-enhanced increase of $1,25(OH)_2D_3$ synthesis in chicks (Tanaka *et al.*, 1976, 1978; Pike *et al.*, 1978). In the immature quail testosterone was not required to demonstrate an estrogen effect (Baksi and Kenny, 1977).

Testosterone has been found to augment the increased plasma levels of $25(OH)D_3$ in male and female rats during ultraviolet irradiation (Ohata *et al.*, 1977). Estrogens had no effect and neither testosterone nor estrogen increased $25(OH)D_3$ levels without irradiation.

H. Summary

The influence of gonadal steroids on mineral metabolism is most obvious during sex steroid deficiency states. A characteristic example is in the postmenopausal woman where one observes an accelerated decrease in bone mass along with a slight elevation of the serum calcium concentration and increased urinary calcium and hydroxyproline excretion. Although decreased skeletal matrix formation may contribute to the decrease in skeletal mass, enhanced mineral resorption appears to be a major factor in the subsequent loss of bone. Since estrogen antagonizes the effects of parathyroid hormone on bone, the relative estrogen deficiency in the postmenopausal women probably leads to an increased skeletal sensitivity to parathyroid hormone and increased skeletal resorption. Estrogen administration can also increase intestinal calcium absorption in the postmenopausal woman. This effect may be mediated through an increased formation of $1,25(OH)_2D_3$. The improvement in calcium absorption would decrease parathyroid hormone secretion and therefore decrease skeletal resorption.

III. THYROID HORMONE

A. Mode of Action

The molecular basis for thyroid hormone action is in considerable dispute. A large body of evidence has been gathered in support of the concept that hormonal action initiates at the nuclear level (Oppenheimer *et al.*, 1976). This is based upon demonstration of specific high affinity binding sites in nuclei for triiodothyronine, the correlation of the number of nuclear sites in various tissues with the known effects of thyroid hormone on these tissues, the correlation between the relative biological potency of thyroid hormone analogs and the affinity of nuclear binding, and the limited number of nuclear sites that could modulate hormone response. As yet there is no convincing evidence that a specific cytosol-binding protein transports the hormone to the nucleus in a manner analogous to those of steroid hormones.

Other mechanisms of thyroid hormone action that have been proposed include activation of mitochondria, enhanced sensitivity of adrenergic receptors, and stimulation of Na,K-ATPase. It is conceivable that one or more of these mechanisms might be a secondary phenomenon to that of nuclear transcription.

B. Interaction with Bone

The effects of thyroid hormone on bone have been extensively documented since the first description of bone disease in a patient with hyperthyroidism by von Recklinghausen (1891). In this initial report and subsequent studies histologic examination of bone in hyperthyroidism has consistently revealed evidence of increased bone resorption mediated by osteoclasts, particularly in cortical bone (Hunter, 1930; Askanazy and Rutishauser, 1933; Follis, 1953; Adams *et al.*, 1967; Bordier *et al.*, 1967; Meunier *et al.*, 1972; Bressot *et al.*, 1976; Mosekilde *et al.*, 1977b). An increase in fibrovascular bone marrow is also a feature of hyperthyroid bone disease. The presence of increased osteoclastic bone resorption and fibrous bone marrow are characteristic of the lesions of osteitis fibrosa in patients with hyperparathyroidism. However, there are morphological differences which allow separation of the two disorders. In hyperthyroidism, osteoclastic activity on cortical bone surfaces is greater than on trabecular bone surfaces (Meunier *et al.*, 1972; Mosekilde *et al.*, 1977a), whereas in hyperparathyroidism trabecular osteoclastic activity is much greater. Another feature that aids in distinguishing the two osteopathies is the size of the periosteocytic lacunae, an index of osteocytic osteolysis. In primary hyperparathyroidism the lacunae are increased in size, whereas in hyperthyroidism they are normal (Meunier *et al.*, 1972; Mosekilde *et al.*, 1977b).

Numerous foci of osteoblasts are often found near sites of osteoclastic activity. Because Follis (1953) noted osteoid seams in six patients, he felt that osteomalacia was a complication of thyrotoxicosis. Quantitative morphometry of bone from thyrotoxic patients has now clearly shown that this is not so (Bordier *et al.*, 1967; Bressot *et al.*, 1976; Mosekilde *et al.*, 1977b). Although there is an increased percentage of bone surface covered by osteoid, the osteoid thickness is not increased and the total volume of osteoid is normal or only slightly increased.

Studies of tetracycline labeling of bone indicate that the calcification rate of bone is increased (Bressot *et al.*, 1976; Mosekilde *et al.*, 1977b).

Even though bone resorption and bone formation have been shown by histologic means to have increased in hyperthyroidism, the degree of bone resorption appears to predominate in most patients. This is reflected by a decrease in both cortical and trabecular bone (Meunier *et al.*, 1972; Bressot *et al.*, 1976; Mosekilde *et al.*, 1977b).

Surgical treatment of hyperthyroidism (Meunier *et al.*, 1972) and antithyroid medication (Mosekilde and Melsen, 1978) have both led to an increase in bone mass.

The histologic abnormalities in hyperthyroidism are reflected by the radiologic features of the disorder. Most commonly there is evidence of decreased bone mass as manifested by increased radiolucency of the vertebral bodies, patchy demineralization of the cranial bones and a "flaky" appearance of the cortices in the phalanges, pelvis, and long bones (Meunier *et al.*, 1972). In general, the radiologic manifestations of osteoporosis in thyrotoxicosis are difficult to distinguish from those of osteoporosis of other causes. The occurrence of pseudofractures is extremely rare in hyperthyroidism (Meunier *et al.*, 1972); only two instances have been reported. Another uncommon finding specific to the hyperthyroidism of Grave's disease is the presence of periosteal overgrowth of the hands and feet (Gimlette, 1960; Kinsella and Back, 1968). This has been termed thyroid achropachy. Clubbing of the fingers and toes may be prominent in some patients. The pathogenesis of this interesting manifestation of Grave's disease is unknown, but is always associated with exophthalmos and usually with pretibial myxedema. It does not appear to arise from the increased secretion of thyroid hormones, since it typically occurs after treatment of the disease or after spontaneous remission.

Biochemical evidence of increased bone turnover in hyperthyroidism was first reported by Krane and colleagues (1956). After injection of radiocalcium they found that the specific activity of the labeled calcium in serum and urine declined more rapidly in patients with hyperthyroidism than in normal subjects. In addition there was an increased exchangeable pool of calcium and rates of calcium resorption from and deposition in bone were increased. These observations were confirmed in human (Bordier *et al.*, 1967) and animal studies (Aubert *et al.*, 1964).

Further evidence of increased bone resorption is provided by studies of urinary and serum hydroxyproline levels (Dull and Henneman, 1963; Kivirikko *et al.*, 1965; Mosekilde *et al.*, 1978). This amino acid, which is almost unique to collagen, has been an excellent marker of bone matrix resorption in a variety of bone diseases. Excretion of this amino acid is often increased in hyperthyroidism and, since serum levels have been found to be increased, a direct effect of thyroid hormone on renal excretion of hydroxyproline cannot account for the hydroxyprolinuria (Kivirikko *et al.*, 1965). Because increased turnover of skin collagen could also contribute to the amount of hydroxyproline excreted, Askenasi and Demeester-Mirkine (1975) measured a more specific marker of bone collagen resorption, the glucosyl-galactosyl-hydroxylysine/galactosyl-hydroxylysine urinary ratio. In normocalcemic hyperthyroid subjects the ratio was 1.5, virtually identical to normal. In two patients who were hypercalcemic, the ratio was less than one. This would indicate that a significantly greater proportion of the hydroxylysine had its origin in bone.

Elevation of serum alkaline phosphatase concentration is common in hyperthyroidism (Cook *et al.*, 1959; Smith *et al.*, 1973; Moseleilde *et al.*, 1978) and correlates reasonably well with urinary hydroxyproline excretion (Smith *et al.*, 1973). The enzyme elevation in most patients probably arises from increased osteoblastic activity. This is supported by the finding that the skeletal isoenzyme of alkaline phosphatase in serum is often increased in patients with hyperthyroidism (Richter and Ohlen, 1971; Cleeve and Brown, 1978). In severe thyrotoxicosis of long duration liver disease may arise and also lead to an elevated serum alkaline phosphatase.

The skeletal manifestations of hypothyroidism depend to a great extent on the age of onset of the disorder. In children, hypothyroidism characteristically leads to an arrest of growth, manifested radiologically by increased density of the provisional zone of calcification and a delay in the appearance of ossification of epiphyseal centers (Krane and Goldring, 1978). Less commonly it leads to a generalized osteopetrosis or marble bone disease (Braid, 1951; Fanconi and Girardet, 1952; Jeune and Béraud, 1955; Breton *et al.*, 1958; Jeune and Muller, 1959; Andersen, 1961; Royer and Mathieu, 1962; Schmidt, 1962; Tümay *et al.*, 1962). In some of the osteopetrotic patients, hypercalcemia, nephrocalcinosis, or soft tissue calcification was present (Braid, 1951; Fanconi and Giardet, 1952; Schmidt, 1962; Tümay *et al.*, 1962). In adult onset hypothyroidism, radiologic changes are not seen, but quantitative morphometry of bone has revealed a markedly decreased area of cancellous bone undergoing resorption (Bordier *et al.*, 1967). This was associated with an increase in cancellous bone volume. Radiocalcium kinetic studies in hypothyroidism have demonstrated a decreased calcium pool and low rates of bone resorption and formation (Krane *et al.*, 1956; Bordier *et al.*, 1967). Decreased collagen turnover is reflected by low levels of urinary hydroxyproline excretion (Kivirikko *et al.*, 1965). Serum alkaline phosphatase concentration may be low in children, probably as a result of decreased osteoblastic activity (Talbot, 1939).

The effects of excessive secretion of thyroid hormones on bone appear to be direct, since *in vitro* studies indicate that thyroxine and triiodothyronine can stimulate osteoclastic bone resorption (Mundy *et al.*, 1976) and increased bone resorption can be produced by thyroid hormone administration to parathyroidectomized dogs (Adams and Jowsey, 1967). As discussed in the section on thyroid hormone interaction with parathyroid hormone, the modulation of intracellular cyclic AMP concentration may be an important effect of thyroid hormone.

C. Interaction with Kidney

It has not been demonstrated that thyroid hormone has direct effects on renal handling of divalent cations and phosphate, but calcium and phosphate excretion are altered in abnormal thyroid states. Hypercalciuria is a frequent feature of hyperthyroidism but rarely leads to renal calculi formation or nephrocalcinosis (Bradley *et al.*, 1974). It is likely that the hypercalciuria results from increased mobilization of bone mineral (Krane *et al.*, 1956) and suppression of parathyroid hormone secretion (Buckle *et al.*, 1969; Bouillon and DeMoor, 1974; Burman *et al.*, 1976; Rude *et al.*, 1976; Mosekilde and Christensen, 1977). Both of these factors probably account for the hyperphosphatemia often found in hyperthyroidism (Fujita *et al.*, 1958; Cook *et al.*, 1959; Parsons and Anderson, 1964). Parathyroid hormone suppression leads to hyperphosphatemia as a result of increased renal tubular reabsorption of phosphate, a finding well documented in patients with hyperthyroidism (Harden *et al.*, 1964; Parsons and Anderson, 1964; Bijvoet and Majoor, 1965; Malamos *et al.*, 1969). In hypothyroidism there is a reduction of glomerular filtration (Bradley *et al.*, 1974) and generally less calcium is excreted in the urine than normal. However, there are documented cases of hypercalciuria and nephrocalcinosis in children (Naylor, 1955; Royer *et al.*, 1958; Jeune and Muller, 1959; Lang, 1960; Royer and Mathieu, 1962; Schmidt, 1962; Tümay *et al.*, 1962; Job *et al.*, 1963). This appears to occur as a consequence of intestinal hyperabsorption of calcium. Hypothyroidism is associated with a reduced renal tubular reabsorption of phosphate (Nordin and Fraser, 1956; Adams *et al.*, 1968) and a decreased tubular maximum for phosphate (Malamos *et al.*, 1969). Despite this, patients often have a normal or only slightly low serum phosphate concentration (Aub *et al.*, 1929; Adams *et al.*, 1968; Malamos *et al.*, 1969). It is possible that a reduction in glomerular filtration rate and intestinal hyperabsorption of phosphate counterbalance the renal phosphate leak.

D. Interaction with Intestine

Studies in both animals and man indicate a striking influence of thyroid hormone on intestinal absorption of calcium. Although an excess of thyroid hormone is generally associated with increased metabolic activity, in the hyperthyroid state intestinal calcium absorption is usually reduced (Cook *et al.*, 1959; Finkelstein and Schacter, 1962; Friedland *et al.*, 1965; Adams *et al.*, 1967; Krawitt, 1967; Noble and Matty, 1967; Williams *et al.*, 1967; Bordier *et al.*, 1967; Shafer and Gregory, 1972; Singhelakis *et al.*, 1974; Swaminathan and

Care, 1975; Haldimann *et al.*, 1980). The converse has been found in most studies of hypothyroidism (Jeune and Muller, 1959; Lang, 1960; Lowe *et al.*, 1962; Royer and Mathieu, 1962; Lekkerkerker *et al.*, 1971; Lekkerkerker and Doorenbos, 1973), although in two rat studies increased calcium absorption was not found (Winter *et al.*, 1970; Hehrmann *et al.*, 1973). The increased intestinal absorption of calcium observed in hypothyroid children may contribute to the hypercalcemia found in some patients (Braid, 1951; Johnson and White, 1952; Naylor, 1955; Royer *et al.*, 1958; Jeune and Muller, 1959; Schmidt, 1962; Job *et al.*, 1963; Pretorius and Potgieter, 1971). In adults with hypothyroidism, hypercalcemia has been reported in only three patients (Lowe *et al.*, 1962; Adams *et al.*, 1968). There may be two reasons for the effects of thyroid hormone on intestinal calcium absorption. The hyperthyroid state is associated with a reduced intestinal transit time (Middleton, 1971). This could account for some calcium malabsorption. In turn the prolonged intestinal transit time noted in hypothyroidism could explain the more efficient absorption of calcium in this condition (Middleton, 1971).

A second possibility is that thyroid hormone might play a role in vitamin D metabolism. This is discussed in Section II,G.

E. Interaction with Parathyroid Hormone

There is little evidence that thyroid hormone acts directly on parathyroid hormone secretion. In patients with mild or frank hypercalcemia, the concentration of parathyroid hormone in the circulation is low (Buckle *et al.*, 1969; Bouillon and DeMoor, 1974; Burman *et al.*, 1976; Rude *et al.*, 1976; Mosekilde and Christensen, 1977). In three studies of normocalcemic hyperthyroid patients (Bouillon and DeMoor, 1974; Manderlier *et al.*, 1974; Castro *et al.*, 1975) parathyroid hormone concentration was normal but in one study (Bommer *et al.*, 1976) the levels were elevated in 15 out of 20 patients. Adult hypothyroid patients have been found to have high normal or elevated concentrations of parathyroid hormone, usually in the presence of a normal calcium concentration (Adams *et al.*, 1968; Bouillon and DeMoor, 1974; Castro *et al.*, 1975; Bouillon *et al.*, 1980). Further evidence of suppressed parathyroid hormone levels in hyperthyroid patients is provided by the finding of increased renal tubular reabsorption of phosphate in many patients (Bortz *et al.*, 1961; Harden *et al.*, 1964; Parsons and Anderson, 1964; Bijvoet and Majoor, 1965; Malamos *et al.*, 1969). Hyperphosphatemia is another possible manifestation of the secondary hypoparathyroidism of hyperthyroidism (Fujita *et al.*, 1958; Cook *et al.*, 1959; Parsons and Anderson, 1964). Bommer and colleagues (1976) feel that hyperphosphatemia is not a consequence of suppressed parathyroid function, since they observed hyperphosphatemia in the absence of hypercalcemia or low concentrations of parathyroid hormone. In hypothyroidism, hypophosphatemia is seldom found but tubular reabsorption of phosphate is decreased (Adams *et al.*, 1968); this presumably reflects an increased concentration of parathyroid hormone in the circulation.

The peripheral metabolism of parathyroid hormone could conceivably influence hormone levels in the circulation of patients with hyperthyroidism or hypothyroidism by altering the rate of parathyroid hormone clearance. No studies have been reported that bear on this aspect of the interaction of parathyroid with thyroid hormone.

The coexistence of primary hyperparathyroidism and hyperthyroidism may lead to confusion in the differential diagnosis of hypercalcemia (Parfitt and Dent, 1970; Richards, 1970; Bergdahl, 1977) unless plasma levels of parathyroid hormone are shown to be elevated in hypercalcemic patients with both disorders (Burman *et al.*, 1976). The reversal of hypercalcemia by appropriate therapy of the hyperthyroidism provides definitive evidence of thyrotoxic hypercalcemia. Persistence of the hypercalcemic state after the patient is euthyroid strongly suggests the presence of primary hyperparathyroidism or another hypercalcemic disorder.

The sensitivity of patients with thyroid disease to exogenous parathyroid hormone has been examined in three studies (Harrison *et al.*, 1964; Castro *et al.*, 1975; Guttler *et al.*, 1977). In each study patients with hyperthyroidism were found to be more responsive to the hormone than normal subjects or hypothyroid patients. Serum calcium concentrations rose to higher levels in two studies (Harrison *et al.*, 1964; Castro *et al.*, 1975). Excretion of hydroxyproline and phosphate in the urine also were greater in hyperthyroid patients (Castro *et al.*, 1975). Urinary cyclic AMP excretion was greater in response to parathyroid extract in hyperthyroid patients than in normal subjects and was less in hypothyroid patients than in the normal group (Guttler *et al.*, 1977). The greater effect of parathyroid hormone on serum calcium concentration and urinary hydroxyproline in hyperthyroidism could be explained by a high prevailing rate of bone resorption (see section on bone) and/or by relatively low levels of endogenous parathyroid hormone in the circulation. The latter factor could also explain the greater phosphaturic and cyclic AMP responses. In the hypothyroid patients a decreased rate of bone resorption and/or a relatively larger concentration of circulating parathyroid hormone could explain the insensitivity to exogenous parathyroid hormone. It is possible that peripheral responsiveness to parathyroid hormone in states of abnormal thyroid function is an important factor in determining the secretory rate of the parathyroid glands. The study of urinary cyclic AMP excretion in thyroid hormone excess or deficiency states (Guttler *et al.*, 1977) suggests that the hormone modulates end-organ activity by an unknown interaction with membrane-bound adenylate cyclase. The *in vitro* observation that thyroid hormone can inhibit bone cyclic nucleotide phosphodiesterase (Marcus, 1975) provides an alternate or complementary explanation for thyroid hormone action. Since propranolol can reverse the hypercalcemia of thyrotoxicosis (Rude *et al.*, 1976) thyroid hormone may act on bone through β-adrenergic modulation of intracellular cyclic AMP concentration.

F. Interaction with Calcitonin

A direct effect of thyroid hormone on calcitonin secretion has not been demonstrated, although antithyroid drugs have been reported to decrease the rate of secretion of calcitonin in pigs (Duncan and Care, 1967). In contrast to this study, Peng and colleagues have found that in rats iodine deficiency (Peng *et al.*, 1976) or propylthiouracil (Peng *et al.*, 1977) induces goiter formation, C-cell hyperplasia, and hypersecretion of calcitonin. Hypercalcemia has been noted in iodine deficient rats and may be primarily responsible for the stimulation of calcitonin (Clark *et al.*, 1978). The measurement of serum calcitonin concentrations in hyperthyroidism by sensitive techniques has not been reported but in a few patients with Grave's disease, the concentration of calcitonin in the thyroid gland was low (Aliapoulos *et al.*, 1966; Mazzuoli *et al.*, 1966).

The hypocalcemic effect of calcitonin is enhanced in patients with hyperthyroidism (Bijvoet *et al.*, 1968; Martin and Melick, 1969) and in rats treated with thyroid hormone (Milhaud *et al.*, 1967; Cherny *et al.*, 1970). A similar enhancement of calcitonin-induced hypocalcemia has been found in hypothyroid (thyroidectomized) rats (Talmage and Kennedy, 1969) and athyreotic children (Milhaud, 1968; Lambertz *et al.*, 1969). The sensitivity to calcitonin in the absence of the thyroid gland probably can be attributed to calcitonin deficiency.

G. Interaction with Vitamin D

In three studies of patients with thyrotoxicosis, plasma 25(OH)D levels were significantly lower than normal (Hunstein *et al.*, 1977; Mosekilde *et al.*, 1977a; Velentzas *et al.*, 1977). In one study the concentration was below the lower limit of normal in 11 of 12 patients who had elevated plasma alkaline phosphatase concentrations (Hunstein *et al.*, 1977). In three subsequent studies normal 25(OH)D levels were reported (Cleeve and Brown, 1978; Kaptein *et al.*, 1979; Bouillon *et al.*, 1980). The significance of these findings and of the lowered levels of this hepatic metabolite of vitamin D in certain patients remain unknown. In one study in patients with hypothyroidism, normal levels were reported. In two studies decreased levels of serum $1,25(OH)_2D$ were reported (Kaptein *et al.*, 1979; Bouillon *et al.*, 1980). It is not known whether these results reflect a direct action of thyroid hormone on production rate or metabolic clearance rate of the vitamin D metabolite, effects of blood phosphate and parathyroid hormone on production rate, or a combination of these influences. Elevated levels of $1,25(OH)_2D$ were found in one study of patients with hypothyroidism (Bouillon *et al.*, 1980). The precise mechanism which accounts for this has also not been determined.

Hypersensitivity to vitamin D as manifested by hypercalcemia has been observed in several hypothyroid children (Royer and Mathieu, 1962; Job *et al.*, 1963; Wilkins, 1965; Pretorius and Potgieter, 1971) as well as in hypothyroid dogs (Handovsky and Goormaghtigh, 1937). Resistance to the effect of vitamin D on reducing fecal calcium excretion was found in two adult hyperthyroid patients (Cook *et al.*, 1959). However, several other studies suggest that sensitivity to vitamin D may be present in some patients with hyperthyroidism. In a rare case of hypoparathyroidism and hyperthyroidism, vitamin D requirements for the control of hypocalcemia were reduced when the patient developed hyperthyroidism (Rothenberg and Redleaf, 1959). Further indirect evidence of a role of vitamin D in patients with hyperthyroidism is provided by the observation that corticosteroid therapy can suppress the hypercalcemia of thyrotoxicosis in some patients (Sataline *et al.*, 1962; Harper and Hughes, 1970; Richards, 1970).

H. Summary

Thyroid hormone has been demonstrated to have profound effects on mineral metabolism. A direct effect on bone accounts for increased bone turnover in patients with hyperthyroidism and reduced bone turnover in hypothyroid patients. Hypercalcemia may occur in hyperthyroidism when the rate of bone resorption exceeds that of bone formation and is accompanied by reduced levels of serum parathyroid hormone, hyperphosphatemia, an elevated renal threshold for phosphate excretion, increased urinary hydroxyproline and hypercalciuria. An impairment in intestinal calcium absorption has also been noted, probably resulting from decreased intestinal transport time and reduced $1,25(OH)_2D$ levels. Hypothyroidism in children produces marked impairment of growth at the epiphyses. Rarely, hypercalcemia and/or hypercalciuria may occur in hypothyroid patients. This may occur as a result of increased intestinal calcium absorption and a reduced exchangeable calcium pool.

IV. GROWTH HORMONE

A. Mode of Action

Growth hormone is the major hormonal regulator of growth. Its effects include anabolism of cartilage and bone, lipolysis, and a decrease in glucose tolerance. The growth-promoting influence of growth hormone appear to be effected through the intermediary action of somatomedin as discussed in Section IV,B.

The mechanism by which growth hormone acts on fat and carbohydrate metabolism is less clear. A relationship with the adenylate cyclase-cyclic AMP system has been suggested (Goodman and Schwartz, 1974).

B. Interaction with Bone

Growth hormone is a necessary factor for normal growth and development. Although growth hormone plays no role in fetal growth, its absence in childhood results in a growth rate only one-third to one-half that of normal (Daughaday, 1977). Excess growth hormone will result in accelerated linear growth in childhood leading to gigantism and to bony overgrowth in the adult (Daughaday, 1974).

Growth hormone has no direct effect either on cartilage (Salmon and Daughaday, 1957) or on bone (Canalis *et al.*, 1977b) *in vitro*. All anabolic effects on the skeleton appear to be mediated through the intermediary action of the somatomedins. The somatomedins are a group of peptides that circulate bound to another growth hormone-dependent carrier protein (Daughaday, 1977). These peptides appear to be synthesized and released by the liver since serum somatomedin activity falls following partial hepatectomy in the rat (Uthne and Uthne, 1972) and is low in cirrhosis (Wu *et al.*, 1974). In addition, perfusion of rat liver with growth hormone increases somatomedin activity (McCanoghey and Sledge, 1970; Phillips *et al.*, 1976). The action of somatomedin is to enhance the incorporation of proline into collagen, uridine into RNA, and thymidine into DNA (Salmon and duVall, 1970; Raisz *et al.*, 1976). There is good correlation between the rise in serum somatomedin activity and the growth response in hypopituitary children with growth hormone (Daughaday and Parker, 1963). The mechanism by which somatomedin acts on its target cells is unclear. Unlike many peptide hormones, it does not appear to act by stimulating an increase in cyclic AMP. Somatomedin has been found to decrease the basal level and parathyroid hormone-induced increase in chondrocyte adenylate cyclase (Tell *et al.*, 1973).

Although growth hormone is probably the major regulator of somatomedin production, other factors may influence its metabolism. Low levels of somatomedin are seen in fasting (Daughaday and Kipnis, 1966), protein-calorie malnutrition (Grant *et al.*, 1973; Beaton, 1976), and renal failure (Saenger *et al.*, 1974; Lewy and New, 1975). Insulin (Daughaday *et al.*, 1976) and prolactin (Francis and Hill, 1975) have been reported to increase somatomedin production. Modification of the end-organ response to the effect of somatomedin may be present on an inherited basis as in the Laron dwarf (Daughaday *et al.*, 1969) or during starvation (Salmon, 1975).

Growth hormone increases the skeletal uptake of radioactive calcium in the rat (Ulrich *et al.*, 1952) and dog (Harris and Heaney, 1969), and of stable strontium in man (Eisenberg and Gordan, 1961). Similarly, in acromegaly the skeletal uptake of radioactive calcium is increased (Haymovitz and Horwith, 1964; Aloia *et al.,* 1972; Montz *et al.,* 1973). When measured simultaneously, both bone accretion and resorption are increased in patients with acromegaly (Bell and Bartter 1967; Aloia *et al.,* 1972) and during growth hormone therapy (Haas *et al.,* 1976), as determined by radioactive calcium kinetic studies. Microradiographic studies have also indicated that bone formation and resorption are increased in acromegaly (Roelfsema *et al.,* 1970; Riggs *et al.,* 1972b), although one study demonstrated normal bone formation (Aloia *et al.,* 1972). High bone turnover in acromegaly or with growth hormone therapy is also suggested by the finding of increased urinary excretion of hydroxyproline (Jasin *et al.,* 1962; Smiley and Ziff, 1964; Wright *et al.,* 1965; Aloia *et al.,* 1976; Haas *et al.,* 1976).

The growth hormone-induced changes in bone formation and resorption may not be closely coupled throughout cortical and trabecular bone. Quantitative morphometry has generally shown a net increase in periosteal new bone formation, while in some studies resorption appears to predominate in intracortical or Haversian bone (Frost, 1966; Kruse and Kuhlencordt, 1975). Endosteal bone resorption is increased in man (Frost, 1966; Riggs *et al.,* 1972b), but the dog has been reported to have a net increase in endosteal bone formation in response to growth hormone (Harris *et al.,* 1972).

Osteoporosis was thought to be a manifestation of acromegaly (Daughaday, 1974), based on radiographic findings of skeletal rarefaction (Scriver and Bryan, 1935). The lack of an increased incidence of compression fractures of the spine in acromegalic patients and a number of morphometric and kinetic studies of bone in acromegaly do not support this concept. Eisenberg and Gordan (1961) demonstrated an increase in the miscible calcium pool in acromegaly through the use of stable strontium. These findings were confirmed by radiocalcium kinetic studies in which exchangeable calcium was found to be either increased (Haymovitz and Horwith, 1964; Aloia *et al.,* 1972; Montz *et al.,* 1973) or normal (Bell and Bartter, 1967). In addition, bone mineral content has been found to be normal (Doyle, 1967; Montz *et al.,* 1973), while bone density (Roelfsema *et al.,* 1970; Haas *et al.,* 1976) as well as bone mass (Riggs *et al.,* 1972b) have been reported to be normal or increased. Quantitative microradiographic studies demonstrated cortical and trabecular bone thickness to be normal or increased (Roelfsema *et al.,* 1970; Aloia *et al.,* 1972). Similar studies by Riggs *et al.* (1972b) also demonstrated an increase in cortical bone thickness, but found trabecular bone thickness to be decreased.

C. Interaction with Kidney

Acromegaly is associated with hypercalciuria, which decreases to normal with treatment of the pituitary tumor (Scriver and Bryan, 1935; Bauer and Aub, 1941;

Harrison *et al.*, 1960; Molinatto *et al.*, 1961; Nadarajah *et al.*, 1968; Sjöberg, 1969; Sigurdsson *et al.*, 1973a). In addition, growth hormone administration has been observed to result in an increase in urinary calcium excretion (Ikkos *et al.*, 1958; Hutchings *et al.*, 1959; MRC, 1959; Beck *et al.*, 1960; Henneman *et al.*, 1960; Hanna *et al.*, 1961; Karam *et al.*, 1961; Forbes *et al.*, 1962; Wright *et al.*, 1965; Melvin *et al.*, 1967; Bryson *et al.*, 1972). The exact cause of the hypercalciuria is unclear. The administration of growth hormone to dogs was observed to have no effect on renal calcium or phosphate clearance, renal blood flow, or glomerular filtration rate over a 2-hr period following its administration (Westby *et al.*, 1977). This suggests that acute changes in the plasma growth hormone concentration do not influence calcium or phosphate homeostasis. In contrast, the glomerular filtration rate and renal plasma flow have been shown to be high in acromegaly (Heller *et al.*, 1954; Ikkos *et al.*, 1956; Gershberg *et al.*, 1957) and following chronic exogenous growth hormone administration in man (Corvilain *et al.*, 1962) and dog (White *et al.*, 1949; Davis *et al.*, 1954; Corvilain *et al.*, 1964). As discussed below, growth hormone therapy may be associated with enhanced intestinal calcium absorption. This could contribute to the increased urinary calcium excretion. A recent study has shown a significant positive correlation between intestinal calcium absorption and renal calcium excretion (Sigurdsson *et al.*, 1973a). It is also clear that the hypercalciuria that occurs under the influence of growth hormone may be in excess of that which can be accounted for by increased intestinal calcium absorption (Scriver and Bryan, 1935; Bauer and Aub, 1941; Ikkos *et al.*, 1958; Beck *et al.*, 1960; Nadarajah *et al.*, 1968; Bryson *et al.*, 1972). This suggests another effect of growth hormone on the kidney and/or bone. Fraser *et al.* (1960) found that parathyroidectomy prevented the hypercalciuric effect of growth hormone in rats, a finding which suggests that the hypercalciuria might be related to increased parathyroid hormone secretion. More recently, however, an increase in urinary calcium excretion following growth hormone administration was seen in hypoparathyroid patients (Hernandez *et al.*, 1967; Bryson *et al.*, 1972). An effect of growth hormone in decreasing renal tubular citrate concentration has been suggested as playing a role in the hypercalciuria (Karam *et al.*, 1961). As discussed above, increased bone turnover with increased skeletal calcium resorption also may be a contributing factor in the hypercalciuria.

Although early studies suggested growth hormone caused increased urinary phosphate excretion (Scriver and Bryan, 1935; Bauer and Aub, 1941), subsequent investigations have generally indicated a reduced urinary phosphate excretion (MRC, 1959; Gershberg, 1960; Henneman *et al.*, 1960; Corvilain *et al.*, 1962; Forbes *et al.*, 1962; Bryson *et al.*, 1972). The phosphate excretion index has either been normal or decreased (Camanni *et al.*, 1968; Nadarajah *et al.*, 1968). The mechanism for decreased renal phosphate excretion appears to include a direct effect of growth hormone on the kidneys, since parathyroidectomy does not alter this effect in man (Bryson *et al.*, 1972) or dog (Corvilain *et *al.*, 1964). As indicated earlier, the increased tubular reabsorption of phosphate is associated with an increased serum phosphate concentration and positive phosphate balance.

D. Interaction with Intestine

Increased intestinal absorption of calcium and/or low fecal calcium excretion have been found in some patients with acromegaly (Bauer and Aub, 1941; Hanna *et al.*, 1961; Sigurdsson *et al.*, 1973a) or following exogenous growth hormone administration (Beck *et al.*, 1957; Ikkos *et al.*, 1958; Henneman *et al.*, 1960; Hanna *et al.*, 1961; Bryson *et al.*, 1972; Sigurdsson *et al.*, 1973a). In sheep, growth hormone also appears to enhance intestinal calcium absorption (Braithwaite, 1975). However, in some patients growth hormone produces no change or an increase in fecal calcium excretion (Scriver and Bryan, 1935; Ikkos *et al.*, 1958; Forbes *et al.*, 1962; Melvin *et al.*, 1967; Bryson *et al.*, 1972). A number of studies have also shown negative calcium balance in acromegaly or during growth hormone therapy (Scriver and Bryan, 1935; Bauer and Aub, 1941; Ikkos *et al.*, 1959; Beck *et al.*, 1960; Hanna *et al.*, 1961; Bell and Bartter, 1967; Nadarajah *et al.*, 1968), although many reports of a positive calcium balance have also been published (Scriver and Bryan, 1935; Shorr *et al.*, 1953; Beck *et al.*, 1957; Hutchings *et al.*, 1959; Henneman *et al.*, 1960; Pearson *et al.*, 1960; Nadarajah *et al.*, 1968; Sjöberg *et al.*, 1969; Montz *et al.*, 1973). These conflicting results may be related to the amount of dietary calcium ingested, since increasing dietary calcium intake from low to high levels may convert a negative calcium balance to a positive balance (Scriver and Bryan, 1935; Pearson *et al.*, 1960). Other possible contributing factors toward a negative calcium balance include increased intestinal calcium secretion (Heaney and Skillman, 1964) and hypercalciuria.

Growth hormone deficiency produced by hypophysectomy resulted in decreased intestinal calcium absorption in rats, which returned toward normal with growth hormone therapy (Finkelstein and Schachter, 1962; Mainoya, 1975b). When calcium transport was corrected for intestinal weight, however, no change in intestinal calcium absorption was seen in hypophysectomized rats (Krawitt *et al.*, 1977). Under similar experimental conditions, while hypophysectomy did not prevent the increase in active calcium transport seen in response to a low calcium diet, there was a significant decrease in intestinal calcium absorption when compared to normal rats (Kimberg *et al.*, 1961). In these studies, a comparable defect in glucose transport was not seen; this suggests that the defect in calcium absorption is not secondary to a nonspecific effect of hypophysectomy on the intestine. As discussed below, hypophysectomy in the rat results in decreased levels of $1,25(OH)_2D_3$ in the blood and could account for decreased intestinal calcium absorption (Spanos *et al.*, 1978).

Growth hormone may also increase intestinal magnesium absorption (Hanna *et al.*, 1961) and cause a positive magnesium balance (Henneman *et al.*, 1960; Hanna *et al.*, 1961; Forbes *et al.*, 1962).

Phosphate balance is usually positive under the influence of growth hormone (Scriver and Bryan, 1935; Shorr *et al.*, 1953; Beck *et al.*, 1957; Ikkos *et al.*, 1958; Hutchings *et al.*, 1959; MRC, 1959; Beck *et al.*, 1960; Henneman *et al.*, 1960; Forbes *et al.*, 1962; Braithwaite, 1975). Although fecal phosphate has been found to be decreased in some studies (Beck *et al.*, 1957; Henneman *et al.*, 1960; Forbes *et al.*, 1962; Braithwaite, 1975), the major factor in the positive phosphate balance is the increased renal reabsorption of phosphate as discussed above.

E. Interaction with Parathyroid Hormone

The serum calcium concentration is usually within the normal range in patients with acromegaly, although frank elevations have been reported (Molinatti *et al.*, 1961; Summers *et al.*, 1966; Nadarajah *et al.*, 1968; Brown and Singer, 1969; Aloia *et al.*, 1975). The cause of hypercalcemia in many patients may be related to an inherited predisposition for the development of multiple endocrine neoplasias. Primary hyperparathyroidism and acromegaly may coexist in this syndrome (Wermer, 1954). In two investigations it was noted that following successful treatment of the pituitary disease an elevated serum calcium concentration fell to normal in 12 patients (Nadarajah *et al.*, 1968; Brown and Singer, 1969). This is consistent with the hypothesis that growth hormone has a direct stimulatory effect on the parathyroid glands (Harrison *et al.*, 1960; Summers *et al.*, 1966). Hypophysectomy in the rat has been observed to result in a reduction in parathyroid gland size (Salzer, 1971; Fontaine *et al.*, 1978) and a decrease in serum immunoreactive parathyroid hormone concentration (Spanos *et al.*, 1978), although the serum calcium concentrations remained normal. The administration of bovine growth hormone to rats increased the serum calcium and immunoreactive parathyroid hormone concentrations as well as the weight of the parathyroid glands in one study (Lancer *et al.*, 1976). However, in another study human growth hormone raised the serum calcium concentration in rats, but with morphological evidence of decreased parathyroid gland function (Altenahr and Kampf, 1976). The morphologic changes were thought to be secondary to the hypercalcemia. The hyperphosphatemic and hypercalciuric effects of growth hormone may secondarily enhance parathyroid hormone secretion, although it has been observed that the hypercalciuric effect of growth hormone in the rat is prevented by parathyroidectomy (Fraser and Harrison, 1960). Measurement of the serum immunoreactive parathyroid hormone concentration in acromegaly has revealed an elevation in only one of six patients studied (Aloia *et al.*, 1975) and no change was seen following chronic growth hormone therapy to children

(Gertner *et al.*, 1979; Chipman *et al.*, 1980). Other indirect evidence of an interrelationship of growth hormone with parathyroid hormone is the observation that human growth hormone therapy shortens the recovery time of the blood calcium concentration following EDTA-induced hypocalcemia (Gershberg *et al.*, 1967).

F. Interaction with Calcitonin

The effect of growth hormone on calcitonin secretion and action has not been fully evaluated. Hypophysectomy in the rat resulted in a reduction in the size of parafollicular cell nuclei, cytoplasm, and granules (Salzer, 1971). In these rats calcium infusion resulted in prolonged hypercalcemia, a finding suggestive of calcitonin deficiency.

G. Interaction with Vitamin D

Recent studies have demonstrated an effect of growth hormone on vitamin D metabolism. Spencer and Tobiassen (1977) found that hypophysectomy decreased the amount of labeled $1,25(OH)_2D_3$ in the serum and intestinal mucosa in the rat following administration of labeled $25(OH)D_3$. An increase in the levels of $24,25(OH)_2D_3$ was seen, reciprocal to the decrease in $1,25(OH)_2D_3$. Fontaine *et al.* (1978) have also observed an increase in the conversion of $25(OH)D_3$ to $24,25(OH)_2D_3$ in the hypophysectomized rat. Growth hormone administration to the hypophysectomized rat partially reversed these changes. In other studies, hypophysectomized rats were shown to have a fall in plasma $1,25(OH)_2D_3$ concentration that returned to normal with the administration of human growth hormone (Spanos *et al.*, 1978; Pavlovitch *et al.*, 1978). Patients with acromegaly were found to have increased levels of plasma $1,25(OH)_2D$ and $24,25(OH)_2D$ which returned toward normal with bromocriptine therapy (Eskildsen *et al.*, 1979). The effect of growth hormone on vitamin D metabolism may not be direct, however, as growth hormone did not stimulate the formation of $1,25(OH)_2D_3$ *in vitro* (Bilke *et al.*, 1980).

The effect of growth hormone on intestinal calcium absorption may not be mediated only by an effect on vitamin D metabolism. The administration of growth hormone to growth hormone deficient children in two studies have shown that while an increase in growth, renal phosphate threshold, and fractional intestinal calcium absorption was seen, there was no change in plasma immunoreactive parathyroid hormone, 25(OH)D, $24,25(OH)_2D$, or urinary cyclic AMP (Gertner *et al.*, 1979; Chipman *et al.*, 1980). The level of $1,25(OH)_2D$ remained unchanged in one study (Gertner *et al.*, 1979) while falling in the other (Chipman *et al.*, 1980). In addition, growth hormone was demonstrated to increase intestinal calcium transport in the rat by a mechanism other than its influence on vitamin D metabolism (Aloia and Yeh, 1980).

H. Summary

Growth hormone has a major influence on mineral metabolism, effected primarily through the intermediary action of the somatomedins. Growth hormone deficiency leads to dwarfism in the growing child, and an excess results in acromegaly and gigantism in the adult and child, respectively. Growth hormone causes an increase in both bone formation and resorption. While resorption may predominate in trabecular bone in man, bone acretion appears to predominate in the periosteal region. Bone mass during states of growth hormone excess is usually either normal or increased. A tendency toward hypercalcemia and hypercalciuria may result from increased bone resorption or through an increased intestinal calcium absorption. The enhanced absorption of dietary calcium may result from an effect of growth hormone on intestinal calcium transport or through an effect on vitamin D metabolism.

In addition to the above, growth hormone also raises the serum phosphate concentration. This is primarily due to an increase in the renal tubular phosphate threshold.

V. PROLACTIN

Prolactin, a peptide hormone of the anterior pituitary gland, is important in the development of the mammary gland and in milk formation. It occurs in males, but its function is unknown. Large amounts of exogenous prolactin can simulate certain effects of growth hormone, including nitrogen retention. Some studies have suggested that prolactin plays a role in sodium and water metabolism, but this has not been a consistent finding. Studies of the mode of action of prolactin indicate that hormone binding to receptor sites on plasma membranes of mammary cells does not activate adenylate cyclase (Turkington *et al.*, 1973). Despite this, there is an increase of protein kinase activity and phosphorylated proteins in the cells.

A role of prolactin in mineral metabolism has been suggested by recent animal studies. During lactation there is an increased requirement for calcium that appears to be met by an increase in intestinal calcium absorption (Toverud *et al.*, 1976). It now appears that this adaptation is mediated by an increase in circulating levels of $1,25(OH)_2D_3$, since levels of this vitamin D metabolite are up to fourfold greater in lactating than in normal rats (Boass *et al.*, 1977) and are twice normal in postpartum women (Kumar *et al.*, 1979). The rise in the concentration of $1,25(OH)_2D3$ may be related to prolactin secretion, at least in part, since exogenous prolactin administration increases chick renal 25-hydroxycholecalciferol-1α-hydroxylase activity (Spanos *et al.*, 1976) and circulating levels of the metabolite in the chicken (Spanos *et al.*, 1976; Bikle *et al.*, 1980). Ample evidence has been obtained that exogenous prolactin increases active transport of calcium in the rat intestine (Finkelstein and Schachter, 1962;

Mainoya, 1975a,b). It is also possible that the rise in blood prolactin concentration found during pregnancy may contribute to the increased intestinal calcium absorption found in pregnant women (Heany and Skillman, 1971). This hypothesis is supported by the report of increased plasma $1,25(OH)_2D3$ levels in pregnant women (Kumar *et al.*, 1979). However, other recent studies indicate that an effect of prolactin on vitamin D metabolism may be species-specific. Patients with high blood levels of prolactin due to pituitary tumors do not have elevation of circulating $1,25(OH)_2D$ (Adams *et al.*, 1979; Kumar *et al.*, 1979). Also prolactin failed to stimulate vitamin D metabolism in a study done in vitamin D-deficient rats (Matsumoto *et al.*, 1979).

Exogenous prolactin (10 μg/hr) infused into normal, parathyroidectomized, or thyroparathyroidectomized rats raises plasma calcium concentration even in starved animals. In contrast, higher doses of prolactin (50 μg/hr) reduce plasma calcium in intact rats (Robinson *et al.*, 1975). Injection of fish pituitary extracts into hypophysectomized hypocalcemic killifish produces a hypercalcemic effect also felt to represent a prolactin response (Pang *et al.*, 1978).

Injected prolactin has been shown to increase urinary calcium excretion in some (McAlister and Welbourn, 1962; Beck *et al.*, 1964: Robinson *et al.*, 1975) but not all subjects (Lipsett and Bergenstal, 1960; McAlister and Welbourn, 1962). Urinary calcium excretion in patients with endogenous hyperprolactinemia was not increased in one study (Hipkin *et al.*, 1978).

It would appear that prolactin also interacts with mineral metabolism as a consequence of an effect on serum estradiol levels. In a study of young amenorrheic hyperprolactinemic women serum estradiol levels were either at postmenopausal levels or at the levels found during the follicular phase of the menstrual cycle (Klibanski *et al.*, 1980). Bone density was reduced in these patients as compared to age-matched normal subjects and there was a positive correlation between serum estradiol concentrations and bone density.

VI. INSULIN

A. Mode of Action

Insulin has profound effects not only on carbohydrate metabolism but also on fat and protein metabolism. The control of blood sugar is modulated by the action of insulin to increase glucose transport into liver (by stimulating glucokinase), adipose cells, and muscle, by stimulation of glycogen synthesis in liver and muscle and by suppressing liver gluconeogenesis. Insulin influences fat metabolism by increasing lipogenesis in the liver and by decreasing lipolysis and stimulating fatty acid synthesis in adipose cells. The effect of insulin on protein metabolism is critical in that it stimulates increased amino acid uptake and protein synthesis in muscle and inhibits proteolysis in the liver. It is an anabolic hormone and is essential for normal growth. Insulin does not appear to activate membrane-bound adenylate cyclase as an initiating step in its biological actions. It is likely that the action of insulin is initiated by binding to receptors on cell membranes, but the details of the subsequent messengers that are activated by the hormone have yet to be elucidated (Czech, 1977).

B. Interaction with Bone

In vitro studies indicate that insulin can influence bone metabolism directly. Insulin enhances the incorporation of pyrimidine nucleosides into intracellular nucleotide and RNA pools in isolated bone cells (Peck and Messinger, 1970). An increase in membrane transport of amino acids in fetal rat calvaria has also been observed (Hahn *et al.*, 1971). The effect on amino acid membrane transport can be blocked by either puromycin or cycloheximide, suggesting that this phenomenon is mediated by synthesis of a membrane carrier protein. Bone collagen synthesis was increased by insulin in cultures of fetal rat or chick bone (Perlish *et al.*, 1973; Canalis *et al.*, 1977a) and newborn rat bone (Wettenhall *et al.*, 1969; Schwartz *et al.*, 1970). This could be demonstrated at concentrations as low as $10^{-9}M$, a level only twice that of the normal rat serum concentration (Canalis *et al.*, 1977a). The increase in collagen synthesis does not appear to reflect a generalized stimulation of cell growth, since collagen synthesis was found to be greater than noncollagen protein synthesis.

In vivo studies in rats have also provided strong evidence for an effect of insulin on bone metabolism. Diabetic rats have reduced incorporation of calcium and citrate into bone which is corrected by insulin administration (Dixit and Stern, 1979). A reduction in osteoid, a failure to acquire a tetracycline label, reduced numbers of osteoclasts and a reduction of bone alkaline phosphatase has been demonstrated in a second study of diabetic rats (Shires *et al.*, 1981). Insulin has also been shown to stimulate matrix-induced cartilage and bone formation (Weiss and Reddi, 1980).

Evidence to support abnormal metabolic activity of bone in diabetic patients has been minimal. An increase in total serum alkaline phosphatase activity is a feature often found in diabetes mellitus (Heath *et al.*, 1979). This finding has usually been attributed to release of liver or intestinal alkaline phosphatase. In the only study of the activity of the bone isoenzyme, increased activity was found in patients on dietary, drug, and insulin regimens (Štěpán *et al.*, 1980).

The above studies should lead one to expect that insulin deficiency in humans would result in decreased bone mass. This appears to be the case in children with diabetes mellitus. Three studies utilizing the Norland-Cameron Bone-Mineral Analyzer have shown a significant decrease in bone mass of the forearm as compared to sex- and age-matched controls (Levin *et al.*, 1976; Rosenbloom *et al.*, 1977; McNair *et al.*, 1978, 1979). In one study, the greatest abnormality was found in white females (Rosenbloom *et al.*, 1977). Levin *et al.* (1976) commented that the abnormality probably reflects the underlying disease and not the effects of insulin deficiency, since they found no correlation of severity with insulin requirements or duration of the disease. The opposite conclusion was reached by Rosenbloom *et al.* (1977) who found a much lower frequency of decreased bone mass in white females after 5 years of insulin therapy. McNair *et al.* (1978, 1979), in the largest study, found that the loss of bone mass appeared to coincide with the onset of clinical diabetes mellitus and that the deficit was greater in patients whose disease developed before age 20 than after age 25. They also found that the bone mineral content was inversely correlated with the fasting blood glucose, glycosuria, and the insulin requirement. Elevated urinary excretion of calcium was common during the early course of the disease and correlated with the loss of skeletal mineral. No histologic studies of bone from diabetic children have been reported.

Studies in adults with diabetes mellitus have produced quite variable results. Although some patients may have a decreased bone mass (Hernberg, 1952; Levin *et al.*, 1976; Ringe *et al.*, 1976; DeLeeuw and Abs, 1977; McNair *et al.*, 1978), many patients have no demonstrable loss of bone by radiologic (Meema and Reid, 1969; Forgács *et al.*, 1976), ^{125}I photon-absorption (DeLeeuw and Abs, 1977), or histologic evaluation (Kelin and Frost, 1964; DeLeeuw *et al.*, 1976). In fact, it has been shown that an increased bone mass is not an uncommon finding (Kelin and Frost, 1964; Meema and Reid, 1969; DeLeeuw *et al.*, 1976; Forgács *et al.*, 1976; DeLeeuw and Abs, 1977). It is likely that several factors account for the variability in findings of the above studies. The age of onset of diabetes mellitus, the degree of insulin deficiency, the duration of therapy, the type of therapy (insulin versus sulfonylurea compounds), the methods used to evaluate bone mass, and other environmental and genetic influences undoubtedly interact to produce a wide range of bone architecture in the diabetic patient. Despite the recent interest in the bone density of diabetic patients, it is still unclear as to whether these patients are susceptible to fracture. A large survey in Rochester, Minnesota revealed that the risk of skeletal fracture in diabetics was not increased (Heath *et al.*, 1980).

C. Interaction with Kidney

In experimental diabetes (Weber *et al.*, 1976) and in patients with diabetic ketoacidosis (Seldin and Tarail, 1950; Raskin *et al.*, 1978; McNair *et al.*, 1979), hypercalciuria and/or hyperphosphaturia have been noted. It has been suggested that associated metabolic acidosis and osmotic diuresis are responsible for these findings. It is also possible that relative insulin deficiency could account for hyperphosphaturia since phosphate excretion is decreased by insulin infusion in normal subjects (DeFronzo *et al.*, 1975). In the same study urinary calcium excretion was increased during insulin infusion.

D. Interaction with Intestine

A large body of evidence has accumulated that points to a role of insulin in the intestinal transport of calcium in experimental animals. Either alloxan or streptozotocin-induced diabetes in the rat produces reduced duodenal calcium absorption (Schneider and Schedl, 1972, 1977; Schneider *et al.*, 1975, 1976, 1977a), which can be restored by insulin treatment (Schneider *et al.*, 1977a). An associated abnormality in experimental diabetes is a decrease in duodenal calcium-binding protein (Schneider and Schedl, 1977). It has been demonstrated that either $1,25(OH)_2D_3$ or 1α-hydroxycholecalciferol is capable of returning duodenal calcium transport to normal (Schneider *et al.*, 1976). In contrast, vitamin D_3 or $25(OH)D_3$ administration failed to alter calcium transport in this study. These observations provide indirect evidence that decreased calcium transport arises as a result of an abnormality in 1α-hydroxylation of $25(OH)D_3$. Direct evidence of the role of vitamin D in the calcium malabsorption associated with experimental diabetes mellitus was provided by the observation that diabetic rats have serum $1,25(OH)_2D_3$ concentrations one-eighth to one-half that of normal rats (Schneider *et al.*, 1977b; Shires *et al.*, 1981). Insulin treatment restores the concentration to normal. These results do not distinguish between impaired synthesis or increased catabolism as the pathogenesis of the low serum $1,25(OH)_2D_3$ concentration. A study of the synthesis and metabolic clearance of this metabolite in diabetic rats suggested that the action of insulin was to stimulate renal 25-hydroxyvitamin D_3-1α-hydroxylase activity (Spencer *et al.*, 1980). Insulin permitted parathyroid hormone stimulation of $1,25(OH)_2D_3$ production in cultured chick kidney cells but did not have an effect alone (Henry, 1981).

In three studies of experimental diabetes in the rat, parathyroid hormone concentration in the circulation was found to be increased (Schneider *et al.*, 1974; Weber *et al.*, 1976; Schedl *et al.*, 1978). This evidence of secondary hyperparathyroidism is consistent with a homeostatic attempt to stimulate renal 25-hydroxyvitamin D_3 1α-hydroxylase activity and restore intestinal calcium absorption to normal. Inexplicably, low levels of parathyroid hormone were reported in one study of diabetic rats (Shires *et al.*, 1981).

In one study of intestinal magnesium absorption in diabetic rats there was a decrease in duodenal magnesium absorption when expressed per gram dry weight of mucosa (Miller and Schedl, 1976). However, the absorptive capacity of a given segment-length of duodenum was unchanged due to a marked increase of mucosal growth in diabetic animals. This finding contrasts with the studies of calcium absorption in that both specific absorption and segment absorptive capacity of calcium are both reduced. The difference between magnesium and calcium absorption in diabetic rats suggests an inherent difference in the regulation of transport of these divalent cations in the rat.

The relevance of the animal studies to the osteopenia of human diabetes has been challenged by a study comparing 40 healthy subjects with 82 diabetic patients (Heath *et al.*, 1979). No differences in intestinal calcium absorption, serum 1,25$(OH)_2D$ concentration or serum parathyroid hormone concentration were detected.

E. Summary

A number of *in vitro* studies have demonstrated the anabolic effects of insulin on bone. Insulin enhances incorporation of pyrimidine nucleosides into bone cell nucleotide and RNA pools, stimulates membrane transport of amino acids in fetal rat calvaria and stimulates bone collagen synthesis. In children with diabetes mellitus a decrease in bone mass has been observed. This finding is less predictable in adults. Studies in experimental animals have focused on the observation that drug-induced diabetes mellitus produces reduced intestinal calcium absorption that is reversed by insulin treatment. Serum 1,25$(OH)_2D_3$ levels are reduced in the diabetic animals and return to normal after insulin treatment.

VII. GLUCAGON

A. Mode of Action

Glucagon is a peptide hormone whose main physiologic role is the control of blood glucose concentration. The hyperglycemic effect of this hormone is mediated by stimulation of hepatic glycogenolysis and gluconeogenesis. These effects are initiated by binding of glucagon to receptors on hepatic cell plasma membranes and activation of membrane-bound adenylate cyclase (Pohl, 1977).

Evidence that glucagon may be a factor in mineral metabolism is provided by the observation that glucagon administration produces transient hypocalcemia in the dog, rabbit, rat, sheep, and man (Paloyan *et al.*, 1967a,b; Aliapoulios and Morain, 1968; Bowser *et al.*, 1968; Avioli *et al.*, 1969; Barlet, 1969; Birge and Avioli, 1969; Ottenjann and Deyhle, 1969; Pickleman *et al.*, 1969; Tanzer *et al.*, 1970; Williams *et al.*, 1969; Federspil *et al.*, 1970; Hattner *et al.*, 1970; Raman, 1970b; Ulbrych-Jablonska, 1972; Aliapoulios *et al.*, 1973). It has also been suggested that endogenous glucagon release in patients with acute pancreatitis may be primarily responsible for the hypocalcemia encountered in such patients (Paloyan *et al.*, 1976b). Data concerning the mechanism by which glucagon induces hypocalcemia will now be considered.

B. Interaction with Bone

The hypocalcemic effect of glucagon appears to arise primarily from a direct action on the skeleton, although there is also evidence of an indirect action. The known stimulation of calcitonin secretion by glucagon (see Chapter 8, this volume) suggested that the hypocalcemia was due to a decrease in bone resorption mediated by calcitonin. Evidence to support this hypothesis was provided by studies in dogs (Avioli *et al.*, 1969) and rabbits (Pickleman *et al.*, 1969) where thyroidectomy was found to prevent a hypocalcemic response to glucagon. In contrast, four studies in rats clearly indicated that the hypocalcemic response was not dependent on the presence of the thyroid gland (Williams *et al.*, 1969; Hattner *et al.*, 1970; Stern and Bell, 1970; Tanzer *et al.*, 1970). The hypocalcemic response to glucagon in humans is dependent to a great extent on the serum calcium concentration, a larger decrease being found in hypercalcemic patients and a smaller or no decrease being found in normocalcemic subjects (Paloyan *et al.*, 1967a; Birge and Avioli, 1969; Ottenjann and Deyhle, 1969; Federspil *et al.*, 1970; Ulbrych-Jablonska, 1972). Of interest also is the finding that glucagon infusions in normocalcemic or hypocalcemic patients with pancreatitis produce no significant fall in serum calcium concentration (Condon *et al.*, 1975; Robertson *et al.*, 1976). No studies in athyroidal patients have been reported.

A direct effect of glucagon on bone *in vitro* has been reported in two studies. Stern and Bell (1970) found that glucagon inhibited bone resorption in embryonic rat bone cultures stimulated with either parathyroid hormone or dibutyryl-3′,5′-adenosine monophosphate. No effect could be found in unstimulated cultures, an observation opposite to that found with calcitonin (see Chapter 8, this volume). Gozariu *et al.* (1971) reported identical results in a study utilizing newborn rat bone in culture. Kalu *et al.* (1972) studied the effect of administered glucagon on bone collagen metabolism in the thyroparathyroidectomized rat and also concluded that glucagon inhibited parathyroid hormone-induced bone resorption but had little effect in normal rats.

Williams *et al.* (1969) compared the effects of calcitonin and glucagon on ^{47}Ca kinetics and suggested that glucagon produced hypocalcemia by promoting uptake of ^{47}Ca by bone. A subsequent study demonstrated that glucagon administration produced increased femoral weight in control and immobilized rat extremities, although a relative degree of osteoporosis was present in the immobilized extremity (Woodward and Jowsey, 1972). This observation would tend to support the concept of glucagon as an inducer of bone formation. However, Kalu *et al.* (1972) found that glucagon inhibited incorporation of proline into rat bone *in vivo* and Canalis *et al.* (1977a) reported that glucagon inhibited proline incorporation into embryonic rat bone *in vitro*. In man, administration of glucagon may decrease bone resorption and bone formation as evidenced by a rapid decrease in urinary hydroxyproline excretion and plasma alkaline phosphatase concentration in patients with Paget's disease treated with glucagon (Condon, 1971). These effects were not found in a subsequent study, possibly because the glucagon doses administered were somewhat lower (Singer *et al.*, 1978). In general, very large doses of glucagon are required to produce effects on mineral metabolism. This suggests that this hormone may not play an important physiologic role in the regulation of mineral metabolism.

C. Interaction with Kidney

It has been found in the dog that pharmacologic doses of glucagon induce significant increases in urinary calcium excretion (Charbon *et al.*, 1963; Dewonck *et al.*, 1963; Pullman *et al.*, 1967). This has not been confirmed in man (Birge and Avioli, 1969). Since nephrectomy did not abolish the hypocalcemic effect of glucagon in any species studied (Avioli *et al.*, 1969; Williams *et al.*, 1969; Tanzer *et al.*, 1970; Aliapoulios *et al.*, 1973), it is unlikely that the hypocalcemic effect is dependent on renal calcium excretion.

Glucagon administration also produces hypophosphatemia of a significant degree (Avioli *et al.*, 1969; Tanzer *et al.*, 1970; Aliapoulios *et al.*, 1973). Increased renal excretion of inorganic phosphate has been found after glucagon administration in dogs and humans (Staub *et al.*, 1957; Elrick *et al.*, 1958; Charbon *et al.*, 1963; Pullman *et al.*, 1967). In two studies undertaken in nephrectomized rats, contradictory results were obtained concerning the role of the kidney in glucagon-induced hypophosphatemia. Tanzer *et al.* (1970) found that prior nephrectomy did not alter the hypophosphatemic response, whereas Aliapoulios *et al.* (1973) observed a diminution in hypophosphatemia following nephrectomy.

D. Interaction with Intestine

Little is known of the effect of glucagon on intestinal transport of calcium. A study in rats demonstrated that removal of the entire gastrointestinal tract, but not the stomach alone, decreased the hypocalcemic effect of glucagon (Aliapoulios *et al.*, 1973). In this study, intestinal transport of calcium was not assessed, so that the possibility of a direct effect of glucagon on calcium transport was not substantiated. A study of the effect of glucagon on colonic radiocalcium excretion in rats revealed that fecal radiocalcium was reduced tenfold in glucagon-treated rats as compared to control rats given systemic ^{45}Ca (Bogdat *et al.*, 1974). The latter study does not support the hypothesis that the intestine is involved in the hypocalcemic response to glucagon.

E. Summary

Glucagon, in pharmacologic doses, is capable of producing transient hypocalcemia in a variety of species. This response is dependent on the presence of the thyroid gland in dogs and rabbits but not in rats. In rats, removal of the entire gastrointestinal tract reduced the hypocalcemic response. *In vitro* studies have demonstrated a direct effect of glucagon on bone resorption. Parathyroid hormone-induced bone resorption was inhibited by glucagon in two studies, although no effect was found on unstimulated bone. The physiologic significance of these observations is unclear.

VIII. GASTROINTESTINAL HORMONES

A. Gastrin

Gastrin is a peptide hormone of considerable structural heterogeneity found in mucosal cells of the gastric antrum, in the D cells of the pancreas and in the mucosa of the small intestine, primarily the proximal duodenum. The hormone is a potent secretagogue of gastric acid and affects esophageal motility, as well as muscle contraction of the stomach, small and large intestine, gallbladder, and uterus. The mode of action of the hormone is unknown; adenylate cyclase activation is not the mediator of its biological effects.

The administration of gastrin to pigs, lambs, and rats produces a significant degree of hypocalcemia (Care *et al.*, 1971; Cooper *et al.*, 1971, 1972; Barlet, 1973; Schulak and Kaplan, 1974, 1975; Kaplan *et al.*, 1977; Krishnamra and Limlomwongse, 1978). Since it was known that gastrin or pentagastrin could stimulate calcitonin release (see Chapter 8, this volume), it was initially thought that the hypocalcemic effect of gastrin was mediated by calcitonin. This speculation was supported by the observations that thyroidectomy abolished the hypocalcemic effect in the pig (Care *et al.*, 1971), in the lamb (Barlet, 1973), and in the rat (Cooper *et al.*, 1972). In subsequent studies in which younger rats were used and/or higher doses of gastrin were administered, the hypocalcemic effect persisted in the absence of the thyroid (Schulak and Kaplan, 1974, 1975; Kaplan *et al.*, 1977; Krishnamra and Limlomwongse, 1978). In the studies of Schulak and Kaplan, prior total gastrectomy or removal of the proximal 75% of the stomach abolished the hypocalcemic effect of gastrin. An increase in gastric calcium excretion has been observed in response to gastrin administration and could, in part, account for the role of the stomach (Krishnamra and Limlomwongse, 1978). Increased fecal calcium excretion after gastrin administration has been found in normal and thyroidectomized sheep (Barlet, 1973). It is not known what was the source of the fecal calcium in this study. Synthetic tetragastrin increased calcium absorption *in vivo* in a rat duodenal loop study (Fujita, 1973). This was found in intact but not parathyroidectomized animals.

Stimulation of endogenous hypergastrinemia by gastric antral exclusion in rats does not result in hypocalcemia (Grimelius *et al.*, 1977). This could be due to the induction of parathyroid hyperplasia observed in the animals. Parathyroid hormone assays were not done in this study. In sheep 1-hr infusions of gastrin failed to stimulate parathyroid hormone secretion (Jaffe *et al.*, 1974).

Gastrin does not increase urinary calcium excretion (Barlet, 1973; Krishnamra and Limlomwongse, 1978) and nephrectomy does not abolish its hypocalcemic effect in rats (Schulak and Kaplan, 1975).

Cholecystokinin-pancreozymin, which contains the same carboxyl-terminal four amino acids as gastrin, is also a hypocalcemic agent in lambs (Barlet and Garel, 1976).

B. Secretin

Secretin, the first hormone to be recognized, is a peptide found in the proximal small intestine. Administration of this hormone results in increased bicarbonate and water secretion by the exocrine pancreas. Secretin also acts on the endocrine pancreas through a stimulatory effect on insulin secretion. The action of the hormone appears to be mediated through activation of adenylate cyclase (Schwartz *et al.*, 1974).

There is no evidence of an effect of endogenous secretin on calcium metabolism, but observation of an increase in serum calcium concentration in a patient with Zollinger-Ellison syndrome given secretin prompted further studies (Isenberg *et al.*, 1972). Infusion of secretin in normal subjects and patients with Zollinger-Ellison syndrome and primary hyperparathyroidism produced a significant increase in total and ionized serum calcium in one study (Isenberg *et al.*, 1973). A subsequent study in normal subjects, duodenal ulcer patients, and patients with primary hyperparathyroidism revealed a rise in total calcium but not ionized calcium concentration during secretin infusion (Schwille *et al.*, 1975). Two other studies in man (J. C. Thompson *et al.*, 1972; Bradley *et al.*, 1975) and one in the rat (Kaplan *et al.*, 1977) failed to demonstrate any significant hypercalcemia due to secretin. It is unclear as to why there is such variability in the results. An elegant *in vitro* study of the effect of secretin on isolated bovine parathyroid cells did demonstrate a simultaneous rise in intracellular cyclic AMP accumulation and parathyroid hormone release (Windeck *et al.*, 1978).

C. Vasoactive Intestinal Polypeptide

Vasoactive intestinal polypeptide (VIP) is a 28-amino-acid putative hormone found in the intestine and nervous system that has been demonstrated to have pharmacologic effects on the cardiovascular, respiratory, and gastrointestinal systems. The gastrointestinal effects of this peptide appear to be mediated by cyclic AMP and include increased fecal loss of water and electrolytes and achlorhydria (Schwartz *et al.*, 1974). These findings are common in a syndrome termed Verner-Morrison Syndrome (Verner and Morrison, 1958), pancreatic cholera, watery diarrhea syndrome, or the syndrome of watery diarrhea, hypokalemia, and achlorhydria. Most of the patients with this syndrome have a pancreatic islet cell tumor. Recent studies have indicated that VIP may be a factor in the pathogenesis of this syndrome, since elevated serum and tissue concentrations of VIP have been found in most patients (Bloom *et al.*, 1973; Rambaud *et al.*, 1975; Gagel *et al.*, 1976; Shields and Haff, 1976; Holdaway *et al.*, 1977; Bloom, 1978; Cooperman *et al.*, 1978). Other diarrheogenic agents such as prostaglandin E have also been implicated in the pathogenesis of this syndrome (Jaffe *et al.*, 1977).

Hypercalcemia has been observed in some patients with the Verner-Morrison syndrome and is reversible when the pancreatic tumor is resected (Verner and Morrison, 1958, 1974; Holdaway *et al.*, 1977). It is not certain whether VIP is responsible for the abnormal calcium homeostasis. In a preliminary report, VIP injection raised serum calcium concentrations by 5% after 10 min in dogs (Makhlouf *et al.*, 1974). However, in the rat VIP caused no detectable hypercalcemia (Kaplan *et al.*, 1977). It has also been reported that prostaglandin E (Jaffe *et al.*, 1977) and parathyroid hormone (Hirose *et al.*, 1975) may be involved in the pathogenesis of the hypercalcemia. Since there also are patients with hypercalcemia and low serum PTH concentrations (Rambaud *et al.*, 1975; Gagel *et al.*, 1976; Holdaway *et al.*, 1977) and patients with elevated plasma prostaglandin E levels who are normocalcemic (Rambaud *et al.*, 1975), further studies will be required to determine the pathogenesis of hypercalcemia in this syndrome.

D. Summary

The gastrointestinal hormones gastrin, secretin, and vasoactive intestinal peptide have all been reported to exert an influence on extracellular fluid calcium concentration. Gastrin administration to a variety of species produces transient hypocalcemia. Secretin has been reported to raise the serum calcium concentration in two studies, but other studies have failed to confirm the hypercalcemic effect. Hypercalcemia is sometimes found in patients with the syndrome of watery diarrhea, hypokalemia, and achlorhydria. These patients usually harbor a pancreatic tumor and have elevated serum and tumor vasoactive intestinal peptide concentrations. The physiologic significance of the above observations is unknown.

IX. EPINEPHRINE

Epinephrine, the catecholamine primarily synthesized in the adrenal medulla, interacts with beta adrenergic receptors in numerous organs and thereby influences the regulation of blood flow, blood glucose and free fatty acid concentrations, renal sodium reabsorption, bowel, and bladder tone and body temperature. These actions of epinephrine are associated with activation of adenylate cyclase.

Interest in the role of epinephrine in mineral metabolism has existed for more than 50 years since it was first recognized that epinephrine could influence calcium concentration in the circulation (Kenny, 1964). As Kenny has pointed out, the early studies produced conflicting results, with both hypercalcemia and hypocalcemia reported to have resulted from epinephrine administration. Studies during the past 15 years have to some extent helped clarify the complex interaction between epinephrine and extracellular calcium regulation.

Administration of epinephrine or other β-adrenergic agonists causes an acute increase in parathyroid hormone (see Chapter 6, this volume) and calcitonin (see Chapter 8) secretion in several species including man. In intact animals there is usually no detectable change in blood calcium concentration after β-adrenergic stimulation (Kenny, 1964; Morey and Kenny, 1964; Wells and Lloyd, 1968; Fischer *et al.*, 1973; Hsu and Cooper, 1975; Kukreja *et al.*, 1975; Blum *et al.*, 1978; Harney *et al.*, 1978; Metz *et al.*, 1978), although a small degree of hypocalcemia has sometimes been reported (Phillippo *et al.*, 1970; Fischer *et al.*, 1973; Vora *et al.*, 1978). A simultaneous rise in calcitonin secretion may prevent a hypercalcemic response (Harney *et al.*, 1978). In parathyroidectomized animals β-adrenergic agonists can elevate blood calcium concentration, whether or not the thyroid gland is present (Kenny, 1964; Morey and Kenny, 1964; Wells and Lloyd, 1968; Hsu and Cooper, 1975). This suggests that calcitonin secretion is not solely responsible for blocking a parathyroid-induced hypercalcemic response to epinephrine in intact animals. It may be that a prevailing normal rate of bone resorption in intact animals does not permit the hypercalcemic action of β-adrenergic stimulation to be expressed.

There are 15 case reports of patients with pheochromocytoma and hypercalcemia in whom adrenalectomy was reported to reverse the hypercalcemic state (Swinton *et al.*, 1972; Kukreja *et al.*, 1973; Bouillon *et al.*, 1974; Finlayson and Casey, 1975; Ghose *et al.*, 1976; Gray and Gillon, 1976; Kalager *et al.*, 1977; Atuk *et al.*, 1979). Parathyroid hormone concentrations in the circulation were measured in eight patients and found to be elevated or inappropriately detectable in seven patients. In no patient was an arteriovenous gradient of parathyroid hormone concentration measured in an attempt to localize the site of abnormal parathyroid hormone secretion. Also no tumor was examined for parathyroid hormone content. In a group of ten normocalcemic patients with pheochromocytoma, serum parathyroid hormone concentrations were normal (Miller *et al.*, 1975). In man it seems unlikely that a chronic excess of catecholamines in the circulation leads to hypercalcemia. The hypercalcemia reversed by adrenalectomy in patients with pheochromocytoma appears to result from ectopic secretion of parathyroid hormone or other hypercalcemic agents.

The hypercalcemic effect of epinephrine in parathyroidectomized animals probably can be explained by a direct effect of the hormone on bone. A renal mechanism is ruled out by the observation that epinephrine increases urinary calcium in parathyroidectomized rats (Morey and Kenny, 1964). A gastrointestinal effect also is unlikely since rats that have fasted for 18–24 hr still manifest hypercalcemia (Hsu and Cooper, 1975). Consistent with the hypothesis of a direct skeletal action of epinephrine are the observations that cyclic 3′5′ adenosine monophosphate content is increased by epinephrine in isolated bone cells (Peck *et al.*, 1974; Rodan and Rodan, 1974) and in fetal rat calvaria (Chase and Aurbach, 1970). It has yet to be reported that epinephrine increases bone resorption *in vitro*. This information is needed to help establish the mechanism by which β-adrenergic agonists can increase extracellular calcium concentration.

X. ERYTHROPOIETIN

Erythropoietin is a glycoprotein with a molecular weight of approximately 60,000. It is thought to be synthesized by the kidney and/or by the liver in response to a renal factor and to be released into the circulation in response to blood loss or a lowering of plasma oxygen tension. The hormone acts to stimulate erythropoiesis and release red cells from the bone marrow into the systemic circulation (Gordon, 1973).

Perris and Whitfield (1971) observed that acute blood loss in rats resulted in significant hypercalcemia beginning 24 hr after induction of hemorrhage. The hypercalcemia persisted for several days and returned to normal coincident with correction of the anemia. Thyroparathyroidectomy prior to hemorrhage prevented the hypercalcemic response and also the rapid restoration of red cell mass. Since significant hypocalcemia occurred during the initial 24 hr after hemorrhage, it was hypothesized that an overshoot of parathyroid hormone secretion in response to the early hypocalcemia might explain the transient hypercalcemia. However, subsequent studies utilizing exogenous erythropoietin in rats suggest a role of this hormone in calcium homeostasis (Hunt and Perris, 1973). Exogenous hormone administered subcutaneously produced a rise of plasma calcium concentration of the order of 1 mg/dl. This hypercalcemic effect was abolished by prior parathyroidectomy. Since parathyroid hormone levels were not measured, it is not known whether erythropoietin is capable of stimulating parathyroid hormone secretion or whether it potentiates the peripheral actions of the hormone.

There is little evidence to support the role of erythropoietin in the physiology or pathophysiology of calcium homeostasis in man. In one unconfirmed study of children with congenital heart disease and elevated hematocrits, ionized calcium concentrations were elevated (Putnam, 1972).

XI. SUMMARY

Many hormones whose principal actions are not directed towards mineral metabolism do contribute in a minor or even major fashion to mineral homeostasis. These hormones may act directly on the skeleton, intestine, and kidney or may influence the function of these organs by interacting with the major hormonal regulators of mineral metabolism.

Steroid hormones have a profound effect on the skeleton. An excess of endogenous cortisol or pharmacologic doses of glucocorticosteroids may produce a marked deficit in bone mass. Deficiency of estrogens or testosterone also contributes to the development of osteoporosis.

Thyroid hormone directly influences bone metabolic activity. In hyperthyroidism hypercalcemia and/or osteoporosis may occur when the rate of bone resorption exceeds that of bone formation. The main skeletal manifestation of hypothyroidism is failure of epiphyseal development leading to short stature.

Growth hormone, through the intermediary action of somatomedin, is the critical hormonal regulator of growth. Dwarfism and gigantism or acromegaly may result from deficiency or excess of the hormone, respectively. Growth hormone also induces an increase in intestinal calcium absorption and may produce hypercalcemia, possibly by a stimulation of $1,25(OH)_2D$ production.

Prolactin may be responsible for the increased intestinal calcium absorption found in lactating women and perhaps in pregnant women. Prolactin also is capable of stimulating $1,25(OH)_2D$ production in animals.

The pancreatic hormones insulin and glucagon affect mineral homeostasis in differing degrees. Insulin is required for normal bone development in children. In animals, insulin deficiency results in decreased intestinal calcium absorption in association with low levels of $1,25(OH)_2D_3$. Glucagon, in pharmacologic doses, produces transient hypocalcemia, but its physiologic role is unknown.

Gastrin, secretin, and vasoactive intestinal peptide have been shown to alter the extracellular calcium concentration in animals but the physiologic role of these gastrointestinal hormones is not clear.

Epinephrine can produce hypercalcemia in parathyroidectomized animals, but this has not been demonstrated in man.

Erythropoietin has been reported to raise the serum calcium concentration in rats. Prior parathyroidectomy prevents the response. Definitive studies in man are lacking.

REFERENCES

Adams, N. D., Garthwaite, T. L., Gray, R. W., Hagen, T. C. and Lemann, J., Jr. (1979). The interrelationships among prolactin, 1,25-dihydroxyvitamin D, and parathyroid hormone in humans. *J. Clin. Endocrinol. Metab.* **49,** 628–630.

Adams, P., and Jowsey, J. (1967). Bone and mineral metabolism in hyperthyroidism: An experimental study. *Endocrinology (Baltimore)* **81**, 735–740.

Adams, P. H., Jowsey, J., Kelly, P. J., Riggs, B. L., Kinney, V. R., and Jones, J. D. (1967). Effects of hyperthyroidism on bone and mineral metabolism in man. *Q. J. Med.* [N.S.] **36**, 1–15.

Adams, P., Chalmers, T. M., Riggs, B. L., Jr., and Jones, J. D. (1968). Parathyroid function in spontaneous primary hypothyroidism. *J. Endocrinol.* **40**, 467–475.

Aitken, J. M., Hart, D. M., and Smith, D. A. (1971). The effect of long-term mestranol administration on calcium and phosphorus homeostasis in oophorectomized women. *Clin. Sci.* **41**, 233–236.

Aitken, J. M., Armstrong, E., and Anderson, J. B. (1972). Osteoporosis after oophorectomy in the mature female rat and the effect of oestrogen and/or progestogen replacement therapy in its prevention. *J. Endocrinol.* **55**, 79–87.

Aitken, J. M., Hart, D. M., and Lindsay, R. (1973a). Osteoporosis after oophorectomy for non-malignant disease in premenopausal women. *Br. Med. J.* **2**, 325–328.

Aitken, J. M., Hart, D. M., Anderson, J. B., Lindsay, R., Smith, D. A., and Speirs, C. F. (1973b). Oestrogen replacement therapy for prevention of osteoporosis after oophorectomy. *Br. Med. J.* **3**, 515–518.

Albright, F., Smith, D. H., and Richardson, A. M. (1941). Postmenopausal osteoporosis. *JAMA, J. Am. Med. Assoc.* **116**, 2465–2474.

Aliapoulios, M. A., and Morain, W. D. (1968). Comparative hypocalcemic and hypophosphatemic effects of glucagon and thyrocalcitonin. *Surg. Forum* **19**, 379–380.

Aliapoulios, M. A., Voelkel, E. F., and Munson, P. L. (1966). Assay of human thyroid gland for thyrocalcitonin activity. *J. Clin. Endocrinol. Metab.* **26**, 897–901.

Aliapoulios, M. A., Morain, W. D., and Kacoyanis, G. P. (1973). Glucagon as a hypocalcemic and hypophosphatemic agent in the rat. *Gastroenterology* **65**, 912–918.

Aloia, J. F., Roginsky, M. S., Jowsey, J., Dombrowski, C. S., Shukla, K., and Cohn, S. H. (1972). Skeletal metabolism and body composition in acromegaly. *J. Clin. Endocrinol. Metab.* **35**, 543–551.

Aloia, J. F., Roginsky, M., Ellis, K., Shukla, K., and Cohn, S. (1974). Skeletal metabolism and body composition in Cushing's Syndrome. *J. Clin. Endocrinol. Metab.* **39**, 981–985.

Aloia, J., Powell, D., Mendizibal, E., and Roginsky, M. (1975). Parathyroid function in acromegaly. *Horm. Res.* **6**, 145–149.

Aloia, J. F., Zanzi, I., Ellis, K., Jowsey, J., Roginsky, M., Wallach, S., and Cohn, S. H. (1976). Effects of growth hormone in osteoporosis. *J. Clin. Endocrinol. Metab.* **43**, 992–999.

Aloia, J. F., Zanzi, I., Vaswani, A., Ellis, K., and Cohn, S. H. (1977). Combination therapy for osteoporosis. *Metab. Clin. Exp.* **26**, 787–792.

Aloia, J. F., and Yeh, J. K. (1980). Growth hormone and intestinal calcium transport in the rat. *Metab. Bone Dis. and Rel. Res.* **2** 251–255.

Altenahr, E., and Kampf, E. (1976). Parathyroid function in rats treated with growth hormone. *Virchows Arch. A: Pathol. Anat. Histol.* **371**, 363–371.

Anderson, H. J. (1961). Studies of hypothyroidism in children. *Acta Paediatr. Scand.* **50**; Suppl. **125**, 11–107.

Anderson, I. A. (1950). Postmenopausal osteoporosis, clinical manifestations and the treatment with oestrogens. *Q. J. Med.* [N.S.] **19**, 67–69.

Anderson, J., and Foster, J. B. (1959). The effect of cortisone on urinary phosphate excretion in man. *Clin. Sci.* **18**, 437–439.

Armbrecht, H. J., Zenser, T. V., and Davis, B. B. (1980). Effect of age on the conversion of 25-hydroxyvitamin D_3 to 1,25dihydroxyvitamin D_3 by kidney of rat. *J. Clin. Invest. 1118–1123.*

Askanazy, M., and Rutishauser, E. (1933). Die Knochen der Basedow-kranken. *Virchows Arch. Pathol. Anat. Physiol.* **291,** 653–681.

Askenasi, R., and Demeester-Mirkine, N. (1975). Urinary excretion of hydroxy-lysylglycosides and thyroid function. *J. Clin. Endocrinol Metab.* **40,** 342–344.

Atkins, D., and Peacock, M. (1975). A comparison of the effects of the calcitonins, steroid hormones, and thyroid hormones on the response of bone to parathyroid hormone in tissue culture. *J. Endocrinol.* **64,** 573–583.

Atkins, D., Zanelli, J. M., Peacock, M., and Nordin, B. E. C. (1972). The effect of oestrogens on the response of bone to parathyroid hormone in vitro. *J. Endocrinol.* **54,** 107–117.

Atuk, N. O., McDonald, T., Wood, T., Carpenter, J. T., Walzak, M. P., Donaldson, M., and Gillenwater, J. Y. (1979). Familial pheochromocytoma, hypercalcemia, and von Hippel-Lindau disease. *Medicine* **58,** 209–218.

Au, W. (1976). Cortisol stimulation of parathyroid hormone secretion by rat parathyroid glands in organ culture. *Science* **193,** 1015–1017.

Aub, J. C., Bauer, W., Heath, C., and Ropes, M. (1929). Studies of calcium and phosphorus metabolism. III. The effects of thyroid hormone and thyroid disease. *J. Clin. Invest.* **7,** 97–137.

Aubert, J. P., Cherian, A. G., Moukhtar, M. S., and Milhaud, G. (1964). Etude du metabolisme du calcium chez le rat a l'aide de calcium 45. V. La thyroparathyroidectomie et l'effet de la thyroxine et da la parathormone. *Biochem. Pharmacol.* **13,** 31–44.

Avioli, L., McDonald, J. E., and Lee, S. W. (1965). The influence of age on the intestinal absorption of ^{47}Ca in women and its relation to ^{47}Ca absorption in postmenopausal osteoporosis. *J. Clin. Invest.* **44,** 1960–1967.

Avioli, L. V., Birge, S. J., Scott, S., and Shieber, W. (1969). Role of the thyroid gland during glucagon induced hypocalcemia in the dog. *Am. J. Physiol.* **216,** 939–945.

Baksi, S. N., and Kenny, A. D. (1977). Vitamine D_3 metabolism in immature Japanese quail: Effects of ovarian hormone. *Endocrinology (Baltimore)* **101,** 1216–1220.

Baksi, S. N., and Kenny, A. D. (1977). Vitamin D_3 metabolism in immature Japanese quail: Effects dihydroxy vitamin D_3 in the rat? *Life Sci.* **22,** 787–792.

Barlet, J. (1969). Etude de l'influence du glucagon et de l'arginine sur la calcémie du lapin et de la brebis. *C. R. Hebd. Seances Acad Sci.* **269,** 621–624.

Barlet, J. P. (1973). The influence of gastrin on the fecal and urinary excretion of water, calcium, magnesium and inorganic phosphorus in sheep. *Horm. Metab. Res.* **5,** 124–128.

Barlet, J. P., and Garel, J. M. (1976). Effect of an intravenous injection of cholecystokinin-pancreozymin on plasma calcium and calcitonin levels in newborn lambs. *J. Endocrinol.* **70,** 151–152.

Barrett, A. J., Sledge, C. B., and Dingle, J. T. (1966). Effect of cortisol on the synthesis of chondritin sulphate by embryonic cartilage. *Nature (London)* **211,** 83–84.

Bauer, W., and Aub, J. C. (1941). Studies of calcium and phosphorus metabolism. XVI. The influence of the pituitary gland. *J. Clin. Invest.* **20,** 295–301.

Baxter, J. D. (1976). Glucocorticoid hormone action. *Pharmacol. Ther.* **2,** 605–69.

Beaton, G. R. (1976). Studies on serum somatomedin activity and cartilage responsiveness in the regulation of growth. Thesis, Faculty of Science, University of Witwatersrand, Johannesberg, South Africa.

Beck, J. C., McGarry, E. E., Dyrenfurth, I., and Venning, E. H. (1957). Metabolic effects of human and monkey growth hormone in man. *Science* **125,** 884–885.

Beck, J. C., McGarry, E. E., Dyrenfurth, I., Morgen, R. O., Bird, E. D., and Venning, E. H. (1960). Primate growth hormone studies in man. *Metab. Clin. Exp.* **9,** 699–737.

Beck, J. C., Gonda, A., Hamid, M. A., Morgen, R. O., Rubinstein, D., and McGarry, E. E. (1964). Some metabolic changes induced by primate growth hormone and purified ovine prolactin. *Metab. Clin. Exp.* **13,** 1108–1134.

Becks, H., Simpson, M. E., Marx, W., Li, C. H., and Evans, H. M. (1944). Antagonism of pituitary adrenocorticotropic hormone (ACTH) to the action of growth hormone on the osseous system of of hypophysectomized rats. *Endocrinology (Baltimore)* **34,** 311–316.

Bell, N. H., and Bartter, F. C. (1967). Studies of ^{47}Ca metabolism in acromegaly. *J. Clin. Endocrinol. Metab.* **27,** 178–184.

Bergdahl, L. (1977). Hyperparathyroidism in thyrotoxicosis. *Am. J. Surg.* **133,** 206–210.

Bergenstal, D. M., and Lipsett, M. B. (1960). Metabolic effects of human growth hormone and growth hormone of other species in man. *J. Clin. Endocrinol. Metab.* **20,** 1427–1436.

Berlyne, G. M., Ben-Ari, J., Kushelevsky, A., Idelman, A., Galinsky, D., Hirsh, M., Shainkin, R., Yagil, R., and Zlotnik, M. (1974). The aetiology of senile osteoporosis: Secondary hyperparathyroidism due to renal failure. *Q. J. Med.* [N.S.] **175,** 505–521.

Bijvoet, O. L. M., and Majoor, C. L. H. (1965). The renal tubular reabsorption of phosphate in thyrotoxicosis. *Clin. Chim. Acta* **11,** 181–183.

Bijvoet, O. L. M., van der Sluys Veer, J., and Jansen, A. P. (1968). Effects of calcitonin on patients with Paget's disease, thyrotoxicosis, or hypercalcemia. *Lancet* **1,** 876–881.

Bikle, D. D., Spencer, E. M., Burke, W. H., and Rost, C. R. (1980). Prolactin but not growth hormone stimulates 1,25-dihydroxyvitamin D_3 production by chick renal preparations in vitro. *Endocrinology* **107,** 81–84.

Birge, S. J., and Avioli, L. V. (1969). Glucagon-induced hypocalcemia in man. *J. Clin. Endocrinol. Metab.* **29,** 213–218.

Blodgett, F. M., Burgin, L., Iezzoni, D., Gribetz, D., and Talbot, N. B. (1956). Effects of prolonged cortisone therapy on the statural growth, skeletal maturation and metabolic status of children. *N. Engl. J. Med.* **254,** 636–641.

Bloom, S. R. (1978). Vasoactive intestinal peptide, the major mediator of the WDHA (pancreatic cholera) syndrome: Value of measurement in diagnosis and treatment. *Am. J. Dig. Dis.* [N.S.] **23,** 373–376.

Bloom, S. R., Polak, J. M., and Pearse, A. G. E. (1973). Vasoactive intestinal polypeptide and watery diarrhea syndrome. *Lancet* **2,** 14–16.

Blum, J. W., Fischer, J. A., Hunziker, W. H., Binswanger, V., Picotti, G. B., DaPrada, M., and Guillebeau, A. (1978). Parathyroid hormone response to catecholamines and to changes in extracellular calcium in cows. *J. Clin. Invest.* **61,** 1113–1122.

Blunt, J. W., Jr., Plotz, C. M., Lattes, R., Howes, E. L., Meyer, K., and Ragan, C. (1950). Effect of cortisone on experimental fractures in the rabbit. *Proc. Soc. Exp. Biol. Med.* **73,** 678–681.

Boass, A., Toverud, S., McCain, T. A., Pike, J. W., and Haussler, M. R. (1977). Elevated serum levels of 1 α, 25-dihydroxycholecalciferol in lactating rats. *Nature (London)* **267,** 630–632.

Bogdat, J., Jedrychowski, A., Tarnowski, A., Dura, K., and Marszalek, Z. (1974). Effect of glucagon on radiocalcium excretion by the colon in rats after intracardial administration of ^{45}Ca. *Can. J. Physiol. Pharmacol.* **52,** 1230–1232.

Bogdonoff, M. D., Shock, N. W., and Parson, J. (1954). The effects of stilbesterol on the retention of nitrogen, calcium, phosphorus, and potassium in aged males with and without osteoporosis. *J. Gerontol.* **9,** 262–275.

Bohr, H. H., and Dawids, S. G. (1964). The effect of cortisone and anabolic steriods on the retention of radioactive calcium and strontium in rats. *Acta Endocrinol. (Copenhagen)* **47,** 223–230.

Bommer, J., Ritz, E., and Gegenbach, E. (1976). Parathyroid activity in hyperthyroidism. *Proc. Eur. Symp. Calcif. Tissues, 11th, 1976*. pp. 288–293.

Bordier, P., Matrajt, H., Miravet, L., and Hioco, D. (1965). Mesure histologique de la resorption osseuse dan l'ostéoporose: Etude préliminaire. *In* "Calcified Tissues" (L. J. Richelle and M. J. Dallenagne, eds.), pp. 39–50. Collection des Colloques de l'Université de Liège.

Bordier, P., Miravet, L., Matrajt, H., Hioco, D., and Ryckewaet, A. (1967). Bone changes in adult patients with abnormal thyroid function (with special reference to ^{45}Ca kinetics and quantitative histology.) *Proc. R. Soc. Med.* **60,** 26–28.

Bortz, W., Eisenberg, E., Bowers, C. Y., and Pont, M. (1961). Differentiation between thyroid and parathyroid causes of hypercalcemia. *Ann. Intern. Med.* **54,** 610–619.

Bouillon, R., and DeMoor, P. (1974). Parathyroid function in patients with hyper- or hypothyroidism. *J. Clin. Endocrinol. Metab.* **38,** 999–1004.

Bouillon, R., DeMoor, P., and Nagant de Deuxchaines, C. (1974). Pheochromocytoma and hyperparathyroidism. *Ann. Intern. Med.* **81,** 131.

Bouillon, R., Muls, E., and De Moor, P. (1980). Influence of thyroid function on the serum concentration of 1,25-dihydroxyvitamin D_3. *J. Clin. Endocrinol. Metab.* **51,** 793–797.

Bowser, E. N., Henderson, W. J., and Williams, G. A. (1968). Glucagon-induced hypocalcemia in the rat. *J. Lab. Clin. Med.* **72,** 857.

Bradley, E. L., III, Wenger, J., Smith, R. B., III, and Galambos, J. T. (1975). Serum calcium responses to exogenous secretin. *Arch. Surg. (Chicago)* **110,** 1221–1223.

Bradley, S. E., Stephan, F., Coelho, J. B., and Reville, P. (1974). The thyroid and the kidney. *Kidney Int.* **6,** 346–365.

Braid, F. (1951). Hypothyroidism in childhood. *Br. Med. J.* **1,** 1169–1176.

Braithwaite, G. D. (1975). The effect of growth hormone on calcium metabolism in the sheep. *Br. J. Nutr.* **33,** 309–314.

Braithwaite, G. D., Glascock, R. F., and Raizuddin, S. (1972). The effect of hexoestrol on calcium metabolism in the sheep. *Br. J. Nutr.* **28,** 269–273.

Bressot, C., Courpron, P., Edouward, C., and Meunier, P. (1976). Les hypogonadismes. *In* "Histomorphometric des Ostéopathies Endocieniennes," pp. 173–179. Association Corporative des Etudiants en Medecine de Lyon.

Breton, A., Vandendorf, F., Dubois, R., and Bubois, O. (1958). A propos d'un cas de myxoedème avec condensation osseuse. *Pediatric* **13,** 100.

Bronner, F., Richelle, L. J., Saville, P. D., Nicholas, J. A., and Cobb, J. R. (1963). Quantitation of Calcium Metabolism in Postmenopausal Osteoporosis and in Scoliosis. *J. Clin. Invest.* **42,** 898–905.

Brown, D. M., Jowsey, J., and Bradfor, D. S. (1974). Osteoporosis in ovarian dysgenesis. *J. Pediatr.* **84,** 816–820.

Brown, J., and Singer, F. R. (1969). Calcium metabolism in acromegaly. *Br. Med. J.* **2,** 50.

Bryson, M. F., Forbes, G. B., Amirhakimi, G. H., and Reina, J. C. (1972). Metabolic response to growth hormone administration with particular reference to the occurrence of hypercalcuria. *Pediatr. Res.* **6,** 743–751.

Buckle, R. M., Mason, A. M. S., and Middleton, J. E. (1969). Thyrotoxic hypercalcemia treated with porcine calcitonin. *Lancet* **1,** 1128–1130.

Bullamore, J. R., Gallagher, J. C., Wilkenson, R., and Nordin, B. E. C. (1970). Effect of age on calcium absorption. *Lancet* **2,** 535–537.

Burckhardt, P., Ruedi, B., and Felber, J. P. (1975). Estrogen-induced tetany in idiopathic hypoparathyroidism. *Horm. Res.* **6,** 321–328.

Burkhart, J. M., and Jowsey, J. (1967). Parathyroid and thyroid hormone in the development of immobilization osteoporosis. *Endocrinology* **81,** 1053–1062.

Burman, K. D., Monchik, J. M., Earll, J. M., and Wartofsky, L. (1976). Ionized and total serum calcium and parathyroid hormone in hyperparathyroidism. *Ann. Intern. Med.* **84,** 668–671.

Camanni, F., Massara, F., Losana, O., and Molinatti, G. M. (1968). Increased renal tubular reabsorption of phosphorus in acromegaly. *J. Clin. Endocrinol. Metab.* **28,** 999–1005.

Canalis, E. M., Dietrich, J. W., Maina, D. M., and Raisz, L. G. (1977a). Hormonal control of bone collagen synthesis in vitro. Effects of insulin and glucagon. *Endocrinology (Baltimore)* **100,** 668–674.

Canalis, E. M., Hintz, R. L., Dietrich, J. W., Maina, D. M., and Raisz, L. G. (1977b). Effect of somatomedin and growth hormone on bone collagen synthesis in vitro. *Metab. Clin. Exp.* **26,** 1079–1087.

Canas, F. M., Bergstrom, W. H., and Churgin, S. J. (1967). Effects of the adrenal on calcium homeostasis in the rat. *Metab. Clin. Exp.* **16,** 670–675.

Caniggia, A., and Gennari, C. (1972). Sites and modes of action of an estrogen-gestation combination on calcium and phosphate metabolism in postmenopausal osteoporosis. *Clin. Orthop. Relat. Res.* **85,** 184–192.

Caniggia, A., and Gennari, C. (1973). Effect of 25-hydroxycholecalciferol (25-HCC) on intestinal absorprion of ^{47}Ca in four cases of iatrogenic Cushing's syndrome. *Helv. Med. Acta* **37,** 221–225.

Caniggia, A., Gennari, C., Bianchi, V., and Guideri, R. (1963). Intestinal absorption of ^{45}Ca in senile osteoporosis. *Acta Med. Scand.* **173,** 613–617.

Caputo, C. B., Meadows, D., and Raisz, L. G. (1976). Failure of estrogens and androgens to inhibit bone resorption in tissue culture. *Endocrinology (Baltimore)* **98,** 1065–1068.

Care, A. D., Bates, R. F. L., Swaminathan, R., and Ganguli, P. C. (1971). The role of gastrin as a calcitonin secretagogue. *J. Endocrinol.* **51,** 735–741.

Castro, J. H., Genuth, S. M., and Klein, L. (1975). Comparative response to parathyroid hormone in hyperthyroidism and hypothyroidism. *Metal., Clin. Exp.* **24,** 839–848.

Charbon, G. A., Hoekstra, M. H., and Kool, D. S. (1963). The influence of glucagon on the urinary excretion of water, sodium, potassium, calcium, magnesium, chloride and inorganic phosphate. *Acta Physiol. Pharmacol. Neerl.* **12,** 48–56.

Chase, L. R., and Aurbach, G. D. (1970). The effect of parathyroid hormone in the concentration of adenosine 3′,5′-monophosphate in skeletal tissue in vitro. *J. Biol. Chem.* **245,** 1520–1526.

Chen, T. L., Aronow, L., and Feldman, D. (1977). Glucocorticoid receptors and inhibition of bone cell growth in primary culture. *Endocrinology (Baltimore)* **100,** 619–628.

Cherny, S. N., Chausmer, A. B., Bellavia, J. V., and Wallach, S. (1970). Interactions of thyroxine and thyrocalcitonin in the rat. *Endoctrinology (Baltimore)* **86,** 1337–1346.

Chestnut, C. H., Nelp, W. B., Baylink, D. J., and Denney, J. D. (1977). Effect of methandrostenolone on postmenopausal bone wasting as assessed by changes in total bone mineral mass. *Metab., Clin. Exp.* **26,** 267–277.

Chipman, J. J. Zerwekh, J., Nicar, M., Marks, J., and Pak, C. Y. C. (1980). Effect of growth hormone administration: Reciprocal changes in serum 1-alpha-25-dihydroxyvitamin D and intestinal calcium absorption. *J. Clin. Endocrinol. Met.* **51,** 321–324.

Christiansen, C., Christensen, M. S., and Transbol, I. (1981). Bone mass in postmenopausal women after withdrawal of oestrogen/gestagen replacement therapy. *Lancet* **1,** 459–461.

Christiansen, C., Christensen, M. S., McNair, P., Hagen, C., Stocklund, K., and Transbol, I. (1980). Prevention of early postmenopausal bone loss: controlled 2-year study in 315 normal females. *Eur. J. Clin. Invest.* **10,** 273–279.

Christy, N. P., and Shaver, J. C. (1974). Estrogens and the kidney. *Kidney Int.* **6,** 366–376.

Clark, I., Geoffroy, R. F., and Bowers, W. (1959). Effects of adrenal cortical steroids on calcium metabolism. *Endocrinology (Baltimore)* **64,** 849–856.

Clark, O. H., Rehfield, S. J., Castner, B., Stroop, J., Loken, H. F., and Deftos, L. J. (2978). Iodine deficiency produces hypercalcemia and hypercalcitonemia in rats. *Surgery* **83,** 626–632.

Cleeve, H. J. W., and Brown, I. R. F. (1978). Plasma 25-hydroxyvitamin D and alkaline phosphatase isoenzymes in hyperthyroidism. *Ann. Clin. Biochem.* **15,** 320–323.

Collins, E. J., Garrett, E. R., and Johnston, R. L. (1962). Effect of adrenal steroids on radio-calcium metabolism in dogs. *Metab. Clin. Exp.* **II,** 716–726.

Condon, J. R. (1971). Glucagon in the treatment of Paget's disease of bone. *Brit. Med. J.* **4,** 719–721.

Condon, J. R., Ives, D., Knight, M. J., and Day, J. (1975). The aetiology of hypocalcaemia in acute pancreatitis. *Br. J. Surg.* **62,** 115–118.

Cook, P. B., Nassim, J. R., and Collins, J. (1959). The effects of thyrotoxicosis upon the metabolism of calcium, phosphorus, and nitrogen. *Q. J. Med.* [N.S.] **28,** 505–529.

Cooper, C. W., Schwesinger, W. H., Mahgoub, A. M., and Ontjes, D. A. (1971). Thyrocalcitonin: Stimulation of secretion by pentagastrin. *Science* **172,** 1238–1240.

Cooper, C. W., Biggerstaff, C. R., Wiseman, C. W., and Carlone, M. F. (1972). Hypocalcemic effect of pentagastrin and related gastrointestinal hormonal peptides in the rat. *Endocrinology (Baltimore)* **91,** 1455–1461.

Cooperman, A. M., DeSantis, D., Winkelman, E., Farmer, R., Eversman, J., and Said, S. (1978). Watery diarrhea syndrome. Two unusual cases and further evidence that VIP is a humoral mediator. *Ann. Surg.* **187,** 325–328.

Corvilain, J., Abramow, M., and Bergans, A. (1962). Some effects of human growth hormone on renal hemodynamics and on tubular phosphate transport in man. *J. Clin. Invest.* **41,** 1230–1235.

Corvilain, J., Abramow, J., and Bergans, A. (1964). Effect of growth hormone on tubular transport of phosphate in normal and parathyroidectomized dogs. *J. Clin. Invest.* **43,** 1608–1612.

Currie, G. N., and Black, D. L. (1972). Effects of estrogen on thyrocalcitonin activity in male and female rabbits. *Acta Endocrinol. (Copenhagen)* **71,** 55–61.

Curtiss, P. H., Jr., Clark, W. S., and Herndon, C. H. (1954). Vertebral fractures resulting from prolonged cortisone and corticotropin therapy. *JAMA, J. Am. Med. Assoc.* **156,** 467–469.

Czech, M. P. (1977). Molecular basis of insulin action. *Annu. Rev. Biochem.* **46,** 359–384.

Daughaday, W. H. (1974). Pituitary tumors. *In* "Textbook of Endocrinology" (R. H. Williams, ed.), 5th ed., pp. 64–75. Saunders, Philadelphia, Pennsylvania.

Daughaday, W. H. (1977). Hormonal regulation of growth hormone by somatomedin and other tissue growth factors. *Clin. Endocrinol. Metab.* **6,** 117–135.

Daughaday, W. H., and Kipnis, D. M. (1966). The growth-promoting and anti-insulin actions of somatotropin. *Recent Prog. Horm. Res.* **22,** 49–99.

Daughaday, W. H., and Mariz, I. K. (1962). Conversion of proline-U-C^{14} to labelled hydroxyproline by rat cartilage in vitro: Effects of hypophysectomy, growth hormone, and cortisol. *J. Lab. Clin. Med.* **59,** 741–751.

Daughaday, W. H., and Parker, M. L. (1963). Sulfation factor measurement as an aid in the recognition of pituitary dwarfism. *J. Clin. Endocrinol. Metab.* **23,** 638–650.

Daughaday, W. H., Laron, Z., Pertzelan, A., and Heins, J. N. (1969). Defective sulfation factor generation: A possible etiological link in dwarfism. *Trans. Assoc. Am. Physicians* **82,** 129–140.

Daughaday, W. H., Phillips, L. S., and Mueller, M. C. (1976). The effects of insulin and growth hormone on the release of somatomedin by the isolated rat liver. *Endocrinology* **98,** 1214–1219.

Davies, M., Mawer, E. B., and Adams, P. H. (1977). Vitamin D metabolism and the response to 1,25-Dihydroxycholecalciferol in osteoporosis. *J. Clin. Endocrinol. Metab.* **45,** 199–208.

Davis, J. O., Howell, D. S., Laqueur, G. L., and Pierce, E. C. (1954). Renal hemodynamic function, electrolyte metabolism and water exchange in adrenalectomized-hypophysectomized dogs. *Am. J. Physiol.* **176,** 411–418.

Davis, M. E., Strandjord, N. M., and Lanzl, L. H. (1966). Estrogens and the aging process. *JAMA, J. Am. Med. Assoc.* **197,** 129–134.

Deding, A., Tougaard, L., Jensen, M. K., and Rodbro, P. (1977). Bone changes during prednisone treatment. *Acta Med. Scand.* **202,** 253–255.

DeFronzo, R. A., Cooke, C. R., Andres, R., Faloona, G. R., and Davis, P. (1975). The effect of insulin on renal handling of sodium, potassium, calcium, and phosphate in man. *J. Clin. Invest.* **55,** 845–855.

Deftos, L. J., Weisman, M. H., Williams, G. W., Karph, D. B., Frumar, A. M., Davidson, B. J. Parthemore, J. G., and Judd, H. L. (1980). Influence of age and sex on plasma calcitonin in human beings. *N. Engl. J. Med.* **302,** 1351–1353.

deGiuseppe, L., and Rindi, G. (1969). Influence of adrenal cortex on thyrocalcitonin content of the rat thyroid. *Experientia* **25,** 1099–1100.

DeLeeuw, I., and Abs, R. (1977). Bone mass and bone density in maturity-type diabetics measured by the ^{125}I photon-absorption technique. *Diabetes* **26,** 1130–1135.

DeLeeuw, I., Mulkens, N. Vertommen, J., and Abs, R. (1976). A histomorphometric study on the trabecular bone of diabetic subjects. *Diabetologia* **12,** 385–386.

DeLorme, M. L., Digioia, Y., Fandard, J., Mercerom, R., Raymond, J. Y., and Klotz, H. P. (1976). Estrogenes et calcitonine. *Ann. Endocrinol.* **37,** 503–504.

Demartini, F., Grokoest, A. W., and Ragan, C. (1952). Pathological fractures in patients with rheumatoid arthritis treated with cortisone. *JAMA, J. Am. Med. Assoc.* **149,** 750–752.

Dewonck, G., Bacq., Z. M., and Barac, G. (1963). Influence du glucagon sur l'excrétion urinaire du calcium chez le chien. *C. R. Seances Soc. Biol. Ses Fil.* **157,** 897–899.

Dixit, P. K., and Stern, A. M. K. (1979). Effect of insulin on the incorporation of citrate and calcium into the bones of alloxan-diabetic rats. *Calcif. Tiss. Intl.* **27,** 227–232.

Doyle, F. H. (1967). Nonparathyroid endocrine bone disease. *Proc. R. Soc. Med.* **60,** 25–32.

Dull, T. A., and Henneman, P. H. (1963). Urinary hydroxyproline as an index of collagen turnover in bone. *N. Engl. J. Med.* **268,** 132–134.

Duncan, T., and Care, A. D. (1967). The effect of anti-thyroid drugs on thyrocalcitonin secretion. *Br. J. Surg.* **54,** 196–198.

Edelstein, S., and Noff, O. (1977). The functional metabolism of Vitamin D in rats treated with cortisol. *FEBS. Lett.* **82,** 115–117.

Eisenberg, E., and Gordon, G. S. (1961). Skeletal dynamics in man measured by non-radioactive strontium. *J. Clin. Invest.* **40,** 1809–1825.

Eliel, L. P., Thomsen, C., and Chanes, R. (1965). Antagonism between parathyroid extract and adrenal cortical steroids in man. *Endoctrinology (Baltimore)* **25,** 457–464.

Eliel, L. P., Palmiere, G. M. A., Thompson, J. S., Bird, P. C., and Hawrylko, J. (1971). The relationships between adrenal cortical steroids, parathyroid extract and calcitonin. *Pediatrics* **47,** 229–238.

Elrick, H., Huffman, E. R., Hlad, C. J., Jr., Whipple, N., and Staub, A. (1958). Effects of glucagon on renal function in man. *J. Clin. Endocrinol. Metab.* **18,** 813–824.

Epker, B. N. (1970). Studies on bone turnover and balance in the rabbit. *Clin. Orthop. Relat. Res.* **72,** 315–326.

Eskildsen, P. C., Lund, Bi., Sorensen, O. H., Lund, Bi., Bishop, J. E., and Norman, A. W. (1979). Acromegaly and vitamin D metabolism: effect of bromocriptine treatment. *J. Clin. Endocrinol. Met.* **49,** 484–486.

Fanconi, G., and Girardet, P. (1952). Chronische hypercalcaemie, Kombiniet mit osteosklerose, hyperazotamie, minderwuchs and kongenitalen missbildungen. *Helv. Paediatr. Acta* **7,** 314–334.

Favus, M. J., Kimberg, D. V., Millar, G. N., and Gershon, E. (1973a). Effects of cortisone administration on the metabolism and localization of 25-hydroxycholecalciferol in the rat. *J. Clin. Invest.* **52,** 1328–1335.

Favus, M. J., Walling, M. W., and Kimberg, D. V. (1973b). Effects of 1,25-Dihydroxycholecalciferol on intestinal calcium transport in cortisone treated rats. *J. Clin. Invest.* **52,** 1680–1685.

Federspil, G., Conte, N., Trisotto, A., and Scandellari, C. (1970). Action hypocalcemiante du glucagon chez l'homme:données préliminaires. *Ann. Endocrinol.* **31,** 728–734.

Feher, J. J., and Wasserman, R. H. (1978). Suppresion of intestinal vitamin D dependent calcium-binding protein and calcium absorption in chicks given cortisol. *Fed. Proc., Fed. Am. Soc. Exp. Biol.* **37,** 332.

Feldman, D., Dziak, R., Koehler, R., and Stern, P. (1975). Cytoplasmic glucocorticoid binding proteins in bone cells. *Endocrinology (Baltimore)* **96,** 29–36.

Finkelstein, J. D., and Schachter, D. (1962). Active transport of calcium by intestine: Effects of hypophysectomy and growth hormone. *Am. J. Physiol.* **203,** 873–880.

Finlayson, J. F., and Casey, J. H. (1975). Hypercalcemia and multiple pheochromocytomas. *Ann. Intern. Med.* **82,** 810–811.

Fischer, F., and Hastrup, B. (1954). Cortisone and calcium balance (Effect of calcium, vitamin D, and methylandrostenediol). *Acta Endocrinol. (Copenhagen)* **16,** 141–148.

Fischer, J. A., Blum, J. W., and Binswanger, V. (1973). Acute parathyroid hormone response to epinephrine in vivo. *J. Clin. Invest.* **52,** 2434–2440.

Follis, R. H., Jr. (1951). The pathology of the osseous changes in Cushing's syndrome in an infant and in adults. *Bull. Johns Hopkins Hosp.* **88,** 440–448.

Follis, R. H., Jr. (1953). Skeletal changes associated with hyperthyroidism. *Bull. Johns Hopkins Hosp.* **92,** 405–411.

Fontaine, O., Pavlovitch, H., and Balsan, S. (1978). 25-hydroxycholecalciferol metabolism in hypophysectomized rats. *Endocrinology (Baltimore)* **102,** 1822–1826.

Forbes, A. P., Jacobsen, J. G., Carroll, E. L., and Pechet, M. M. (1962). Studies of growth arrest in gonadal dysgenesis: Response to exogenous human growth hormone. *Metab., Clin. Exp.* **11,** 56–75.

Forgács, S., Rosinger, A., and Vertes, L. (1976). Diabetes mellitus and osteoporosis. *Endokrinologie* **67,** 343–350.

Foster, G. V., Dorsey, N. K., and Zacur, H. A. (1977). Sex related differences in the regulation of plasma calcium in the rat. *Proc. 59th Annu. Meet. Endocr. Soc.*, p. 69.

Fox, J., Care, A. D., and Marshall, D. H. (1978). Reversal of betamethasone-induced inhibition of intestinal calcium absorption by 1-alpha-hydroxycholecalciferol. *J. Endocrinol.* **78,** 187–194.

Fox, J., Bunnett, N. W., Farrar, A. R., and Care, A. D. (1981). Stimulation by low phosphorus and low calcium diets of duodenal absorption of phosphate in betamethasone-treated chicks. *J. Endocrinol.* **88,** 147–153.

Francis, M. J. O., and Hill, O. J. (1975). Prolactin-stimulated production of somatomedin by rat liver. *Nature (London)* **255,** 167–168.

Frantz, A. G., and Rabkin, M. T. (1964). Human Growth Hormone. *N. Engl. J. Med.* **271,** 1375–1381.

Fraser, R., and Harrison, M. (1960). The effect of growth hormone on urinary calcium excretion. *Ciba Found. Colloq. Endocrinol.* **13,** 135–155.

Fraser, R., Harrison, M., and Ibbertson, K. (1960). The rate of calcium turnover in bone. *Q. J. Med.* [N.S.] **29,** 85–111.

Friedland, J. A., Williams, G. A., Bowser, E. N., Henderson, W. J., and Hoffeins, E. (1965). Effect of hyperthyroidism on intestinal absorption of calcium in the rat. *Proc. Soc. Exp. Biol. Med.* **120,** 20–23.

Frost, H. M. (1966). Bone dynamics in metabolic bone disease. *J. Bone J. Surg., Am. Vol.* **48-A,** 1192–1203.

Fucik, R. F., Kukreja, S. C., Hargis, G. K., Bowser, E. N., Henderson, W. J., and Williams, G. A. (1975). Effect of glucocorticoids on function of the parathyroid glands in man. *J. Clin. Endocrinol. Metab.* **40,** 152–155.

Fujita, T. (1973). Effect of tetragastrin on calcium absorption from rat duodenal loop in vivo. *Endocrinol. Jpn.* **20,** 407–410.

Fujita, T., Ishii, J., and Shizume, K. (1958). Parathyroid function in hyperthyroidism. *Endocrinol. Jpn.* **5,** 273–276.

Gagel, R. F., Costanza, M. E., DeLellis, R. A., Norton, R. A., Bloom, S. R., Miller, H. H., Voci, A., and Nathanson, L. (1976). Streptozotocin-treated Verner-Morrison syndrome. Plasma vasoactive intestinal peptide and tumor responses. *Arch. Intern. Med.* **136,** 1429–1435.

Gallagher, J. C., and Nordin, B. E. C. (1972). Treatment with estrogens of primary hyperparathyroidism in postmenopausal women. *Lancet* **1,** 503-507.

Gallagher, J. C., and Wilkinson, R. (1973). The effect of ethinyloestradiol on calcium and phosphorus metabolism of postmenopausal women with primary hyperparathyroidism. *Clin. Sci. Mol. Med.* **45,** 785-802.

Gallagher, J. C., Aaron, J., Norsman, A., Wilkinson, R., and Nordin, B. E. C. (1973a). Corticosteroid osteoporosis. *Clin. Endocrinol. Metab.* **2,** 355-365.

Gallagher, J. C., Aaron, J., Norsman, A., Marshall, D. H., Wilkinson, R., and Nordin, B. E. C. (1973b). The Crush Fracture syndrome in postmenopausal women. *Clin. Endocrinol. Metab.* **2,** 293-315.

Gallagher, J. C., Riggs, B. L., Eisman, J., Hamstra, A., Arnaud, S. B., and DeLuca, H. F. (1979). Intestinal calcium absorption and serum vitamin D metabolites in normal subjects and osteoporotic patients. *J. Clin. Invest.* **64,** 729-736.

Gallagher, J. C., Riggs, B. L., and DeLuca, H. F. (1980). Effect of estrogen on calcium absorption and vitamin D metabolites in postmenopausal osteoporosis. *J. Clin. Endocrinol. Met.* **51,** 1359-1364.

Gertner, J. M., Horst, R. L., Broadus, A. E., Rasmussen, H., and Gerel, M. (1979). Parathyroid function and vitamin D metabolism during human growth hormone replacement. *J. Clin. Endocrinol. Met.* **49,** 185-188.

Gershberg, H. (1960). Metabolic and renotropic effects of human growth hormone in disease. *J. Clin. Endocrinol. Metab.* **20,** 1107-1119.

Gershberg, H., Heinemann, H. O., and Stumpf, H. H. (1957). Renal function studies and autopsy report in a patient with gigantism and acromegaly. *J. Clin. Endocrinol. Metab.* **17,** 377-385.

Gershberg, H., Hecht, A., Javier, Z. (1967). Growth hormone and blood calcium homeostasis. *J. Clin. Endocrinol. Metab.* **27,** 1492-1494.

Ghose, R. R., Jemmett, J., Winsey, H. S., and Woodhead, J. S. (1976). Phaeochromocytoma and hypercalcemia. *Postgrad. Med. J.* **52,** 593.-595.

Gimlette, T. M. D. (1960). Thyroid acropachy. *Lancet* **1,** 22-24.

Goepfert, H. G., Smart, C. R., and Rochlin, D. B. (1966). Metastatic parathyroid carcinoma and hormonal chemotherapy. *Ann. Surg.* **164,** 917-920.

Goldsmith, R. S., Siemsen, A. W., Mason, A. D., Jr., and Forland, M. (1965). Primary role of plasma hydrocortisone concentration in the regulation of the normal forenoon pattern of urinary phosphate excretion. *J. Clin. Endocrinol. Metab.* **25,** 1649-1659.

Goodman, H. M., and Schwartz, J. (1974). Growth hormone and lipid metabolism. *In* "Handbook of Physiology" (R. O. Greep, E. B. Astwood, E. Knobil, W. H. Sawyer, and S. R. Geiger, eds.), Sec. 7, Vol. IV, pp. 221-223. Am. Physiol. Soc., Washington, D.C.

Gordan, G. S., and Eisenberg, E. (1963). The effect of oestrogens, androgens, and corticoids on skeletal kinetics in man. *Proc. R. Soc. Med.* **56,** 31-33.

Gordan, G. S., Picchi, J., and Roof, B. S. (1973). Antifracture efficacy of long-term estrogens for osteoporosis. *Trans. Assoc. Am. Physicians* **86,** 326-332.

Gordon, A. S. (1973). Erythropoietin. *Vitamin Horm. (N.Y.)* **31,** 106-174.

Gorski, J., and Gannon, F. (1976). Current models of steroid hormone action: A critique. *Annu. Rev. Physiol.* **38,** 425-450.

Gozariu, L., Minne, H., and Ziegler, R. (1971). Rat bone osteolysis in vitro: Inhibitory effect of glucagon and cortisol. *Horm. Metab. Res.* **3,** 225-226.

Grant, D. B., Hambley, J., Becker, D., and Pimstone, B. L. (1973). Reduced sulphation factor in undernourished children. *Arch. Dis. Child.* **48,** 596-600.

Gray, R. S., and Gillon, J. (1976). Normotensive pheochromocytoma with hypercalcemia: Correction after andrenalectomy. *Br. Med. J.* **1,** 378.

Grimelius, L., Johansson, H., Lundqvist, G., Olazabal, A., Polak, J. H., and Pearse, A. G. E. (1977). The parathyroid glands in experimentally induced hypergastrinemia in the rat. *Scand. J. Gastroenterol.* **12,** 739–744.

Guleke, P. (1911). Experimentelle untersuchungen über tetanic. *Langenbecks Arch. Klin. Chir.* **94,** 496.

Guttler, R. B., Croxson, M. S., DeQuattro, V. L., Warren, D. W., Otis, C. L., and Nicoloff, J. T. (1977). Effects of thyroid hormone on plasma adenosine 3′,5′-monophosphate production in man. *Metab., Clin. Exp.* **26,** 1155–1162.

Haas, H. G., Dambacher, M. A., Göschke, H., Guncaga, J., Lauffenburger, T., Lentner, C., Olah, H. J., and Wacker, H. R. (1976). Growth hormone in osteoporosis. *Calcif. Tissue Res.* **21,** 467–468.

Hahn, T. J., Downing, S. J., and Phang, J. M. (1971). Insulin effect on amino acid transport in bone: Dependence on protein synthesis and Na^+. *Am. J. Physiol.* **220,** 1717–1723.

Hahn, T. J., Halstead, L. R., and Haddad, J. G., Jr. (1977). Serum 25-hydroxyvitamin D concentrations in patients receiving chronic corticosteroid therapy. *J. Lab. Clin. Med.* **90,** 399–404.

Hahn, T. J., Baran, D. T., and Halstead, L. R. (1979b). Alteration in mineral and vitamin D metabolism produced by subacute prednisone administration in man. *Proc. 61st Ann. Meet. Endocr. Soc.* p. 195.

Hahn, T. J., Halstead, L. R., Teitelbaum, S. L., and Hahn, B. V. (1979a). Altered mineral metabolism in glucocorticoid-induced osteopenia. *J. Clin. Invest.* **64,** 655–665.

Hall, B. D., MacMillan, D. R., and Bronner, F. (1969). Vitamin D-resistant rickets and high fecal endogenous calcium output. *Am. J. Clin. Nutr.* **22,** 448–457.

Handovsky, H., and Goormaghtigh, N. (1937). D_2-vitamin, schilddrüse and arteriosklerose. *Arch. Int. Pharmacodyn. Ther.* **56,** 376–418.

Hanna, S., Harrison, M. T., MacIntyre, I., and Fraser, R. (1961). Effects of growth hormone on calcium and magnesium metabolism. *Br. Med. J.* **2,** 12–15.

Haldimann, B., Kaptein, E. M., Singer, F. R., Nicoloff, J. T., and Massry, S. G. (1980). Intestinal calcium absorption in patients with hyperthyroidism. *J. Clin. Endocrinol. Metab.* **51,** 995–997.

Hansson, C. G. (1967). The parathyroids in corticosteroid-treated male rats. *Acta Endocrinol. (Copenhagen)* **55,** 247–255.

Harden, R. McG., Harrison, M. T., Alexander, W. D., and Nordin, B. E. C. (1964). Phosphate excretion and parathyroid function in thyrotoxicosis. *J. Endocrinol.* **28,** 281–288.

Harney, A. N., Kukreja, S. C., Hargis, G. K., Johnson, P. A., Bowser, E. N., and Williams, G. A. (1978). Effect of long-term administration of epinephrine and propranolol on serum calcium, parathyroid hormone, and calcitonin in the rat. *Proc. Soc. Exp. Biol. Med.* **159,** 266–269.

Harper, P. S., and Hughes, R. O. (1970). Severe hypercalcemia from hyperthyroidism with unusual features. *Br. Med. J.* **1,** 213–214.

Harris, W. H., and Heaney, R. P. (1969). Effect of growth hormone on skeletal mass in adult dogs. *Nature (London)* **223,** 403–404.

Harris, W. H., Heaney, R. P., Jowsey, J., Cockin, J., Atkins, C., Graham, J., and Weinberg, E. H. (1972). Growth hormone: The effect on skeletal renewal in the adult dog. I. Morphometric studies. *Calcif. Tissue Res.* **10,** 1–13.

Harrison, H. E., and Harrison, H. C. (1960). Transfer of Ca^{45} across intestinal wall in vitro in relation to action of vitamin D and cortisol. *Am. J. Physiol.* **199,** 265–271.

Harrison, M. T., Joplin, G. F., and Hartog, M., and Fraser, R. (1960). Acromegaly treated by needle-implantation of ^{198}Au seeds into the pituitary gland, showing changes in growth, carbohydrate, and calcium metabolism. *Proc. R. Soc. Med.* **53,** 869–871.

Harrison, M. T., Harden, R. McG., and Alexander, W. D. (1964). Some effects of parathyroid hormone in thyrotoxicosis. *J. Clin. Endocrinol. Metab.* **24,** 214–217.

Hartog, M., Gaafar, M. A., and Fraser, R. (1964). Effect of corticosteroids on serum growth hormone. *Lancet* **2,** 376–378.

Hattner, R. S., Bernstein, D. S., Aliapoulios, M. A., George, B., and Rose, E. (1970). The hypocalcemic activity of glucagon: Demonstration of independence from endogenous calcitonin secretion in the rat. *Acta Endocrinol. (Copenhagen)* **64,** 726–736.

Haussler, M. R., and McCain, T. A. (1978). Circulatory 1,25-Dihydroxyvitamin D in Health and Disease: An update. *Clin. Res.* **26,** 128A.

Haymovitz, A., and Horwith, M. (1964). The miscible calcium pool in metabolic bone disease—in particular, acromegaly. *J. Clin. Endocrinol. Metab.* **24,** 4–14.

Heaney, R. P., and Skillman, T. G. (1964). Secretion and excretion of calcium by the human gastrointestinal tract. *J. Lab. Clin. Med.* **64,** 29–41.

Heaney, R. P., and Skillman, T. G. (1971). Calcium metabolism in normal human pregnancy. *J. Clin. Endocrinol. Metab.* **33,** 661–670.

Heaney, R. P., and Whedon, G. D. (1958). Radiocalcium studies of bone formation rate in human metabolic bone disease. *J. Clin. Endocrinol. Metab.* **18,** 1246–1267.

Heaney, R. P., Recker, R. R., and Saville, P. D. (1974). Calcium balance and calcium requirements in middle-aged women. *Clin. Res.* **22,** 649A.

Heaney, R. P., Recker, R. R., and Saville, P. D. (1978a). Menopausal changes in calcium balance performance. *J. Lab. Clin. Med.* **92,** 953–963.

Heaney, R. P., Recker, R. R., and Saville, P. D. (1978b). Menopausal changes in bone remodeling. *J. Lab. Clin. Med.* **92,** 964–970.

Heath, H., III, Lambert, P. W., Service, F. J., and Arnaud, S. B. (1979). Calcium homeostasis in diabetes mellitus. *J. Clin. Endocrinol. Metab.* **49,** 462–466.

Heath, H., III, Melton, L. J., III, and Chu, C.-P. (1980). Diabetes mellitus and risk of skeletal fracture. *New Engl. J. Med.* **303,** 567–570.

Heath, H., and Sizemore, G. W. (1977). Plasma calcitonin in normal man. *J. Clin. Invest.* **60,** 1135–1140.

Hehrmann, R., Hagemann, J., Montz, R., and Jentsch, E. (1973). Differential action of parathyroid hormones on effective intestinal absorption of calcium. *Acta Endocrinol. (Copenhagen)* **73,** 489–498.

Heller, B. I., Smith, R. E., and Lubin, R. I. (1954). Renal functional status in patients with acromegaly. *J. Clin. Med.* **44,** 811.

Henneman, P. H., and Wallach, S. (1957). The use of androgens and estrogens and their metabolic effects. *Arch. Intern. Med.* **100,** 715–723.

Henneman, P. H., Forbes, A. P., Moldawer, M., Dempsey, E. F., and Carroll, E. L. (1960). Effects of human growth hormone in man. *J. Clin. Invest.* **39,** 1223–1238.

Henry, H. L. (1978). Response of 25-hydroxyvitamin D_3 metabolism by cultured chick kidney cells to 1,25-dihydroxyvitamin D_3, estradiol and parathyroid hormone. *Proc. 60th Annu. Meet. Endocr. Soc.* p. 233.

Henry, H. L. (1981). Insulin permits parathyroid hormone stimulation of 1,25-dihydroxyvitamin D_3 production in cultured kidney cells. *Endocrinology* **108,** 733–735.

Hernandez, G. R., Balsan, S., and Royer, P. (1967). Action de l'hormone de croissance humaine sur la calciurie. *Ann. Pediatr. Fenn.* **14,** 298–306.

Hernberg, C. A. (1952). The bone structure in alloxan-induced diabetes mellitus in rats. *Acta Med. Scand.* **142,** 274–277.

Hernberg, C. A. (1960). Treatment of postmenopausal osteoporosis with oestrogens and androgens. *Acta Endocrinol. (Copenhagen)* **34,** 51–59.

Hillyard, C. J., Stevenson, J. C., and MacIntyre, I. (1978). Relative deficiency of plasma-calcitonin in normal women. *Lancet* **1,** 961–962.

Hinde, F., and Phillippo, M. (1968). The effect of oestrogen on the response to thyrocalcitonin in the rat. *J. Physiol. (London)* **194,** 43.

Hipkin, L. J., Davis, J. C., and Diver, M. J. (1978). Urinary calcium excretion in hyperprolactinemia. *J. Endocrinol.* **77,** 143–144.

Hirose, S., Kabayashi, K., Kajikawa, K., Sawabu, N., and Takeuchi, J. (1975). A case of watery diarrhea, hypokalemia, and hypercalcemia associated with nonulcerogenic islet cell tumor of the pancreas. *Am. J. Gastroenterol.* **61,** 382–391.

Holdaway, I. M., Evans, M. C., and Clarke, E. D. (1977). Watery diarrhea syndrome with eposodic hypercalcemia. *Aust. N.Z.J. Med.* **7,** 63–65.

Hollo, I., Boross, M., and Szucs, J. (1971). Sex hormone deficiency and calcitonin sensitivity. *Lancet* **1,** 1205–1206.

Horsman, A., Simpson, M., Kirby, P. A., and Nordin, B. E. C. (1977). Nonlinear bone loss in oophorectomized women. *Br. J. Radiol.* **50,** 504–507.

Horsman, A., Nordin, B. E. C., and Crilly, R. G. (1979). Effect on bone of withdrawal of oestrogen therapy. *Lancet* **2,** 33.

Hosking, D. J., and Chamberlain, M. J. (1973). Osteoporosis and long-term corticosteroid therapy. *Br. Med. J.* **3,** 125–127.

Hossain, M., Smith, D. A., and Nordin, B. E. C. (1970). Parathyroid activity and postmenopausal osteoporosis. *Lancet* **1,** 809–811.

Hsu, W. H., and Cooper, C. W. (1975). Hypercalcemic effect of catecholamines and its prevention by thyrocalcitonin. *Calcif. Tissue Res.* **19,** 125–137.

Hunstein, W., Gless, K. H., Schmidt-Gayk, H., Mittelstaedt, G. V., and Hüfner, M. (1977). Alkaline phosphatase and plasma-25-OH-vitamin D in hyper thyroidism. *Horm. Metab. Res.* **9,** 532–533.

Hunt, N. H., and Perris, A. D. (1973). Erythropoietin-induced changes in plasma calcium and bone marrow mitosis in the rat. *J. Endocrinol.* **56,** 47–57.

Hunter, D. (1930). The significance of clinical medicine of studies in calcium and phosphorus metabolism. *Lancet* **1,** 947–957.

Hutchings, J. J., Escamilla, R. F., Deamer, W. C., and Li, C. H. (1959). Metabolic changes produced by human growth hormone (LI) in a pituitary dwarf. *J. Clin. Endocrinol Metab.* **19,** 759–769.

Iannaccone, A., Gabrilove, J. L., Brahms, S. A., and Soffer, L. J. (1960). Osteoporosis in Cushing's syndrome. *Ann. Intern. Med.* **52,** 570–586.

Igarashi, M., Hayash, Y., and Karube, S. (1974). Effect of estriol on bone collagen of rats with experimental osteoporosis. *Endocrinol. Jpn.* **21,** 387–391.

Ikkos, D., Ljunggren, H., and Luft, R. (1956). Glomerular filtration rate and renal plasma flow in acromegaly. *Acta Endrocrinol. (Copenhagen)* **21,** 226–236.

Ikkos, D., Luft, R., and Gemzell, C. A. (1958). The effect of human growth hormone in man. *Lancet* **1,** 720–721.

Ikkos, D., Luft, R., and Gemzell, C. A. (1959). The effect of human growth hormone in man. *Acta Endocrinol. (Copenhagen)* **32,** 341–361.

Ingbar, S. H., Kass, E. H., Burnett, C. H., Relman, A. S., Burrows, B. A., and Sisson, J. H. (1951). The effects of ACTH and cortisone on the renal tubular transport of uric acid, phosphorus, and electrolytes in patients with normal renal and adrenal function. *J. Lab. Clin. Med.* **38,** 533–541.

Ireland, P., and Fordtran, J. S. (1973). Effect of dietary calcium and age on jejunal calcium absorption in humans studied by intestinal perfusion. *J. Clin. Invest.* **52,** 2672–2681.

Isaksson, B., and Lindholm, B. (1965). Studies on cortisone-induced osteoporosis. *Am. J. Clin. Nutr.* **16,** 287–291.

Isenberg, J. I., Walsh, J. H., Passaro, E., Jr., Moore, E. W., and Grossman, M. J. (1972). Unusual effect of secretin on serum gastrin, serum calcium and gastric acid secretion in a patient with suspected Zollinger-Ellison syndrome. *Gastroenterology* **62,** 626–631.

Isenberg, J. I., Brickman, A. S., and Moore, E. W. (1973). The effect of secretin on serum calcium in man. *J. Clin. Endocrinol. Metab.* **37,** 30–33.

Jaffe, B. M., Peskin, G. W., and Kaplan, E. L. (1974). Relationship of serum gastrin to parathyroid hormone secretion in sheep. *Metab., Clin. Exp.* 307–310.

Jaffe, B. M., Kopen, D. F., DeSchryver-Kecskemeti, K., Gingerich, R. L., and Greiden, M. (1977). Indomethacin-responsive pancreatic cholera. *N. Engl. J. Med.* **297,** 817–821.

Jasin, H. E., Fink, C. W., Wise, W., and Ziff, M. (1962). Relationship between urinary hydroxyproline and growth. *J. Clin. Invest.* **41,** 1928–1935.

Jaworski, Z. F., Brown, E. M., Fedoruk, S., and Setiz, H. (1963). A method for the study of calcium absorption by the human gut using a standard dose of calcium labelled with calcium. *N. Engl. J. Med.* **269,** 1103–1111.

Jee, W. S. S., Park, H. Z., Roberts, W. E., and Kenner, G. H. (1970). Cortocosteroid and bone. *Am. J. Anat.* **129,** 477–480.

Jett, S., Wu, K., Duncan, H., and Frost, H. M. (1970). Adrenalcorticosteroid and salicylate actions on human and canine haversian bone formation and resorption. *Clin. Orthop. Relat. Res.* **68,** 301–315.

Jeune, M., and Béraud, C. (1955). Ostéopétrose myxoedémateuse. *Arch. Fr. Pediatr.* **12,** 368–382.

Jeune, M., and Muller, J. M. (1959). L'ostéopétrose myxoedémateuse. Hyperdesification généralisée du squelette au cours du myxoedéme congénital. *Pediatrie* **14,** 43–62.

Job, J. C., Ribierre, M., and Badoual, J. (1963). Hypercalcémie, hypercalciurie et diminution du pouvoir concentrateur de rein. Au cours du traitement de l'hypothyroidie congenitale. *Arch. Fr. Pediatr.* **20,** 1033–1050.

Joly, R., Chapuy, M. C., Alexandre, C., and Meunier, P. J. (1980). Osteoporoses a haut niveau de remodelage et fonction parathyroidienne. *Path. Biol.* **7,** 417–424.

Johnson, F., and White, H. (1952). Cretinism and marble bones. *Case Rep. Child. Mem. Hosp. (Chicago)* **10,** 2030.

Jorgenson, H. (1973). Hypercalcemia in adrenalcortical insufficiency. *Acta Med. Scand.* **193,** 175–179.

Jowsey, J. (1966). Quantitative microradiography. *Am. J. Med.* **40,** 485–491.

Jowsey, J., and Raisz, L. G. (1968). Experimental osteoporosis and parathyroid activity. *Endocrinology (Baltimore)* **82,** 385–396.

Jowsey, J., and Riggs, B. L. (1970). Bone formation in hypercortisonism. *Acta Endocrinol. (Copenhagen)* **63,** 21–28.

Jowsey, J., Kelly, P. J., Riggs, B. L., Bianco, A. J., Jr., Scholz, D. A., and Gershan-Cohen, J. (1965). Quantitative microradiographic studies of normal and osteoporotic bone. *J. Bone Jt. Surg., Am. Vol.* **47-A,** 785–806.

Kalager, T., Glück, E., Heimann, P., and Myking, O. (1977). Phaeochromocytoma with ectopic calcitonin production and parathyroid cyst. *Br. Med. J.* **3,** 21.

Kalu, D. N., Hillyard, C., and Foster, G. V. (1972). Effect of glucagon on bone collagen metabolism in the rat. *J. Endocrinol.* **55,** 245–252.

Kaplan, E. L., North, P. T., Norberg, H. P., Schulak, J. A., and Hill, B. J. (1977). Evidence for a role of the stomach in serum calcium regulation. *J. Surg. Res.* **22,** 237–241.

Kaptein, E. M., Singer, F. R., Nicoloff, J. T., Bishop, J. E., and Norman, A. W. (1979). Plasma 1α, 25-dihydroxycholecalciferol is decreased in hyperthyroidism. *Clin. Res.* **27,** 269A (Abstr.).

Karam, J., Harrison, M. T., Hartog, M., and Fraser, R. (1961). Renal citrate and urinary calcium excretion—the effects of growth hormone contrasted with those of sodium fluoroacetate. *Clin. Sci.* **21,** 265-272.

Katz, A. I., and Lindheimer, M. D. (1977). Actions of hormone on the kidney. *Annu. Rev. Physiol.* **39,** 97-134.

Kelin, M., and Frost, H. M. (1964). Cortical area of diabetic rib. *Henry Ford Hosp. Med. Bull.* **12,** 547-555.

Kenny, A. D. (1964). Effect of catecholamines on serum calcium in intact and parathyroidectomized rats. *Naunyn-Schmiedeberg's Arch. Exp. Pathol. Pharmakol.* **248,** 144-152.

Kenny, A. D. (1966). Hypercalciuric response to acute parathyroidectomy in rats: Effect of adrenalectomy. *Endocrinology (Baltimore)* **78,** 880-883.

Kenny, A. D. (1976). Vitamin D metabolism:physiological regulation in egg-laying Japanese quail. *Am. J. Physiol.* **230,** 1609-1615.

Kimberg, D. V., Schachter, D., and Schenker, H. (1961). Active transport of calcium by intestine: Effects of dietary calcium. *Am. J. Physiol.* **200,** 1256-1262.

Kimberg, D. V., Baerg, R. D., Gershon, E., and Graudusius, R. T. (1971). Effect of cortisone treatment on the active transport of calcium by the small intestine. *J. Clin. Invest.* **50,** 1309-1321.

Kinsella, R. A., Jr., and Back, D. K. (1968). Thyroid acropachy. *Med. Clin. North Am.* **52,** 393-398.

Kisch, B. (1924). Experimentelle unter suchunger uben die Funktion der Nebennieren. *Klin. Wochenschr.* **3,** 1661-1663.

Kivirikko, K. I., Laitenen, O., and Lamberg, B. A. (1965). Value of urine and serum hydroxyproline in the diagnosis of thyroid disease. *J. Clin. Endocrinol. Metab.* **25,** 1347-1352.

Kleeman, C. R., Levi, J., and Better, O. (1975). Kidney and adrenocortical hormones. *Nephron* **15,** 261-278.

Klein, M., Villanueva, A. R., and Frost, H. M. (1965). A quantitative histological study of rib from 18 patients treated with adrenal cortical steroids. *Acta Orthop. Scand.* **35,** 171-184.

Klein, R. G., Arnaud, S. B., Gallagher, J. C., DeLuca, H. F., and Riggs, B. L. (1977). Intestinal calcium absorption in exogenous hypercortisonism. *J. Clin. Invest.* **60,** 253-259.

Klibanski, A., Neer, R. M., Beitins, I. Z., Ridgway, E. C., Zervas, N. T., and McArthur, J. W. (1980). Decreased bone density in hyperprolactinemic women. *New Engl. J. Med.* **303,** 1511-1514.

Kowalewski, K., Heron, F., and Russell, J. C. (1971). Effect of sex hormones on the metabolism of collegan and ^{45}Ca by the bone of young gonadectomized rats. *Acta Endocrinol. (Copenhagen)* **67,** 740-755.

Krane, S. M., and Goldring, S. R. (1978). Hypothyroidism: Skeletal system. *In* "The Thyroid" (S. C. Werner and S. H. Ingbar, eds.), pp. 892-900. Harper & Row, Hagerstown, Maryland.

Krane, S. M., Brownell, G. L., Stanbury, J. B., and Corrigan, H. (1956). The effect of thyroid disease on calcium metabolism in man. *J. Clin. Invest.* **35,** 874-887.

Krawitt, E. L. (1967). Duodenal calcium transport in hyperthyroidism. *Proc. Soc. Exp. Biol. Med.* **125,** 417-419.

Krawitt, E. L. (1972). The role of intestinal transport proteins in cortisonemediated suppression of Ca^{2+} absorption. *Biochim. Biophys. Acta* **274,** 179-188.

Krawitt, E. L., Kunin, A. S., Sampson, H. W., and Bacon, B. F. (1977). Effect of hypophysectomy on calcium transport by rat duodenum. *Am. J. Physiol.* **232,** E229-E233.

Krieger, D. T., and Glick, S. M. (1972). Growth hormone and cortisol responsiveness in Cushing's syndrome. *Am. J. Med.* **52,** 25-40.

Krishnamra, N., and Limlomwongse, L. (1978). The influence of gastrin on plasma calcium, bile and gastric calcium secretions in the rat. *Proc. Soc. Exp. Biol. Med.* **158,** 40-44.

Kruse, H.-P., and Kuhlencordt, F. (1975). On an attempt to treat primary and secondary osteoporosis with human growth hormone. *Horm. Metab. Res.* **7,** 488–491.

Kukreja, S. C., Hargis, G. K., Rosenthal, I. M., and Williams, G. A. (1973). Pheochromocytoma causing excessive parathyroid hormone production and hypercalcemia. *Ann. Intern. Med.* **79,** 838–840.

Kukreja, S. C., Hargis, G. K., Bowser, E. N., Henderson, W. J., Fisherman, E. W., and Williams, G. A. (1975). Role of adrenergic stimuli in parathyroid hormone secretion in man. *J. Clin. Endocrinol. Metab.* **40,** 478–481.

Kukreja, S. C., Bowser, E. N., Hargis, G. K., Henderson, W. J., and Williams, G. A. (1976). Mechanisms of glucocorticoid-induced osteopenia: Role of parathyroid glands. *Proc. Soc. Exp. Biol. Med.* **152,** 358–361.

Kumar, R., Abboud, C. F., and Riggs, B. L. (1980). The effect of elevated prolactin levels on plasma 1,25-dihydroxyvitamin D and intestinal absorption of calcium. *Mayo Clin. Proc.* **55,** 51–53.

Kumar, R., Cohen, W. R., Silva, P., and Epstein, F. H. (1979). Elevated 1,25-dihydroxyvitamine D plasma levels in normal human pregnancy and lactation. *J. Clin. Invest.* **63,** 342–344.

Laake, H. (1960). The action of corticosteroids on the renal reabsorption of calcium. *Acta Endocrinol. (Copenhagen)* **34,** 60–64.

Lafferty, F. W., Spencer, G. E., and Pearson, O. H. (1964). Effects of androgens, estrogens and high calcium intakes on bone formation and resorption in osteoporosis. *Am. J. Med.* **36,** 515–528.

Lamberg, B. A., and Torsti, P. (1964). The dependence of calcium excretion on adrenal steroids. *Acta Med. Scand.* **412,** 193–203.

Lambertz, J., Job, J.-C., Milhaud, G., Boigne, J.-M., and Rossier, A. (1969). Effets de la thyrocalcitonine de porc chez l'enfant normal et dans quelques affections thyroïdiennes et troubles du métabolisme phosphos-calcique. *Arch. Fr. Pediatr.* **26,** 445–469.

Lancer, S. R., Bowser, E. N., Hargis, G. K., Williams, G. A. (1976). The effect of growth hormone on parathyroid function in rats. *Endocrinology (Baltimore)* **98,** 1289–1293.

Landau, R. L., and Kappas, A. (1965). Anabolic hormones in hyperparathyroidism. *Ann. Intern. Med.* **62,** 1223–1233.

Lang, K. (1960). Untersuchungen zum calcium stoffwechsel bei der hypothyreose im kindesalter. *Monatsschr. Kinderheilkd.* **108,** 395–398.

Lavender, A. R., and Pullman, T. N. (1963). Changes in inorganic phosphate excretion induced by renal arterial infusion of calcium. *Am. J. Physiol.* **205,** 1025–1032.

Leeksma, C. H. W., DeGraeff, J., and DeCock, J. (1957). Hypercalcemia in adrenal insufficiency. *Acta Med. Scand.* **156,** 455–458.

Lekkerkerker, J. F. F., and Doorenbos, H. (1973). The influence of thyroid hormone on calcium absorption from the gut in relation to urinary calcium excretion. *Acta Endocrinol. (Copenhagen)* **73,** 672–680.

Lekkerkerker, J. F. F., Van Woudenberg, F., Beekhuis, H., and Doorenbus, H. (1971). Enhancement of calcium absorption in hypothyroidism. Observations with a new method measuring calcium absorption. *Isr. J. Med. Sci.* **7,** 399–400.

Levin, M. E., Boisseau, V. C., and Avioli, J. V. (1976). Effects of diabetes mellitus on bone mass in juvenile and adult-onset diabetes. *N. Engl. J. Med.* **294,** 241–245.

Liskova-Kiar, M. (1979). Mode of action of cortisol on bone resorption in fetal rat fibulae cultured *in vitro*. *Am. J. Anat.* **156,** 63–76.

Lewy, J. E., and New, M. I. (1975). Growth in children with renal failure. *Am. J. Med.* **58,** 65–68.

Lindgren, U., Lindholm, S., and Sarby, B. (1978). Short-term effects of 1-alpha-hydroxyvitamin D_3 in patients on corticosteroid treatment and in patients with senile osteoporosis. *Acta Med. Scand.* **204,** 89–92.

Lindsay, R., Sweeney, A., and Hart, D. M. (1976). Osteoporosis. *Lancet* **1,** 417.
Lindsay, R., Hart, D. M., Forrest, C., and Baird, C. (1980). Prevention of spinal osteoporosis in oophorectomised women. *Lancet* **2,** 1151–1154.
Lindsay, R., Coutts, J. R. T., and Hart, D. M. (1977). The effect of endogenous oestrogen on plasma and urinary calcium and phosphate in oophorectomized women. *Clin. Endocrinol. (Oxford)* **6,** 87–93.
Lindsay, R., Hart, D. M., Purdie, D., Ferguson, M. M., Clark, A. S., and Kraszewski, A. (1978a). Comparative effects of oestrogen and a progestogen on bone loss in postmenopausal women. *Clin. Sci. Mol. Med.* **54,** 193–195.
Lindsay, R., MacLean, A., Kraszewski, A., Hart, D. M., Clark, A. C., and Garwood, J. (1978b). Bone response to termination of oestrogen treatment. *Lancet* **1,** 1325–1327.
Lineberry, M. D., and Waite, L. C. (1978). Calcitonin responses in intact and adrenalcalcitomized rats. *Life Sci.* **22,** 511–518.
Lipsett, M. B., and Bergenstahl, D. M. (1960). Lack of effect of human growth hormone and ovine prolactin on cancer in man. *Cancer Res.* **20,** 1172–1178.
Liskova, R. F. (1976). Influence of estrogens on bone resorption in organ culture. *Calcif. Tissue Res.* **22,** 207–218.
Loeb, R. F. (1932). Chemical changes in the blood in Addison's disease. *Science* **76,** 420–421.
Lowe, C. E., Bird, E. D., and Thomas, W. C., Jr. (1962). Hypercalcemia in myxedema. *J. Clin. Endocrinol. Metab.* **22,** 261–267.
Lukert, B. P., and Adams, J. S. (1976). Calcium and phosphorus homeostasis in man. *Arch. Intern. Med.* **136,** 1249–1253.
Lukert, B. P., Stanbury, S. W., and Mawer, E. B. (1973). Vitamin D and intestinal transport of calcium: Effects of prednisolone. *Endocrinology (Baltimore)* **93,** 718–722.
Lund, B., Sorenson, O. H., and Christensen, A. B. (1975). 25-Hydroxycholecalciferol and fractures of the proximal femur. *Lancet* **2,** 300–302.
McAllen, M. (1970). Long term side effects of corticosteroids. *Respiration* **27,** 250–259.
McCalister, A., and Welbourn, R. B. (1962). Stimulation of mammary cancer by prolactin and the clinical response to hypophysectomy. *Br. Med. J.* **1,** 1669–1670.
McConaghey, P., and Sledge, C. B. (1970). Production of "Sulphation Factor" by the perfused liver. *Nature (London)* **225,** 1249–1250.
McConkey, B., Fraser, G. M., and Bligh, A. S. (1962). Osteoporosis and purpura in rheumatoid disease: Prevalence and relation to treatment with corticosteroids. *Q. J. Med.* [N.S.] **124,** 419–427.
McNair, P., Madsbad, S., Christiansen, C., Faber, O. K., Transbol, I., and Binder, C. (1978). Osteopenia in insulin treated diabetes mellitus. *Diabetologia* **15,** 87–90.
McNair, P., Madsbad, S., Christensen, M. S., Christiansen, C., Faber, O. K., Binder, C., and Transbol, I. (1979). Bone mineral loss in insulin-treated diabetes mellitus: Studies on pathogenesis. *Acta Endocrinol. (Copenhagen)* **90,** 463–472.
Mainoya, J. R. (1975a). Further studies on the action of prolactin on fluid and ion absorption by the rat jejunum. *Endocrinology (Baltimore)* **96,** 1158–1164.
Mainoya, J. R. (1975b). Effects of bovine growth hormone, human placental lactogen and ovine prolactin on intestinal fluid and ion transport in the rat. *Endocrinology (Baltimore)* **96,** 1165–1170.
Makhlouf, G. M., Said, S., and Yau, W. M. (1974). Interplay of vasoactive intestinal peptide and synthetic VIP fragments with secretin and octapeptide of cholecystokinin on pancreatic and biliary secretion. *Gastroenterology* **66,** 737.
Malamos, B., Sfikakis, P., and Pandos, P. (1969). The renal handling of phosphate in thyroid disease. *J. Endocrinol.* **45,** 269–273.
Manderlier, T., Bergans, A., Brauman, J., Brauman, H., and Corvilain, J. (1974). Etude de la fonction parathyroïdienne dans l'hyperthyroïdie. *Ann. Endocrinol.* **35,** 185–188.

Manolagas, S. C., Anderson, D. C., and Lumb, G. A. (1979). Glucocorticoids regulate the concentration of 1,25-dihydroxycholecalciferol receptors in bone. *Nature (London)* **277,** 314–315.

Marcus, R. (1975). Cyclic nucleotide phosphodiesterase from bone: Characterization of the enzyme and studies of inhibition by thyroid hormones. *Endocrinology (Baltimore)* **96,** 400–408.

Margargal, L. E., Margargal, H., and Reidenbert, M. M. (1969). Effects of steroid hormones on the parathyroid hormone dose-response curve. *J. Pharmacol. Exp. Ther.* **169,** 138–141.

Martin, T. J., and Melick, R. A. (1969). The acute effects of porcine calcitonin in man. *Australas. Ann. Med.* **18,** 258–263.

Massry, S. G., and Coburn, J. W. (1973). The hormonal and non-hormonal control of renal excretion of calcium and magnesium. *Nephron* **10,** 66–112.

Massry, S. G., Friedler, R. M., and Coburn, J. W. (1973). Excretion of phosphate and calcium. *Arch. Intern. Med.* **131,** 828–852.

Matiasevic, D., and Gershberg, H. (1966). Studies on hydroxyproline excretion and corticosteroid-induced dwarfism. *Metab., Clin. Exp.* **15,** 720–729.

Matsumoto, T., Horiuchi, N., Suda, T., Takahashi, H., Shimazawa, E., and Ogata, E. (1979). Failure to demonstrate stimulatory effect of prolactin on vitamin D metabolism in vitamin D deficient rats. *Metabolism* **28,** 925–927.

Mazzuoli, G. F., Coen, G., Antonozzi, I., Terrenato, L., Zuliani, A., and Ceccorini, E. (1966). L'attivita calcitoninica della tiroide umane in alcine condizioni di alterato metabolismo del calcio. *Folia Endocrinol.* **19,** 539–546.

Meema, H. E., and Meema, S. (1968). Prevention of postmenopausal osteoporosis by hormone treatment of the menopause. *Can. Med. Assoc. J.* **99,** 248–251.

Meema, H. E., and Reid, D. B. W. (1969). The relationship between skin and cortical bone thickness in old age with special reference to osteoporosis and diabetes mellitus: A roentgenographic study. *J. Gerontol.* **24,** 28–32.

Meema, H. E., Bunker, M. L., and Meema, S. (1965). Loss of compact bone due to menopause. *Obstet. Gynecol.* **26,** 333–342.

Meema, S., Bunker, M. L., and Meema, H. E. (1975). Preventive effect of estrogen on postmenopausal bone loss. *Arch. Intern. Med.* **135,** 1436–1440.

Melick, R. A. (1966). Calcium-47 kinetics in osteoporosis. *Australas. Ann. Med.* **15,** 318–325.

Melvin, K. E. W., Wright, A. D., Hartog, M., Antcliff, A. C., Copestake, A. M., and Fraser, T. R. (1967). Acute metabolic response to human growth hormone in different types of dwarfism. *Br. Med. J.* **3,** 196–199.

Metz, S. A., Deftos, L. J., Baylink, D. J., and Robertson, R. P. (1978). Neuroendocrine modulation of calcitonin and parathyroid hormone in man. *J. Clin. Endocrinol. Metab.* **47,** 151–159.

Meunier, P. J., Bianchi, G. G. S., Edouard, C. M., Bernard, J. C., Coupron, P., and Vignon, G. E. (1972). Bony manifestations of thyrotoxicosis. *Orthop. Clin. North Am.* **3,** 745–774.

Meunier, P. J., Coupron, P., Edouard, C., Bernard, J., Bringuier, J., and Vignon, G. (1973). Physiological senile involution and pathological rarefaction of bone. *Clin. Endocrinol. Metabl.* **2,** 239–256.

Meyer, R. A., Jr., and Brinkley, H. J. (1972). Effects of adrenalectomy on the response of mice to parathyroid hormone and thyrocalcitonin. *J. Pharmacol. Exp. Ther.* **181,** 171–175.

MIddleton, W. R. J. (1971). Progress report. Thyroid hormones and the gut. *Gut* **12,** 172–177.

Milhaud, G. (1968). Utilization of thyrocalcitonin in man in normal and pathological conditions. *In* "Parathyroid Hormone and Thyrocalcitonin (Calcitonin)" (R. V. Talmage and L. F. Bélanger, eds.), pp. 86–99. Excerpta Medica, Amsterdam.

Milhaud, G., Tsien-Ming, L., and Mouthtar, M. S. (1967). Synergic et antagonisme de la thyroxine, de la parathormone et de la thyrocalcitonine sur la calcémie et la phosphatemie. *C. R. Hebd. Seances Acad. Sci.* **264,** 846–849.

Miller, D. L., and Schedl, H. P. (1976). Effects of diabetes on intestinal magnesium absorption in the rat. *Am. J. Physiol.* **231,** 1039–1042.

Miller, S. S., Sizemore, G. W., Sheps, S. G., and Tyce, G. M. (1975). Parathyroid function in patients with pheochromocytoma. *Ann. Intern. Med.* **82,** 372–375.

Miravet, L., Carre, M., Ayigbede, O., and Rasmussen, H. (1975). The effect of prednisolone upon intestinal metabolism and action of 25-hydroxy and 1,25-dihydroxyvitamin D_3. *In* "Vitamin D and Problems Related to Uremic Bone Disease" (A. W. Norman, K. Schaefer, H. G., Grigoleit, D. von Herroth, and E. Ritz, eds.), pp. 59–65. de Gruyter, Berlin.

Molinatti, G. M., Camanni, F., and Olivetti, M. (1960). A study on the metabolism of calcium in the hyperadrenocortical syndrome. *Acta Endocrinol. (Copenhagen)* **34,** 323–334.

Molinatti, G. M., Camanni, F., Losana, O., and Olivetti, M. (1961). Changes in the metabolism of calcium and phosphorus in the various phases of acromegaly and following the implantation of the pituitary gland with ^{90}Y. *Acta Endocrinol. (Copenhagen)* **36,** 161–179.

Montz, R., Hehrman, R., Delling, G., Kuhlencordt, F., Nowakowski, H., and Schneider, C. (1973). ^{47}Calcium kinetics in endocrine osteopathies. *Acta Endocrinol. (Copenhagen)* **177,** 113.

Morey, E. R., and Kenny, A. D. (1964). Effects of catecholamines on urinary calcium and phosphorus in intact and parathyroidectomized rats. *Endocrinology* **75,** 78–85.

Morimoto, S., Tsuji, M., Okada, Y., Onishi, T., and Kumahara, Y. (1980). The effect of oestrogens on human calcitonin secretion after calcium infusion in elderly female subjects. *Clin. Endocrinol.* **13,** 135–143.

Morris, H. G., Jorgensen, J. R., and Jenkins, S. A. (1968a). Plasma growth hormone concentration in corticosteroid-treated children. *J. Clin. Invest.* **47,** 427–435.

Morris, H. G., Jorgensen, J. R., Elrick, H., and Goldsmith, R. E. (1968b). Metabolic effects of human growth hormone in corticosteroid-treated children. *J. Clin. Invest.* **47,** 436–451.

Mosekilde, L., and Christensen, M. S. (1977). Decreased parathyroid function in hyperthyroidism: Interrelationships between serum parathyroid hormone, calcium-phosphorus metabolism and thyroid function. *Acta Endocrinol. (Copenhagen)* **84,** 566–575.

Mosekilde, L., and Melsen, F. (1978). Effect of antithyroid treatment on calcium-phosphorus metabolism in hyperthyroidism. II. Bone histomorphometry. *Acta Endocrinol. (Copenhagen)* **87,** 751–758.

Mosekilde, L., Lund, B., Sorensen, O. H., Christensen, M. S., and Melsen, F. (1977a). Serum 25-hydroxycholecalciferol in hyperthyroidism. *Lancet* **1,** 806–807.

Mosekilde, L., Melsen, F., Bagger, J. P., Myhre-Jensen, O., and Sorensen, N. S. (1977b). Bone changes in hyperthyroidism. *Acta Endocrinol. (Copenhagen)* **85,** 515–525.

Mosekilde, L., Christensen, M. S., Melson, F., and Sorensen, N. S. (1978). Effect of antithyroid treatment on calcium-phosphorus metabolism in hyperthyroidism. I. Chemical quantities in serum and urine. *Acta Endocrinol. (Copenhagen)* **87,** 743–750.

MRC (1959). The effectiveness in man of human growth hormone. *Lancet* **1,** 7–12.

Munck, O. (1964). Osteoporosis due to malabsorption of calcium responding favorably to large doses of vitamin D. *Q. J. Med.* [N.S.] **33,** 209–221.

Mundy, G. R., Shapiro, J. L., Bandelin, J. G., Canalis, E. M., and Raisz, L. G. (1976). Direct stimulation of bone resorption by thyroid hormones. *J. Clin. Invest.* **58,** 529–534.

Myers, W. P. L., and Lawrence, W., Jr. (1958). Studies on the influence of cortisone on serum calcium homeostasis. *J. Clin. Invest.* **37,** 919.

Myers, W. P. L., and Lawrence, W. (1961). The adrenal glands and calcium metabolism. *J. Clin. Invest.* **40,** 1065–1066.

Nadarajah, A., Hartog, M., Redfern, G., Thalassinos, N., Wright, A. D., Joplin, G. F., and Fraser, R. T. (1968). Calcium metabolism in acromegaly. *Br. Med. J.* **4,** 797–801.

Nassim, J. R., Saville, P. D., and Mulligan, L. (1956). The effect of stilbestrol on urinary phosphate excretion. *Clin. Sci.* **15,** 367–371.

Naylor, J. M. (1955). A case of hypothyroidism with nephrocalcinosis. *Arch. Dis. Child.* **30,** 165–168.

Noble, H. M., and Matty, A. J. (1967). The effect of thyroxine on the movement of calcium and inorganic phosphate through the small intestine of the rat. *J. Endocrinol.* **37,** 111–117.

Nordin, B. E. C. (1959). Investigation of bone metabolism with ^{47}Ca-a preliminary report. *Proc. R. Soc. Med.* **52,** 351–353.

Nordin, B. E. C. (1971). Clinical significance and pathogenesis of osteoporosis. *Br. Med. J.* **1,** 571–576.

Nordin, B. E. C., and Fraser, R. (1956). The indirect assessment of parathyroid function. *Bone Struct. Metab., Ciba Found. Symp., 1955* pp. 222–232. Churchill, London.

Nordin, B. E. C., MacGregor, J., and Smith, D. A. (1966). The incidence of osteoporosis in normal women: Its relation to age and the menopause. *Q. J. Med.* [N.S.] **35,** 25–38.

Nutik, G., and Cruess, R. L. (1974). Estrogen receptors in bone: An evaluation of the uptake of estrogen into bone cells. *Proc. Soc. Exp. Biol. Med.* **146,** 265–268.

Ogata, E., Shimazawa, E., Suzuki, H., Yoshitoshi, Y., Asano, H., and Ando, H. (1970). Androgens and enhancement of hypocalcemic response to thyrocalcitonin in rats. *Endocrinology (Baltimore)* **87,** 421–426.

Ohata, M., Sakagami, Y., and Fujita, T. (1977). Elevation of serum 25-hydroxycalciferol levels in androgen-treated and ultraviolet-irradiated rats. *Endocrinol. Jpn.* **24,** 519–521.

Oikarinen, A. (1977). Effect of cortisol acetate on collagen biosynthesis and on the activities of prolylydroxylase, lyslhydroxylase, collagen galactosyltransferase and collagen glucosyltransferase in chick embryo tendon cells. *Biochem. J.* **164,** 533–539.

O'Malley, B. W. (1971). Mechanisms of action of steroid hormones. *N. Engl. J. Med.* **284,** 370–377.

Oppenheimer, J. H., Schwartz, H. L., Surks, M. I., Koerner, D., and Dillman, W. H. (1976). Nuclear receptors and the initiation of thyroid hormone action. *Recent Prog. Horm. Res.* **32,** 322–354.

Orimo, H. O., Fujita, T., and Yoshikawa, M. (1972). Increased sensitivity of bone to parathyroid hormone in ovariectomized rats. *Endocrinology (Baltimore)* **90,** 760–770.

Ottenjann, R., and Deyhle, P. (1969). Uber den einfluss von glucagon auf serum-calcium and magensekretion. *Klin. Wochenschr.* **47,** 388–389.

Paloyan, E., Paloyan, D., and Harper, P. V. (1967a). Glucagon-induced hypocalcemia. *Metab., Clin. Exp.* **16,** 35–39.

Paloyan, E., Paloyan, D., and Harper, P. V. (1967b). The role of glucagon hypersecretion in the relationship of pancreatitis and hyperparathyroidism. *Surgery* **62,** 167–173.

Pang, P. K. T., Schreibman, M. P., Balbontin, E., and Pang, R. K. (1978). Prolactin and pituitary control of calcium regulation in the killifish, Fundulus heteroclitus. *Gen. Comp. Endocrinol.* **36,** 306–316.

Parfitt, A. M., and Dent, C. E. (1970). Hyperthyroidism and hypercalcemia. *Q. J. Med.* [N.S.] **39,** 171–187.

Parsons, V., and Anderson, J. (1964). The maximum renal tubular reabsorptive rate for inorganic phosphate in thyrotoxicosis. *Clin. Sci.* **27,** 313–318.

Parsons, V., Veall, N., and Butterfield, W. J. H. (1968). The clinical use of orally administered ^{47}Ca for the investigation of intestinal calcium absorption. *Calcif. Tissue Res.* **2,** 83–92.

Parthemore, J. G., and Deftos, L. J. (1978). Calcitonin secretion in normal human subjects. *J. Clin. Endocrinol. Metab.* **47,** 184–188.

Pavlovitch, H., Fontaine, O., and Balson, S. (1978). Effect of growth hormone on the metabolism of 25-hydroxycholecalciferol in hypophysectomized rats on a diet without vitamin D and low in calcium. *J. Endocrinol.* **79,** 277–281.

Peacock, M., Taylor, G. A., and Norman, A. W. (1977). Action of vitamin D metabolites and analogous, parathyroid hormone, calcitonin and steroid sex hormones on bone in tissue culture. *In* "Vitamin D: Biochemical Chemical, and Clinical Aspects Related to Calcium Metabolism" (A. W. Norman, K. Schaefer, J. W. Coburn, H. F. DeLuca, D. Fraser, H. G. Rogoleit, and D. von Herroth, eds.), pp. 411–413. de Gruyter, Berlin.

Pearson, E., Soroff, H. S., Prudden, J. F., and Schwartz, M. S. (1960). Studies on growth hormone. V. Effect on the mineral and nitrogen balances of burned patients. *Am. J. Med. Sci.* **239,** 17–25.

Pechet, M. M., Bowers, B., and Bartter, F. C. (1959). Metabolic studies with a new series of 1,4-Diene steroids. *J. Clin. Invest.* **38,** 681–701.

Peck, W. A., and Messinger, K. (1970). Nucleoside and ribonucleic acid metabolism in isolated bone cells. Effects of insulin and cortisol in vitro. *J. Biol. Chem.* **245,** 2722–2729.

Peck, W. A., Brandt, J., and Miller, I. (1967). Hydorcortisone-induced inhibition of protein synthesis and uridine incorporation in isolated bone cells in vitro. *Proc. Natl. Acad. Sci. U.S.A.* **57,** 1599–1606.

Peck, W. A., Messinger, K., Brandt, J., and Carpenter, J. (1969). Impaired accumulation of ribonucleic acid precursors and depletion of ribonucleic acid in glucocorticoid-treated bone cells. *J. Biol. Chem.* **244,** 4174–4184.

Peck, W. A., Carpenter, J., and Messinger, K. (1974). Cyclic 3′,5′-adenosine monophosphate in isolated bone cells. II. Responses to adenosine and parathyroid hormone. *Endocrinology (Baltimore)* **94,** 148–153.

Peng, T.-C., Cooper, C. W., Volpert, E. M., and Munson, P. L. (1976). Hypersecretion of thyrocalcitonin and C-cell hyperplasia in rats chronically fed low iodine diet. *Program 58th Annu. Meet. Endocr. Soc.* p. 103.

Peng, T.-C., Cooper, C. W., Elks, M. L., and Garner, S. C. (1977). Thyrocalcitonin in rats chronically treated with propylthiouracil. *Fed. Proc. Fed. Am. Soc. Exp. Biol.* **36,** 985.

Peng, T., and Garner, S. C. (1980). Sex defference in serum calcitonin level in rats as related to feeding, fasting, and age. *Endocrinology* **107,** 289–293.

Perlish, J. S., Bashey, R. I., and Fleischmajer, R. (1973). The in vitro effect of insulin on collagen synthesis in embryonic chick tibia. *Proc. Soc. Exp. Biol. Med.* **142,** 1152–1154.

Perris, A. D., and Whitfield, J. F. (1971). Calcium homeostasis and erythropoietic control in the rat. *Can. J. Physiol. Pharmacol.* **49,** 22–35.

Persky, M., Linsk, J., Isaacs, M., Jenkins, J. P., Rosenbluth, M., and Kupperman, H. S. (1955). Acute effects of intravenous hydrocortisone on glucose and insulin tolerances, and levels of serum and urinary inorganic phosphorus. *J. Clin. Endocrinol. Metab.* **15,** 1247–1256.

Phillippo, M., Bruce, J. B., and Lawrence, C. B. (1970). The effect of adrenaline on calcitonin secretion in conscious sheep. *J. Endocrinol.* **46,** XII–XIII.

Phillips, L. S., Herington, A. C., Karl, I. E., and Daughaday, W. H. (1976). Comparison of somatomedin activity in perfusates of normal and hypophysectomized rat livers with and without added growth hormone. *Endocrinology (Baltimore)* **98,** 606–614.

Pickleman, J. R., Ernst, K., Brown, S., and Paloyan, E. (1969). Glucagon-induced hypocalcemia: Effect of the thyroid gland. *Surg. Forum* **20,** 85–87.

Pike, J. W., Spanos, E., Colston, K. W., MacIntyre, I., and Haussler, M. R. (1978). Influence of estrogen on renal vitamin D hydroxylases and serum 1α,25-$(OH)_2D_3$ in chicks. *Am. J. Physiol.* **235,** E338–E343.

Pohl, S. L. (1977). The glucagon receptor and its relationship to adenylate cyclase. *Fed. Proc., Fed. Am. Soc. Exp. Biol.* **36,** 2115–2118.

Pretorius, P. J., and Potgieter, M.deJ. (1971). Hypothyroidism and hypercalcemia. Report of a cretin showing manifestations of idiopathic infantile hypercalcemia. *S. Afr. Med. J.* **45,** 735–757.

Pullman, T. N., Lavender, A. R., and Aho, I. (1967). Direct effects of glucagon on renal hemodynamics and excretion of inorganic ions. *Metab., Clin. Exp.* **16,** 358–373.

Putnam, J. M. (1972). A routine method for determining plasma ionized calcium and its application to the study of congenital heart disease in children. *Clin. Chim. Acta* **32,** 33–41.

Raisz, L. G. (1965). Bone resorption in tissue culture. Factors influencing the response to parathyroid hormone. *J. Clin. Invest.* **44,** 103–116.

Raisz, L. G., Trummel, C. L., Wener, J. A., and Simmons, H. (1972). Effect of glucocorticoids on bone resorption in tissue culture. *Endocrinology (Baltimore)* **90,** 961–967.

Raisz, L. G., Dietrich, J. W., and Canalis, E. M. (1976). Factors influencing bone formation in organ culture. *Isr. J. Med. Sci.* **12,** 108–114.

Raman, A. (1970a). Effect of adrenalectomy on ionic and total plasma calcium in rats. *Horm. Metab. Res.* **2,** 181–183.

Raman, A. (1970b). The effect of glucagon on plasma calcium ion activity in the monkey. *Q. J. Exp. Physiol. Cogn. Med. Sci.* **55,** 271–274.

Rambaud, J.-C., Modigliani, R., Matuchansky, C., Bloom, S., Said, S., Pessayre, D., and Bernier, J.-J. (1975). Pancreatic cholera. Studies on tumoral secretions and pathophysiology of diarrhea. *Gastroenterology* **69,** 110–122.

Raskin, P., Stevenson, M. R., Barilla, D. E., and Pak, C. Y. C. (1978). The hypercalciuria of diabetes mellitus: Its amelioration with insulin. *Clin. Endocrinol. (Oxford)* **9,** 329–335.

Recker, R. R., Saville, P. D., and Heaney, R. P. (1977). Effect of estrogens and calcium carbonate on bone loss in postmenopausal women. *Ann. Intern. Med.* **87,** 649–655.

Reifenstein, E. C., and Albright, F. (1947). The metabolic effects of steroid hormones in osteoporosis. *J. Clin. Invest.* **26,** 24–56.

Reynolds, J. J. (1966). The effect of hydrocortisone on the growth of chick rudiments in chemically defined medium. *Exp. Cell Res.* **41,** 174–189.

Richards, A. J. (1970). Hypercalcemia in thyrotoxicosis with and without hyperparathyroidism. *Postgrad. Med. J.* **46,** 440–446.

Richter, J., and Ohlen, J. (1971). Hyperthyrose und die Isoenzyme der alkalischen phosphatase. *Dtsch. Med. Wochenschr.* **96,** 196–202.

Riggs, B. L., Jowsey, J., and Kelly, P. J. (1966). Quantitative microradiographic study of bone remodeling in Cushing's syndrome. *Metab., Clin. Exp.* **15,** 773–780.

Riggs, B. L., Jowsey, J., Kelly, P. J., Jones, J. D., and Maher, F. T. (1969). Effect of sex hormones on bone in primary osteoporosis. *J. Clin. Invest.* **48,** 1065–1072.

Riggs, B. L., Jowsey, J., Goldsmith, R. S., Kelly, P. J., Hoffman, D. L., and Arnaud, C. D. (1972a). Short and long-term effects of estrogen and synthetic anabolic hormone in postmenopausal osteoporosis. *J. Clin. Invest.* **51,** 1659–1663.

Riggs, B. L., Randall, R. V., Wahner, Jowsey, J., Kelly, P. J., and Singh, M. (1972b). The nature of the metabolic bone disorder in acromegaly. *J. Clin. Endocrinol. Metab.* **34,** 911–918.

Riggs, B. L., Jowsey, J., Kelly, P. J., Hoffman, D. L., and Arnaud, C. D. (1973). Studies on pathogenesis and treatment in postmenopausal and senile osteoporosis. *J. Clin. Endocrinol. Metab.* **22,** 317–332.

Riggs, B. L., Wahner, H. W., Dunn, W. L., Mazess, R. B., Offord, K. P., and Melton, L. J. (1981). Differential changes in bone mineral density of the appendicular and axial skeleton with aging. *J. Clin. Invest.* **67,** 328-335.

Ringe, J.-D., Kuhlencordt, F. and Kuhnau, J., Jr. (1976). Mineralgehalt des skeletts bei langzeitdiabetikern. *Dtsch. Med. Wschr.* **101,** 280–282.

Roberts, K. E., and Pitts, R. F. (1953). The effects of cortisone and desoxycorticosterone on the renal tubular reabsorption of phosphate and the excretion of titrable acid and potassium in dogs. *Endocrinology (Baltimore)* **52,** 324–330.

Robertson, G. M., Jr., Moore, E. W., Switz, D. M., Sizemore, G. W., and Estep, H. L. (1976). Inadequate parathyroid response in acute pancreatitis. *N. Engl. J. Med.* **294,** 512–516.

Robinson, C. J., Mahajan, K. K., and Harrobin, D. F. (1975). Some effects of prolactin on calcium metabolism. *J. Endocrinol.* **65,** 27P.

Rodan, S. V., and Rodan, G. A. (1974). The effect of parathyroid hormone and thyrocalcitonin on the accumulation of cyclic adenosine 3′,5′-monophosphate in freshly isolated bone cells. *J. Biol. Chem.* **249,** 3068–3074.

Roelfsema, F., Van der Sluys, J., and Smeenk, D. (1970). Quantitation of bone and bone turnover in biopsy specimens from the iliac crest in acromegaly. *J. Endocrinol.* **48,** lxi.

Rogoff, J. M., and Stewart, G. N. (1928). Studies on adrenal insufficiency. *Am. J. Physiol.* **86,** 25–31.

Root, A. W., Rosenfield, R. L., Bongiovanni, A. M., and Eberlein, W. R. (1967). The plasma growth hormone response to insulin-induced hypoglycemia in children with retardation of growth. *Pediatrics* **39,** 844–851.

Rosenbloom, A. L., Lezotte, D. C., Weber, F. T., Gudat, J., Heller, D. R., Weber, M. L., Klein, S., and Kennedy, B. B. (1977). Diminution of bone mass in childhood diabetes. *Diabetes* **26,** 1052–1055.

Rothenberg, S., and Redleaf, P. D. (1959). Hypoparathyroidism and recurrent hyperthyroidism. *Arch. Intern. Med.* **104,** 783–786.

Royer, P., and Mathieu, H. (1962). Métabolisme du calcium dans l'insuffisance thyroidie e humaine et expérimentale. *Pathol. Biol.* **10,** 1035–1045.

Royer, P., Lestradet, H., and Habib, R. (1958). Les hypercalcemies et les nephrocalcinoses au course du myxoedeme congenital. *Arch. Fr. Pediat.* **15,** 896–919.

Rubin, M. I., and Krick, E. T. (1936). The salt and water metabolism of adrenal insufficiency and partial starvation in rats. *J. Clin. Invest.* **15,** 685–695.

Rude, R. K., Oldham, S. B., Singer, F. R., and Nicoloff, J. T. (1976). Treatment of thyrotoxic hypercalcemia with propranolol. *N. Engl. J. Med.* **294,** 431–433.

Saenger, P., Wiedmann, E., Schwartz, E., Korth-Schutz, S., Lewy, J. E., Riggio, R. R., Rubin, A. L., Stenzel, K. H., and New, M. I. (1974). Somatomedin and growth after renal transplantation. *Pediatr. Res.* **8,** 163–168.

Salmon, W. D. (1975). Interaction of somatomedin and a peptide inhibitor in serum of hypophysectomized and starved pituitary-intact rats. *Adv. Metab. Disord.* **8,** 183–202.

Salmon, W. D., and Daughaday, W. H. (1957). A hormonally controlled serum factor which stimulates sulfate incorporation by cartilage in vitro. *J. Lab. Clin. Med.* **49,** 825–836.

Salmon, W. D., and duVall, M. R. (1970). A serum fraction with "sulfation factor activity" which stimulates in vitro incorporations of leucine and sulfate into protein-polysaccharide complexes, uridine into RNA, and thymidine into DNA of costal cartilage from hypophysectomized rats. *Endocrinology (Baltimore)* **86,** 721–727.

Salzer, G. M. (1971). Hypophyse und hormonelles. Calcium-regulations system. *Acta Endocrinol. (Copenhagen)* **157,** 5–64.

Sataline, L. R., Powell, C., and Hamwi, G. J. (1962). Suppression of the hypercalcemia of thyrotoxicosis by corticosteroids. *N. Engl. J. Med.* **267,** 646–650.

Saville, P. D., and Kharmosh (1967). Osteoporosis of rheumatoid arthritis: Influence of age, sex, and corticosteroids. *Arthritis Rheum.* **10,** 423–430.

Schartum, S., and Nichols, G. (1961). Influence of adrenal glucocorticoids on distribution of calcium and phosphorus between bone and its surrounding fluids. *Proc. Soc. Exp. Biol. Med.* **108,** 228–231.

Schedl, H. P., Heath, H., III, and Wenger, J. (1978). Serum calcitonin and parathyroid hormone in experimental diabetes: Effects of insulin treatment. *Endocrinology (Baltimore)* **103,** 1368–1373.

Schmidt, J. (1962). Osteoporoses myxoedematosa mit nephrolithiasis. *Z. Kinderheilkd.* **86,** 602–618.

Schneider, L. E., and Schedl, H. P. (1972). Diabetes and intestinal calcium absorption in rat. *Am. J. Physiol.* **223,** 1319–1323.

Schneider, L. E., and Schedl, H. P. (1977). Effects of Solanum malacoxylon on duodenal calcium binding protein in the diabetic rat. *Endocrinology (Baltimore)* **100,** 928–933.

Schneider, L. E., Hargis, G. K., Schedl, H. P., and Williams, G. A. (1974). Parathyroid function in the alloxan diabetic rat. *Endocrinology (Baltimore)* **95,** 749–752.

Schneider, L. E., Wasserman, R. H., and Schedl, H. P. (1975). Depressed duodenal calcium absorption in the diabetic rat: Restoration by Solanum malacoxylon. *Endocrinology (Baltimore)* **97,** 649–653.

Schneider, L. E., Omdahl, J., and Schedl, H. P. (1976). Effects of vitamin D and its metabolites on calcium transport in the diabetic rat. *Endocrinology (Baltimore)* **99,** 793–799.

Schneider, L. E., Nowoseilski, L. M., and Schedl, H. P. (1977a). Insulin-treatment of diabetic rats: Effects on duodenal calcium absorption. *Endocrinology (Baltimore)* **100,** 67–73.

Schneider, L. E., Schedl, H. P., McCain, T., and Haussler, M. R. (1977b). Experimental diabetes reduces circulating 1,25-dihydroxyvitamin D in the rat. *Science* **196,** 1452–1454.

Schryver, H. F. (1965). The effect of hydrocortisone on chondroitin sulfate production and loss by embryonic chick tibiotarsi in organ culture. *Exp. Cell Res.* **40,** 610–618.

Schulak, J. A., and Kaplan, E. L. (1974). Gastrin-induced hypocalcemia in thyroparathyroidectomized rats. *Metab., Clin. Exp.* **23,** 1103–1106.

Schulak, J. A., and Kaplan, E. L. (1975). The importance of the stomach in gastrin-induced hypocalcemia in the rat. *Endocrinology (Baltimore)* **96,** 1217–1220.

Schwartz, C. J., Kimberg, D. V., Sheerinke, V., Field, M., and Said, S. (1974). Vasoactive intestinal peptide stimulation of adenylate cyclase and active electrolyte secretion in intestinal mucosa. *J. Clin. Invest.* **54,** 536–544.

Schwartz, E., Echememdia, E., Schiffer, M., and Panariello, V. A. (1969a). Mechanism of estrogenic action in acromegaly. *J. Clin. Invest.* **48,** 260–270.

Schwartz, E., Wiedemann, E., Simm, S., and Schiffer, M. (1969b). Estrogenic antagonism of metabolic effects of administered growth hormone. *J. Clin. Endocrinol. Metab.* **29,** 1176–1181.

Schwartz, P. L., Wettenhall, R. E. H., Troedel, M. A., and Bornstein, J. (1970). A long-term effect of insulin on collagen synthesis by newborn rat bone in vitro. *Diabetes* **19,** 465–466.

Schwille, P. O., Scholz, D., Samberger, N. M., and Kayser, P. E. (1975). Studies on the calcemic effect of intravenous secretin in humans. *Acta Hepato-Gastroenterol.* **22,** 192–200.

Scriver, W. de M., and Bryan, A. H. (1935). Observations upon the calcium and phosphorus metabolism in a case of acromegaly showing marked osteoporosis. *J. Clin. Invest.* **14,** 212–219.

Seeman, E., Kumar, R., Hunder, G. G., Scott, M. Heath, H., and Riggs, B. L. (1980). Production, degradation, and circulating levels of 1,25-dehydroxy-vitamin D in health and in chronic glucocorticoid excess. *J. Clin. Invest.* **66,** 664–669.

Seldin, D. W., and Tarail, R. (1950). The metabolism of glucose and electrolyte in diabetic acidosis. *J. Clin. Invest.* **29,** 552–565.

Selye, H. (1952). Prevention of cortisone overdosage effects with the somatotrophic hormone (STH). *Am. J. Physiol.* **171,** 381–384.

Shafer, R. B., and Gregory, D. H. (1972). Calcium malabsorption in hyperthyroidism. *Gastroenterology* **63,** 235–239.

Shai, F., and Wallach, S. (1973). Interactions of estradiol and calcitonin on the rat skeleton. *Endocrinology (Baltimore)* **93,** 1044–1051.

Sheagren, J. N., Jowsey, J., Bird, D. C., Gurton, M. E., and Jacobs, J. B. (1977). Effect on bone growth of daily versus alternate-day corticosteroid administrations: An experimental study. *J. Lab. Clin. Med* **89,** 120–130.

Shields, C. F., III, and Haff, R. C. (1976). The VIPoma: Further confirmation of VIP as the hormone agent in the WDHA syndrome. *Am. J. Surg.* **132,** 784–786.

Shires, R., Teitelbaum, S. L., Bergfeld, M. A., Fallon, M. D., Slatopolsky, E., and Avioli, L. V. (1981). The effect of streptozotocin-induced chronic diabetes mellitus on bone and mineral homeostasis in the rat. *J. Lab. Clin. Med.* **97,** 231–240.

Shorr, E. (1945). The possible usefulness of estrogens and aluminum hydroxide gels in the management of renal stone. *J. Urol.* **53,** 507–519.

Shorr, E., Carter, A. C., Kennedy, B. J., and Smith, R. W. (1953). Metabolic studies on the effects of crystalline growth hormone (Somatotropin) in man. *Trans. Assoc. Am. Physicians* **66,** 114–128.

Sigurdsson, G., Nunziata, V., Reiner, M., Nadarajah, A., and Joplin, G. F. (1973a). Calcium absorption and excretion in the gut in acromegaly. *Clin. Endocrinol. (Oxford)* **2,** 187–192.

Sigurdsson, G., Woodhouse, N. J. Y., Taylor, S., and Joplin, G. F. (1973b). Stilbesterol diphosphate in hypercalcemia due to parathyroid carcinoma. *Br. Med. J.* **1,** 27–28.

Singer, F. R., Schiller, A. L., Pyle, E. B., and Krane, S. M. (1978). Paget's disease of bone. *In* "Metabolic Bone Disease" (L. V. Avioli and S. M. Krane, eds.), Vol. 2, pp. 489–575. Academic Press, New York.

Singhelakis, P., Alevizaki, C. C., and Ikkos, D. G. (1974). Intestinal calcium absorption in hyperthyroidism. *Metab., Clin. Exp.* **23,** 311–321.

Sjöberg, H. E. (1969). Retention of oral ^{47}calcium in acromegaly. *Horm. Metab. Res.* **1,** 136–138.

Smiley, J. D., and Ziff, M. (1954). Urinary hydroxyproline excretion and growth. *Physiol. Rev.* **44,** 30–44.

Smith, D. A., Fraser, S. A., and Wilson, G. M. (1973). Hyperthyroidism and calcium metabolism. *Clin. Endocrinol. Metab.* **2,** 333–354.

Soffer, L. J., and Bader, R. (1952). Corticotropin and cortisone in acute disseminated lupus erythematosus. *JAMA, J. Am. Med. Assoc.* **149,** 1002–1008.

Sorenson, O. H., and Hindberg, I. (1971). Influence of gonadal hormones on the action of calcitonin in the rat. *Acta Endocrinol. (Copenhagen)* **68,** 585–596.

Soyka, L. F., and Crawford, J. D. (1965). Antagonism by cortisone of the linear growth induced in hypopituitary patients and hypophysectomized rats by human growth hormone. *J. Clin. Endocrinol. Metab.* **25,** 469–475.

Spanos, E., Colston, K. W., Evans, J. M. S., Galante, L. S., MacCauley, S. J., and MacIntyre, I. (1976a). Effects of prolactin on vitamin D metabolism. *Mol. Cell. Endocrinol.* **5,** 163–167.

Spanos, E., Pike, J. W., Haussler, M. R., Colston, K. W., Evans, I. M. A., Goldner, A. M., McCain, T. A., and MacIntyre, I. (1976b). Circulating 1 α, 25-dihydroxyvitamin D in the chicken: Enhancement by injection of prolactin and during egg laying. *Life Sci.* **19,** 1751–1756.

Spanos, E., Colston, K. W., and MacIntyre, I. (1977). Effect of glucocorticoids on vitamin D metabolism. *FEBS Lett.* **75,** 73–76.

Spanos, E., Barrett, D., MacIntyre, I., Pike, J. W., Safilian, E. F., and Haussler, M. R. (1978). Effect of growth hormone on vitamin D metabolism. *Nature (London)* **273,** 246–247.

Spencer, E. M., and Tobiassen, O. (1977). The effects of hypophysectomy on 25-hydroxyvitamin D_3 metabolism in the rat. *In* "Vitamin D_3: Biochemical Chemical, and Clinical Aspects Related to Calcium Metabolism" (A. W. Norman, K. Schaefer, J. W. Coburn, H. F. DeLuca, D. Fraser, H. G. Grigoleit, and D. Von Herrath, eds.), pp. 197–199. de Gruyter, New York.

Spencer, E. M., Khalil, M., and Tobiassen, O. (1980). Experimental diabetes in the rat causes an insulin-reversible decrease in renal 25-hydroxyvitamin D_3-1α hydroxylase activity. *Endocrinology* **107,** 300–305.

Spencer, H., Menczel, J., and Lewin, I. (1964). Metabolic and radioisotope studies in osteoporosis. *Clin. Orthop. Relat. Res.* **35,** 202–219.

Spencer, H., Kramer, L., Osis, D., and Norris, C. (1976). Effect of conventional and newer forms of treatment on calcium absorption in osteoporosis. *Isr. J. Med. Sci.* **12,** 638–651.

Staub, A., Springs, V., Stoll, F., and Elrick, H. (1957). A renal action of glucagon. *Proc. Soc. Exp. Biol. Med.* **94,** 57–60.

Štěpán, J., Havránek, Formán-Ková, J., Škrha, J., Škrha, F., and Pacovský, V. (1980). Bone isoenzyme of serum alkaline phosphatase in diabetes mellitus. *Clin. Chim. Acta* **105,** 75–81.

Stern, P. H. (1969). Inhibition by steroids of parathyroid hormone-induced Ca^{45} release from embryonic rat bone in vitro. *J. Pharmacol. Exp. Ther.* **168,** 211–217.

Stern, P. H., and Bell, N. H. (1970). Effects of glucagon on serum calcium in the rat and on bone resorption in tissue culture. *Endocrinology* **87,** 111–117.

Stevenson, J. C., Abeyasekera, G., Hillyard, C. J., Phang, K. G., MacIntyre, I., Campbell, S., Townsend, P. T., Young, O., and Whitehead, M. I. (1981). Calcitonin and the calcium-regulating hormones in postmenopausal women: Effect of oestrogens. *Lancet* **1,** 693–695.

Stoerk, H. C., Peterson, A. C., and Jelinek, V. S. (1963). The blood calcium lowering effect of hydrocortisone in parathyroidectomized rats. *Proc. Soc. Exp. Biol. Med.* **114,** 690–695.

Storey, E. (1961). Cortisone-induced bone resorption in the rabbit. *Endocrinology (Baltimore)* **68,** 533–542.

Storey, E. (1963). The influence of adrenal cortical hormones on bone formation and resorption. *Clin. Orthop. Relat. Res.* **30,** 197–216.

Strickland, A. L., Underwood, L. E., Voina, S. J., French, F. S., and VanWyk, J. J. (1972). Growth retardation in Cushing's syndrome. *Am. J. Dis. Child.* **123,** 207–213.

Suki, W. N., Schwettmann, R. S., Rector, F. C., Jr., and Seldin, D. W. (1968). Effect of chronic mineralcorticoid administration on calcium excretion in the rat. *Am. J. Physiol.* **215,** 71–74.

Summers, V. K., Hunter, W. R., Hipkin, L. J., and Davis, J. C. (1966). Hyperparathyroidism in acromegaly. *Lancet* **2,** 601–604.

Swaminathan, R., and Care, A. D. (1975). The effect of thyroxine administration on intestinal calcium absorption and calcium binding protein activity in the chick. *Calcif. Tissue Res.* **17,** 257–261.

Swinton, N. W., Jr., Clerkin, E. P., and Flint, L. D.)1972). Hypercalcemia and familial pheochromocytoma. Correction after adrenalectomy. *Ann. Intern. Med.* **76,** 455–457.

Talbot, N. B. (1939). Influence of thyroid hormone on serum phosphatase. *Endocrinology (Baltimore)* **24,** 872–873.

Talmage, R. V., and Kennedy, J. W., III (1969). Influence of the thyroid on the response of rats to administered calcitonins. *Endocrinology (Baltimore)* **84,** 1026–1031.

Talmage, R. V., and Kennedy, J. W., III (1970). Parathyroid hormone and thyrocalcitonin function in adrenalectomized rats. *Endocrinology (Baltimore)* **86,** 1075–1079.

Talmage, R. V., Park, H., and Jee, W. (1970). Parathyroid hormone and thyrocalcitonin function in cortisol-treated rats. *Endocrinology (Baltimore)* **86,** 1080–1084.

Tanaka, Y., Castillo, L., and DeLuca, H. F. (1976). Control of renal vitamin D hydroxylases in birds by sex hormones. *Proc. Natl. Acad. Sci. U.S.A.* **23,** 2701–2705.

Tanaka, Y., Castillo, L., Wineland, M. J., and DeLuca, H. F. (1978). Synergistic effect of progesterone, testosterone, and estradiol in the stimulation of chick renal 25-hydroxyvitamin D_3 1α-hydroxylase. *Endocrinology* **103,** 2035–2039.

Tanzer, F. S., Kennedy, J. W. III, and Talmage, R. V. (1970). A comparison of the effects of thyrocalcitonin and glucagon on plasma calcium and phosphate. *Proc. Soc. Exp. Biol. Med.* **133,** 500–505.

Taylor, N. B., and Caven, W. R. (1927). Observations upon the serum calcium after adrenalectomy. *Am. J. Physiol.* **81,** 511.

Teitelbaum, S. L., Rosenberg, E. M., Richardson, C. A., and Avioli, L. V. (1976). Histological studies of bone from normocalcemic postmenopausal osteoporotic patients with increased circulatory parathyroid hormone. *J. Clin. Endocrinol. Metab.* **42,** 537–543.

Teitelbaum, T. L., Malone, J. D., and Kahn, A. J. (1981). Glucocorticoid enhancement of bone resorption by rat peritoneal macrophages *in vitro*. *Endocrinology* **108,** 795–799.

Tell, G. P. E., Cuatrecasas, P., VanWyk, J. J., and Hintz, R. L. (1973). Somatomedin: Inhibition of adenylate cyclase activity in subcellular membranes of various tissues. *Science* **180,** 312–315.

Thompson, E. B., and Lippman, M. E. (1974). Mechanism of action of glucocorticoids. *Metab., Clin. Exp.* **23,** 159–202.

Thompson, J. C., Reeder, D. D., Bunchman, H. H., Becker, H. D., and Brandt, E. N., Jr. (1972). Effect of secretin on circulating gastrin. *Ann. Surg.* **176,** 384–393.

Thompson, J. S., and Urist, M. R. (1973). Effects of cortisone on bone metabolism in intact and thyroidectomized rabbits. *Calcif. Tissue Res.* **13,** 197–215.

Thompson, J. S., Palmieri, G. M. A., and Eliel, L. P. (1974). Dissociation of the lowering effect of calcitonin on plasma Ca and P in cortisone-treated nephrectomized rats. *Endocrinology (Baltimore)* **94,** 799–802.

Thompson, J. S., Palmieri, G. M. A., Eliel, L. P., and Cutler, G. A. (1968). Effects of cortisone and adrenalectomy on the responses to thyrocalcitonin. *Endocrinology (Baltimore)* **83,** 470–474.

Thompson, J. S., Palmieri, G. M. A., Eliel, L. P., and Crawford, R. L. (1972). The effects of porcine calcitonin on osteoporosis induced by adrenal cortical steroids. *J. Bone Joint Surg., Am. Vol.* **54-A,** 1490–1500.

Thompson, R. G., Rodriguez, A., Kowarski, A., and Blizzard, R. M. (1972). Growth hormone: Metabolic clearance rates, integrated concentrations and production rates in normal adults and the effect of prednisone. *J. Clin. Invest.* **51,** 3193–3199.

Tibbetts, D. M., and Aub, J. C. (1937). Magnesium metabolism in health and disease. *J. Clin. Invest.* **16,** 511–515.

Toverud, S. V., Harper, C., and Munson, P. L. (1976). Calcium metabolism during lactation: Enhanced effects of thyrocalcitonin. *Endocrinology* **99,** 371–378.

Tümay, S. B., Bilger, M., and Hatemi, N. (1962). Skeletal changes and nephrocalcinosis in a case of athyreosis. *Arch. Dis. Child.* **37,** 543–547.

Turkington, R. W., Majumber, G. C., Kadohama, N., MacIndoe, J. H., and Frantz, W. L. (1973). Hormonal regulation of gene expression in mammary cells. *Recent Prog. Horm. Res.* **29,** 417–455.

Turner, R. T., and Schraer, H. (1977). Estrogen-induced sequential changes in avian bone metabolism. *Calcif. Tissue Res.* **24,** 157–162.

Ulbrych-Jablonska, A. (1972). The hypocalcemic effect of glucagon in cases of hypercalcemia. *Helv. Paediatr. Acta* **27,** 613–615.

Ulrich, F., Reinhardt, W. O., and Li, C. H. (1952). Some aspects of the role of pituitary hormones in calcium metabolism. *Acta Endocrinol. (Copenhagen)* **10,** 117–127.

Uthne, K., and Uthne, T. (1972). Influence of liver resection and regeneration on somatomedin activity in sera from normal and hypophysectomized rats. *Acta Endocrinol. (Copenhagen)* **71,** 255–264.

Valentzas, C., Oreopoulos, D. G., From, G., Porret, B., and Raporport, A. (1977). Vitamin-D levels in thyrotoxicosis. *Lancet* **1,** 370–371.

Verbeelen, D., and Fuss, M. (1979). Hypercalcaemia induced by oestrogen withdrawal in vitamin D-treated hypoparathyroidism. *Br. Med. J.* **1,** 522–523.

Verner, J. V., and Morrison, A. B. (1974). Non-B islet tumors and the syndrome of watery diarrhea, diarrhea and hypokalemia. *Am. J. Med.* **25,** 374–380.

Verner, J. V., and Morrison, A. B. (1974). Non-B islet tumors and the syndrome of water diarrhea, hypokalemia, and hypochlorhydria. *Clin. Gastroenterol.* **3,** 595–608.

Villanueva, A., Frost, H., Ilnicki, L., Frame, B., Smith, R., and Arnstein, R. (1966). Cortical bone dynamics measured by means of tetracycline labeling in 21 cases of osteoporosis. *J. Lab. Clin. Med.* **68,** 599–616.

von Recklinghausen, F. C. (1891). Die fibrose oder deformierende Ostitis, die Osteomalazie und die osteoplastische Karzinose in ihren gegenseittigen Beziehungen. *In* "Festschrift R. Virchow," pp. 1–89. Reener, Berlin.

von Werder, K., Hane, S., and Forsham, P. H. (1971). Suppression of the hypotalalamo-pituitary-adrenal axis and growth hormone release with dexamethasone. *Horm. Metab. Res.* **3,** 171–174.

Vora, N. M., Williams, G. A., Hargis, G. K., Bowser, E. N., Kawahara, W., Jackson, B. L., Henderson, W. J., and Kukreja, S. C. (1978). Comparative effect of calcium and of the adrenergic system on calcitonin secretion in man. *J. Clin. Endocrinol. Metab.* **46,** 567–571.

Wajchenberg, B. L., Quintao, E. R., Liberman, B., and Cintra, A. B. U. (1965). Antagonism between adrenal steroids and parathyroid hormone. *J. Clin. Endocrinol. Metab.* **25,** 1677–1681.

Wajchenberg, B. L., Pereira, V. G., Kieffer, J., and Ursic, S. (1969). Effect of dexamethasone on calcium metabolism and ^{47}Ca kinetics in normal subjects. *Acta Endocrinol. (Copenhagen)* **61,** 173–192.

Wallach, S., and Henneman, P. H. (1959). Prolonged estrogen therapy in postmenopausal women. *JAMA, J. Am. Med. Assoc.* **171,** 1637–1642.

Walser, M., Robinson, B. H. B., and Duckett, J. W. (1963). The hypercalcemia of adrenal insufficiency. *J. Clin. Invest.* **42,** 456–465.

Weber, C. J., Hardy, M. A., Williams, G. A., Lerner, R. L., and Reemtsma, K. (1976). Pancreatic islet transplantation and hyperparathyroidism in diabetic rats. *Surg. Forum* **27,** 317–320.

Weisbrode, S. E., and Capen, C. C. (1976). Ultrastructural evaluation of the interaction of glucocorticoids and vitamin D on bone cells in thyroparathyroidectomized rats. *Am. J. Pathol.* **84,** 457–463.

Weiss, N. S., Ure, C. L., Ballard, J. H., Williams, A. R., and Daling, J. R. (1980). Decreased risk of fractures of the hip and lower forearm with postmenopausal use of estrogen. *N. Engl. J. Med.* **303,** 1195–1198.

Wells, H., and Lloyd, W. (1968). Inhibition of the hypocalcemic action of thyrocalcitonin by theophylline and isoproterenol. *Endocrinology (Baltimore)* **82,** 468–474.

Weiss, R. E., and Reddi, A. H. (1980). Influence of experimental diabetes and insulin on matrix-induced cartilage and bone differentiation. *Am. J. Physiol.* **238,** E200–E207.

Wermer, P. (1954). Genetic aspects of adenomastosis of endocrine glands. *Am. J. Med.* **16,** 363–371.

Westby, G. R., Goldfarb, S., Goldberg, M., and Agus, Z. S. (1977). Acute effects of bovine growth hormone on renal calcium and phosphorus excretion. *Metab., Clin. Exp.* **26,** 525–530.

Wettenhall, R. E. H., Schwartz, P. L., and Bornstein, J. (1969). Actions of insulin and growth hormone on collagen and chondroitin sulfate synthesis in bone organ cultures. *Diabetes* **18,** 280–284.

White, H. L., Heinbecker, P., and Rolf, D. (1949). Enhancing effects of growth hormone on renal function. *Am. J. Physiol.* **157,** 47–51.

Wilkins, L. (1965). "The Diagnosis and Treatment of Endocrine Disorders in Childhood and Adolescence," 3rd ed., p. 82. Thomas, Springfield, Illinois.

Williams, G. A., Bowser, E. N., and Henderson, W. J. (1967). Calcium-47 absorption in rats with induced hyperthyroidism. *Isr. J. Med. Sci.* **3,** 639–642.

Williams, G. A., Bowser, E. N., and Henderson, W. J. (1969). Mode of hypocalcemic action of glucagon in the rat. *Endocrinology (Baltimore)* **85,** 537–541.

Williams, G. A., Peterson, W. C., Bowser, E. N., Henderson, W. J., Hargis, G. K., and Martinez, N. J. (1974). Interrelationship of parathyroid and adrenocortical function in calcium homeostasis in the rat. *Endocrinology (Baltimore)* **95,** 707–712.

Windeck, R., Brown, E. M., Gardner, D. G., and Aurbach, G. D. (1978). Effect of gastrointestinal hormones on isolated bovine parathyroid cells. *Endocrinology (Baltimore)* **103,** 2020–2026.

Winter, M., Morava, E., and Simon, G. (1970). The role of the thyroid in the intestinal effects of vitamin D on rachitic rats. *J. Endocrinol.* **48,** 541–544.

Woessner, J. F. (1969). Inhibition by oestrogen of collagen breakdown in the involuting rat uterus. *Biochem. J.* **112,** 637–645.

Wong, G. (1979). Basal activities and hormone responsiveness of osteoclast-like and osteoblast-like bone cells are regulated by glucocorticoids. *J. Biol. Chem.* **54,** 6337–6340.

Woodward, A. H., and Jowsey, J. (1972). The effect of glucagon on immobilization osteoporosis in rats. *Endocrinology (Baltimore)* **90,** 1399–1401.

Wright, J. C., Brasel, J. A., Aceto, T., Finkelstein, J. W., Kenny, F. M., Spaulding, J. S., and Blizzard, R. M. (1965). Studies with human growth hormone (HGH). An attempt to correlate metabolic response during short-term administration with linear growth during prolonged therapy. *Am. J. Med.* **38,** 499–516.

Wu, A., Grant, D. B., Hambley, J., and Levi, A. J. (1974). Reduced serum somatomedin activity in patients with chronic liver disease. *Clin. Sci. Mol. Med.* **47,** 359–366.

Wu, K., and Frost, H. M. (1969). Bone formation in osteoporosis. *Arch. Pathol.* **88,** 508–510.

Wu, K., Jett, S., and Frost, H. M. (1967). Bone resorption rates in rib in physiological, senile, and postmenopausal osteoporosis. *J. Lab. Clin. Med.* **69,** 810–818.

Yasumura, S. (1976). Effect of adrenal steroids on bone resorption in rats. *Am. J. Physiol.* **230,** 90–93.

Yasumura, S., Ellis, K. J., and Conn, S. H. (1976). Effect of hydrocortisone on total body calcium in rats. *J. Lab. Clin. Med.* **88,** 834–840.

Yatvin, M. B., Wannemacher, R. W., Jr., and Brown, N. V. (1966). Effects of cortisone on thyroid protein metabolism in euthyroid and thiouracil-treated rats. *Endocrinology (Baltimore)* **79,** 1079–1086.

Young, M. M., and Nordin, B. E. C. (1967). Effects of natural and artificial menopause on plasma and urinary calcium and phosphorus. *Lancet* **2,** 118–120.

Young, M. M., Jasani, C., Smith, D. A., and Nordin, B. E. C. (1968). Some effects of ethinyl oestradiol on calcium and phosphorus metabolism in osteoporosis. *Clin. Sci.* **34,** 411–417.

Index

D

E

F

G

I

K

L

M

N

O

P

T

U

V